Clinical Progress in Neuroinflammation

Clinical Progress
in Neuroinflammation

Editor: Charlie Romero

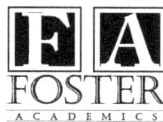

FA
FOSTER
ACADEMICS

www.fosteracademics.com

www.fosteracademics.com

FA FOSTER
ACADEMICS

Cataloging-in-Publication Data

Clinical progress in neuroinflammation / edited by Charlie Romero.
 p. cm.
Includes bibliographical references and index.
ISBN 978-1-63242-900-1
1. Nervous system--Diseases. 2. Inflammation. 3. Nervous system--Degeneration. I. Romero, Charlie.
RC346 .C55 2020
616.8--dc23

Foster Academics,
118-35 Queens Blvd., Suite 400,
Forest Hills, NY 11375, USA

ISBN 978-1-63242-900-1 (Hardback)

Contents

Preface

This book was inspired by the evolution of our times; to answer the curiosity of inquisitive minds. Many developments have occurred across the globe in the recent past which has transformed the progress in the field.

The inflammation of the nervous tissue is termed as neuroinflammation. It is generally regarded as a chronic inflammation. It is initiated as a response to infection, aging, toxic metabolites, traumatic brain injury, spinal cord injury or autoimmunity. Microglia are activated in response to such stimuli in the central nervous system. The class of proteins called cytokines regulate inflammation, cell signaling and other cell processes such as cell growth and survival. Neuroinflammation is strongly associated with several neurodegenerative diseases, such as Alzheimer's disease, multiple sclerosis and Parkinson's disease. Drug therapy and exercise are some potential treatment strategies for the management of neuroinflammation. This book is a valuable compilation of topics, ranging from the basic to the most complex advancements in neuroinflammation. It presents this complex subject in the most comprehensible and easy to understand language. This book, with its detailed analyses and data, will prove immensely beneficial to professionals and students involved in neurology at various levels.

This book was developed from a mere concept to drafts to chapters and finally compiled together as a complete text to benefit the readers across all nations. To ensure the quality of the content we instilled two significant steps in our procedure. The first was to appoint an editorial team that would verify the data and statistics provided in the book and also select the most appropriate and valuable contributions from the plentiful contributions we received from authors worldwide. The next step was to appoint an expert of the topic as the Editor-in-Chief, who would head the project and finally make the necessary amendments and modifications to make the text reader-friendly. I was then commissioned to examine all the material to present the topics in the most comprehensible and productive format.

I would like to take this opportunity to thank all the contributing authors who were supportive enough to contribute their time and knowledge to this project. I also wish to convey my regards to my family who have been extremely supportive during the entire project.

Editor

Microglia prevent peripheral immune cell invasion and promote an anti-inflammatory environment in the brain of APP-PS1 transgenic mice

M. S. Unger[1,2], P. Schernthaner[1,2], J. Marschallinger[1,2,3], H. Mrowetz[1,2] and L. Aigner[1,2*]

Abstract

Background: Undoubtedly, neuroinflammation is a major contributor to Alzheimer's disease (AD) progression. Neuroinflammation is characterized by the activity of brain resident glial cells, in particular microglia, but also by peripheral immune cells, which infiltrate the brain at certain stages of disease progression. The specific role of microglia in shaping AD pathology is still controversially discussed. Moreover, a possible role of microglia in the interaction and recruitment of peripheral immune cells has so far been completely ignored.

Methods: We ablated microglia cells in 12-month-old WT and APP-PS1 transgenic mice for 4 weeks using the CSF1R inhibitor PLX5622 and analyzed its consequences to AD pathology and in particular to peripheral immune cell infiltration.

Results: PLX5622 treatment successfully reduced microglia numbers. Interestingly, it uncovered a treatment-resistant macrophage population (Iba1$^+$/TMEM119$^-$). These cells strongly expressed the phagocytosis marker CD68 and the lymphocyte activation, homing, and adhesion molecule CD44, specifically at sites of amyloid-beta plaques in the brains of APP-PS1 mice. In consequence, ablation of microglia significantly raised the number of CD3$^+$/CD8$^+$ T-cells and reduced the expression of anti-inflammatory genes in the brains of APP-PS1 mice.

Conclusion: We conclude that in neurodegenerative conditions, chronically activated microglia might limit CD3$^+$/CD8$^+$ T-cell recruitment to the brain and that local macrophages connect innate with adaptive immune responses. Investigating the role of peripheral immune cells, their interaction with microglia, and understanding the link between innate and adaptive immune responses in the brain might be a future directive in treating AD pathology.

Keywords: Alzheimer's disease, Microglia, TMEM119, Macrophages, T-cells

Background

Alzheimer's disease (AD) is an age-related human neurodegenerative disease with a complex pathology leading to a progressive and detrimental cognitive decline (reviewed in [1]). Among the major histopathological hallmarks, i.e. amyloid-beta plaque and neurofibrillary tangle formation (reviewed in [2–6]), neuroinflammation is described as an important contributor to AD pathology (reviewed in [7–9]).

Microglia, the brains resident immune cells, are a key element in inflammatory processes of the central nervous system (CNS) and are mediating chronic neuroinflammation and aggravation of AD pathology (reviewed in [8, 10, 11]). Indeed, genome-wide association studies linked microglia (dys-) functions to AD [12, 13], and therefore, modulation of microglia phenotypes and functions is a promising target for possible treatment options (reviewed in [10, 14]). Besides the creation of a disease-stage-specific pro- or anti-inflammatory environment, one of the main functions of microglia is to phagocytose and degrade dying cells, cellular debris, and toxic molecules (reviewed in [15]), as for example amyloid-beta along AD pathology (reviewed in

* Correspondence: ludwig.aigner@pmu.ac.at
[1]Institute of Molecular Regenerative Medicine, Paracelsus Medical University, Strubergasse 21, 5020 Salzburg, Austria
[2]Spinal Cord Injury and Tissue Regeneration Center Salzburg (SCI-TReCS), Paracelsus Medical University, Salzburg, Austria
Full list of author information is available at the end of the article

[16, 17] and [18]). While the initial immune response to amyloid-beta is described as beneficial because it counteracts plaque formation [19], chronically activated microglia stir disease progression through the secretion of pro-inflammatory cytokines and neurotoxic factors (reviewed in [20]). Ultimately, microglia cells might become dysfunctional along brain aging and in neurodegenerative conditions and switch their phenotype into a senescent state with impaired phagocytosis (reviewed in [21]). In summary, microglia have multiple and extremely disease-stage-specific roles and functions in AD pathology.

Besides the brain's innate immune system, i.e. the resident microglia, peripheral macrophages (reviewed in [22, 23]) as well as cells from the adaptive immune system are increasingly recognized as being involved in AD pathology [24–26]. Macrophages, i.e. bone marrow-derived monocytes, infiltrate the brains of transgenic AD mice [27] and participate in amyloid clearance (reviewed in [28–30]). Moreover, T-cell lymphocyte populations infiltrate the brains of transgenic AD mice in high numbers [25, 31] and were detected in human AD post-mortem brains [32–34]. The exact function of lymphocyte subsets and their contribution to AD pathology is completely unknown ([24, 25, 36] and reviewed in [35]). We recently identified a CD45[+]/CD8[+] T-cell lymphocyte population present in the brains of transgenic APP-PS1 mice that are placed in close proximity to microglia suggesting that microglia might be involved in the recruitment of T-cells to the brain and that these two cell populations might interact and influence each other [37]. In order to experimentally address these hypotheses, we ablated microglia cells from 12-month-old WT and APP-PS1 transgenic mice for 4 weeks using the colony stimulating factor 1 receptor (CSF1R) inhibitor PLX5622 and analyzed its consequences on behavior, on amyloid plaque pathology, on the recruitment of peripheral immune cells from the innate and adaptive immune system, i.e. macrophages and T-cells, and on the expression of typical pro-inflammatory, anti-inflammatory, and phagocytosis specific-genes.

Methods
Compounds
PLX5622 was provided by Plexxikon Inc. and formulated in AIN-76A standard chow by Research Diets Inc. at 1200 mg/kg, as previously described [38, 39].

Animals
Female and male APP Swedish PS1 dE9 mice (reviewed in [40, 41]) expressing a chimeric mouse/human mutant amyloid precursor protein (Mo/HuAPP695swe) and a mutant human presenilin 1 (PS1-dE9) both directed to CNS neurons under the prion protein promoter (available by Jackson Laboratory, http://www.jax.org/strain/005864) were used. Mice were housed at the Paracelsus Medical University Salzburg in groups under standard conditions at a temperature of 22 °C and a 12-h light/dark cycle with ad libitum access to standard food and water. Animal care, handling, genotyping, and experiments were approved by local ethical committees (BMWFW-66.019/0032-WF/V/3b/2016).

For this study, 12-month old animals were used and treated for 28 days with PLX5622 chow. Age-matched non-transgenic mice, derived from the breeding of APP Swedish PS1 dE9 (herein abbreviated as APP-PS1) were used as control animals (WT). All animals were adapted to control chow 2 weeks before introducing the PLX5622 chow. Thus, there were 4 experiment groups: WT and APP-PS1 mice which received control chow, and WT and APP-PS1 mice which received the PLX5622 chow for a total of 28 days (see Fig. 1a).

Behavioral tests
All behavior tests were performed in a special animal experiment room at the animal facility of the Paracelsus Medical University under constant light and environmental conditions. After 21 days of PLX5622 treatment, behavioral tests were performed as previously published [42]. All behavior tests were conducted at the same day time and camera tracked using EthoVision tracking system (EthoVision XT 9.0.726, Noldus).

Morris water maze
Morris water maze (MWM) is a standard cognitive behavior test for spatial learning and memory function [43, 44]. MWM was performed on six consecutive days, starting on day 23 of the PLX5622 treatment. The maze consisted of a 108-cm round white pool that was filled with 22 °C warm water up to 1 cm above a transparent plastic platform that was placed in the southwest quadrant of the arena. The 10×10 cm platform was hidden under the water surface and was visually not detectable for the animals. Every mouse was put in the maze for 60 s, and the activity (e.g. latency to platform, swim speed, distance moved) until the mouse reached the platform was recorded. If the mouse does not reach the platform after 60 s, it was manually cued to the platform for orientation before it was taken out of the maze. Each mouse had to perform four trials per day for five consecutive days. Every trial per day started at four different visually marked entry points (square, triangle, circle, moon), and the entry points to the maze were randomly shuffled over the 5 days to avoid any learning effects caused by memory of the entry point. After each trial, the animals had 1 h to rest before starting a new trial. On the first day, the platform was emphasized with a flag to help the mice to find the platform and the data from day 1 were therefore excluded from the analysis. On the sixth day, the mice were additionally tested for spatial memory by removing the platform. The mice had 60 s to search the original spatial location of the platform.

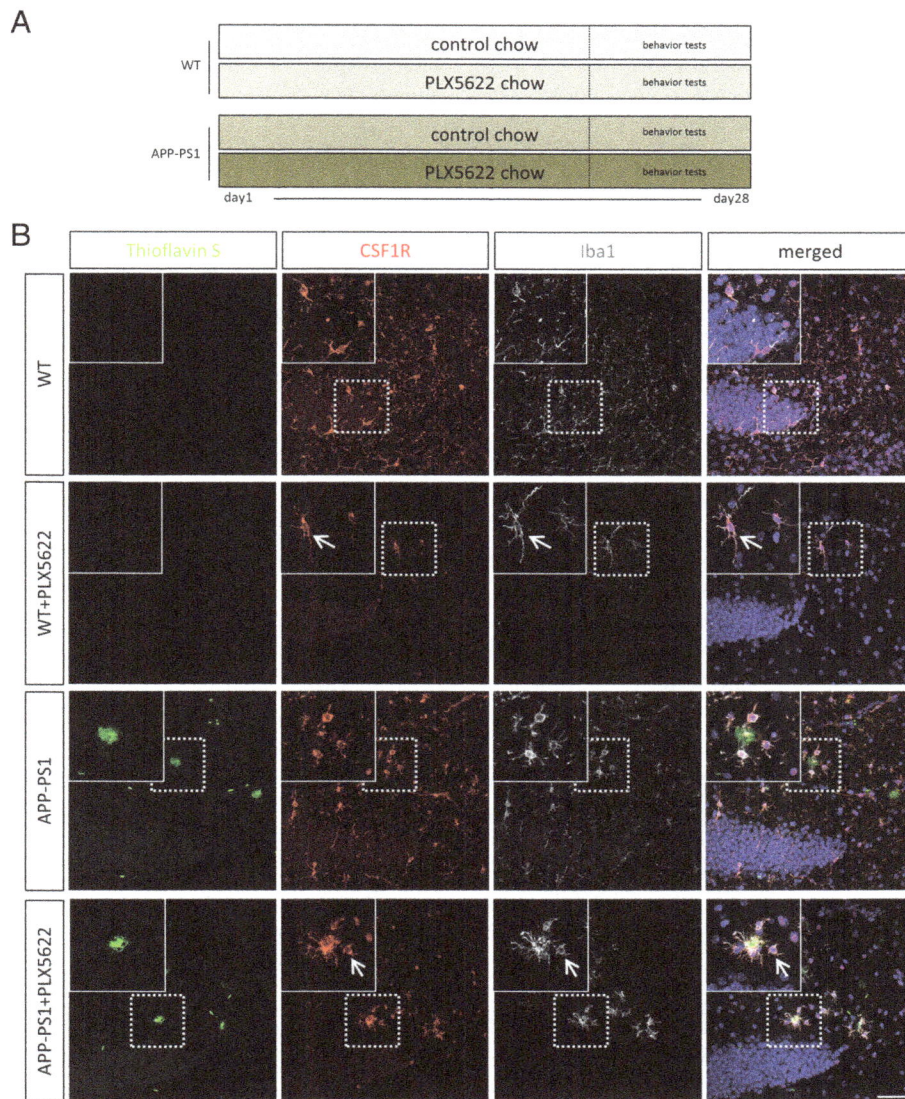

Fig. 1 Experimental set up and expression of CSF1R in mouse hippocampus: 12-month-old WT and APP-PS1 animals were treated for a total of 28 days with PLX5622 or control chow followed by behavior tests after 20 days of treatment (**a**). Qualitative immunohistochemical staining for CSF1R receptor (red) showed high-receptor expression in Iba1[+] cells (white) in all studied groups (**b**). ThioflavinS was used to stain amyloid plaques (green), and Dapi (blue) was used as nucleus stain. Scale: 50 μm

Perfusion and tissue sectioning

After 28 days of treatment, the mice were anesthetized by intraperitoneal injection of a ketamine (20.5 mg/ml, Richter Pharma), xylazine (5.36 mg/ml, Chanelle), and acepromacine (0.27 mg/ml, VANA GmbH) mixture. Afterwards, their thoracic cavity was opened with an incision caudal to the sternum. Animals were manually perfused through the left ventricle with ice cold HBSS containing 15 mM HEPES (all from Thermofisher) and 0.5% glucose (Sigma) to wash out the blood. Afterwards, mice were decapitated, and brains were extracted from the skull. One total brain hemisphere was immersed in 4% paraformaldehyde (in 0.1 M sodium phosphate solution, pH = 7.4) at 4 °C for

2 days for fixation before being washed in PBS and transferred into 30% sucrose for cryoprotection. When fully soaked with sucrose, brain hemispheres were cut in 40 μm slices on dry ice using a sliding microtome (Leika) dividing one brain hemisphere in representative tenths of the brain. Sections were stored at − 20 °C in cryoprotectant solution (ethylene glycol, glycerol, 0.1 M phosphate buffer pH 7.4, 1:1:2 by volume). The other brain hemisphere was further processed for RNA extraction or flow cytometric analysis.

Flow cytometric analysis

For analysis of microglia and T-cells, one total brain hemisphere per mouse was mechanically chopped with a razor blade and homogenized in 2 mL ice cold HBSS with 15 mM HEPES (all from Thermofisher), 0.5% glucose (Sigma), DNAse I (1:20, Worthington) and RNAsin (1:250, Promega) using a glass homogenizer. Cells were passed through a 100-μm cell strainer and rinsed two times with 2 mL ice cold HBSS (with 15 mM HEPES and 0.5% glucose). Cell suspensions were centrifuged at 340 g for 7 min at 4 °C. Myelin was removed by resuspending the cell pellet in 30% Percoll (Sigma) solution and centrifugation at 950 g for 20 min at 4 °C. Supernatant was carefully removed, and pellets containing cells of interest were diluted in HBSS followed by centrifugation at 300 g for 10 min at 4 °C. Pellets were resuspended in PBS containing fixable viability dye (1:2000, eBioscience #65–0865) for 3 min at RT and transferred to round-bottom polystyrene tubes (Corning). After centrifugation for 5 min at 300 g, cell pellets were dissolved in FACS buffer (PBS with 2% BSA and 2 mM EDTA) containing Rat Anti-Mouse CD16/CD32 Fc-Block (1:100, BD Biosciences, #553141) for 5 min at RT. Samples were centrifuged at 300 g for 5 min, and pellets dissolved in FACS buffer containing primary fluorescent-labeled antibodies. Antibody incubation was performed for 15 min at RT. Samples were washed in FACS buffer two times and centrifuged at 400 g for 5 min. Finally, cell pellets were resuspended in 500 μl FACS buffer with RNAsin (1:250, Promega #N2115) and filtered with a 30-μm cell strainer followed by flow cytometric analysis using LSR Fortessa flow cytometer (BD) with BD FACSDiva software (8.0.1, BD). The following primary antibodies were used: CD11b-PE (1:100, eBioscience #12–0112-82), CD45-PE/Cy7 (1:100, BioLegend #103114), CD3-APC (1:100, eBioscience #17–0032), CD4-eFluor450 (1:100, eBioscience #48–0041), CD8a-FITC (1:100, eBioscience #11–0081).

Single stains were performed for compensations with isolated microglia cells from APP-PS1 mouse brains for viability dye eFluor780, CD11b-PE, and CD45-PE/Cy7 and with PBMCs collected from whole mouse blood drawn from the heart for CD3-APC, CD4-eFluor450, and CD8a-FITC. As gating strategy cells of interest were taken, and cell doublets were discriminated. Single cells negative for viability dye eFluor780 were counted as living cells and gated for CD11b-PE expression for microglia analysis. CD11b-positive cell populations were further gated for CD45 expression and divided into a low (microglia) and high population (CNS/peripheral macrophages) as published by several research groups [45–48]. Total cell numbers for CD11b+, CD11b+/CD45low, and CD11b+/CD45high were measured from total brain hemispheres and calculated for 1×10^6 living cells in each sample. For T-cell analysis in the brain, single-living cells were gated for CD3-APC and CD45-PE/Cy7 expression and further analyzed for CD4-eFluor450 and CD8-FITC expression. Total

cell numbers for CD3+, CD3+/CD4+, and CD3+/CD8+ were measured and calculated for 1×10^5 living cells in each sample. Flow cytometric data analysis and graphs were done with Kaluza analysis software (1.3 Beckman Coulter).

Fluorescence immunohistochemistry (IHC)

Fluorescence immunohistochemistry of mouse tissue was performed on free-floating sections as previously described [49, 50]. Antigen retrieval was performed depending on the used primary antibodies by steaming the sections for 15–20 min in citrate buffer (pH = 6.0, Sigma). The following primary antibodies were used: rabbit or goat anti-Iba1 (1:1000 or 1:500, Abcam), rabbit anti-Iba1 (1:300, Wako), rabbit anti-CSF1R (1:200, Cell Signaling), rabbit anti-TMEM119 (1:300, Abcam) and rat anti-CD44 (1:500, BioLegend), rat anti-CD8 (1:100, eBioscience), rabbit anit-Zap70 (1:400, Cell Signaling), rat anti-MHCII (1:100, eBioscience), rat anti-CD68 (1:250, Serotec/Bio-Rad), rat anti-CD4 (1:100, eBioscience), and goat anti-PCNA (1:300, Santa Cruz).

Sections were extensively washed in PBS and incubated for 3 h at RT in secondary antibodies all diluted 1:1000. The following secondary antibodies were used: donkey anti-goat Alexa Fluor 488, donkey anti-rabbit Alexa Fluor 568 or Alexa Fluor 647 (all Invitrogen/Life Technologies), donkey anti-goat Alexa Fluor 647 (Jackson Immuno Research), donkey anti-rat Alexa Fluor 488, donkey anti-goat Alexa Fluor 568, goat anti-rat Alexa Fluor 568 (all Molecular Probes), and donkey anti-rat Alexa Fluor 647 (Dianova).

Nucleus counterstaining was performed with 4′,6′-diamidino-2-phenylindole dihydrochloride hydrate (DAPI 1 mg/ml, 1:2000, Sigma). For amyloid-beta plaque staining, ThioflavinS (1 mg/ml, 1:625, Sigma) was added to the secondary antibody solution. Tissue sections were additionally treated with 0.2% Sudan Black (Sigma) in 70% ethanol for 1–2 min to reduce the autofluorescence in tissues from old animals [51]. After this treatment, the sections were extensively washed in PBS and mounted onto microscope glass slides (Superfrost Plus, Thermo Scientific). Brain sections were cover slipped semi-dry in ProLong Gold Antifade Mountant (Life technologies) or Fluorescence Mounting Medium (Dako).

Confocal microscopy and image processing

For imaging, the Confocal Laser Scanning Microscopes LSM700 and LSM710 from Zeiss were used and gratefully provided by the microscopy core facility of SCI-TReCS (Spinal Cord Injury and Tissue Regeneration Center Salzburg). Images were taken with the ZEN 2011 SP3 or SP7 (black edition) software (all from Zeiss). Quantitative analysis was done using × 20 magnification with 0.5 or 0.6 zoom, and for qualitative analysis, images were taken in × 20, × 40, or × 63 oil magnification. Images were taken as confocal z-stacks and combined to merged maximum intensity projections. For 3D reconstruction, images were processed at the LSM 710 using the Zen 2011 SP7 (black edition) software.

All images were edited and processed with the ZEN 2012 (blue edition) software (version 1.1.2.0) and Microsoft PowerPoint.

RNA isolation and gene expression analysis

To detect mRNA levels of microglia, anti-inflammatory, pro-inflammatory, and phagocytosis-relevant genes in different brain regions of 12-month-old mice, the total RNA was extracted from mouse hippocampus and cortex. After manual perfusion, animals were decapitated and the tissue of interest was dissected of one brain hemisphere. Brain samples were immediately transferred to RNA later (Sigma) and stored at -80 °C. Tissues were homogenized in 1 ml Trizol (TRI°Reagent; Sigma). For phase separation, 150 µl of 1-bromo-3-chloropropane (Sigma) were added, vortexed, and centrifuged (15 min at 12,000×g at 4 °C). After transferring the aqueous phase into a new tube, 1 µl GlycoBlue™ (Invitrogen) and 500 µl 2-Propanol p.A. (Millipore) were added and vortexed. To obtain RNA, samples were centrifuged (10 min at 12,000×g at 4 °C). The pellet was washed with 1 ml 75% ethanol, dried and resuspended in a 30-µl RNase-free water (pre-warmed to 55 °C). cDNA was synthesized using the iScript Reverse Transcription Supermix (Bio-Rad). Quantitative gene expression analyses were performed using TaqMan RT-PCR technology. Technical duplicates containing 10 ng of reverse transcribed RNA were amplified with the GoTAQ Probe qPCR Master Mix (Promega) using a two-step cycling protocol (95 °C for 15 s, 60 °C for 60 s; 40 cycles, Bio-Rad CFX 96 Cycler). The following validated exon-spanning gene expression assays were employed; from a set of three validated candidate housekeepers, the two best fitting were chosen for the present experiments (PSMD4, Mm.PT.56.13046188; Heatr3 Mm.PT.56.8463 165; both Integrated DNA Technologies). Quantification analyses were performed with qBase Plus (Biogazelle) using geNorm algorithms for multi-reference gene normalization. Bars are represented as mean with SD ($n = 6$–8/group). Used Primer for analyzed genes: Arg1 (Mm00475988_m1), H2-Aa (Mm00439211_m1), MRC1 (Mm00485148_m1), Nos2 (Mm00440485_m1), TNF (Mm00443258_m1), and Marco (Mm00440265_m1, all from Thermofisher); CCL2 (Mm.PT.56a.42151692), IL-1ß (Mm.PT.56a.41616450), IL-6 (Mm.PT.56a.10005 566), TGFß (Mm.PT.56a.11254750), INF (Mm.PT.56a.41 152792), IL-10 (Mm.PT.58.13531087), CD33 (Mm.PT.5 8.12829132), Trem2 (Mm.PT.58.7992121), TMEM119 (Mm.PT.58.6766267), and AIF1 (Mm.PT.56a.7014816, all from Integrated DNA Technologies).

Data analysis
Behavioral testing

The data of the behavioral tests were collected with EthoVision XT (version 9.0.72) software from Noldus. MWM was divided in spatial learning which consisted of the first 5 days and spatial memory analysis on the sixth day. For learning assessment, the swim speed, the total distance the animals moved, and the latency from the arena entry to the platform were calculated and plotted as learning curves with mean and standard error of the mean (SEM). To assess the spatial memory, the cumulative durations the animals spent in the platform quadrant were calculated.

Fluorescence immunohistochemistry (IHC)

For quantitative analysis, comparable images of the hippocampus (dentate gyrus) and the cortex from four different brain slices of each animal were taken with the LSM700 or LSM710 confocal fluorescence microscope at $\times 20$ magnification with 0.5 or 0.6 zoom. In each image, the total number of Iba1 positive cells, Iba1$^+$/ThioflavinS$^+$ doublepositive cells, the number of ThioflavinS positive amyloid-beta plaques, as well as the area of the plaques were assessed. The percentage of Iba1$^+$/ThioflavinS$^+$positive cells from the total number of Iba1 positive cells was calculated. Furthermore, the total number of Iba1$^+$/TMEM119$^+$ double positive and Iba1$^+$/TMEM119$^-$ cells was counted. Again, the ratio of Iba1$^+$/TMEM119$^+$ and Iba1$^+$/TMEM119$^-$ cells from the total number of Iba1-positive cells was calculated in percentage (all analysis $n = 6$/group). For further characterization Iba1$^+$/TMEM119$^+$/CD68$^+$ and Iba1$^+$/TMEM119$^-$/CD68$^+$ cells were counted ($n = 3$/group). Only cells with visible somata and nuclei were taken for analysis.

For semi-quantitative analysis of CD44 expression, staining was performed at the same time for all groups and the percentage area of CD44 staining was calculated. Four confocal z-stacks of areas from the cortex and the hippocampus of each animal were taken ($n = 3$/group) with constant illumination and detection settings at $\times 20$ magnification and 0.5 zoom. For every image, maximum intensity projections were generated and the threshold for the respective staining was manually set. The number of particles (bigger than 1 µm^2) and the particle areas [square micrometers] were calculated using the ImageJ tool "Analyze particles." The total tissue area [in square micrometers] of each image was calculated, and the area percentage (area of stained particles/field of view) was calculated. The counting and measuring procedures were done manually using ImageJ software (1.44p).

Qualitative analysis for the CSF1R staining and the CD44 staining was performed, taking images of the hippocampus and cortex from all four study groups. The images were adjusted in color, size, brightness, and contrast using the ZEN lite 2012 software (version 1.1.2.0) and Microsoft PowerPoint.

Colocalization analysis was done using Imaris Software (9.1.2, Bitplane). Four confocal images of the hippocampus or cortex per animal were taken at ×40 magnification and 0.6 zoom and processed with the "Coloc" tool of the Imaris software. Colocalization channels were created for ThioflavinS and Iba1 as well as ThioflavinS and TMEM119 after setting manually the threshold for overlapping signals. The percentage (%) of dataset colocalized for the entire z-stack was calculated in APP-PS1 and APP-PS1 PLX5622-treated animals. For analysis of specifically macrophage plaque uptake, the percentage of ThioflavinS TMEM119 colocalization was subtracted from the total percentage of ThioflavinS Iba1 colocalization dataset (% of dataset colocalized ThioflavinS$^+$/Iba1$^+$/TMEM119$^-$; $n = 3$/group).

Quantification of CD8$^+$ T-cell numbers in the total brain section was performed using a Virtual Slide Microscope VS120 with the Olympus VS-ASW.L100 software (both from Olympus). Four total sagittal brain sections of one-tenth brain hemisphere per animal (12-month-old WT and APP-PS1 mice) were scanned at ×20 magnification ($n = 5$/genotype). The total number of CD8$^+$ cells was manually counted using Fiji software (ImageJ 1.51 h) and OlyVIA software (2.9, Olympus). The corresponding area (square micrometer) of the total sagittal section, the cortex, and the dorsal hippocampus was measured and multiplied by 40 to obtain the tissue volume represented in cubic micrometer (μm^3). To assess cell densities, the total number of counted cells per animal was divided by the corresponding tissue volume and represented as cells/cubic millimeter (cells/mm^3).

Statistics

For statistical analysis, the Prism 5–7 software (GraphPad) was used. The data were tested for normal distribution with the Kolmogorov-Smirnov test and were tested for outliers using Grubb's test. Comparing two groups, the unpaired Student's t test was used. Welch's correction was performed when variances were significantly different. If more than two groups were compared, one-way analysis of variance (ANOVA) was used and for behavioral learning assessment over time, two-way ANOVA was performed. For the one-way ANOVA, the Tukey's multiple comparison test was used as a post-hoc test, and for the two-way ANOVA, the Bonferroni or Tukey's multiple comparison post-test was performed. For gene expression data analysis two-way ANOVA with Tukey's multiple comparison was used. The data were depicted as mean and standard deviation (SD) with a 95% confidence interval or as mean with standard error of the mean (SEM) as indicated in the figure legends. p values of $p < 0.0001$ and $p < 0.001$ were considered extremely significant (**** or ***), $p < 0.01$ very significant (**), and $p < 0.05$ significant (*).

Results

CSF1R inhibition with PLX5622 diminished microglia but revealed a PLX5622-resistant population in the brains of APP-PS1 mice

To analyze the relevance of microglia in amyloid plaque pathology and CNS inflammation, we ablated these cells for a total of 28 days using the colony stimulating factor 1 receptor (CSF1R) inhibitor PLX5622 in 12-months-old APP-PS1 mice and WT littermate controls (Fig. 1a). We have chosen APP-PS1 mice with the age of 12 months, because at this stage, these animals already have massive amyloid-beta plaque formation in the hippocampus and cortex, high levels of microgliosis, and microglia activation as well as alterations in microglia cytokine production [52, 53]. The CSF1R is a cytokine receptor highly expressed on microglia and macrophages [54], and microglia survival in the adult brain strictly depends on CSF1R signaling [55]. As a consequence, inhibition of CSF1R in mice using pharmacological inhibitors such as PLX3397 leads to a total loss of about 99% of microglia cells in the brain [56]. Moreover, as a functional consequence, PLX5622-mediated ablation of microglia slightly alleviated the cognitive deficits in 3xTg-AD and 5xfAD transgenic mouse models of AD [38, 39]. Of note, peripheral macrophages and myeloid cells are less receptive to PLX5622-mediated depletion [39, 57, 58].

CSF1R is widely and exclusively expressed in Iba1$^+$ cells, i.e. microglia and macrophages, of the hippocampus (Fig. 1b) and cortex (Additional file 1: Figure S1) of 12-month-old WT and APP-PS1 animals. Iba1$^+$ cells co-expressed CSF1R, and in APP-PS1 mice, these cells clustered primarily at sites of amyloid plaques (Fig. 1b, APP-PS1 insert). After 28 days of treatment with PLX5622 (Fig. 1a) a few randomly distributed Iba1$^+$ cells were observed in WT animals (Fig. 1b, WT + PLX5622 insert), while in PLX5622-treated APP-PS1 mice, the remaining Iba1$^+$ cells were observed mainly at sites of amyloid-beta plaques (Fig. 1b, APP-PS1 + PLX5622 insert). The Iba1$^+$ cells detected in the brains of PLX5622-treated WT and of APP-PS1 animals did co-express CSF1R (Fig. 1b, arrow), but seem to be resistant to the PLX5622 treatment, a fact that has been noticed also by others [39]. Similar results were observed in the cortex (Additional file 1: Figure S1).

The 28-day PLX5622 treatment largely depleted the hippocampus and cortex of Iba1$^+$ cells in both genotypes (Fig. 2a, b). Interestingly, APP-PS1 animals started out having higher numbers of Iba1$^+$ cells compared to WT animals, and PLX5622-mediated Iba1 cell depletion in APP-PS1 animals was less efficient compared to WT animals. While 82.35% of Iba1 cells were ablated in WT hippocampus, only 70.04% of the cells were ablated in the APP-PS1 hippocampus (Fig. 2c). In the WT cortex, 92.12% of Iba1 cells were ablated, while in the APP-PS1

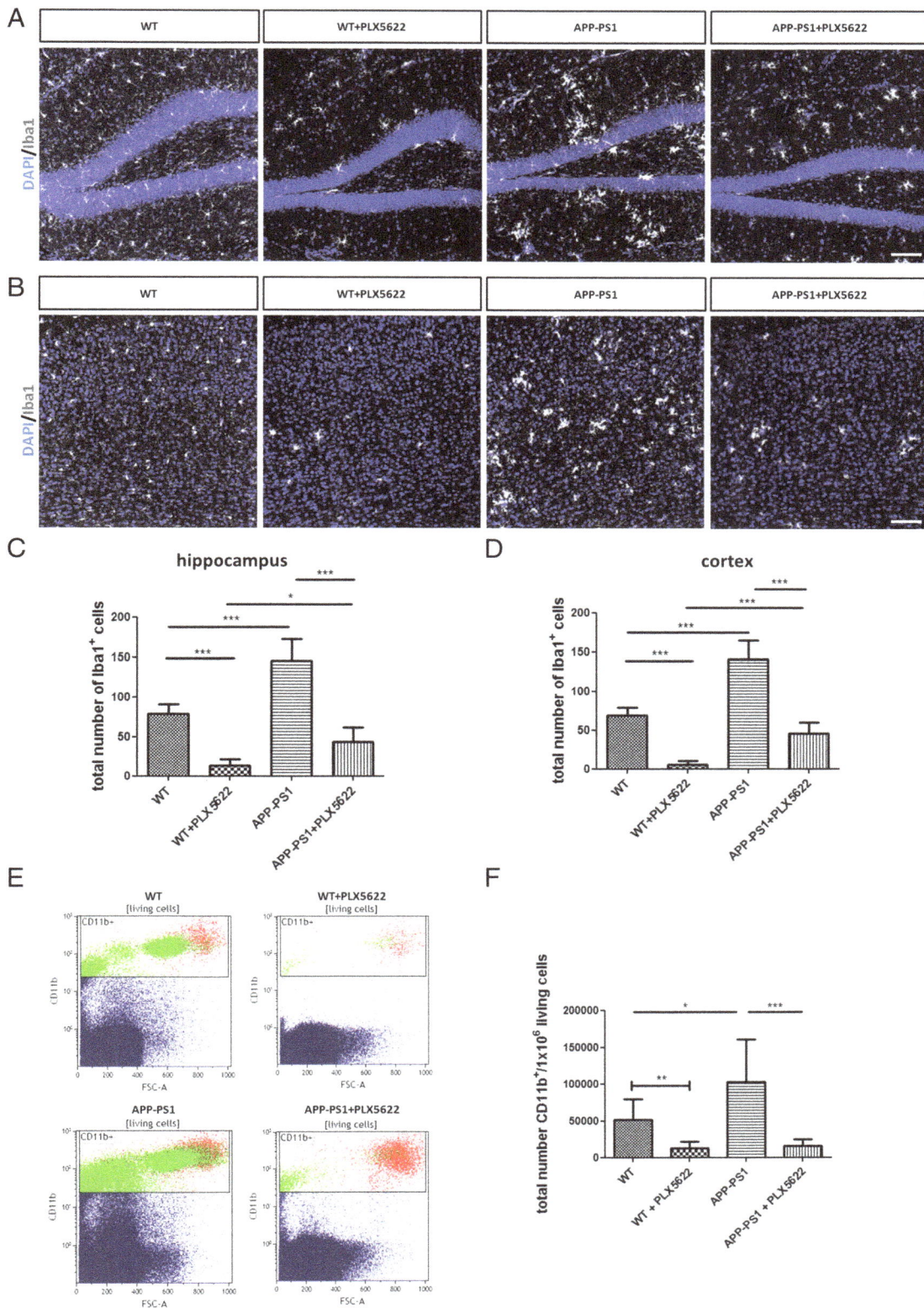

Fig. 2 (See legend on next page.)

(See figure on previous page.)
Fig. 2 Immunohistochemical and flow cytometric analysis of microglia/macrophage cells in the brains of WT and APP-PS1 animals treated with PLX5622. Staining for Iba1 (white) in the hippocampus (**a**) and the cortex (**b**) revealed significantly reduced numbers of Iba1$^+$ cells in brains of WT and APP-PS1 mice treated with PLX5622. Surprisingly, higher numbers of Iba1$^+$ cells were observed in both brain regions of APP-PS1 animals before treatment and higher numbers of Iba1$^+$ cells remained resistant to PLX5622 application compared to WT animals (**c, d**). After 28 days of treatment, microglia were mechanically isolated from total brain hemispheres, stained for CD11b, and quantitatively analyzed via flow cytometry. Representative flow cytometric dot plots of single-living CD11b$^+$ cells isolated from total brain hemispheres (**e**). Both WT and APP-PS1 animals treated with PLX5622 had highly reduced numbers of CD11b$^+$ cells, and surprisingly APP-PS1 animals had significantly higher numbers of isolated CD11b$^+$ cells compared to WT animals (**f**). Dapi (blue) was used as nucleus stain. One-way ANOVA with Tukey's multiple comparison test (**c, d** $n = 6$/group and **f** $n = 8$–9/group) and unpaired Student's t test with Welch's correction was performed comparing only WT with WT + PLX5622 (**f**, $n = 8$–9/group). Scale: 100 μm (**a, b**)

cortex, Iba1 cell ablation was 67.77% (Fig. 2d). The remaining Iba1$^+$ cells in the APP-PS1 animals were especially gathered around amyloid-plaques (Fig. 1b, APP-PS1 + PLX5622). Next, we used flow cytometry analysis of all CD11b-positive cells to quantify the effects of the PLX5622 treatment on the microglia/macrophage population (Fig. 2e). First, the total number of CD11b$^+$ cells isolated was significantly higher in the brains of APP-PS1 compared to WT mice (Fig. 2f). This was specifically seen in female APP-PS1 mice compared to female WT and compared to male APP-PS1 animals (Additional file 4: Figure S4, A-C). Second, after 28 days of PLX5622 treatment, the population of CD11b$^+$ cells was largely diminished but not completely erased in the brains of WT and APP-PS1 animals (Fig. 2e, f). In summary, microglia/macrophage depletion by PLX5622 treatment was efficient but not complete, and it identified a PLX5622-resistant microglia/macrophage population clustering at amyloid-beta plaques in the brains of APP-PS1 mice.

PLX5622 treatment and microglia ablation did neither modulate plaque pathology nor improve cognition in APP-PS1 mice

Since microglia cells are highly involved in amyloid-beta clearance, we assumed that a lack of microglia might increase the plaque burden in APP-PS1 mice. Surprisingly, there was neither a change in plaque numbers nor in plaque size in the hippocampus or cortex of APP-PS1 PLX5622-treated mice (Fig. 3a–f). These data suggest that the depleted microglia might not have been a major contributor to amyloid plaque degradation at this stage of disease pathology or that the remaining PLX5622 resistant Iba1$^+$ cells in APP-PS1 mice are highly efficient in amyloid phagocytosis and able to compensate the low numbers of microglia thereby keeping the plaque load at the same level. Another explanation might be that the 28-day treatment was just too short for a modulation of plaque pathology.

Next, we were interested in the consequences of the microglia depletion on cognitive function using the Morris water maze (MWM) test (Additional file 2: Figure S2). For behavior data analysis, mixed gender was used, since only minor sex differences were observed in the animals

(Additional file 3: Figure S3). We analyzed the total distance the animals traveled to reach the platform from day 2 to day 5. Despite a similar swimming speed of all animals (Additional file 2: Figure S2A), APP-PS1 mice had significant learning deficits and required longer distances to reach the platform compared to WT mice (Additional file 2: Figure S2B). PLX5622 treatment had no impact on learning behavior in WT mice (Additional file 2: Figure S2C), and microglia ablation did not improve cognitive deficits in APP-PS1 animals (Additional file 2: Figure S2D, E). For analysis of spatial memory, the platform was removed on day 6 and the time the animals spent in the original platform quadrant was measured. Memory deficits were not observed in APP-PS1 compared to WT mice, and PLX5622 treatment did not alter memory function in the APP-PS1 animals. In contrast, PLX5622-treated WT mice spent less time in the platform quadrant when compared only to their respective controls (Additional file 2: Figure S2F), indicating that microglia might contribute to memory function in the healthy CNS.

APP-PS1 brains are colonized by macrophages closely located to amyloid-beta plaques and are less susceptible to PLX5622 treatment

Triggered by the lack of PLX5622-mediated alterations in plaque pathology and the lack of effects on learning and memory, we focused on the identity and activity of the PLX5622 treatment-resistant Iba1$^+$ and CD11b$^+$ cells in the APP-PS1 mice. As Iba1 and CD11b are expressed by CNS resident microglia and by infiltrating macrophages, we first aimed to distinguish between these two cell populations by flow cytometry and by immunohistochemistry. Total mouse brain hemispheres were homogenized, and microglia/macrophage cells were isolated and quantified by flow cytometric analysis using antibodies against CD11b and CD45, where the microglia population is defined by being CD11b$^+$/CD45^{low} and the macrophage population by being CD11b$^+$/CD45^{high} [45–48]. In APP-PS1 mouse brains, the number of microglia (CD11b$^+$/CD45^{low}, green) was slightly but significantly higher compared to WT animals (Fig. 4h, i). This was specifically observed in female APP-PS1 mice compared to female WT mice (Additional file 4: Figure S4D). PLX5622 treatment drastically reduced this cell

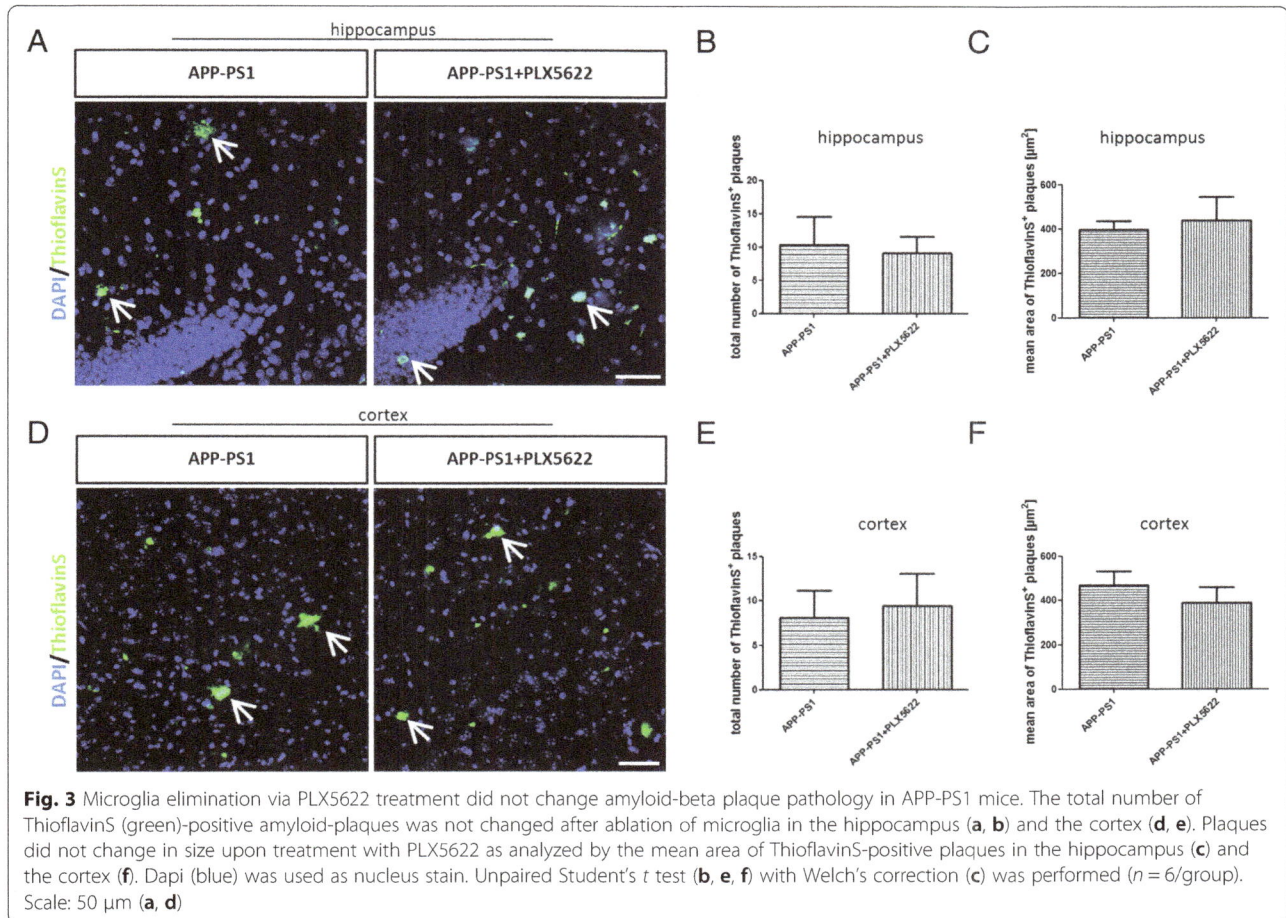

Fig. 3 Microglia elimination via PLX5622 treatment did not change amyloid-beta plaque pathology in APP-PS1 mice. The total number of ThioflavinS (green)-positive amyloid-plaques was not changed after ablation of microglia in the hippocampus (**a**, **b**) and the cortex (**d**, **e**). Plaques did not change in size upon treatment with PLX5622 as analyzed by the mean area of ThioflavinS-positive plaques in the hippocampus (**c**) and the cortex (**f**). Dapi (blue) was used as nucleus stain. Unpaired Student's t test (**b**, **e**, **f**) with Welch's correction (**c**) was performed ($n = 6$/group). Scale: 50 μm (**a**, **d**)

population in both genotypes (Fig. 4h, i). Similarly, the macrophage population (CD11b$^+$/CD45^{high}) was significantly larger in the brains of APP-PS1 mice compared to WT animals (Fig. 4j) and higher in female APP-PS1 mice compared to female WT mice (Additional file 4: Figure S4G). PLX5622 treatment diminished this cell population, however, with less efficacy compared to the CD11b$^+$/CD45^{low} microglia population (Fig. 4j). Also, female and male APP-PS1 mice had higher numbers of CD11b$^+$/CD45^{high} cells compared to female and male WT mice; PLX5622 treatment did not decrease this cell numbers in male animals of both genotypes (Additional file 4: Figure S4H). Additionally, female APP-PS1 compared to male APP-PS1 mice had higher numbers of CD11b$^+$/CD45^{low} and CD11b$^+$/CD45^{high} cell populations (Additional file 4: Figure S4F, I).

To analyze the microglia and macrophage populations in more detail, we performed immunohistochemical analysis using the recently identified microglia-specific marker TMEM119, which in combination with Iba1 immunohistochemistry nicely distinguishes microglia (Iba1$^+$/TMEM119$^+$) from macrophages (Iba1$^+$/TMEM119$^-$) in brain sections [48]. The immunohistochemical characterization and

quantitative analysis of Iba1$^+$/TMEM119$^+$ and Iba1$^+$/TMEM119$^-$ cells in the hippocampus (Fig. 4k) and in the cortex (Additional file 5: Figure S5) revealed that WT and APP-PS1 animals had similar amounts of Iba1$^+$/TMEM119$^+$ microglia cells and that this population was largely reduced by the PLX5622 treatment (Fig. 4l). In contrast to WT animals, which had only few Iba1$^+$/TMEM119$^-$ macrophages, APP-PS1 animals contained a higher number of these cells in the hippocampus (Fig. 4m) and cortex (Additional file 5: Figure S5C). Iba1$^+$/TMEM119$^-$ macrophages colonized mainly areas at sites of ThioflavinS-positive plaques (Fig. 4k, arrow). PLX5622 treatment only slightly diminished this population leaving a high number of Iba1$^+$/TMEM119$^-$ macrophages in these brain regions (Fig. 4m). Analyzing the percentage of TMEM119$^+$ and TMEM119$^-$ cell populations in the total Iba1$^+$ cell count revealed a small population of Iba1$^+$ macrophages in PLX5622-treated WT animals. In contrast, in APP-PS1 animals, approximately 50% of the Iba1$^+$ population were macrophages, and most dramatically, in PLX5622-treated APP-PS1 mice, the majority of Iba1$^+$ cells was negative for TMEM119 and therefore presumably macrophages (Fig. 4n). This pool of Iba1$^+$/TMEM119$^-$ macrophages was predominantly observed at sites of

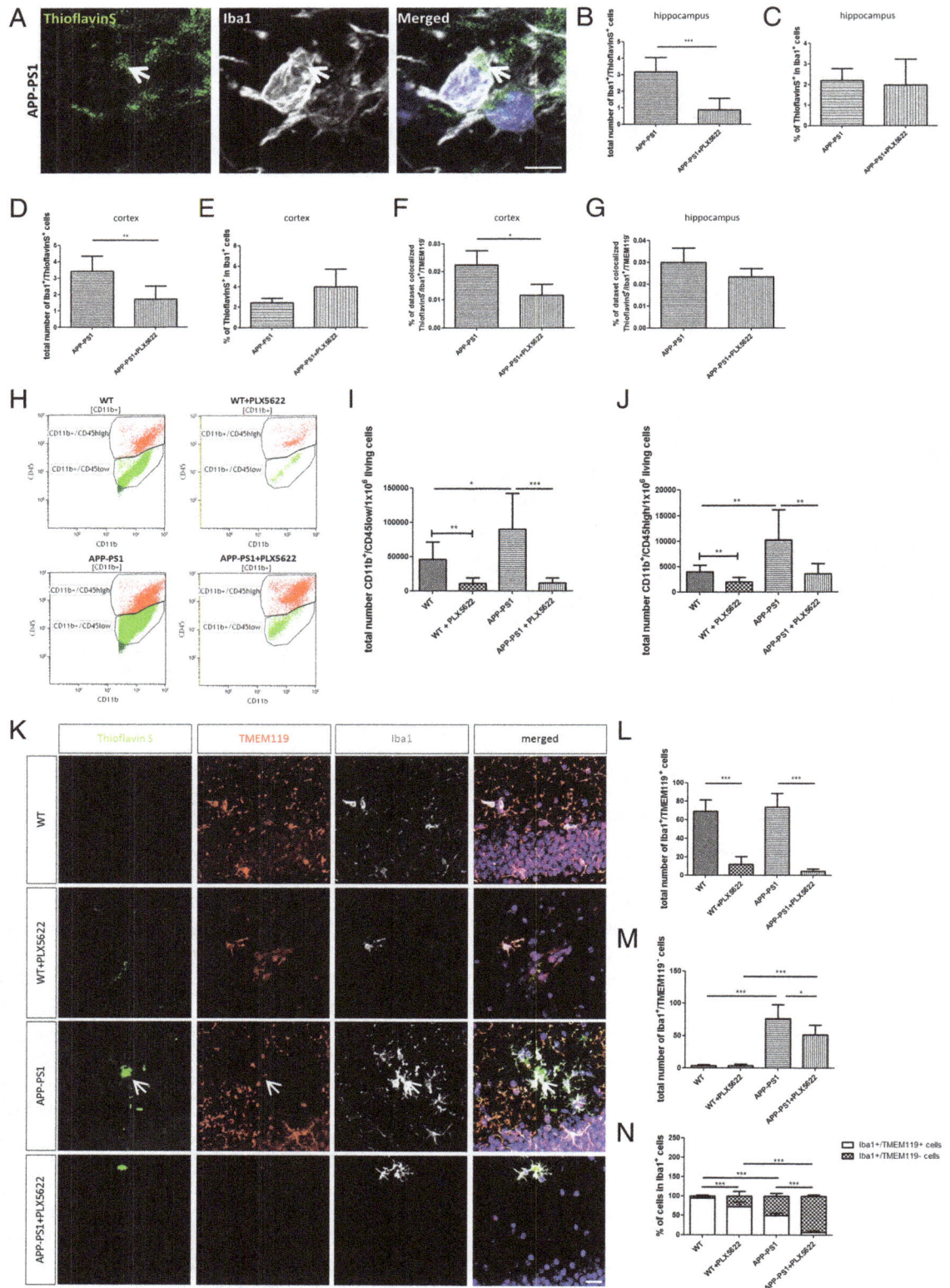

Fig. 4 (See legend on next page.)

(See figure on previous page.)
Fig. 4 Microglia ablation did not alter amyloid-beta phagocytosis and revealed high numbers of macrophages located at sites of plaques resistant to CSF1R inhibition. **a** Representative image of Iba1$^+$ cell at site of plaque with incorporated ThioflavinS$^+$ particle in the hippocampus of APP-PS1 mice. The total number of Iba1$^+$/ThioflavinS$^+$ cells was significantly reduced upon PLX5622 treatment in the hippocampus (**b**) and the cortex (**d**). However, the percentage (%) of Iba1$^+$/ThioflavinS$^+$ cells from total Iba1$^+$ cell counts remained the same in both brain regions of APP-PS1 animals treated with PLX5622 (**c, e**). Colocalization analysis with ThioflavinS was performed to analyze the plaque uptake by ThioflavinS$^+$/Iba1$^+$/TMEM119$^-$ cells. There was no observed increase in the amount of engulfed plaque material, represented by the percentage of dataset colocalized with ThioflavinS; however, in the cortex, the percentage of dataset colocalized was significantly reduced in microglia-ablated APP-PS1 mice (**f**). This was not seen in the hippocampus (**g**). Mechanically isolated CD11b$^+$ cells were further characterized by their CD45 expression via flow cytometric analysis (**h**) to distinguish microglia (CD11b$^+$/CD45^{low}, green) from macrophage populations (CD11b$^+$/CD45^{high}, red). Besides strongly reduced CD11b$^+$/CD45^{low} microglia numbers in WT and APP-PS1 animals treated with PLX5622, APP-PS1 mice revealed significantly increased numbers of CD11b$^+$/CD45^{low} microglia compared to WT animals (**i**). Analysis of CD11b$^+$/CD45^{high} macrophages revealed significantly increased numbers of CD11b$^+$/CD45^{high} cells in APP-PS1 compared to WT and treatment with PLX5622 reduced this cell population in WT and APP-PS1 mice (**j**). Using the newly identified microglia marker TMEM119 for detailed immunohistochemical analysis in the hippocampus revealed strong co-localization of Iba1$^+$ (white) cells with TMEM119 (red) in WT and WT animals treated with PLX5622; however, Iba1$^+$ cells at sites of plaques (green) in APP-PS1 animals and APP-PS1 treated with PLX5622 did not express TMEM119 (**k**, arrow). Quantitative analysis of Iba1$^+$/TMEM119$^+$ revealed a significant reduction upon PLX5622 treatment in WT and APP-PS1 mice (**l**). Surprisingly, APP-PS1 animals had increased numbers of Iba1$^+$/TMEM119$^-$ cells that were more resistant to PLX5622 treatment than in WT animals (**m**). (**n**) Calculation of the percentage of Iba1$^+$/TMEM119$^+$ and Iba1$^+$/TMEM119$^-$ cells from the total Iba1$^+$ cell population. ThioflavinS was used to stain amyloid plaques (green), and Dapi (blue) was used as nucleus stain. Unpaired Student's t test (**b, c, d** $n = 6$/group; **f, g** $n = 3$/group; **j** comparing WT with WT + PLX5622 $n = 8–9$/group;) with Welch's correction (**e** $n = 6$/group; **i** comparing WT with WT + PLX5622 $n = 8–9$/group) and one-way ANOVA with Tukey's multiple comparison test (**i, j** $n = 8–9$/group; **l, m, n** $n = 6$/group) was performed. Scale: 5 μm (**a**), 20 μm (**k**)

amyloid-plaques in APP-PS1 brains and microglia-ablated APP-PS1 brains. Very similar findings were observed in the cortex (Additional file 5: Figure S5). In summary, PLX5622 treatment was highly efficacious to ablate microglia but identified a CSF1R blockage-resistant and plaque-associated Iba1$^+$/TMEM119$^-$ macrophage population in APP-PS1 animals.

Iba1$^+$/TMEM119$^-$ cells expressed the phagocytosis marker CD68 representing a macrophage population presumably involved in amyloid-beta plaque clearance

To determine whether the resistant Iba1$^+$ cells take on new and different roles in plaque phagocytosis depending on the presence or absence of microglia, quantitative co-localization analysis was performed to estimate the engulfed amount of plaque material. We counted the number of Iba1$^+$ cells that had incorporated ThioflavinS-positive particles (Iba1$^+$/ThioflavinS$^+$), as an indicator for phagocytosis, in the hippocampus and cortex of APP-PS1 mice and APP-PS1 mice treated with PLX5622 (Fig. 4a, arrow). PLX5622 treatment did significantly reduce Iba1$^+$/ThioflavinS$^+$ cell numbers in both brain regions (Fig. 4b, d). However, the percentage of Iba1$^+$/ThioflavinS$^+$ cells in the total Iba1$^+$ cell count was the same in PLX5622 and control treated in APP-PS1 mice, indicating that the principal capacity of the Iba1$^+$ cells to phagocytose was unaffected by the treatment (Fig. 4c, e). Taken together, this suggests that the PLX5622-resistant Iba1$^+$ cell population might be able to compensate the PLX5622 mediated deficiency of phagocytosing microglia in the APP-PS1 mouse brains.

We next analyzed the PLX5622-resistant Iba1$^+$ cell population in more detail and estimated the amount of engulfed plaque material, discriminating between macrophages and microglia. The percentage of ThioflavinS colocalized with Iba1, i.e. microglia and macrophages, and colocalized with TMEM119 (microglia) was calculated using Imaris software. There was no general increase in plaque uptake in PLX5622-resistant cells; moreover, in the hippocampus of microglia-ablated APP-PS1 brains, the percentage of colocalization was very similar compared to not-ablated APP-PS1 brains (Fig. 4g). However, PLX5622-resistant Iba1$^+$ cells in the cortex (Fig. 4f) showed a significant decrease in colocalization with ThioflavinS upon microglia depletion. Given the fact that there were no alterations in plaque pathology after microglia ablation, we conclude that PLX5622-resistant cells contribute to plaque phagocytosis. However, phagocytotic activity was not elevated in these cells upon microglia ablation in the brains of APP-PS1 mice.

We further investigated the activity/inflammatory state of microglia (Iba1$^+$/TMEM119$^+$) and macrophages (Iba1$^+$/TMEM119$^-$) in the hippocampus (Fig. 5) and cortex (Additional file 6: Figure S6) of WT and APP-PS1 mice by staining for CD68, a classical macrophage and microglia activation marker that is involved in cellular phagocytosis. WT and APP-PS1 mice had the same numbers of CD68$^+$ microglia that were equally affected and reduced by the PLX5622 treatment (Fig. 5a). APP-PS1 mice had significantly more CD68$^+$ macrophages in the brain compared to WT animals, the latter showing barely any CD68$^+$ macrophages (Fig. 5b). PLX5622 treatment reduced this population in APP-PS1 mice, but higher numbers of CD68$^+$ macrophages remained in PLX5622-treated APP-PS1 compared to treated WT mice (Fig. 5b). High expression of CD68 was detected in macrophages at sites of amyloid plaques in APP-PS1 mice (Fig. 5c). Besides CD68, the amyloid

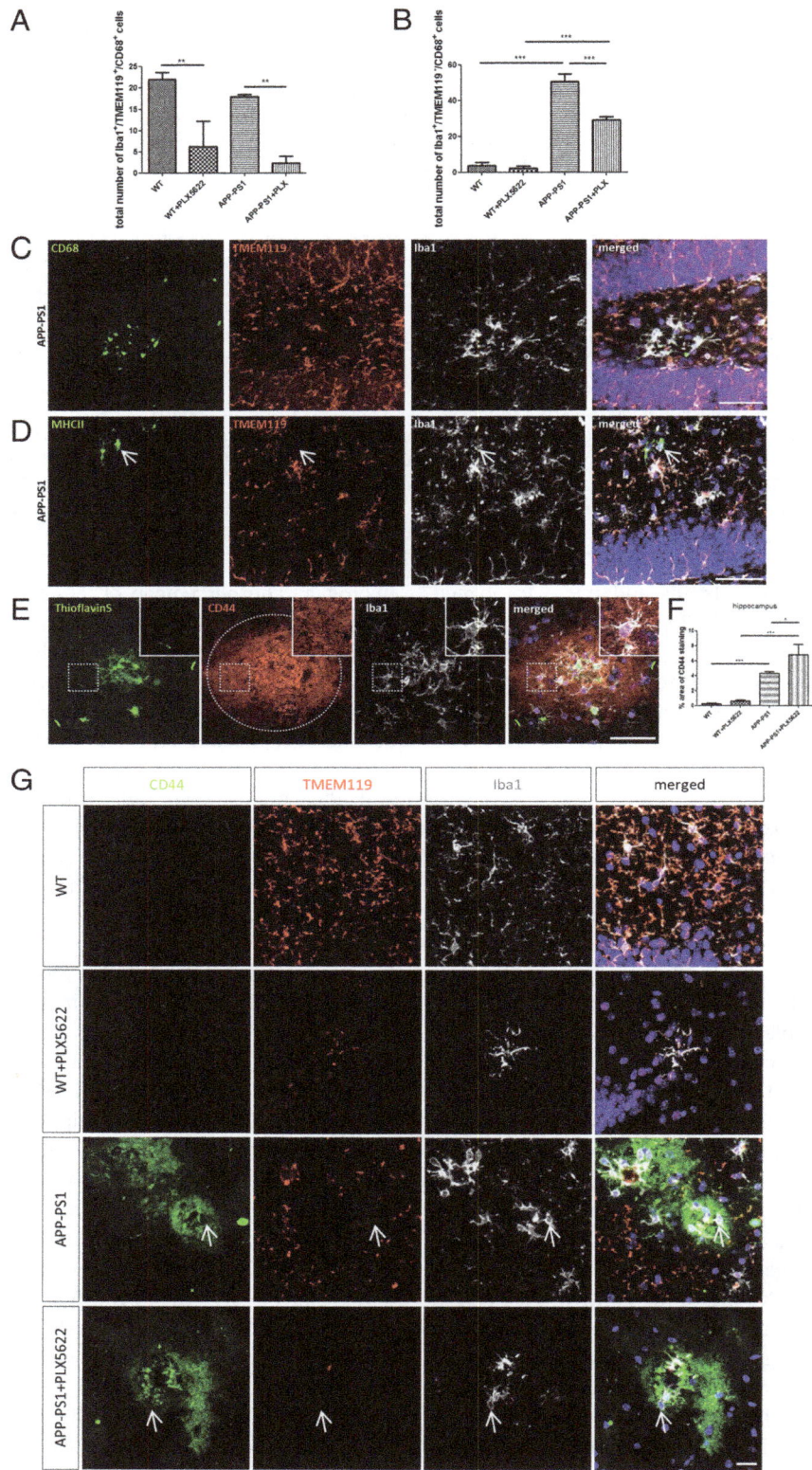

Fig. 5 (See legend on next page.)

(See figure on previous page.)
Fig. 5 Iba1+/TMEM119− cells represent a CD68+ macrophage population with peripheral origin highly involved in amyloid-beta phagocytosis. Analysis of CD68 expression in the hippocampus revealed significantly reduced numbers of Iba1+/TMEM119+/CD68+ cells in APP-PS1 and WT animals upon PLX5622 treatment (**a**). Surprisingly, higher numbers of Iba1+/TMEM119−/CD68+ cells were found in APP-PS1 animals compared to WT, although these numbers were slightly reduced in APP-PS1 animals by PLX5622 treatment (**b**). Representative image of CD68 expression in Iba1+/TMEM119− cells located at sites of plaque in APP-PS1 mice (**c**). Strong MHCII expression was seen sporadically in Iba1+/TMEM119− cells in APP-PS1 mice (**d**, arrow). Accumulation of CD44 staining (red) was observed extracellularly around amyloid depositions (green) as indicated by the doted ellipse, and CD44 staining was seen on Iba1+ cells at sites of plaques (**e**, insert). Quantification of percentage (%) area of CD44 staining in hippocampal brain regions revealed barely any staining in WT and WT + PLX5622-treated animals; however, in APP-PS1 and APP-PS1 PLX5622-treated mice, significantly higher expression of CD44 was observed compared to WT controls (**f**). Detailed immunohistochemical analysis revealed increased staining for CD44 at sites of amyloid deposition in areas colonized with Iba1+/TMEM119− cells in APP-PS1 and APP-PS1 PLX5622-treated mice (**g**, arrow). ThioflavinS was used to stain amyloid plaques, and Dapi (blue) was used as nucleus stain. One-way ANOVA with Tukey's multiple comparison test (**a**, **b**, **f** $n = 3$/group) was performed. Scale: 50 μm (**c**, **d**, **e**), 20 μm (**g**)

plaque-associated macrophage population in the APP-PS1 mice sporadically co-localized with MHCII (Fig. 5d) further supporting the macrophage identity of these cells and indicating that these cells are probably involved in antigen presentation. Similar findings were observed in the cortex (Additional file 6: Figure S6).

To further substantiate the peripheral origin of Iba1+/TMEM119− macrophage cells characterized in this work, we used CD44 as recently described marker to distinguish between resident and infiltrating immune cells in the brain [46]. Surprisingly, we found very prominent staining for CD44 in APP-PS1 and APP-PS1 PLX5622-treated mice around amyloid-beta plaques in the hippocampus (Fig. 5e) and the cortex (Additional file 6: Figure S6E). CD44 was localized extracellularly around the amyloid plaques and at Iba1+ cells closely attached to amyloid plaques (Fig. 5e, insert). Quantification of CD44 staining revealed barely any CD44 staining in WT or WT PLX5622-treated mice; however, CD44 staining was significantly higher in the hippocampus (Fig. 5f) and cortex (Additional file 6: Figure S6F) of APP-PS1 and APP-PS1 PLX5622-treated mice. Triple staining with Iba1 and TMEM119 revealed intense staining for CD44 at sites of plaques, where Iba1+/TMEM119− cells were located (Fig. 5g, arrow). Very similar findings were observed in cortical brain regions (Additional file 6: Figure S6). These data further suggest that Iba1+/TMEM119− cells have peripheral origin and that the extracellular adhesion molecule CD44 might play a pivotal role in leukocyte homing from the periphery to the CNS and to the sites of inflammation in AD.

Elevated levels of CD8+ T-cells in brains of APP-PS1 mice and increased CD8+ T-cell homing to microglia-ablated APP-PS1 mouse brains

Apparently, lymphocytes are one of the biggest peripheral immune cell populations observed in the CNS of healthy adult mice [46]. Besides, T-cells are reported to enter the brain parenchyma of AD-transgenic mice [31]. We recently identified a specific T-cell population highly associated and presumably interacting with resident microglia in the brains of APP-PS1-transgenic mice [37]. Here, we first

quantified the number of CD8+ T-cells present in the brains of WT and of APP-PS1 mice via histology in total sagittal brain sections. While the numbers did not differ for the total brain, there was a significantly higher number of CD8+ T-cells in the cortex of APP-PS1 mice compared to WT controls (Fig. 6a). To address now the question, if T-cell infiltration is microglia dependent, we made further use of the present PLX5622-mediated microglia depletion experiment and analyzed the numbers and identity of T-cells in the brain of WT and APP-PS1 mice where microglia cells were ablated. We first isolated T-cells from total brain hemispheres of WT and APP-PS1 mice revealing no difference in the number of CD3+, CD3+/CD4+, or CD3+/CD8+ T-cells in APP-PS1 mice compared to WT (Fig. 6b–e) confirming the histology data from above. A gender-specific analysis of the flow cytometric data revealed increased CD3+, CD3+/CD4+, and CD3+/CD8+ T-cell numbers in female compared to male APP-PS1 mice (Additional file 7: Figure S7C, F, I), and increased cell numbers were found in female APP-PS1 mice when specifically compared to female WT mice (Additional file 7: Figure S7A, D, G). Surprisingly, ablation of microglia caused a significant increase in the numbers of CD3+, more specifically CD3+/CD8+ T-cells, exclusively in brains of APP-PS1 and not WT mice treated with PLX5622 (Fig. 6b, c, e). CD4+ T-cells were slightly but not significantly increased in PLX5622-treated APP-PS1 mice. Microglia ablation apparently allowed specifically CD3+/CD8+ T-cell homing to the APP-PS1 brain. Vice versa, this let suggest that microglia in APP-PS1 mice might somehow inhibit specifically CD3+/CD8+ T-cell recruitment to the brain. To test if the herein observed increase in CD8+ T-cell numbers might arise from proliferation of brain resident T-cells, we additionally stained for expression of the proliferation cell nuclear antigen (PCNA). CD8+ T-cells in the brain of PLX5622-treated or untreated APP-PS1 animals did not show expression of PCNA indicating no clonal expansion and no local generation of these cells in the brain (Additional file 8: Figure S8). To investigate the CD8+ T-cells in the context of microglia in more detail, we analyzed their spatial relation to Iba1+

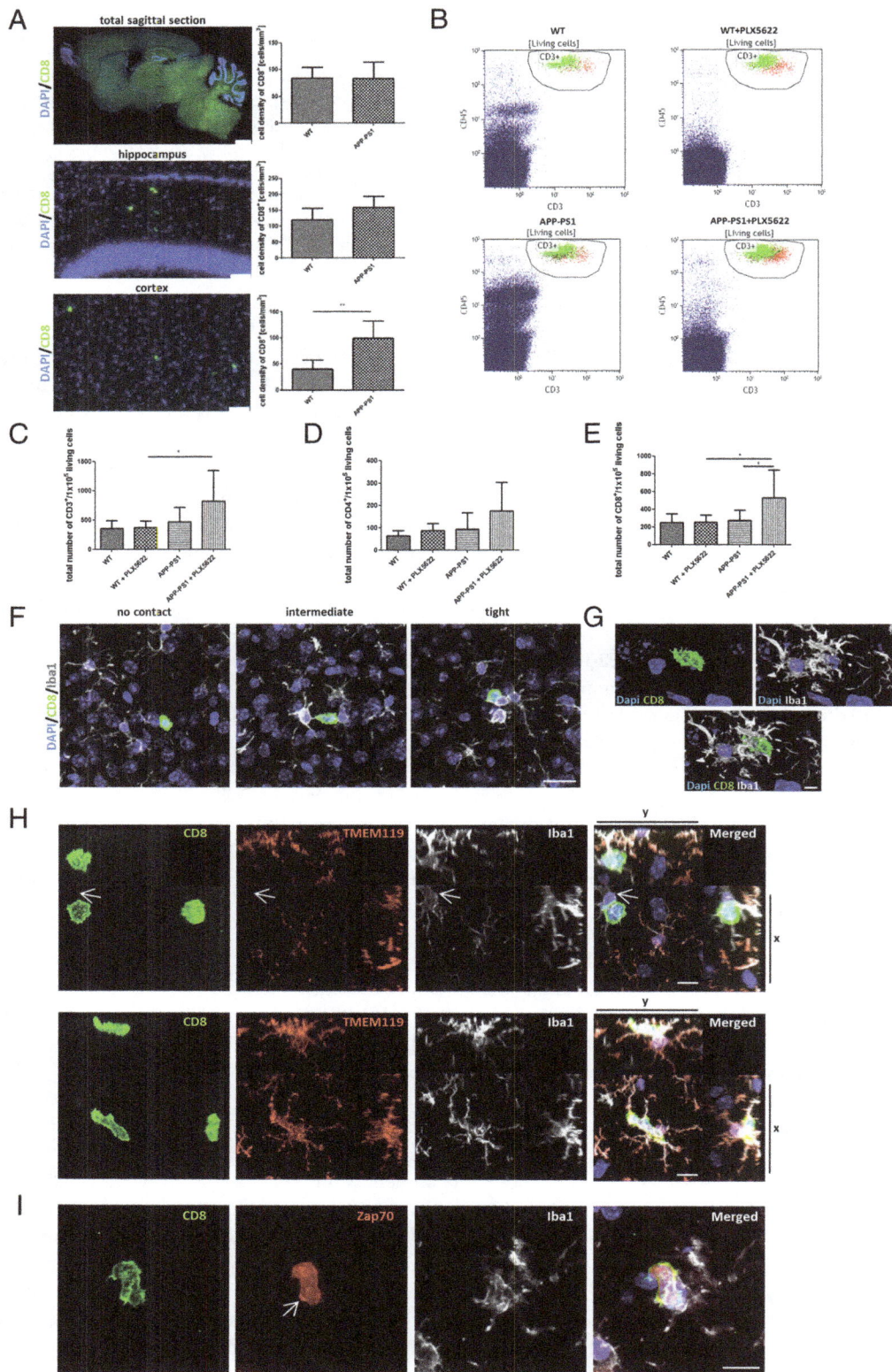

Fig. 6 (See legend on next page.)

(See figure on previous page.)

Fig. 6 Microglia ablation in APP-PS1 mice resulted in increased CD3$^+$/CD8$^+$ T-cell numbers in the brain, and CD8$^+$ T-cell numbers were highly increased in cortical brain regions of APP-PS1 mice interacting with Iba1$^+$/TMEM119$^+$ and Iba1$^+$/TMEM119$^-$ cells. Detailed immunohistochemical analysis of CD8$^+$ T-cell numbers (green) in brains of APP-PS1 mice revealed similar CD8$^+$ T-cell numbers compared to WT when analyzing total sagittal brain sections; however, CD8$^+$ T-cell numbers were significantly increased in cortical brain regions of APP-PS1 mice compared to WT (**a**). T-cells were mechanically isolated from total brain hemispheres and quantitatively analyzed by flow cytometry after ablation of microglia cells (**b**, gated for single-living CD45$^+$/CD3$^+$ cells; CD4$^+$ red, CD8$^+$ green). The total number of CD45$^+$/CD3$^+$ T-cells was significantly increased in APP-PS1 mice treated with PLX5622 compared to WT-treated mice (**c**). CD3$^+$/CD4$^+$ T-cell numbers trend to be increased in APP-PS1 mice treated with PLX5622 (**d**). CD3$^+$/CD8$^+$ T-cell numbers were significantly increased in APP-PS1 mice treated with PLX5622 compared to APP-PS1 and WT PLX5622-treated mice (**e**). CD8$^+$ T-cells in APP-PS1 mice were located directly in the brain parenchyma and observed in different interaction types with Iba1$^+$ cells (white), showing either no contact, intermediate, or very tight interaction with brains Iba1$^+$ cells (**f**). Performing confocal microscopy, we observed very tight cell to cell interactions with Iba1$^+$ cells (**g**) and orthogonal projections showed CD8$^+$ T-cells associated with Iba1$^+$/TMEM119$^+$ and as well with Iba1$^+$/TMEM119$^-$ cells in APP-PS1 mice (arrow, **h**). CD8$^+$ T-cells that tightly associated to Iba1$^+$ cells showed high expression of Zap70 (red) at sites of the cell membrane, indicating immune synapse formation, and activation of the T-cell receptor complex (arrow, **i**). Dapi (blue) was used as nucleus stain. One-way ANOVA with Tukey's multiple comparison test (**c**, **d**, **e** $n = 8$–9/group) and unpaired Student's t test (**a**, $n = 5$/group) was performed. Scale: 1 mm and 50 μm (**a**), 20 μm (**f**), 10 μm (**h**, **i**), 5 μm (**g**)

cells in APP-PS1 brains. CD8$^+$ T-cells were in different proximities and interactions with Iba1$^+$ cells. They either had barely any cell to cell contact, some interaction at the level of the cellular processes, or a very close and tight interaction with Iba1$^+$ cells (Fig. 6f). In the latter, high magnification of confocal z-stacks and 3D reconstruction revealed very close cell to cell communication of CD8$^+$ T-cells with Iba1$^+$ cells (Fig. 6g). To address the question if CD8$^+$ T-cells are interacting only with microglia or as well with the herein described macrophage population in APP-PS1 mice, we performed triple staining with Iba1 and TMEM119 and could demonstrate that CD8$^+$ T-cells form tight interaction with both cell types (Fig. 6h).

To further confirm this immune cell interaction present in APP-PS1 brains, we stained for Zap70, an essential kinase for T-cell receptor function and immune synapse formation. CD8$^+$ T-cells in the brain were mostly positive for Zap70, and Zap70 staining was very prominent on the cell membrane and clustered at sites of interaction with Iba1$^+$ cells (Fig. 6i, arrow) suggesting a functional interaction between the two cell types. Besides CD8$^+$ T-cells, we qualitatively analyzed the brains of APP-PS1 mice for CD4$^+$ T-cells via histology. As expected from the flow cytometric data, CD4$^+$ T-cells were observed less frequently than CD8$^+$ T-cells, even though they did express the immune synapse marker Zap70 (Additional file 9: Figure S9). In summary, microglia ablation resulted in increased CD3$^+$/CD8$^+$ T-cell homing to sites of inflammation specifically in the brain of APP-PS1 mice, suggesting that the present microglia in APP-PS1 mice might block adaptive immune responses along AD pathology.

Microglia depletion has profound consequences on gene transcription of pro- and anti-inflammatory and phagocytosis-relevant genes in the brain

To analyze the herein described rather complex cellular effects of PLX5622 treatment on the brain's immunological micro-environment, we performed mRNA expression analysis of genes specific for microglia, for a pro- or anti-inflammatory micro-milieu, and for phagocytosis (Fig. 7a, b). In APP-PS1 compared to WT mice, expression of the microglia genes AIF1 (=Iba1) and TMEM119 was only slightly higher in the hippocampus (Fig. 7a) but significantly (about two-fold) higher in the cortex (Fig. 7b) correlating with the histological and flow cytometric findings (Fig. 2). Along this line, APP-PS1 brains had higher expression levels of the phagocytosis-relevant genes Trem2 and CD33. APP-PS1 brains showed a more pronounced elevation of some pro-inflammatory (H2-Aa = MHCII, IL-1beta, CCL2), as well as some anti-inflammatory (IL10, TGF-beta) genes in the cortex compared to the hippocampus. The 28-day PLX5622 treatment resulted in a highly diminished but not completely erased expression of AIF1 and TMEM119 in the hippocampus and cortex in both genotypes, which again correlates with the histological and flow cytometric findings. The pro-inflammatory genes H2-Aa and IL6 were significantly lower in the hippocampus of APP-PS1 and WT animals after treatment with PLX5622. This effect was less pronounced in the cortex. Moreover and surprisingly, gene expression levels of CCL2 and of IL-1beta were higher in the PLX5622-treated APP-PS1 cortex compared to control-treated and compared to WT cortex. The elevated expression of CCL2 is especially of interest, as it is known to be a major chemoattractant for monocytes and might explain the prominent presence of monocytes after PLX5622 treatment in the APP-PS1 brains. Microglia ablation affected also the gene expression of the anti-inflammatory molecules MRC1 (=CD206) and TGFbeta. In the hippocampus, MRC1 and TGFbeta gene expression was massively reduced upon PLX5622 treatment in WT and APP-PS1 animals. This effect was even more pronounced in the cortex, where also IL10 expression was almost completely erased by the PLX5622 treatment. PLX5622 treatment led to an enormous reduction in Trem2 expression, however more effective in WT than in APP-PS1 mice. CD33 was also massively lower in PLX5622-treated WT and APP-PS1 mice compared to the

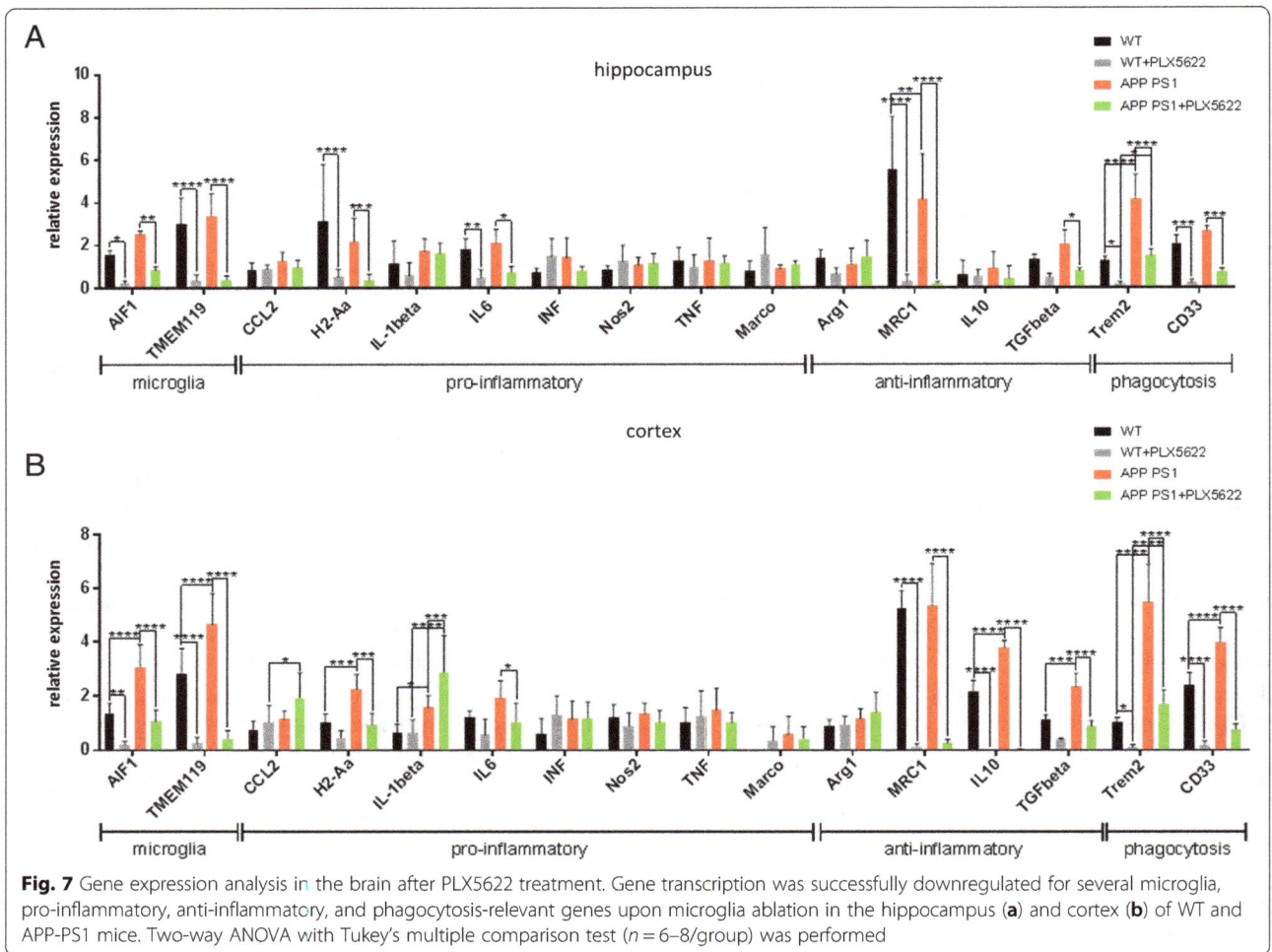

Fig. 7 Gene expression analysis in the brain after PLX5622 treatment. Gene transcription was successfully downregulated for several microglia, pro-inflammatory, anti-inflammatory, and phagocytosis-relevant genes upon microglia ablation in the hippocampus (**a**) and cortex (**b**) of WT and APP-PS1 mice. Two-way ANOVA with Tukey's multiple comparison test ($n = 6$–8/group) was performed

control animals. In summary, APP-PS1 mice had a higher expression of microglia- and phagocytosis-specific genes compared to WT animals, as well as an alteration in the pattern of pro-inflammatory as well as anti-inflammatory proteins. PLX5622 treatment resulted in diminished expression of the microglia- and phagocytosis-specific genes in WT as well as APP-PS1 brains and, except for a higher expression of CCL2 and of IL-1beta in the cortex, resulted in a reduction of the expression of some pro-inflammatory but mainly and more pronounced in the reduction of anti-inflammatory cytokine expression.

Discussion

In the present work, we demonstrate that a 28-day treatment with PLX5622 resulted in massive reduction of microglia cell numbers and a decrease of microglia-related gene expression in the brains of WT and APP-PS1 mice. Furthermore, we show that APP-PS1 mice harbor a specific Iba1+/TMEM119− and CD68+ macrophage population resistant to CSF1R treatment presumably involved in plaque clearance. Ablation of microglia revealed the existence of

these cells at sites of amyloid plaques, and colonization by macrophages appeared with a strong CD44 staining at sites of amyloid-plaques, which together with the elevated CCL2 expression points towards a milieu that is highly attractive for peripheral immune cells. Indeed, microglia depletion in APP-PS1 animals increased the number of CD3+/CD8+ T-cells specifically in the brains of APP-PS1 mice. These T-cells expressed the immune synapse marker Zap70 and additionally were in close association with remaining microglia and macrophages. Therefore, we assume that in AD pathology, microglia restrain the brain from an adaptive immune response and act in that sense primarily anti-inflammatory. In their absence, macrophages might function as important linchpin and connect innate to adaptive immune responses by recruiting T-cells to the AD brain. Overall, microglia depletion led to a diminished expression of anti-inflammatory cytokines in the APP-PS1 mice shifting the balance towards a pro-inflammatory milieu.

Over the past years, there is emerging evidence that the brain is not immunologically isolated from the peripheral immune system (reviewed in [59, 60]). The brain and its specific compartments, i.e., the meninges and choroid plexus, but also the brain parenchyma itself is highly immune-competent and harbors a diversity of peripheral-derived immune cells comparable to the blood [46]. Bone marrow-derived monocytes and macrophages were observed to infiltrate the brains of transgenic AD mice [27] and are controversially discussed to participate in amyloid clearance (reviewed in [28–30] and [61]). Even though infiltration of macrophages in brains of transgenic AD mice was already observed by others ([27], reviewed in [23]), the clear presence of Iba1$^+$ cells lacking the microglia-specific marker TMEM119 (Iba1$^+$/TMEM119$^-$) located at sites of amyloid plaques in transgenic AD mouse brains is to our knowledge not yet reported. Here, we show for the first time a specific TMEM119$^-$ macrophage population colonizing at sites of the amyloid plaques in APP-PS1 mice. The recently identified specific microglia marker TMEM119 developed by Bennet et al. [48] allowed us to clearly distinguish the microglia population from the macrophage population in the transgenic AD brains. TMEM119 reliably stains microglia in the human brain, while macrophages (Iba1$^+$/CD68$^+$) at sites of necrotic lesion in human multiple sclerosis (MS) brains do not express TMEM119 [62]. How microglia cells can be distinguished from peripheral-derived macrophage populations in the brain and how these two cell types differ from their genetic profile and marker expression is currently discussed [63, 64]. For example, only microglia and not macrophages fully regain their cellular identity, when transplanted in the brain of microglia-deficient mice. Bennett et al. demonstrated that brain environment and microglia ontogeny are crucial for keeping cellular identity and characteristics. However, macrophages of different peripheral origin transplanted to the microglia-depleted brain are able to engraft and become a microglia-like cell population, still keeping specific ontogeny markers, but hard to distinguish from brain resident microglia cells [63]. To what extend macrophages that once entered the brain can turn into microglia cells or keep their cellular identity and if this has any functional consequences especially under neurodegenerative conditions is still scarce [64]. Nevertheless, the herein presented data are in line with the current literature and show the spatial presence of this non-microglia population in the brain at sites of inflammation in the APP-PS1 transgenic mice.

There are various reports on microglia depletion targeting the CSF1R receptor in mice [38, 39, 55, 56, 65, 66]. In these studies, CSF1R signaling is either blocked using small molecular inhibitors [55, 56], CSF1R$^{-/-}$ knockout mice [67, 68], or genetically modified inducible microglial reporter mice, where transient microglia ablation is achieved by diphtheria toxin injections [65] or by ganciclovir administration in suicide gene herpes simplex virus thymidine kinase (HSVTK)-carrying mice

(reviewed in [69] and [70]). Microglia ablation specifically in AD mice resulted in several beneficial effects on AD pathology such as a reduction in dendritic spine and neuronal loss as well as behavioral alterations, e.g. improvement in contextual memory [38, 39]. However, although neuroinflammation was highly dampened in these microglia-ablated mice, amyloid plaque pathology was not altered by CSF1R inhibition [38, 39]. Prokop et al., who conditionally ablated microglia cells with ganciclovir treatment using a CD11b-HSVTK transgenic AD mouse model, analyzed the capability of peripheral myeloid cells in repopulating the brain and their potential in amyloid-beta plaque phagocytosis. They demonstrated that after microglia depletion, the brains were nearly completely exchanged by peripheral myeloid cells and the overall amyloid-beta burden was unchanged in repopulated brains [61]. These data are in line with our data, indicating that peripheral-derived macrophages might compensate functions of microglia.

Besides monocytes/macrophages, lymphocytes resemble a big proportion of peripheral immune cells [46, 71]. Specifically, T-cells are reported to infiltrate the CNS in higher numbers during normal brain aging ([71], reviewed in [72]) and under pathological conditions as for example after viral infections (reviewed in [73]). Also, under neurodegenerative conditions such as Parkinsons's disease (PD) [74], amyotrophic lateral sclerosis (ALS) (reviewed in [75]), stroke (reviewed in [76]), and autoimmune diseases such as MS and its animal model experimental autoimmune encephalomyelitis (reviewed in [77]), increased numbers of lymphocytes were observed in the brain. Contribution of lymphocytes to AD is less evident; however, there are few reports on mostly CD3$^+$/CD4$^+$ T-cells or regulatory T-cells (Tregs) infiltrating the brains of transgenic AD mice with already advanced pathology [31, 36]. The presence of T-cells was first mentioned in human AD brains in 1988 [32, 33]. In terms of their functional relevance, increased CD3$^+$ T-cell numbers were recently reported to correlate with Tau pathology rather than amyloidosis in humans [34]. The exact functional role of T-cells in the context of AD is not known at all, and ablation of the complete T-cell population (CD3$^+$ cells) [78], of regulatory T-cells (Treg) [25, 36]), or immuno-deficiency in AD mice showed rather conflicting results [24]. Therefore, it is still under debate, if T-cells are beneficial or detrimental in AD pathology.

In the present work, we could demonstrate that CD8$^+$ T-cells form tight cell to cell contact with microglia and macrophages in the brain of transgenic AD mice and that this interaction is highlighted by the formation of an immune synapse as indicated by translocation of Zap70 to the T-cell surface [79]. Zap70 is an essential kinase for T-cell receptor (TCR) signaling and important for the formation of immune synapses upon interaction of T-cells with antigen presenting cells (APC) [80, 81]. Indeed, this is the first presentation of a direct microglia (as an APC) -T-cell interaction in vivo in the context of AD. Our data strengthens the hypothesis that the adaptive immune system is highly involved in AD pathology and crosstalks with innate immune processes in the brain. In our study, we primarily focused on CD8[+] T-cell populations. Normally, CD8[+] T-cells have cytotoxic effector function eliminating infected target cells or tumor cells (reviewed in [82]); their role in neurodegenerative diseases is unclear but might open new research avenues and treatment options for AD. We demonstrate that after microglia depletion, high numbers of CD3[+]/CD8[+] T-cells were recruited to the brain, specifically in the APP-PS1 animals, assuming that under healthy conditions, T-cell recruitment is kept at a certain baseline level. Since WT mice do not harbor high amounts of macrophages in the brain, the herein described remaining Iba1[+]/TMEM119[−] macrophages at sites of plaques in the APP-PS1 mice might be responsible for the increased T-cell homing.

A key molecule probably responsible for leukocyte homing to the brain is CD44. CD44 is the major surface hyaluronan (HA) receptor originally expressed on lymphocytes and epithelial cells, and its primary function is to mediate interaction of immune cells with the endothelium [83]. CD44 is involved in intercellular adhesion and in cell signaling. In the CNS, CD44 is expressed by glial cells and neurons including their dendritic and axonal processes (reviewed in [84]). In human AD patients, increased CD44 gene expression in lymphocytes was observed, implicating strong participation of CD44 in peripheral immune responses along AD pathology [85]. Furthermore, astrocytes in human AD brains were described to express CD44 [86], and an astrocytoma cell line exposed to amyloid-beta increased CD44 expression in vitro [87]. Additionally, CD44 is highly involved in leukocyte trafficking to inflamed tissue ([88], reviewed in [89]) and is upregulated after activation of T-cells, remaining on the surface of memory T-cells [90]. CD44 is a key molecule that directs T-cells to the sites of inflammation [91]. Most recently, Korin et al. showed by high-dimensional CyTOF mass cytometry that peripheral-derived immune cells in the brain can be distinguished from brain resident immune cells by expression of CD44. Brain resident myeloid cells (CD11b[+]) that were positive for CD44 lacked the expression of TMEM119, and the authors therefore claimed that CD44 can be used in the brain to detect infiltrating immune cells and distinguish them from brain resident cells [46]. In agreement with this data, we observed increased staining for CD44 around amyloid-beta plaques, strongly suggesting that high amounts of extracellular

CD44 might be involved in leukocyte attraction to the plaques. To understand the exact function of CD44 and its role in AD pathology, further studies have to be performed.

The treatment with PLX5622 did reduce microglia numbers and lowered the expression of some pro-inflammatory genes but strongly diminished the expression of anti-inflammatory genes in certain brain regions as previously reported by others [39]. Thus, our data suggest that microglia cells might be responsible for creating an inflammatory milieu in the brain in the context of AD. We showed increased expression of genes for pro-inflammatory molecules (H2-Aa = MHCII, IL-1beta) and anti-inflammatory molecules (IL10, TGFbeta) specifically in the cortex of APP-PS1 mice compared to WT animals. Whereas microglia ablation highly reduced the anti-inflammatory gene transcripts or decreased them at least to WT levels, a pro-inflammatory signature by CCL2 and IL-1beta remained in the microglia-ablated cortex of APP-PS1 mice (Fig. 7b). CCL2 is also referred to as monocyte chemoattractant protein 1 (MCP1), a strong chemoattractant for monocytes and memory T-cells (reviewed in [92]) and has been identified as a blood-derived aging factor [93]. In human genome-wide association studies of prodromal AD [94] and AD patients with mild cognitive impairment (MCI), high amounts of CCL2 were detected in the CSF and CCL2 levels correlated with a faster rate of cognitive decline in the analyzed patient cohort [95]. CCL2 can be produced by a variety of cells including endothelial cells, fibroblasts, astrocytes, and microglia but also by monocyte/macrophages (reviewed in [96]). High levels of CCL2 gene transcripts remained specifically in the cortex of APP-PS1 microglia-ablated brains indicating that CCL2 is not exclusively produced by microglia. A possible explanation might be that the remaining macrophage population itself produces high amounts of CCL2 to attract the herein described CD8[+] T-cell population and to further link the innate with the adaptive immune response in the brain.

Nevertheless, our herein performed gene expression analysis has its limitations. Gene expression was analyzed from total hippocampal and cortical brain regions, and therefore it cannot be excluded that other cell populations, e.g. astrocytes, might compensate microglia-dependent loss of signal molecules. Furthermore, microglia cell death itself might cause changes in gene expression. However, since microglia cells are specifically killed with PLX5622 treatment in WT and APP-PS1 mice, the observed reduction in microglia and inflammatory-specific genes highly suggests microglia cells as the main producer of inflammation in the CNS. Our gene expression analysis illustrated increased gene expression of anti-inflammatory molecules IL-10 and TGFbeta in APP-PS1 cortex samples (Fig. 7b). Chakrabarty et al. showed that an anti-inflammatory treatment with IL10 resulted in decreased amyloid-beta phagocytosis, increased plaque burden, and impaired memory function in transgenic AD mice [19]. In line with this data, Guillot-Sestier et al. showed elevated IL10 signaling pathways in human AD brains and analysis of a transgenic AD mouse model with IL10 knockdown (APP/PS1 + IL10$^{-/-}$) demonstrated mitigation of various AD characteristics and again promotes microglia amyloid-beta phagocytosis in these mice [97]. If this hypothesis holds, a fine-tuned shift from anti-inflammatory microglia towards a more pro-inflammatory phenotype might be a beneficial AD treatment option to be validated and is discussed in the field [98].

Conclusion

Our data suggest that microglia in the brains of APP-PS1 transgenic mice promote an anti-inflammatory milieu and limit T-cell recruitment to the brain, therefore restricting adaptive immune responses in the brain. Ablation of microglia cells revealed a macrophage population present at sites of amyloid plaques highly involved in amyloid-beta clearance and presumably playing a key element in linking innate with adaptive immune responses along AD pathology. The presence of peripheral myeloid and lymphoid cell populations in the brain and their interaction with microglia is fascinating and strengthens the idea that the development of AD pathology is no longer brain restricted but also driven by the adaptive immune system. Further investigations on the functional relevance of each corresponding immune cell population and their interaction with microglia in the brain are necessary. Understanding the immune cell interactions present in the brain during the cause of AD might allow new treatment options for AD pathology.

Additional files

Additional file 1: Figure S1. Qualitative immunohistochemical staining for CSF1R receptor (red) in mouse brain cortex showed high expression in Iba1$^+$ cells (white) in all studied groups. ThioflavinS was used to stain amyloid plaques (green) and Dapi (blue) was used as nucleus stain. Scale: 50 μm. (TIF 3837 kb)

Additional file 2: Figure S2. Microglia ablation has no impact on learning behavior and did not improve learning deficits in APP-PS1 animals. Morris Water Maze (MWM) test for spatial learning and memory was performed and the total distance the animals moved to reach the platform was calculated as measure for learning improvement. (A) All animals moved with the same swim speed. There was a significant difference between the total distances traveled to reach the platform from day 2 to day 5 in APP-PS1 mice compared to WT animals (B). In WT mice PLX5622 treatment has no impact on the total distance the animals moved to reach the platform (C). Microglia ablation in APP-PS1 mice did not improve learning deficits compared to untreated APP-PS1 mice (D) or WT PLX5622 treated mice (E). Spatial memory was tested on day 6 after platform removal and the duration of the animals in the original

platform quadrant was measured (F). There was no significant differences comparing all 4 groups, however WT PLX5622 treated mice spent decreased time in the original platform quadrant when only compared to WT mice (F). Representative track visualization of the total distances traveled at day 5 in MWM test (G). Data are shown as mean with SEM (A-F). Two-way ANOVA with Bonferroni Post-test was performed (A-E, n = 9/group) and One-way ANOVA with Tukey's Multiple Comparison test or Unpaired Student's T-test were performed comparing only WT with WT + PLX5622 (F, n = 9/group). (TIF 536 kb)

Additional file 3: Figure S3. Behavioral data of the Morris Water Maze test were analyzed for gender specific differences: Microglia ablation had no sex-specific impact on learning behavior in female (A) or male (B) WT mice and there was no gender-specific difference in the total distance WT mice moved to reach the platform (C). APP-PS1 female (D) and male (E) mice traveled higher distances to reach the platform compared to female and male WT mice, however no gender differences were observed in APP-PS1 mice (F). Microglia ablation in APP-PS1 mice did not improve learning deficits in female or male mice compared to either untreated APP-PS1 mice (G, H) or WT PLX5622 treated mice of corresponding gender (J, K). There was no difference in the distance moved between female and male WT mice treated with PLX5622 (I). Female and male APP-PS1 microglia ablated mice showed no sex difference in the distance moved to reach the platform (L). Spatial memory was tested on day 6 after platform removal and the duration of the animals in the original platform quadrant was measured. A trend for reduced memory of the spatial platform location was observed in female WT PLX5622 and female APP-PS1 PLX5622 treated mice compared to respective controls (M), but no significant difference was observed in male PLX5622 treated animals (N). Comparison of the duration in the platform quadrant in female versus male mice for the single studied groups showed a significant reduction in spatial memory in male APP-PS1 mice compared to female APP-PS1 mice (O). Data are shown as mean with SEM (A-O). Two-way ANOVA with Bonferroni Post-test (A-L, n = 4-5/group), One-way ANOVA with Tukey's Multiple Comparison test (M, N, n = 4-5/group) and Unpaired Student's T-test for comparison of female versus male in the respective groups (O, n = 4-5/group) were performed. (TIF 867 kb)

Additional file 4: Figure S4. Detailed analysis for gender-specific differences of flow cytometric data from brain isolated microglia/macrophage populations: PLX5622 treatment reduced CD11b$^+$ cell numbers in the brain of female (A) and male (B) animals, however specifically female APP-PS1 mice had higher numbers of CD11b$^+$ cells compared to female WT mice. Gender-specific differences were observed in APP-PS1 mice, where the females had higher numbers of CD11b$^+$ cells compared to male APP-PS1 mice (C). Similar results were obtained from microglia cell numbers (CD11b$^+$/CD45^{low}) of APP-PS1 mice with increased numbers of microglia in female APP-PS1 compared to female WT mice and compared to male APP-PS1 animals (D-F). Macrophage numbers (CD11b$^+$/CD45^{high}) where significantly increased in female APP-PS1 compared to female WT mice and were reduced upon PLX5622 treatment in both genotypes (G). Also male APP-PS1 mice had increased numbers of CD11b$^+$/CD45^{high} cells compared to male WT mice, however PLX5622 treatment did not reduce macrophage numbers in male animals of both genotypes (H). Higher numbers of macrophages were already detected in the brains of female APP-PS1 mice compared to male APP-PS1 animals (I). One-way ANOVA with Tukey's Multiple Comparison test (A, B, D, E, G, H n = 4-5/group) and Unpaired Student's T-test (A, C, D, F, G, H, I) with Welch's correction (B, E) for comparison of only two groups were performed (n = 4-5/group). (TIF 727 kb)

Additional file 5: Figure S5. Using the newly identified microglia specific marker TMEM119 for detailed immunohistochemical analysis in the cortex revealed strong co-localization of Iba1$^+$ (white) cells with TMEM119 (red) in WT and WT animals treated with PLX5622 (A). However, Iba1$^+$ cells at sites of plaques (green) in APP-PS1 and PLX5622 treated APP-PS1 animals did not express TMEM119. Quantitative analysis of Iba1$^+$/TMEM119$^+$ revealed a significant reduction in Iba1$^+$/TMEM119$^+$ cell numbers upon PLX5622 treatment in WT and APP-PS1 mice (B). Surprisingly, APP-PS1 animals had increased numbers of Iba1$^+$/TMEM119$^-$ cells that were more resistant to PLX5622 treatment than in WT animals (C). Calculation of the percentage of Iba1$^+$/TMEM119$^+$ and Iba1$^+$/

TMEM119⁻ cells from the total Iba1⁺ cell population (D). ThioflavinS was used to stain amyloid plaques (green) and Dapi (blue) was used as nucleus stain. One-way ANOVA with Tukey's Multiple Comparison Test (B, C, D $n = 6$/group) was performed. Scale: 20 μm (A). (TIF 1310 kb)

Additional file 6: Figure S6. Iba1⁺/TMEM119⁻ cells represent a CD68⁺ macrophage population with peripheral origin highly involved in amyloid-beta phagocytosis. Analysis of CD68 expression in the cortex revealed significantly reduced numbers of Iba1⁺/TMEM119⁺/CD68⁺ cells in APP-PS1 and WT animals upon PLX5622 treatment (A). Surprisingly, higher numbers of Iba1⁺/TMEM119⁻/CD68⁺ cells were found in APP-PS1 animals compared to WT, although these numbers were slightly reduced in APP-PS1 animals by PLX5622 treatment (B). Representative image of CD68 expression in Iba1⁺/TMEM119⁻ cells located at sites of plaque in APP-PS1 mice (C). Strong MHCII expression was seen sporadically in Iba1⁺/TMEM119⁻ cells in APP-PS1 mice (D, arrow). Accumulation of CD44 staining (red) was observed extracellularly around amyloid depositions (green) as indicated by the dotted ellipse and CD44 staining was seen on Iba1⁺ cells at sites of plaques (E, insert). Quantification of percentage (%) area of CD44 staining in hippocampal brain regions revealed barely any staining in WT and WT + PLX5622 treated animals, however in APP-PS1 and APP-PS1 + PLX5622 treated mice significantly higher expression of CD44 was observed compared to WT or WT + PLX5622 animals (F). Detailed immunohistochemical analysis revealed increased staining for CD44 at sites of amyloid deposition in areas colonized with Iba1⁺/TMEM119⁻ cells in APP-PS1 and APP-PS1 PLX5622 treated mice (G, arrow). ThioflavinS was used to stain amyloid plaques and Dapi (blue) was used as nucleus stain. One-way ANOVA with Tukey's Multiple Comparison Test (A, B, F $n = 3$/group) was performed. Scale: 50 μm (C, D, E), 20 μm (G). (TIF 4515 kb)

Additional file 7: Figure S7. Flow cytometric data of brain isolated T-cells were analyzed for gender-specific differences: (A) Female APP-PS1 mice had significantly increased numbers of CD3⁺ T-cells when compared specifically to female WT mice, however this was not seen in male mice (B). (C) Female APP-PS1 mice had increased numbers of CD3⁺ T-cells compared to male APP-PS1 mice. (D) The number of CD3⁺/CD4⁺ T-cells was significantly increased in female APP-PS1 compared to female WT mice, whereas male mice of both genotypes had the same cell numbers in the brain (E). (F) APP-PS1 female mice had higher numbers of CD3⁺/CD4⁺ T-cells compared to male APP-PS1 mice. (G) There was a trend for higher CD3⁺/CD8⁺ T-cell numbers in the brain of female APP-PS1 mice compared to female WT mice, however this was not seen in male animals (H). (I) Female APP-PS1 mice had higher numbers of CD3⁺/CD8⁺ T-cells compared to male APP-PS1 animals. PLX5622 treatment in APP-PS1 mice of both sexes showed an increase in the number of CD3⁺, CD3⁺/CD4⁺ and CD3⁺/CD8⁺ T-cells in the brain. One-way ANOVA with Tukey's Multiple Comparison Test (A, B, D, E, G, H, $n = 3$–5/group) and Unpaired Student's T-test (A, C, D, F, G, I) for comparison of only two groups were performed ($n = 3$–5/group). (TIF 743 kb)

Additional file 8: Figure S8. Immunohistochemical staining for proliferating cell nuclear antigen (PCNA) to analyze the proliferative activity of CD8⁺ T-cells in APP-PS1 and microglia ablated APP-PS1 brains. CD8⁺ T-cells in the hippocampus (A) and cortex (B) of APP-PS1 mice were not observed to proliferate (arrows). Interestingly, after microglia ablation in APP-PS1 mice, no increase in proliferative activity was detected, suggesting CD8⁺ T-cells to rather infiltrate the brain than being locally generated. Dapi (blue) was used as nucleus stain. Scale: 50 μm (A, B). (TIF 4664 kb)

Additional file 9: Figure S9. Immunohistochemical analysis for CD4⁺ T-cells and Zap70 expression in APP-PS1 mouse brains. CD4⁺ T-cells were observed less frequently than CD8⁺ T-cells in hippocampal (A) and cortical (B) brain regions and expressed the T-cell receptor kinase Zap70 (arrow). Dapi (blue) was used as nucleus stain. Scale: 50 μm (A, B). (TIF 2033 kb)

Abbreviations
AD: Alzheimer's disease; AIF1: Allograft inflammatory factor 1; ALS: Amyotrophic lateral sclerosis; APC: Antigen presenting cell; APP-PS1: APP Swedish PS1 dE9; Arg1: Arginase 1; CCL2: Chemokine (C-C motif) ligand 2 or monocyte chemoattractant protein 1; CD11b: Integrin alpha M;

CD3: Cluster of differentiation 3, T-cell co-receptor; CD33: Cluster of differentiation 33, sialic acid binding Ig-like lectin 3; CD4: Cluster of differentiation 4, transmembrane glycoprotein; CD44: Cluster of differentiation 44, receptor for hyaluronic acid; CD45: Cluster of differentiation 45, protein tyrosine phosphatase receptor type C; CD68: Cluster of differentiation 68; CD8: Cluster of differentiation 8, transmembrane glycoprotein; CNS: Central nervous system; CSF1R: Colony stimulating factor 1 receptor; H2-Aa: Histocompatibility 2, class II antigen A, alpha; HA: Hyaluronan; HSVTK: Herpes simplex virus thymidine kinase; Iba1: Ionized calcium-binding adapter molecule 1; IL10: Interleukin 10; IL-1beta: Interleukin 1 beta; IL6: Interleukin 6; INF: Interferon; Marco: Macrophage receptor with collagenous structure; MHCII: Major histocompatibility complex 2; MRC1: Mannose receptor C-Type 1; MS: Multiple sclerosis; MWM: Morris water maze; Nos2: Nitric oxide synthase 2; PD: Parkinson's disease; TCR: T-cell receptor; TGFbeta: Transforming growth factor beta; TMEM119: Transmembrane protein 119; TNF: Tumor necrosis factor; Treg: Regulatory T-cells; Trem2: Triggering receptor expressed on myeloid cells 2; WT: Wild type

Acknowledgments
The authors thank the flow cytometry and microscopy core facility of SCI-TReCS (Spinal Cord Injury and Tissue Regeneration Center Salzburg). Furthermore, we thank Plexxikon Inc. and Research Diets Inc. for providing PLX5622 and AIN-76A chow. Additionally, we want to thank Dominika Jakubecova and Pia Zaunmair for their help with the animals, and Prof. Michael T. Heneka for providing additional tissue of the APP-PS1 mice.

Funding
This work was supported by the FWF Special Research Programme (SFB) F44 (F4413-B23) "Cell Signaling in Chronic CNS Disorders", by the FWF Hertha-Firnberg Postdoctoral Programme no. T736-B24, PMU-FFF A-15/01/017-MAR, and through funding from the European Union's Seventh Framework Programme (FP7/2007-2013) under grant agreement no. HEALTH-F2-2011-278850 (INMiND).
Funding bodies did not influence the design of the study and collection, analysis, interpretation of data, and writing of the manuscript.

Authors' contributions
MU conducted the experiment and behavioral tests, performed flow cytometric and histological analysis, and wrote the manuscript. PS helped with behavioral testing and histological analysis together with HM, who additionally performed gene expression analysis. JM helped with microglia and T-cell isolation from the brains and was involved in the experimental design of the study. LA is the principle investigator and was involved in the experimental designs, in critical revision and drafting of the manuscript. All authors read and approved the final manuscript.

Competing interests
The authors declare that they have no competing interests.

Author details
[1]Institute of Molecular Regenerative Medicine, Paracelsus Medical University, Strubergasse 21, 5020 Salzburg, Austria. [2]Spinal Cord Injury and Tissue Regeneration Center Salzburg (SCI-TReCS), Paracelsus Medical University, Salzburg, Austria. [3]Department of Neurology and Neurological Sciences, Stanford University School of Medicine, Stanford, USA.

References
1. Goedert M, Spillantini MG. A century of Alzheimer's disease. Science. 2006; 314:777–81.
2. Selkoe DJ, Hardy J. The amyloid hypothesis of Alzheimer's disease at 25 years. EMBO Mol Med. 2016;8:595–608.
3. Serrano-Pozo A, Frosch MP, Masliah E, Hyman BT. Neuropathological alterations in Alzheimer disease. Cold Spring Harb Perspect Med. 2011;1: a006189.

4. Meadowcroft MD, Connor JR, Smith MB, Yang QX. MRI and histological analysis of beta-amyloid plaques in both human Alzheimer's disease and APP/PS1 transgenic mice. J Magn Reson Imaging. 2009;29:997–1007.

5. Philipson O, Lord A, Gumucio A, O'Callaghan P, Lannfelt L, Nilsson LN. Animal models of amyloid-beta-related pathologies in Alzheimer's disease. FEBS J. 2010;277:1389–409.

6. Gotz J, Deters N, Doldissen A, Bokhari L, Ke Y, Wiesner A, Schonrock N, Ittner LM. A decade of tau transgenic animal models and beyond. Brain Pathol. 2007;17:91–103.

7. Heneka MT, Carson MJ, El Khoury J, Landreth GE, Brosseron F, Feinstein DL, Jacobs AH, Wyss-Coray T, Vitorica J, Ransohoff RM, et al. Neuroinflammation in Alzheimer's disease. Lancet Neurol. 2015;14:388–405.

8. Heppner FL, Ransohoff RM, Becher B. Immune attack: the role of inflammation in Alzheimer disease. Nat Rev Neurosci. 2015;16:358–72.

9. Wyss-Coray T. Inflammation in Alzheimer disease: driving force, bystander or beneficial response? Nat Med. 2006;12:1005–15.

10. Wyss-Coray T, Rogers J. Inflammation in Alzheimer disease-a brief review of the basic science and clinical literature. Cold Spring Harb Perspect Med. 2012;2:a006346.

11. Krabbe G, Halle A, Matyash V, Rinnenthal JL, Eom GD, Bernhardt U, Miller KR, Prokop S, Kettenmann H, Heppner FL. Functional impairment of microglia coincides with beta-amyloid deposition in mice with Alzheimer-like pathology. PLoS One. 2013;8:e60921.

12. Bradshaw EM, Chibnik LB, Keenan BT, Ottoboni L, Raj T, Tang A, Rosenkrantz LL, Imboywa S, Lee M, Von Korff A, et al. CD33 Alzheimer's disease locus: altered monocyte function and amyloid biology. Nat Neurosci. 2013;16:848–50.

13. Guerreiro R, Wojtas A, Bras J, Carrasquillo M, Rogaeva E, Majounie E, Cruchaga C, Sassi C, Kauwe JS, Younkin S, et al. TREM2 variants in Alzheimer's disease. N Engl J Med. 2013;368:117–27.

14. Bronzuoli MR, Iacomino A, Steardo L, Scuderi C. Targeting neuroinflammation in Alzheimer's disease. J Inflamm Res. 2016;9:199–208.

15. Kettenmann H, Hanisch UK, Noda M, Verkhratsky A. Physiology of microglia. Physiol Rev. 2011;91:461–553.

16. Fu R, Shen Q, Xu P, Luo JJ, Tang Y. Phagocytosis of microglia in the central nervous system diseases. Mol Neurobiol. 2014;49:1422–34.

17. Lee CY, Landreth GE. The role of microglia in amyloid clearance from the AD brain. J Neural Transm (Vienna). 2010;117:949–60.

18. Stalder M, Phinney A, Probst A, Sommer B, Staufenbiel M, Jucker M. Association of microglia with amyloid plaques in brains of APP23 transgenic mice. Am J Pathol. 1999;154:1673–84.

19. Chakrabarty P, Li A, Ceballos-Diaz C, Eddy JA, Funk CC, Moore B, DiNunno N, Rosario AM, Cruz PE, Verbeeck C, et al. IL-10 alters immunoproteostasis in APP mice, increasing plaque burden and worsening cognitive behavior. Neuron. 2015;85:519–33.

20. Heneka MT, Kummer MP, Latz E. Innate immune activation in neurodegenerative disease. Nat Rev Immunol. 2014;14:463–77.

21. Mosher KI, Wyss-Coray T. Microglial dysfunction in brain aging and Alzheimer's disease. Biochem Pharmacol. 2014;88:594–604.

22. Theriault P, ElAli A, Rivest S. The dynamics of monocytes and microglia in Alzheimer's disease. Alzheimers Res Ther. 2015;7:41.

23. Gate D, Rezai-Zaceh K, Jodry D, Rentsendorj A, Town T. Macrophages in Alzheimer's disease: the blood-borne identity. J Neural Transm (Vienna). 2010;117:961–70.

24. Marsh SE, Abud EM, Lakatos A, Karimzadeh A, Yeung ST, Davtyan H, Fote GM, Lau L, Weinger JG, Lane TE, et al. The adaptive immune system restrains Alzheimer's disease pathogenesis by modulating microglial function. Proc Natl Acad Sci U S A. 2016;113:E1316–25.

25. Baruch K, Rosenzweig N, Kertser A, Deczkowska A, Sharif AM, Spinrad A, Tsitsou-Kampeli A, Sarel A, Cahalon L, Schwartz M. Breaking immune tolerance by targeting Foxp3(+) regulatory T cells mitigates Alzheimer's disease pathology. Nat Commun. 2015;6:7967.

26. Pellicano M, Larbi A, Goldeck D, Colonna-Romano G, Buffa S, Bulati M, Rubino G, Iemolo F, Candore G, Caruso C, et al. Immune profiling of Alzheimer patients. J Neuroimmunol. 2012;242:52–9.

27. Stalder AK, Ermini F, Bondolfi L, Krenger W, Burbach GJ, Deller T, Coomaraswamy J, Staufenbiel M, Landmann R, Jucker M. Invasion of hematopoietic cells into the brain of amyloid precursor protein transgenic mice. J Neurosci. 2005;25:11125–32.

28. Zuroff L, Daley D, Black KL, Koronyo-Hamaoui M. Clearance of cerebral Abeta in Alzheimer's disease: reassessing the role of microglia and monocytes. Cell Mol Life Sci. 2017;74:2167–201.

29. Hohsfield LA, Humpel C. Migration of blood cells to beta-amyloid plaques in Alzheimer's disease. Exp Gerontol. 2015;65:8–15.

30. Simard AR, Soulet D, Gowing G, Julien JP, Rivest S. Bone marrow-derived microglia play a critical role in restricting senile plaque formation in Alzheimer's disease. Neuron. 2006;49:489–502.

31. Ferretti MT, Merlini M, Spani C, Gericke C, Schweizer N, Enzmann G, Engelhardt B, Kulic L, Suter T, Nitsch RM. T-cell brain infiltration and immature antigen-presenting cells in transgenic models of Alzheimer's disease-like cerebral amyloidosis. Brain Behav Immun. 2016;54:211–25.

32. Togo T, Akiyama H, Iseki E, Kondo H, Ikeda K, Kato M, Oda T, Tsuchiya K, Kosaka K. Occurrence of T cells in the brain of Alzheimer's disease and other neurological diseases. J Neuroimmunol. 2002;124:83–92.

33. Rogers J, Luber-Narod J, Styren SD, Civin WH. Expression of immune system-associated antigens by cells of the human central nervous system: relationship to the pathology of Alzheimer's disease. Neurobiol Aging. 1988;9:339–49.

34. Merlini M, Kirabali T, Kulic L, Nitsch RM, Ferretti MT. Extravascular CD3+ T cells in brains of Alzheimer disease patients correlate with tau but not with amyloid pathology: an immunohistochemical study. Neurodegener Dis. 2018;18:49–56.

35. McManus RM, Mills KH, Lynch MA. T cells-protective or pathogenic in Alzheimer's disease? J Neuroimmune Pharmacol. 2015;10:547–60.

36. Dansokho C, Ait Ahmed D, Aid S, Toly-Ndour C, Chaigneau T, Calle V, Cagnard N, Holzenberger M, Piaggio E, Aucouturier P, Dorothee G. Regulatory T cells delay disease progression in Alzheimer-like pathology. Brain. 2016;139:1237–51.

37. Unger MS, Marschallinger J, Kaindl J, Klein B, Johnson M, Khundakar AA, Rossner S, Heneka MT, Couillard-Despres S, Rockenstein E, et al. Doublecortin expression in CD8+ T-cells and microglia at sites of amyloid-beta plaques: A potential role in shaping plaque pathology? Alzheimers Dement. 2018;14(8):1022-37. PMID: 29630865. https://doi.org/10.1016/j.jalz.2018.02.017. Epub 2018 Apr 7.

38. Dagher NN, Najafi AR, Kayala KM, Elmore MR, White TE, Medeiros R, West BL, Green KN. Colony-stimulating factor 1 receptor inhibition prevents microglial plaque association and improves cognition in 3xTg-AD mice. J Neuroinflammation. 2015;12:139.

39. Spangenberg EE, Lee RJ, Najafi AR, Rice RA, Elmore MR, Blurton-Jones M, West BL, Green KN. Eliminating microglia in Alzheimer's mice prevents neuronal loss without modulating amyloid-beta pathology. Brain. 2016;139:1265–81.

40. Jankowsky JL, Slunt HH, Ratovitski T, Jenkins NA, Copeland NG, Borchelt DR. Co-expression of multiple transgenes in mouse CNS: a comparison of strategies. Biomol Eng. 2001;17:157–65.

41. Jankowsky JL, Fadale DJ, Anderson J, Xu GM, Gonzales V, Jenkins NA, Copeland NG, Lee MK, Younkin LH, Wagner SL, et al. Mutant presenilins specifically elevate the levels of the 42 residue beta-amyloid peptide in vivo: evidence for augmentation of a 42-specific gamma secretase. Hum Mol Genet. 2004;13:159–70.

42. Rotheneichner P, Romanelli P, Bieler L, Pagitsch S, Zaunmair P, Kreutzer C, Konig R, Marschallinger J, Aigner L, Couillard-Despres S. Tamoxifen activation of Cre-recombinase has no persisting effects on adult neurogenesis or learning and anxiety. Front Neurosci. 2017;11:27.

43. Bromley-Brits K, Deng Y, Song W. Morris water maze test for learning and memory deficits in Alzheimer's disease model mice. J Vis Exp. 2011;(53). PMID:21808223. https://doi.org/10.3791/2920.

44. RGM M. Spatial localization does not require the presence of local cues. Learning and Motivation. 1981;12:239–60.

45. Ford AL, Goodsall AL, Hickey WF, Sedgwick JD. Normal adult ramified microglia separated from other central nervous system macrophages by flow cytometric sorting. Phenotypic differences defined and direct ex vivo antigen presentation to myelin basic protein-reactive CD4+ T cells compared. J Immunol. 1995;154:4309–21.

46. Korin B, Ben-Shaanan TL, Schiller M, Dubovik T, Azulay-Debby H, Boshnak NT, Koren T, Rolls A. High-dimensional, single-cell characterization of the brain's immune compartment. Nat Neurosci. 2017;20:1300–9.

47. Becher B, Antel JP. Comparison of phenotypic and functional properties of immediately ex vivo and cultured human adult microglia. Glia. 1996;18:1–10.

48. Bennett ML, Bennett FC, Liddelow SA, Ajami B, Zamanian JL, Fernhoff NB, Mulinyawe SB, Bohlen CJ, Adil A, Tucker A, et al. New tools for studying microglia in the mouse and human CNS. Proc Natl Acad Sci U S A. 2016; 113:E1738–46.

49. Unger MS, Marschallinger J, Kaindl J, Hofling C, Rossner S, Heneka MT, Van der Linden A, Aigner L. Early changes in hippocampal neurogenesis in transgenic mouse models for Alzheimer's disease. Mol Neurobiol. 2016;53:5796–806.

50. Marschallinger J, Sah A, Schmuckermair C, Unger M, Rotheneichner P, Kharitonova M, Waclawiczek A, Gerner P, Jaksch-Bogensperger H, Berger S,

et al. The L-type calcium channel Cav1.3 is required for proper hippocampal neurogenesis and cognitive functions. Cell Calcium. 2015;58:606–16.

51. Schnell SA, Staines WA, Wessendorf MW. Reduction of lipofuscin-like autofluorescence in fluorescently labeled tissue. J Histochem Cytochem. 1999, 47:719–30.

52. Babcock AA, Ilkjaer L, Clausen BH, Villadsen B, Dissing-Olesen L, Bendixen AT, Lyck L, Lambertsen KL, Finsen B. Cytokine-producing microglia have an altered beta-amyloid load in aged APP/PS1 Tg mice. Brain Behav Immun. 2015;48:86–101.

53. Manocha GD, Floden AM, Rausch K, Kulas JA, BA MG, Rojanathammanee L, Puig KR, Puig KL, Karki S, Nichols MR, et al. APP regulates microglial phenotype in a mouse model of Alzheimer's disease. J Neurosci. 2016;36: 8471–86.

54. Patel S, Player MR. Colony-stimulating factor-1 receptor inhibitors for the treatment of cancer and inflammatory disease. Curr Top Med Chem. 2009;9: 599–610.

55. Elmore MR, Lee RJ, West BL, Green KN. Characterizing newly repopulated microglia in the adult mouse: impacts on animal behavior, cell morphology, and neuroinflammation. PLoS One. 2015;10:e0122912.

56. Elmore MR, Najafi AR, Koike MA, Dagher NN, Spangenberg EE, Rice RA, Kitazawa M, Matusow B, Nguyen H, West BL, Green KN. Colony-stimulating factor 1 receptor signaling is necessary for microglia viability, unmasking a microglia progenitor cell in the adult brain. Neuron. 2014;82:380–97.

57. Mok S, Koya RC, Tsui C, Xu J, Robert L, Wu L, Graeber T, West BL, Bollag G, Ribas A. Inhibition of CSF-1 receptor improves the antitumor efficacy of adoptive cell transfer immunotherapy. Cancer Res. 2014;74:153–61.

58. Kim TS, Cavnar MJ, Cohen NA, Sorenson EC, Greer JB, Seifert AM, Crawley MH, Green BL, Popow R, Pillarsetty N, et al. Increased KIT inhibition enhances therapeutic efficacy in gastrointestinal stromal tumor. Clin Cancer Res. 2014;20:2350–62.

59. Aloisi F, Ria F, Adorini L. Regulation of T-cell responses by CNS antigen-presenting cells: different roles for microglia and astrocytes. Immunol Today. 2000;21:141–7.

60. Gonzalez H, Elgueta D, Montoya A, Pacheco R. Neuroimmune regulation of microglial activity involved in neuroinflammation and neurodegenerative diseases. J Neuroimmunol. 2014;274:1–13.

61. Prokop S, Miller KR, Drost N, Handrick S, Mathur V, Luo J, Wegner A, Wyss-Coray T, Heppner FL. Impact of peripheral myeloid cells on amyloid-beta pathology in Alzheimer's disease-like mice. J Exp Med. 2015;212:1811–8.

62. Satoh J, Kino Y, Asahina N, Takitani M, Miyoshi J, Ishida T, Saito Y. TMEM119 marks a subset of microglia in the human brain. Neuropathology. 2016;36: 39–49.

63. Bennett FC, Bennett ML, Yaqoob F, Mulinyawe SB, Grant GA, Hayden Gephart M, Plowey ED, Barres BA. A combination of ontogeny and CNS environment establishes microglial identity. Neuron. 2018;98:1170–83 e1178.

64. Cronk JC, Filiano AJ, Louveau A, Marin I, Marsh R, Ji E, Goldman DH, Smirnov I, Geraci N, Acton S, et al. Peripherally derived macrophages can engraft the brain independent of irradiation and maintain an identity distinct from microglia. J Exp Med. 2018;215:1627–47.

65. Bruttger J, Karram K, Wortge S, Regen T, Marini F, Hoppmann N, Klein M, Blank T, Yona S, Wolf Y, et al. Genetic cell ablation reveals clusters of local self-renewing microglia in the mammalian central nervous system. Immunity. 2015;43:92–106.

66. Sosna J, Philipp S, Albay R 3rd, Reyes-Ruiz JM, Baglietto-Vargas D, LaFerla FM, Glabe CG. Early long-term administration of the CSF1R inhibitor PLX3397 ablates microglia and reduces accumulation of intraneuronal amyloid, neuritic plaque deposition and pre-fibrillar oligomers in 5XFAD mouse model of Alzheimer's disease. Mol Neurodegener. 2018;13:11.

67. Dai XM, Ryan GR, Hapel AJ, Dominguez MG, Russell RG, Kapp S, Sylvestre V, Stanley ER. Targeted disruption of the mouse colony-stimulating factor 1 receptor gene results in osteopetrosis, mononuclear phagocyte deficiency, increased primitive progenitor cell frequencies, and reproductive defects. Blood. 2002;99:111–20.

68. Ginhoux F, Greter M, Leboeuf M, Nandi S, See P, Gokhan S, Mehler MF, Conway SJ, Ng LG, Stanley ER, et al. Fate mapping analysis reveals that adult microglia derive from primitive macrophages. Science. 2010;330: 841–5.

69. Han J, Harris RA, Zhang XM. An updated assessment of microglia depletion: current concepts and future directions. Mol Brain. 2017;10:25.

70. Varvel NH, Grathwohl SA, Baumann F, Liebig C, Bosch A, Brawek B, Thal DR, Charo IF, Heppner FL, Aguzzi A, et al. Microglial repopulation model reveals a robust homeostatic process for replacing CNS myeloid cells. Proc Natl Acad Sci U S A. 2012;109:18150–5.

71. Ritzel RM, Crapser J, Patel AR, Verma R, Grenier JM, Chauhan A, Jellison ER, LD MC. Age-associated resident memory CD8 T Cells in the central nervous system are primed to potentiate inflammation after ischemic brain injury. J Immunol. 2016;196:3318–30.

72. Gemechu JM, Bentivoglio M. T cell recruitment in the brain during normal aging. Front Cell Neurosci. 2012;6:38.

73. Almolda B, Gonzalez B, Castellano B. Are microglial cells the regulators of lymphocyte responses in the CNS? Front Cell Neurosci. 2015;9:440.

74. Brochard V, Combadiere B, Prigent A, Laouar Y, Perrin A, Beray-Berthat V, Bonduelle O, Alvarez-Fischer D, Callebert J, Launay JM, et al. Infiltration of CD4+ lymphocytes into the brain contributes to neurodegeneration in a mouse model of Parkinson disease. J Clin Invest. 2009;119:182–92.

75. Holmoy T. T cells in amyotrophic lateral sclerosis. Eur J Neurol. 2008;15:360–6.

76. Arumugam TV, Granger DN, Mattson MP. Stroke and T-cells. Neuromolecular Med. 2005;7:229–42.

77. Fletcher JM, Lalor SJ, Sweeney CM, Tubridy N, Mills KH. T cells in multiple sclerosis and experimental autoimmune encephalomyelitis. Clin Exp Immunol. 2010;162:1–11.

78. Laurent C, Dorothee G, Hunot S, Martin E, Monnet Y, Duchamp M, Dong Y, Legeron FP, Leboucher A, Burnouf S, et al. Hippocampal T cell infiltration promotes neuroinflammation and cognitive decline in a mouse model of tauopathy. Brain. 2017;140:184–200.

79. Sloan-Lancaster J, Zhang W, Presley J, Williams BL, Abraham RT, Lippincott-Schwartz J, Samelson LE. Regulation of ZAP-70 intracellular localization: visualization with the green fluorescent protein. J Exp Med. 1997;186:1713–24.

80. James JR, Vale RD. Biophysical mechanism of T-cell receptor triggering in a reconstituted system. Nature. 2012;487:64–9.

81. Wang H, Kadlecek TA, Au-Yeung BB, Goodfellow HE, Hsu LY, Freedman TS, Weiss A. ZAP-70: an essential kinase in T-cell signaling. Cold Spring Harb Perspect Biol. 2010;2:a002279.

82. Andersen MH, Schrama D, Thor Straten P, Becker JC. Cytotoxic T cells. J Invest Dermatol. 2006;126:32–41.

83. Kennel SJ, Lankford TK, Foote LJ, Shinpock SG, Stringer C. CD44 expression on murine tissues. J Cell Sci. 1993;104(Pt 2):373–82.

84. Dzwonek J, Wilczynski GM. CD44: molecular interactions, signaling and functions in the nervous system. Front Cell Neurosci. 2015;9:175.

85. Uberti D, Cenini G, Bonini SA, Barcikowska M, Styczynska M, Szybinska A, Memo M. Increased CD44 gene expression in lymphocytes derived from Alzheimer disease patients. Neurodegener Dis. 2010;7:143–7.

86. Akiyama H, Tooyama I, Kawamata T, Ikeda K, PL MG. Morphological diversities of CD44 positive astrocytes in the cerebral cortex of normal subjects and patients with Alzheimer's disease. Brain Res. 1993;632:249–59.

87. Speciale L, Ruzzante S, Calabrese E, Saresella M, Taramelli D, Mariani C, Bava L, Longhi R, Ferrante P. 1–40 Beta-amyloid protein fragment modulates the expression of CD44 and CD71 on the astrocytoma cell line in the presence of IL1beta and TNFalpha. J Cell Physiol. 2003;196:190–5.

88. Nandi A, Estess P, Siegelman M. Bimolecular complex between rolling and firm adhesion receptors required for cell arrest; CD44 association with VLA-4 in T cell extravasation. Immunity. 2004;20:455–65.

89. McDonald B, Kubes P. Interactions between CD44 and hyaluronan in leukocyte trafficking. Front Immunol. 2015;6:68.

90. Baaten BJ, Li CR, Deiro MF, Lin MM, Linton PJ, Bradley LM. CD44 regulates survival and memory development in Th1 cells. Immunity. 2010;32:104–15.

91. DeGrendele HC, Estess P, Siegelman MH. Requirement for CD44 in activated T cell extravasation into an inflammatory site. Science. 1997; 278:672–5.

92. Xia M, Sui Z. Recent developments in CCR2 antagonists. Expert Opin Ther Pat. 2009;19:295–303.

93. Villeda SA, Luo J, Mosher KI, Zou B, Britschgi M, Bieri G, Stan TM, Fainberg N, Ding Z, Eggel A, et al. The ageing systemic milieu negatively regulates neurogenesis and cognitive function. Nature. 2011;477:90–4.

94. Kauwe JS, Bailey MH, Ridge PG, Perry R, Wadsworth ME, Hoyt KL, Staley LA, Karch CM, Harari O, Cruchaga C, et al. Genome-wide association study of CSF levels of 59 alzheimer's disease candidate proteins: significant associations with proteins involved in amyloid processing and inflammation. PLoS Genet. 2014;10:e1004758.

95. Westin K, Buchhave P, Nielsen H, Minthon L, Janciauskiene S, Hansson O. CCL2 is associated with a faster rate of cognitive decline during early stages of Alzheimer's disease. PLoS One. 2012;7:e30525.

96. Deshmane SL, Kremlev S, Amini S, Sawaya BE. Monocyte chemoattractant protein-1 (MCP-1): an overview. J Interferon Cytokine Res. 2009;29:313–26.

97. Guillot-Sestier MV, Doty KR, Gate D, Rodriguez J Jr, Leung BP, Rezai-Zadeh K, Town T. Il10 deficiency rebalances innate immunity to mitigate Alzheimer-like pathology. Neuron. 2015;85:534–48.

98. Michaud JP, Rivest S. Anti-inflammatory signaling in microglia exacerbates Alzheimer's disease-related pathology. Neuron. 2015;85:450–2.

2

Complement-dependent bystander injury to neurons in AQP4-IgG seropositive neuromyelitis optica

Tianjiao Duan[1,2], Alex J. Smith[1] and Alan S. Verkman[1*]

Abstract

Background: Aquaporin-4-immunoglobulin G (AQP4-IgG) seropositive neuromyelitis optica spectrum disorder (herein called NMO) is an autoimmune disease of the central nervous system in which AQP4-IgG binding to AQP4 on astrocytes results in complement-dependent astrocyte injury and secondary inflammation, demyelination, and neuron loss. We previously reported evidence for a complement bystander mechanism for early oligodendrocyte injury in NMO. Herein, we tested the hypothesis that complement bystander injury, which involves diffusion to nearby cells of activated soluble complement components from complement-injured astrocytes, is a general phenomenon that may contribute to neuronal injury in NMO.

Methods: Primary cocultures of rat astrocytes and cortical neurons were established to study complement-dependent cell death after exposure to AQP4-IgG and complement. In animal experiments, AQP4-IgG was delivered to adult rats by intracerebral injection. Cell cultures and rat brain were studied by immunofluorescence.

Results: In primary astrocyte-neuron cocultures, addition of AQP4-IgG and complement resulted in death of neurons nearby astrocytes. Deposition of complement membrane attack complex C5b-9 was seen on neurons nearby astrocytes, whereas C1q, the initiating protein in the complement pathway, was seen only on astrocytes. Neuron death was not seen with a complement inhibitor, with C1q- or C6-depleted complement, in pure neuron cultures exposed to AQP4-IgG and complement or in cocultures exposed to an astrocyte toxin. Intracerebral injection in rats of AQP4-IgG and a fixable dead cell fluorescent marker produced death of neurons near astrocytes, with C5b-9 deposition. Neuron death was not seen in rats receiving a complement inhibitor or in AQP4-IgG-injected AQP4 knockout rats.

Conclusion: These results support a novel mechanism for early neuron injury in NMO and provide evidence that complement bystander injury may be a general phenomenon for brain cell injury following AQP4-IgG-targeted astrocyte death.

Keywords: NMO, Aquaporin-4, Astrocyte, Neuron, Complement

Background

Aquaporin-4-immunoglobulin G (AQP4-IgG) seropositive neuromyelitis optica spectrum disorder (herein called NMO) is an autoimmune demyelinating disease of the central nervous system. NMO pathogenesis involves binding of AQP4-IgG autoantibodies to water channel AQP4 on astrocytes, resulting in complement- and cell-mediated astrocyte injury, inflammation, demyelination, and neuron

loss [1–3]. Though demyelination and neuronal injury could be secondary consequences of astrocyte death and an inflammatory response, the rapid disease progression seen in some NMO patients [4, 5] and the rapid pathological changes seen in animal models during in vivo imaging of lesion formation [6, 7] suggest more direct mechanisms by which astrocyte injury produces neuronal injury and neurologic deficit. Several mechanisms have been proposed to account for neuronal injury in NMO, including excitotoxic damage following glutamate release from injured astrocytes [8, 9] and secondary recruitment of granulocytes and cytotoxic T cells [10, 11]. However,

* Correspondence: alan.verkman@ucsf.edu
[1]Departments of Medicine and Physiology, University of California, 1246 Health Sciences East Tower, 513 Parnassus Ave, San Francisco, CA 94143-0521, USA
Full list of author information is available at the end of the article

the role of excitotoxic mechanisms has been controversial [12, 13], and although cellular mechanisms are probably important, they are unlikely to cause the immediate damage to surrounding cells following exposure to AQP4-IgG.

Complement activation is a major effector pathway in NMO. NMO pathology in humans shows centrovascular deposition of activated complement [14–16], and early clinical trials data support the efficacy of a complement inhibitor [17, 18]. Complement-dependent NMO pathology is also seen in experimental animal models of NMO produced by passive transfer of AQP4-IgG [6, 7, 19]. We recently reported evidence for complement bystander injury to oligodendrocytes, in which complement activation following AQP4-IgG binding to AQP4 on astrocytes results in killing of nearby oligodendrocytes by a bystander mechanism involving local diffusion of activated, soluble complement components, leading to formation of the complement membrane attack complex (MAC) on oligodendrocytes [20]. Complement bystander injury has been reported before in Rasmussen's encephalitis [21], cerebral artery smooth muscle cells [22], and on cells surrounding amyloid plaques in postmortem samples from Alzheimer's patients [23]. Low expression of CD59, a membrane-anchored complement regulator protein that inhibits MAC formation on target cells [24, 25], appears to be important for complement bystander injury, probably because of the limited transfer of soluble, metastable C5b67 from the primary target cell to nearby bystander cells. Neurons have been reported to express low levels of endogenous complement inhibitors, including CD59 [26–28], and are therefore potential targets for bystander damage.

Here, we tested the hypothesis that complement bystander injury is a general pathogenic mechanism in NMO, accounting not only for early oligodendrocyte injury and demyelination, but also for direct neuronal injury. This study was motivated by in vivo pilot experiments in rat brain in which neurons were identified as being frequently injured, along with oligodendrocytes, soon after intracerebral AQP4-IgG injection. Here, experiments done in astrocyte-neuron cocultures and in rat brain show that AQP4-IgG and complement do not injure neurons directly, but kill neurons in close proximity to astrocytes by a complement bystander mechanism.

Methods
Materials
Recombinant purified AQP4-IgG (rAb-53) [29, 30] was provided by Dr. Jeffrey Bennett (University of Colorado, Aurora, CO). Fc hexamer Fc-μTP-L309C was as described [31]. Chemicals were purchased from Sigma-Aldrich (St. Louis, MO) unless specified otherwise. Sprague-Dawley rats were purchased from Charles River Laboratories (Wilmington, MA) and bred at UCSF.

$AQP4^{-/-}$ rats for control studies were generated by CRISPR/Cas9 as reported [32]. All animal procedures were approved by the University of California, San Francisco Animal Care and Use Committee (IACUC).

Cell culture
Primary cortical neuron cultures were generated from the brains of embryonic day 18 (E18) Sprague-Dawley rats (timed-pregnant, Charles River Laboratories, Wilmington, MA), as described [33, 34], with modification. Briefly, the cerebral hemispheres were isolated and cortical tissue was placed in cold Hank's balanced salt solution (HBSS, pH 7.2; Invitrogen, Camarillo, CA) without Ca^{2+} and Mg^{2+}. After removal of the meninges, tissue was diced, incubated for 10 min in 0.25% trypsin-EDTA at 37 °C, and triturated with an 18-gauge needle. The single-cell suspension was passed through a 70-μm nylon strainer (Falcon, Corning, NY) and centrifuged. The tissue pellet was resuspended in Neurobasal medium containing 2% B27-supplement and 0.5 mM Glutamax (Gibco, Grand Island, NY). Cells were plated on PDL-coated 12-well plates at the density of 2×10^5/ml. After 5–7 days in culture, neurons were used for experiments.

Primary astrocyte cultures were generated from cerebral cortex of neonatal wild-type and $AQP4^{-/-}$ rats at day 1 post-birth (P1), as described [35, 36]. Briefly, the cerebral hemispheres were isolated and cortical tissue was minced and incubated for 10 min at 37 °C in 0.25% trypsin-EDTA. Dissociated cells were centrifuged at 500g for 5 min and resuspended in Dulbecco's modified Eagle medium (DMEM) containing 10% FBS and 1% penicillin/streptomycin in T75 flasks. After cell confluence (8–10 days), flasks were shaken in a rotator at 180 rpm overnight to purify astrocytes. The medium was replaced with DMEM containing 3% FBS and 0.25 mM dibutyryl cAMP to induce differentiation. Cultures were maintained for up to an additional 2 weeks. For cocultures, astrocytes were plated on neurons and cocultured in neuron medium overnight before experiments. The neuron:astrocyte ratios of cocultures were from 5:1 to 20:1.

Complement-dependent cytotoxicity
Specified concentrations of AQP4-IgG (or control human IgG, Thermo Fisher Scientific, Rockford, IL) and human complement (Innovative Research, Novi, MI) were added in Hank's buffer, and cells were incubated at 37 °C for specified times. In some experiments, cells were exposed to serum of an AQP4-IgG seropositive NMO patient who met the revised diagnostic criteria for clinical disease. A fixable dead-cell stain (amine-reactive dye, Invitrogen, Eugene, OR) at 1:1000 dilution was added 30 min prior to cell fixation. In some experiments, C1q- or C6-deficient human complement

(Innovative Research, Novi, MI) was used instead of normal complement. In some experiments, the astrocyte toxin α-aminoadipic acid (Santa Cruz Biotechnology, Dallas, TX) at 2 mM was added to astrocyte-neuron cocultures for 75 min.

For live-cell real-time imaging, astrocyte-neuron cocultures were grown on 6-well plates and imaged by phase-contrast optics using a 20×, 0.45 NA objective lens on a Nikon Eclipse Ti microscope equipped with an environmental chamber at 37 °C and 5% CO_2. Ethidium homodimer-1 (1 μM, Invitrogen, Eugene, OR) was added to the culture medium prior to image acquisition. Transmitted light (phase-contrast) and red fluorescence images were obtained sequentially every 2 min for a 30-min baseline period and then for 2 h following addition of 20 μg/ml AQP4-IgG and 2% complement.

Rat studies

AQP4-IgG was delivered to adult wild-type or AQP4$^{-/-}$ rats by intracerebral injection. Rats were anesthetized with ketamine (100 mg/kg) and xylazine (10 mg/kg) and mounted on a stereotaxic frame. Following a midline scalp incision, a 1-mm-diameter burr hole was drilled 0.5 mm anterior and 3.5 mm lateral to the bregma for insertion of a glass pipette with a 40-μm-diameter tip to a depth of 3 mm. AQP4-IgG (or control IgG, each 15 μg) together with 6 μM fixable dead cell dye ethidium homodimer-1 (EH-1) was infused in a volume of 3 μl over 6 min by pressure injection. The glass pipette was kept in place for 10 min before withdrawal to prevent leaking. In some studies, the Fc hexamer Fc-μTP-L309C (50 mg/kg, iv) or MK801 (10 mg/kg, ip) was administered 2 h or 30 min, respectively, before intracerebral injection of AQP4-IgG. At 90 min, rats were deeply anesthetized and transcardiacally perfused with 200 ml heparinized PBS and 200 ml of 4% paraformaldehyde (PFA) in PBS. Brains were removed and post-fixed for 4 h in 4% PFA and cryoprotected in 20% sucrose for cutting 7-μm-thick sections on a cryostat.

Immunofluorescence

Following treatments, cell cultures were rinsed in PBS, fixed with 4% PFA for 15 min, and then blocked with 1% BSA and 0.2% Triton-X100 in PBS for 1 h. Cultures were incubated at room temperature for 2 h, and brain sections were incubated at 4 °C overnight with antibodies against AQP4 (1:200, Santa Cruz Biotechnology), GFAP (glial fibrillary acidic protein, 1:1000; Millipore), MAP2 (microtubule-associated protein 2, 1:100, Thermo Fisher Scientific), NeuN (Neuronal Nuclei, 1:200; Millipore), C1q (1:50, Abcam, Cambridge, MA), C5b-9 (1:100, Santa Cruz Biotechnology), or CD59 (5 μg/ml, Lifespan Bioscience), followed by the appropriate species-specific Alexa Fluor-conjugated secondary antibody for 1 h

(5 μg/ml each, Invitrogen). In some control studies, phosphatidylinositol-specific phospholipase C (PI-PLC) (0.5 U/ml, Invitrogen) was added 1 h prior to experiments to release the extracellular portion of glycophosphoinositol (GPI)-anchored membrane protein CD59. AQP4-IgG was detected using Alexa Fluor-conjugated anti-human IgG. Sections were mounted with VectaShield (Vector Laboratories, Burlingame, CA), and immunofluorescence was visualized on a Nikon confocal microscope using a 20×/0.5 N.A., 60×/1.25 N.A., or 100×/1.4 N.A. oil objective lens.

Results

Characterization of astrocyte-neuron cocultures

An astrocyte-neuron coculture model was established with the goal of having relatively few, well-separated astrocytes with many surrounding neurons in order to facilitate imaging of bystander injury to neurons. Figure 1a shows staining for GFAP (astrocyte marker) and MAP2 (neuron marker) in pure astrocyte and neuron cultures and in cocultures generated using different cell ratios. The astrocyte cultures were fully differentiated using dibutyryl-cAMP for these studies, and astrocyte-neuron cocultures were generated as described under the "Methods" section. A neuron:astrocyte cell ratio of 20:1, which showed relatively few and well-separated astrocytes, was used for subsequent experiments.

Figure 1b (top panels) shows that the individual astrocyte and neuron cultures were > 95% pure as seen by GFAP and MAP2 immunofluorescence with DAPI costaining. AQP4 and CD59 immunofluorescence showed, as expected, AQP4 expression only on astrocytes, with AQP4-deficient astrocytes generated from AQP4$^{-/-}$ rats as control (Fig. 1b, lower panels). CD59 was expressed on astrocytes, with little expression seen on neurons. The control for CD59 immunofluorescence was treatment with the enzyme PI-PLC, which cleaves the extracellular CD59 antigen from its membrane-spanning domain. In astrocyte-neuron cocultures, CD59 expression was seen on astrocytes and not on neurons (Fig. 1c). At 1 h following incubation with AQP4-IgG, AQP4-IgG was seen on astrocytes but not neurons as detected using a fluorescent anti-human IgG secondary antibody (Fig. 1d). Therefore, astrocytes but not neurons are the target of the pathogenic NMO anti-AQP4 autoantibody.

Complement bystander killing of neurons in astrocyte-neuron cocultures

Complement-dependent cytotoxicity was produced by incubation of astrocyte-neuron cocultures with AQP4-IgG and human complement. A fixable dead cell stain was included in order to visualize dead cells. In pure astrocyte and neuron cultures, > 60% of astrocytes were stained with dead cell dye following 2 h exposure to

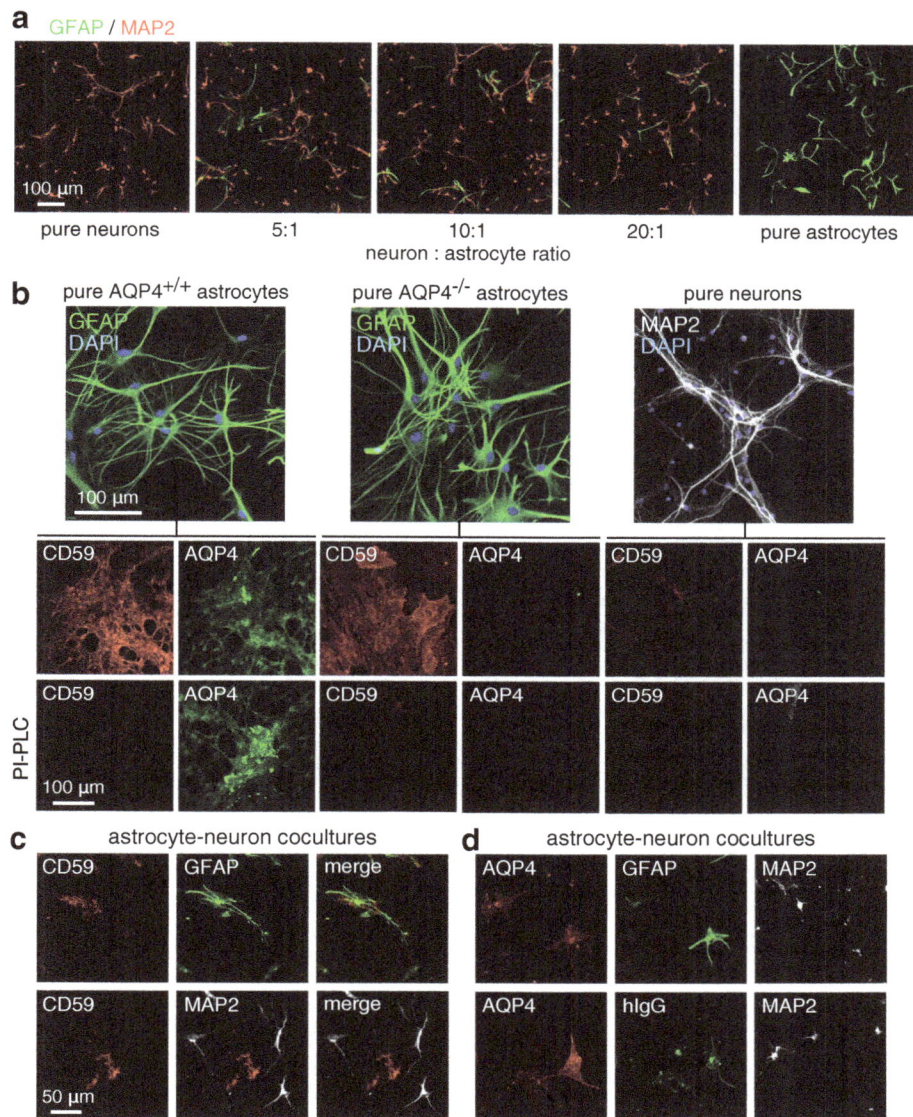

Fig. 1 Characterization of rat astrocyte-neuron cocultures. **a** GFAP and MAP2 immunofluorescence of pure neuron cultures, pure astrocyte cultures, and astrocyte-neuron cocultures at indicated cell ratios. **b** (top panels) GFAP or MAP2 immunofluorescence (with DAPI counterstaining) of pure AQP4$^{+/+}$ and AQP4$^{-/-}$ astrocyte cultures and pure neuron cultures. (lower panels) CD59 and AQP4 immunofluorescence. Where indicated (bottom row), cells were incubated with PI-PLC 1 h prior to fixation. **c** CD59 immunofluorescence of astrocyte-neuron cocultures costained with GFAP or MAP2. **d** (upper) AQP4 immunofluorescence of astrocyte-neuron cocultures costained with GFAP and MAP2. (lower) AQP4-IgG (human IgG, hIgG) immunofluorescence (visualized with secondary anti-human IgG antibody) in astrocyte-neuron cocultures following 1 h incubation with 20 µg/ml AQP4-IgG, costained with AQP4 and MAP2. Micrographs representative of studies done of three sets of cultures

AQP4-IgG and complement, whereas < 5% of neurons were stained (Fig. 2a). In the astrocyte-neuron cocultures, dead cell-stained astrocytes were seen (Fig. 2b, yellow filled arrowheads), as well as dead cell-stained neurons (yellow open arrowheads), generally in close proximity to astrocytes. Dead cell-stained neurons were seen near both dead cell-stained and non-stained astrocytes. Figure 2b (right) summarizes the percentage of dead neurons at different distances from the center of

dead astrocytes, showing preferential killing of neurons within 200 µm of dead astrocytes. A similar pattern of dead neurons nearby astrocytes was seen using NMO patient serum instead of the recombinant AQP4-IgG antibody (Fig. 2c).

Time-lapse imaging was done to visualize in real time the injury to astrocytes and neurons following exposure to AQP4-IgG and complement. Phase-contrast and fluorescence imaging was done to visualize all cells and

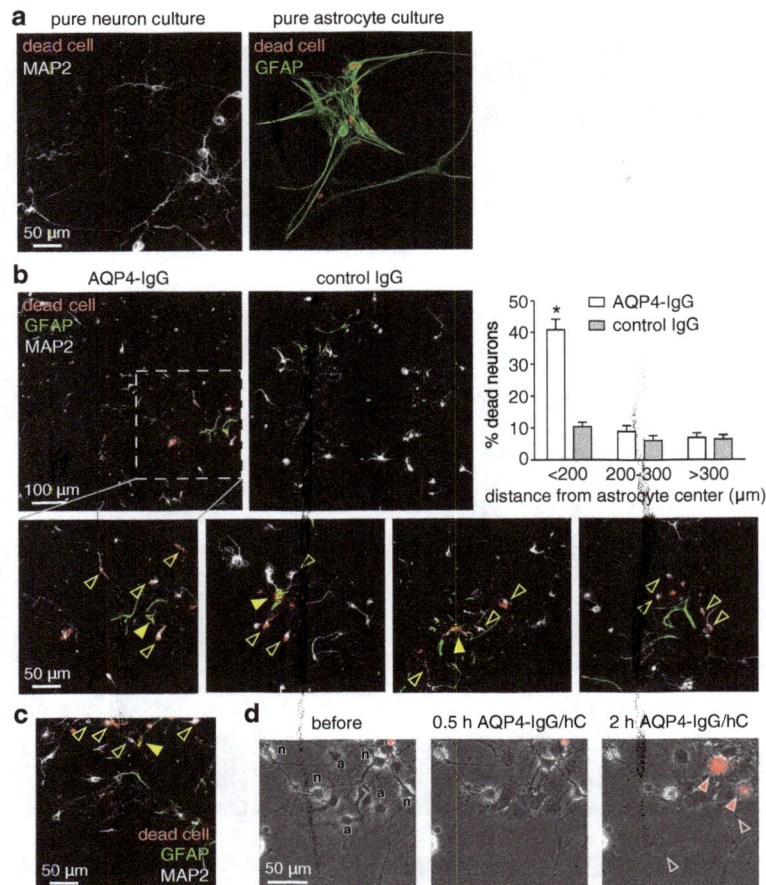

Fig. 2 Complement-mediated neuron injury in astrocyte-neuron cocultures. **a** Complement-dependent cytotoxicity in pure neuron and pure astrocyte cultures following incubation with 20 µg/ml AQP4-IgG and 2% human complement for 2 h, with fixable dead cell marker (reactive amine dye, labeled "dead cell"). Cultures were immunostained for GFAP and MAP2, with dead cells stained red. **b** Cocultures were incubated as in **a** and immunostained for GFAP (green) and MAP2 (gray), with dead cells red. Expanded images (lower panels) showing dead astrocytes (filled yellow arrowheads) and nearby dead neurons (open yellow arrowheads) in representative fields. Bar graph at the right shows percentage of dead neurons at different distances from the center of dead astrocytes (mean ± S.E.M., $n = 6$ cultures, total 32 astrocytes imaged, *$P < 0.01$ comparing AQP4-IgG vs. control IgG). **c** Cocultures were incubated with 1% NMO patient serum and 5% human complement and immunostained as in panel **b**. **d** Panels from time-lapse image sequence (see Additional file 1: Movie 1) showing astrocytes and neurons in coculture before and at 0.5 and 2 h after addition of 20 µg/ml AQP4-IgG and 2% human complement containing dead cell marker ethidium homodimer-1. Labels in the left panel: n, neuron; a, astrocyte. Filled arrowheads point to early damage of neurons in contact with astrocytes, and red color is due to uptake of dead cell marker. Open arrowheads indicate sites of neurite blebbing and degeneration

their injury. Neurons and astrocytes were readily differentiated based on morphological criteria and the weak phase-halo of the very flat astrocytes (Fig. 2d, left panel). Upon addition of AQP4-IgG and complement, astrocytes responded with morphological rearrangements; however, only a subset of cells was damaged severely enough for full membrane permeabilization to occur (not shown). Neurons adjacent to astrocytes showed neurite blebbing and membrane lysis with uptake of ethidium homodimer (Fig. 2d, right panel and Additional file 1: Movie 1).

C5b-9 and C1q immunostaining was done to investigate whether neuronal injury was caused by a complement bystander mechanism, which would predict C5b-9 on both astrocytes and nearby injured neurons, whereas C1q, the initiating complement protein, only on astrocytes. C5b-9 immunofluorescence was seen on many dead cell-stained astrocytes and neurons in the cocultures (Fig. 3a). Figure 3b indicates C5b-9 deposition on astrocytes as well as on neurons near astrocytes, whereas C1q immunofluorescence was seen only on astrocytes. Figure 3c summarizes the percentage of C5b-9 and C1q positive neurons at different distances from C5b-9 and C1q positive astrocytes. These results support a complement bystander mechanism in which C1q binding to AQP4-IgG on astrocytes results in deposition of the cytotoxic C5b-9 complex on both astrocytes and nearby neurons.

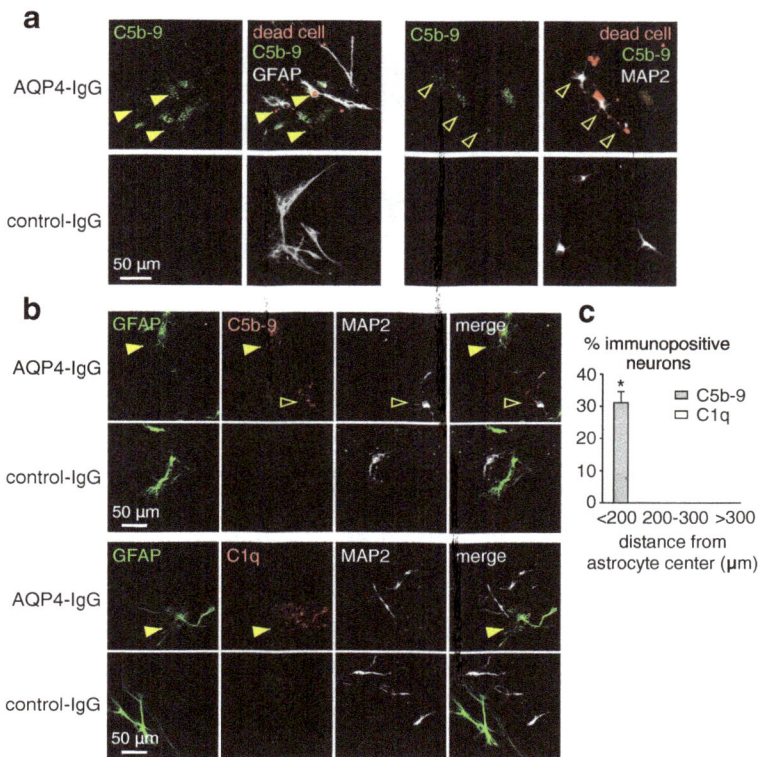

Fig. 3 Evidence for a complement bystander mechanism for AQP4-IgG/complement-induced neuron injury in astrocyte-neuron cocultures. **a** C5b-9 immunofluorescence (green) in astrocyte-neuron cocultures with dead cell stain (red) at 2 h after incubation with 20 µg/ml AQP4-IgG and 2% human complement, immunostained for GFAP or MAP2 (gray). **b** C5b-9 and C1q immunofluorescence of cocultures with cell markers GFAP and MAP2 treated as in **a**. Filled arrowheads indicate C5b-9 or C1q on astrocytes, and open arrowheads show C5b-9 on neurons. **c** Percentage of C5b-9 and C1q positive neurons at different distances from C5b-9 or C1q positive astrocytes (mean ± S.E.M., $n = 6$, *$P < 0.01$ comparing AQP4-IgG vs. control IgG)

Control studies were done to support a complement bystander mechanism for neuron killing in the astrocyte-neuron cocultures. Cocultures incubated with AQP4-IgG and C1q-depleted serum did not show cell killing or C5b-9 deposition, indicating that activation of classic complement pathway is the effector of bystander injury (Fig. 4a (i)). Incubation of cocultures with AQP4-IgG and C6-depleted serum did not produce cytotoxicity, indicating that neuron killing is the consequence of MAC (C5b-9) deposition rather than upstream anaphylotoxins or other mediators (Fig. 4a (ii)). Cytotoxicity was not seen in the presence of a complement inhibitor (Fig. 4a (iii)) or in AQP4-deficient cocultures in which astrocytes were cultured from AQP4$^{-/-}$ rats (Fig. 4a (iv)). In a separate control, cocultures were incubated with the astrocyte-selective toxin α-aminoadipic acid [37, 38] in which the incubation time and toxin concentration were chosen in initial studies to cause killing of many astrocytes but few neurons (in pure cultures). Exposure of pure cultures to 2 mM α-aminoadipic acid for 75 min resulted in ~ 85% astrocyte death and ~ 10% neuron death. Incubation of cocultures with α-aminoadipic acid under these conditions resulted in killing of astrocytes but not neurons (Fig. 4b), suggesting that mediators or other factors released from dying astrocytes are not responsible for neuronal injury.

Complement bystander injury to neurons in a rat model of NMO

To investigate complement bystander injury in vivo, rats were administered AQP4-IgG by intracerebral injection, together with the dead cell dye ethidium homodimer-1 (EH-1) (Fig. 5a). Rats were sacrificed at 90 min, and brains were perfusion-fixed for frozen sections. Figure 5b shows many dead cells near the needle tract in rats receiving AQP4-IgG. In control studies, few or no dead cells were seen with injection of non-NMO human IgG instead of AQP4-IgG, when rats were pre-treated with the Fc hexamer complement inhibitor or when AQP4-IgG was injected in AQP4$^{-/-}$ rats. NeuN immunofluorescence of neurons with GFAP immunofluorescence of astrocytes showed many red-stained dead astrocytes, as well as nearby dead neurons and some

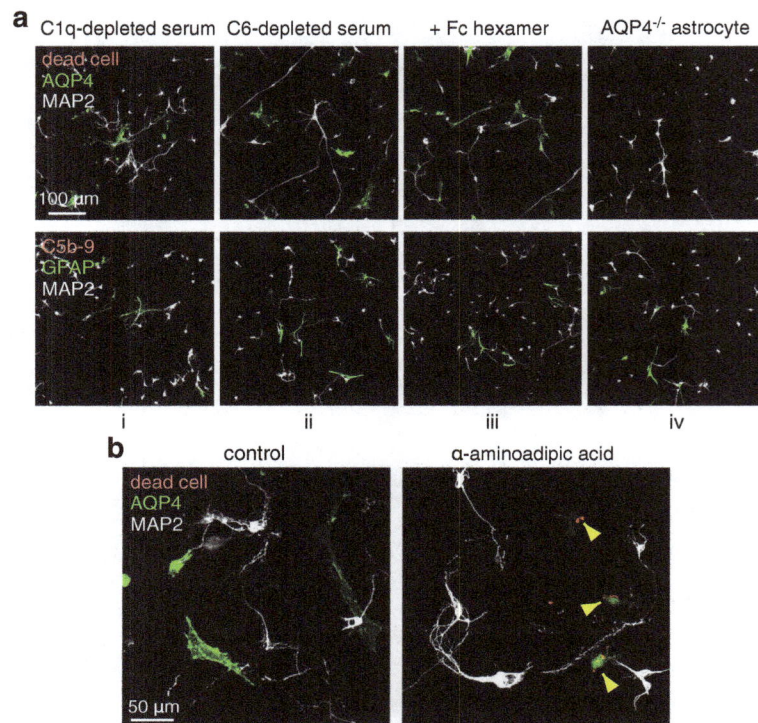

Fig. 4 Control studies supporting a complement bystander mechanism for neuron injury. **a** Astrocyte-neuron cocultures were incubated for 2 h with 20 µg/ml AQP4-IgG and 2% C1q-depleted serum (i) or with 20 µg/ml AQP4-IgG and 2% C6-depleted serum (ii); cocultures were incubated for 2 h with 20 µg/ml AQP4-IgG and 2% human complement that was pre-exposed for 1 h to 1 µg/ml Fc hexamer (complement inhibitor) (iii); AQP4$^{-/-}$ astrocyte-neuron cocultures were incubated for 2 h with 20 µg/ml AQP4-IgG and 2% human complement (iv). GFAP, MAP2, and C5b-9 immunofluorescence as indicated, with dead cells stained red. **b** Direct astrocyte injury caused by α-aminoadipic acid. Cocultures were exposed to 2 mM α-aminoadipic acid for 75 min, with AQP4 and MAP2 immunofluorescence and dead cell stain shown. Filled arrowheads show dead astrocytes. Micrographs representative of three sets of studies done on different cocultures

other cell types not stained with NeuN or GFAP (Fig. 5c). In the area within and just around the needle tract, ∼ 80% of astrocytes were dead (red-stained), with ∼ 55% of dead neurons nearby (within 200 µm) astrocytes (sections from 3 rats examined).

To investigate if excitotoxic mechanisms might contribute to the early neuron injury observed in response to AQP4-IgG, the NMDA receptor antagonist MK801 (10 mg/kg, ip) [39, 40] was injected 30 min before intracerebral injection of AQP4-IgG and EH-1. Figure 5d shows similar EH-1 staining by neurons in the presence and absence of MK801, suggesting minimal contribution of excitotoxicity to neuron cell death in this model.

C5b-9 and C1q immunofluorescence in rats injected with AQP4-IgG and EH-1 showed C5b-9 on dead astrocytes as well as on nearby dead neurons (Fig. 6a). In rats injected with AQP4-IgG (without EH-1), immunofluorescence of C1q, GFAP, and NeuN showed C1q deposition only on astrocytes (Fig. 6b, top panels), whereas C5b-9 was seen on both astrocytes and nearby neurons (Fig. 6b, bottom panels). Figure 6c shows CD59 colocalization with GFAP in astrocytes, but not with NeuN on

neurons in (non-injected) rat brain, which is consistent with the cell culture studies showing CD59 on astrocytes but not neurons.

Discussion

This study reports evidence for complement bystander killing of neurons in astrocyte-neuron cocultures in vitro and in rats in vivo. Astrocyte-neuron cocultures exposed to AQP4-IgG or NMO patient serum and complement showed injury and death in neurons very near astrocytes. Time-lapse imaging revealed early injury to neurons near astrocytes even before gross plasma membrane permeabilization and uptake of the dead cell stain. Neuron death was not seen in the absence of AQP4-IgG or with complement inhibition, with C1q- or C6-depleted serum, or with an astrocyte toxin, implicating a complement-dependent mechanism initiated by AQP4-IgG binding to astrocytes. The deposition of C5b-9 on astrocytes and injured nearby neurons, with C1q deposition only on astrocytes, indicates that activation of the classical complement cascade on astrocytes leads to MAC deposition on both astrocytes and nearby

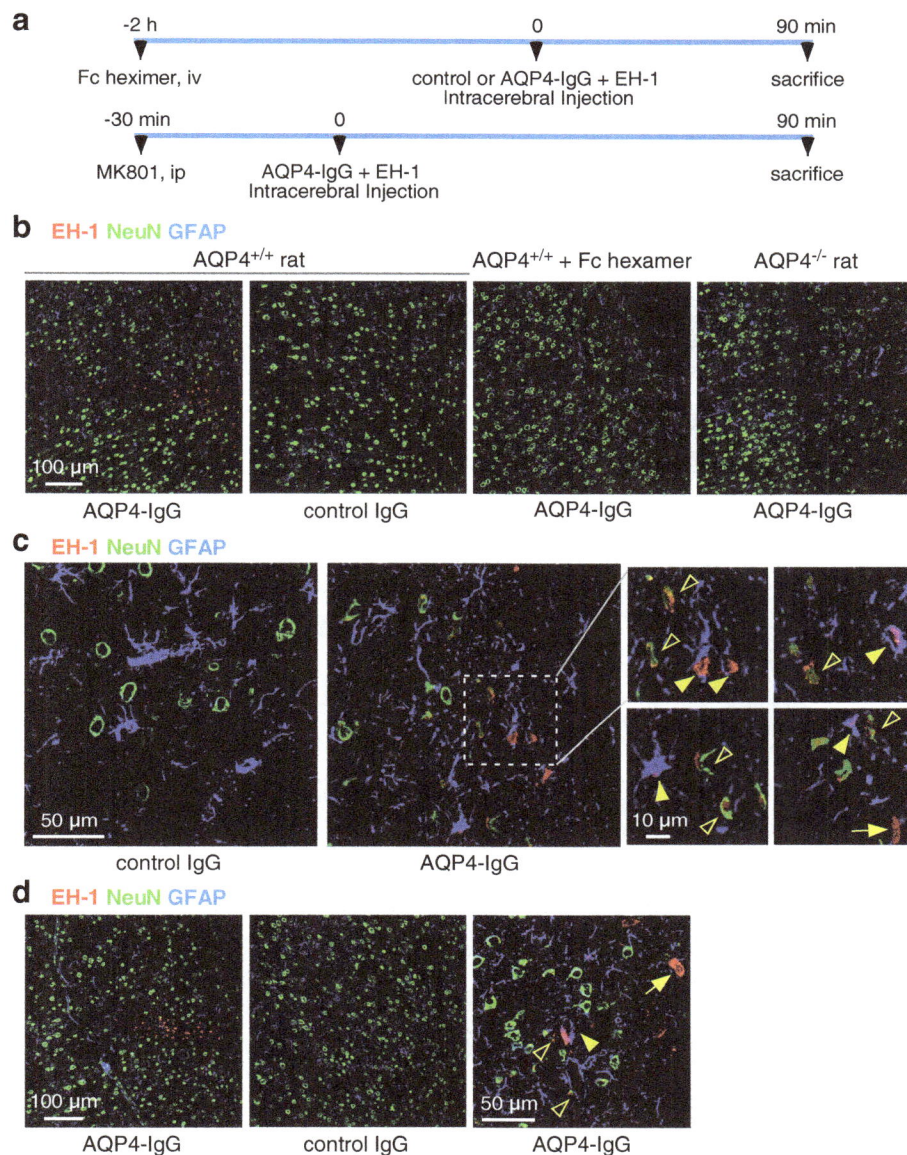

Fig. 5 Complement bystander killing of neurons near astrocytes in rat brain following intracerebral AQP4-IgG injection. **a** AQP4-IgG (15 μg) (or 15 μg control IgG) and dead cell stain EH-1 (6 μM) in a 3-μl volume was injected in cortex and striatum of rat brain, and rats were sacrificed at 90 min. In some studies, rats were injected with Fc hexamer (50 mg/kg, iv) by tail vein 2 h before or MK801 (10 mg/kg, ip) 30 min before intracerebral injection of AQP4-IgG. **b** Low-magnification micrographs showing dead cells (red EH-1 fluorescence), NeuN (green), and GFAP (blue) for studies done in AQP4$^{+/+}$ rats, Fc hexamer-treated AQP4$^{+/+}$ rats, and AQP4$^{-/-}$ rats. **c** High-magnification confocal images of AQP4$^{+/+}$ rat brain at 90 min after injection of AQP4-IgG (or control IgG) and EH-1 showing dead astrocytes and nearby dead injured neurons. Expanded images on the right showing representative fields. Filled arrowheads show dead astrocytes, open arrowheads show nearby dead neurons, and arrow points to a non-neuron, non-astrocyte dead cell. **d** Rats were injected with MK801 (10 mg/kg, ip) 30 min before intracerebral injection of AQP4-IgG (or control IgG) and EH-1. Imaging showing dead cells (red EH-1 fluorescence), NeuN (green), and GFAP (blue). Filled arrowheads show dead astrocytes, open arrowheads show nearby dead neurons, and arrow points to a non-neuron, non-astrocyte dead cell. Representative of micrographs done on sections from three rats

neurons. Astrocyte killing by a selective toxin in the cocultures did not result in neuron killing, indicating the factors released from dead astrocytes are not responsible for neuron killing in the coculture experiments. In rats in vivo, dead neurons near dead astrocytes were seen at 90 min after intracerebral administration of AQP4-IgG, with C5b-9 deposition on astrocytes and neurons, but C1q deposition only on astrocytes. Neuron cytotoxicity was not seen with complement inhibition, with non-NMO human IgG, or in AQP4$^{-/-}$ rats. Though it is not possible to exclude mechanisms other than complement bystander injury to explain the early neuron death

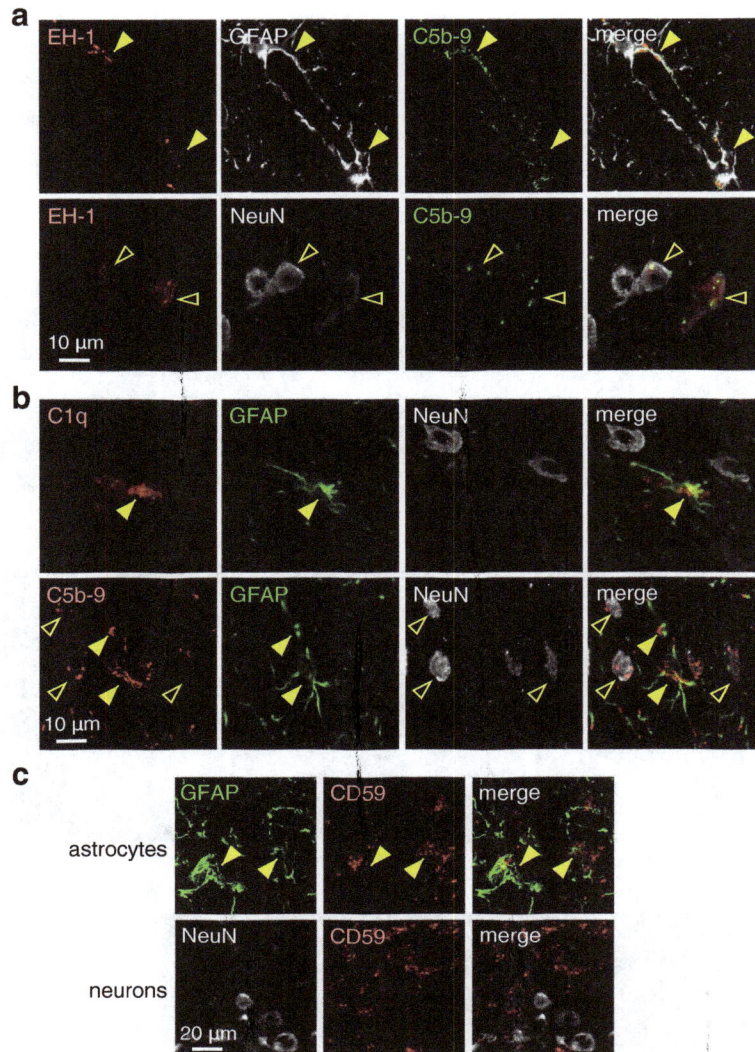

Fig. 6 Evidence for complement bystander killing of neurons in rat brain. **a** Brains were injected with AQP4-IgG and EH-1 and harvested at 90 min as in Fig. 5. High-magnification confocal micrographs showing colocalization of EH-1, GFAP, and C5b-9 (top, filled arrowheads) and EH-1, NeuN, and C5b-9 (bottom, open arrowheads). **b** Brains were injected with AQP4-IgG alone (without EH-1) and harvested at 90 min. C1q colocalization with GFAP and NeuN, and C5b-9 colocalization with GFAP and NeuN (bottom). Filled arrowheads show C5b-9 or C1q deposition on astrocytes, and open arrowheads show C5b-9 on neurons. **c** CD59 immunofluorescence with GFAP or NeuN in control (non-injected) rat. Filled arrowheads indicate CD59 on astrocytes. Representative of micrographs done on sections from three rats

following AQP4-IgG in vivo, similar levels of neuronal damage were observed in control rats and rats treated with the NMDA receptor antagonist MK801, suggesting that excitotoxic mechanisms do not substantially contribute to the observed cell death.

The generality of complement bystander injury in NMO adds to the list of proposed mechanisms linking the AQP4-IgG astrocytopathy to downstream neurological deficit and has potential implications for treatment of NMO. Complement bystander injury to neurons could account for the early and marked neurological deficit seen in some NMO patients, as well as for the rapid early

neuron loss in experimental animal models of NMO. In addition to neuronal injury from a complement bystander mechanism, as reported here, and oligodendrocyte injury as we reported before [20], we speculate that other cell types in the central nervous system may be injured similarly, such as microvascular endothelial cells and pericytes lining the blood-brain barrier in close contact with AQP4-enriched astrocyte foot processes. With regard to NMO therapeutics, early loss of neuron and axons would limit the potential efficacy of remyelination therapeutics [41, 42]. Complement bystander injury would be prevented by inhibition of the classical complement pathway or earlier steps in NMO pathogenesis such as AQP4-IgG binding to AQP4 or by drugs or maneuvers to increase CD59 expression in the secondarily injured cells. Complement bystander injury would be relatively insensitive to drugs acting on more downstream disease pathogenesis mechanisms such as general immunosuppressants.

Though the data here provide strong evidence for complement bystander killing of neurons, several limitations are noted. As human specimens were not studied, the significance of complement bystander injury to neurons in human NMO is uncertain. Even if specimens from humans with active NMO disease were available, it would likely be difficult to identify dead neurons because of their clearance, and the lack of a dead cell stain and defined AQP4-IgG exposure time as in the rat studies here. Though the in vitro cocultures allowed clear-cut interpretation of the immunofluorescence data because of the well-demarcated cell distribution in two dimensions and the specification of precise solution composition, the culture system does not recapitulate many aspects of the central nervous system, such as the blood-brain barrier, the complex three-dimensional network of many different brain cell types, and inflammatory effectors. It is therefore not possible in the in vivo rat studies to exclude contributions from additional mechanisms of early neuronal injury following astrocyte death, such as excitotoxic injury or injury caused by inflammatory mechanisms such as cytokine release by astrocytes or microglial activation.

Conclusions

In conclusion, the evidence here for a complement bystander mechanism for neuronal injury in NMO supports the generality of complement bystander injury to brain cell types implicated in NMO pathology, including neurons, oligodendrocytes, and perhaps microvascular endothelia and other cell types. Bystander injury may also be relevant to cellular injury mechanisms such as leukocyte degranulation following AQP4-IgG-induced antibody-dependent cellular cytotoxicity.

Additional file

Additional file 1: Movie 1. Time-lapse imaging of astrocyte-neuron coculture following addition of AQP4-IgG and complement as in Fig. 2. Cultures were imaged for 30 min before and 2 h following addition of AQP4-IgG and complement. (AVI 4660 kb)

Abbreviations
AQP4: Aquaporin-4; AQP4-IgG: Aquaporin-4-immunoglobulin G; DMEM: Dulbecco's modified Eagle medium; EH-1: Ethidium homodimer-1; GFAP: Glial fibrillary acidic protein; HBSS: Hank's balanced salt solution; hIgG: Non-NMO pooled human IgG; MAP2: Microtubule-associated protein 2; NeuN: Neuronal Nuclei; NMO: Neuromyelitis optica; PFA: Paraformaldehyde; PI-PLC: Phosphatidylinositol-specific phospholipase C

Acknowledgements
We thank Dr. Jeffrey Bennett (Univ. Colorado Denver, Aurora, CO) for providing recombinant monoclonal NMO antibody rAb-53.

Funding
This work was supported by grants EY13574, EB00415, DK72517, and DK101373 from the National Institutes of Health, and a grant from the Guthy-Jackson Charitable Foundation.

Authors' contributions
TJD performed the in vitro and in vivo experiments and analyzed the data. AJS performed live-cell real-time imaging studies. ASV conceived the study and designed the experiments. All authors contributed to the writing and editing and approved the final manuscript.

Competing interests
The authors declare that they have no competing interests.

Author details
[1]Departments of Medicine and Physiology, University of California, 1246 Health Sciences East Tower, 513 Parnassus Ave, San Francisco, CA 94143-0521, USA. [2]Department of Neurology, Second Xiangya Hospital of Central South University, Changsha 410011, Hunan, People's Republic of China.

References
1. Papadopoulos MC, Verkman AS. Aquaporin 4 and neuromyelitis optica. Lancet Neurol. 2012;11:535–44.
2. Jarius S, Paul F, Franciotta D, Waters P, Zipp F, Hohlfeld R, Vincent A, Wildemann B. Mechanisms of disease: aquaporin-4 antibodies in neuromyelitis optica. Nat Clin Pract Neurol. 2008;4:202–14.
3. Jasiak-Zatonska M, Kalinowska-Lyszczarz A, Michalak S, Kozubski W. The immunology of neuromyelitis optica-current knowledge, clinical implications, controversies and future perspectives. Int J Mol Sci. 2016; 17:273.
4. Wingerchuk DM, Hogancamp WF, O'Brien PC, Weinshenker BG. The clinical course of neuromyelitis optica (Devic's syndrome). Neurology. 1999;53: 1107–14.
5. Bruscolini A, Sacchetti M, La Cava M, Gharbiya M, Ralli M, Lambiase A, De Virgilio A, Greco A. Diagnosis and management of neuromyelitis optica spectrum disorders - an update. Autoimmun Rev. 2018;17:195–200.
6. Saadoun S, Waters P, Bell BA, Vincent A, Verkman AS, Papadopoulos MC. Intra-cerebral injection of neuromyelitis optica immunoglobulin G and human complement produces neuromyelitis optica lesions in mice. Brain. 2010;133:349–61.
7. Asavapanumas N, Ratelade J, Verkman AS. Unique neuromyelitis optica pathology produced in naive rats by intracerebral administration of NMO-IgG. Acta Neuropathol. 2014;127:539–51.
8. Marignier R, Nicolle A, Watrin C, Touret M, Cavagna S, Varrin-Doyer M, Cavillon G, Rogemond V, Confavreux C, Honnorat J, Giraudon P. Oligodendrocytes are damaged by neuromyelitis optica immunoglobulin G via astrocyte injury. Brain. 2010;133:2578–91.
9. Hinson SR, Roemer SF, Lucchinetti CF, Fryer JP, Kryzer TJ, Chamberlain JL, Howe CL, Pittock SJ, Lennon VA. Aquaporin-4-binding autoantibodies in patients with neuromyelitis optica impair glutamate transport by down-regulating EAAT2. J Exp Med. 2008;205:2473–81.
10. Sagan SA, Winger RC, Cruz-Herranz A, Nelson PA, Hagberg S, Miller CN, Spencer CM, Ho PP, Bennett JL, Levy M, et al. Tolerance checkpoint bypass permits emergence of pathogenic T cells to neuromyelitis optica autoantigen aquaporin-4. Proc Natl Acad Sci U S A. 2016;113:14781–6.
11. Zeka B, Hastermann M, Hochmeister S, Kogl N, Kaufmann N, Schanda K, Mader S, Misu T, Rommer P, Fujihara K, et al. Highly encephalitogenic aquaporin 4-specific T cells and NMO-IgG jointly orchestrate lesion location and tissue damage in the CNS. Acta Neuropathol. 2015;130:783 98.

12. Ratelade J, Bennett JL, Verkman AS. Evidence against cellular internalization in vivo of NMO-IgG, aquaporin-4, and excitatory amino acid transporter 2 in neuromyelitis optica. J Biol Chem. 2011;286:45156–64.

13. Rossi A, Ratelade J, Papadopoulos MC, Bennett JL, Verkman AS. Neuromyelitis optica IgG does not alter aquaporin-4 water permeability, plasma membrane M1/M23 isoform content, or supramolecular assembly. Glia. 2012;60:2027–39.

14. Lucchinetti CF, Mandler RN, McGavern D, Bruck W, Gleich G, Ransohoff RM, Trebst C, Weinshenker B, Wingerchuk D, Parisi JE, Lassmann H. A role for humoral mechanisms in the pathogenesis of Devic's neuromyelitis optica. Brain. 2002;125:1450–61.

15. Misu T, Fujihara K, Kakita A, Konno H, Nakamura M, Watanabe S, Takahashi T, Nakashima I, Takahashi H, Itoyama Y. Loss of aquaporin 4 in lesions of neuromyelitis optica: distinction from multiple sclerosis. Brain. 2007;130:1224–34.

16. Roemer SF, Parisi JE, Lennon VA, Benarroch EE, Lassmann H, Bruck W, Mandler RN, Weinshenker BG, Pittock SJ, Wingerchuk DM, Lucchinetti CF. Pattern-specific loss of aquaporin-4 immunoreactivity distinguishes neuromyelitis optica from multiple sclerosis. Brain. 2007;130:1194–205.

17. Pittock SJ, Lennon VA, McKeon A, Mandrekar J, Weinshenker BG, Lucchinetti CF, O'Toole O, Wingerchuk DM. Eculizumab in AQP4-IgG-positive relapsing neuromyelitis optica spectrum disorders: an open-label pilot study. Lancet Neurol. 2013;12:554–62.

18. Papadopoulos MC, Bennett JL, Verkman AS. Treatment of neuromyelitis optica: state-of-the-art and emerging therapies. Nat Rev Neurol. 2014;10: 493–506.

19. Kinoshita M, Nakatsuji Y, Kimura T, Moriya M, Takata K, Okuno T, Kumanogoh A, Kajiyama K, Yoshikawa H, Sakoda S. Neuromyelitis optica: passive transfer to rats by human immunoglobulin. Biochem Biophys Res Commun. 2009;386:623–7.

20. Tradtrantip L, Yao X, Su T, Smith AJ, Verkman AS. Bystander mechanism for complement-initiated early oligodendrocyte injury in neuromyelitis optica. Acta Neuropathol. 2017;134:35–44.

21. Whitney KD, McNamara JO. GluR3 autoantibodies destroy neural cells in a complement-dependent manner modulated by complement regulatory proteins. J Neurosci. 2000;20:7307–16.

22. Park CC, Shin ML, Simard JM. The complement membrane attack complex and the bystander effect in cerebral vasospasm. J Neurosurg. 1997;87:294–300.

23. Lee M, Guo JP, Schwab C, McGeer EG, McGeer PL. Selective inhibition of the membrane attack complex of complement by low molecular weight components of the aurin tricarboxylic acid synthetic complex. Neurobiol Aging. 2012;33:2237–46.

24. Zipfel PF, Skerka C. Complement regulators and inhibitory proteins. Nat Rev Immunol. 2009;9:729–40.

25. Piddlesden SJ, Morgan BP. Killing of rat glial cells by complement: deficiency of the rat analogue of CD59 is the cause of oligodendrocyte susceptibility to lysis. J Neuroimmunol. 1993;48:169–75.

26. Singhrao SK, Neal JW, Rushmere NK, Morgan BP, Gasque P. Differential expression of individual complement regulators in the brain and choroid plexus. Lab Investig. 1999;79:1247–59.

27. Singhrao SK, Neal JW, Rushmere NK, Morgan BP, Gasque P. Spontaneous classical pathway activation and deficiency of membrane regulators render human neurons susceptible to complement lysis. Am J Pathol. 2000;157:905–18.

28. Kolev MV, Tediose T, Sivasankar B, Harris CL, Thome J, Morgan BP, Donev RM. Upregulating CD59: a new strategy for protection of neurons from complement-mediated degeneration. Pharmacogenomics J. 2010;10:12–9.

29. Bennett JL, Lam C, Kalluri SR, Saikali P, Bautista K, Dupree C, Glogowska M, Case D, Antel JP, Owens GP, et al. Intrathecal pathogenic anti-aquaporin-4 antibodies in early neuromyelitis optica. Ann Neurol. 2009;66:617–29.

30. Crane JM, Lam C, Rossi A, Gupta T, Bennett JL, Verkman AS. Binding affinity and specificity of neuromyelitis optica autoantibodies to aquaporin-4 M1/M23 isoforms and orthogonal arrays. J Biol Chem. 2011;286:16516–24.

31. Tradtrantip L, Felix CM, Spirig R, Morelli AB, Verkman AS. Recombinant IgG1 Fc hexamers block cytotoxicity and pathological changes in experimental in vitro and rat models of neuromyelitis optica. Neuropharmacology. 2018;133: 345–53.

32. Smith AJ, Yao X, Dix JA, Jin BJ, Verkman AS. Test of the 'glymphatic' hypothesis demonstrates diffusive and aquaporin-4-independent solute transport in rodent brain parenchyma. elife. 2017;6:e27679.

33. Pacifici M, Peruzzi F. Isolation and culture of rat embryonic neural cells: a quick protocol. J Vis Exp. 2012;63:e3965.

34. Brewer GJ. Serum-free B27/neurobasal medium supports differentiated growth of neurons from the striatum, substantia nigra, septum, cerebral cortex, cerebellum, and dentate gyrus. J Neurosci Res. 1995;42:674–83.

35. Yao X, Verkman AS. Marked central nervous system pathology in CD59 knockout rats following passive transfer of Neuromyelitis optica immunoglobulin G. Acta Neuropathol Commun. 2017;5:15.

36. Zhang H, Verkman AS. Aquaporin-4 independent Kir4.1 K$^+$ channel function in brain glial cells. Mol Cell Neurosci. 2008;37:1–10.

37. Brown DR, Kretzschmar HA. The glio-toxic mechanism of alpha-aminoadipic acid on cultured astrocytes. J Neurocytol. 1998;27:109–18.

38. Huck S, Grass F, Hortnagl H. The glutamate analogue alpha-aminoadipic acid is taken up by astrocytes before exerting its gliotoxic effect in vitro. J Neurosci. 1984;4:2650–7.

39. Foster AC, Gill R, Kemp JA, Woodruff GN. Systemic administration of MK-801 prevents N-methyl-D-aspartate-induced neuronal degeneration in rat brain. Neurosci Lett. 1987;76:307–11.

40. McDonald JW, Silverstein FS, Cardona D, Hudson C, Chen R, Johnston MV. Systemic administration of MK-801 protects against N-methyl-D-aspartate- and quisqualate-mediated neurotoxicity in perinatal rats. Neuroscience. 1990;36:589–99.

41. Yao X, Su T, Verkman AS. Clobetasol promotes remyelination in a mouse model of neuromyelitis optica. Acta Neuropathol Commun. 2016;4:42.

42. Dubois-Dalcq M, Ffrench-Constant C, Franklin RJ. Enhancing central nervous system remyelination in multiple sclerosis. Neuron. 2005;48:9–12.

3

Circulating EZH2-positive T cells are decreased in multiple sclerosis patients

Sunny Malhotra[1*], Luisa M. Villar[2], Carme Costa[1], Luciana Midaglia[1], Marta Cubedo[3], Silvia Medina[2], Nicolás Fissolo[1], Jordi Río[1], Joaquín Castilló[1], José C. Álvarez-Cermeño[2], Alex Sánchez[4,5], Xavier Montalban[1] and Manuel Comabella[1*]

Abstract

Background: Recent studies in experimental autoimmune encephalomyelitis, an animal model of multiple sclerosis (MS), suggest an involvement of the histone methyltransferase enhancer of zeste 2 polycomb repressive complex 2 subunit (EZH2) in important processes such as cell adhesion and migration.

Methods: Here, we aimed to expand these initial observations by investigating the role of EZH2 in MS. mRNA expression levels for EZH2 were measured by real-time PCR in peripheral blood mononuclear cells (PBMC) from 121 MS patients (62 untreated and 59 receiving treatment) and 24 healthy controls.

Results: EZH2 expression levels were decreased in PBMC from untreated patients compared to that from controls, and treatment significantly upregulated EZH2 expression. Expression of miR-124 was increased in MS patients compared to controls. Blood immunophenotyping revealed EZH2 expression mostly restricted to CD4+ and CD8+ T cells, and circulating EZH2+ CD4+ and CD8+ T cells were decreased in untreated MS patients compared to controls. CD8+ T cells expressing EZH2 exhibited a predominant central memory phenotype, whereas EZH2+ CD4+ T cells were of effector memory nature, and both T cell subsets produced TNF-α. EZH2+ T cells were enriched in the cerebrospinal fluid compartment compared to blood and were found in chronic active lesions from MS patients. EZH2 inhibition and microarray analysis in PBMC was associated with significant downregulation of key T cell adhesion molecules.

Conclusion: These findings suggest a role of EZH2 in the migration of T cells in MS patients. The observation of TNF-α expression by CD4+ and CD8+ T cells expressing EZH2 warrants additional studies to explore more in depth the pathogenic potential of EZH2+-positive cells in MS.

Keywords: Multiple sclerosis, EZH2, Treatment, Migration, Adhesion molecules

Background

Enhancer of zeste 2 polycomb repressive complex 2 subunit (EZH2) is a histone methyltransferase that serves as the catalytic subunit of the polycomb repressive complex 2, a protein complex that regulates gene expression by methylating nucleosomal histone H3 at lysine 27 (H3K27) on the promoter of its target genes [1]. The identification of a cytosolic methyltransferase EZH2-containing complex suggested that, in addition to its role methylating histones, EZH2 could also be involved in the regulation of extra-nuclear signaling pathways, in particular actin polymerization-dependent processes [2]. Recent investigation on its cytoplasmic role has revealed that EZH2 interacts with cytosolic proteins such as talin and the guanine nucleotide–exchange factor vav1 that link integrin molecules to the actin cytoskeleton, suggesting the potential implication of EZH2 in cell adhesion and migration processes [3]. Interestingly, mice lacking the EZH2 gene exhibited attenuated experimental autoimmune encephalomyelitis (EAE) disease progression due to the inability of EZH2-deficient cells, particularly neutrophils and dendritic cells, to reach the site of inflammation [3]. Taking into consideration the findings of EZH2 in EAE mice and its implication in important processes for the pathogenesis of multiple sclerosis

* Correspondence: sunnymalhotra4u24@gmail.com; manuel.comabella@vhir.org
[1]Servei de Neurologia-Neuroimmunologia, Centre d'Esclerosi Múltiple de Catalunya (Cemcat), Institut de Recerca Vall d'Hebron (VHIR), Hospital Universitari Vall d'Hebron, Universitat Autònoma de Barcelona, Barcelona, Spain
Full list of author information is available at the end of the article

such as cell adhesion and migration, we believe that EZH2 may also be playing a role in multiple sclerosis and contribute to the inflammatory component observed in the central nervous system (CNS) of patients. Hence, the purpose of the present study was to explore the role of EZH2 in the disease by measuring the gene expression levels of EZH2 and associated molecules in peripheral blood cells from untreated and treated multiple sclerosis patients and by characterizing the immune cell populations responsible for EZH2 expression.

Methods

Patients

Initial cohort

Messenger RNA (mRNA) expression levels of EZH2, talin 1 (TLN1), and VAV1 were determined in peripheral blood mononuclear cells (PBMC) from a first cohort of 24 healthy controls (HC) and 62 treatment-naïve multiple sclerosis patients. The case group included 25 patients with relapsing-remitting multiple sclerosis (RRMS), 20 patients with secondary progressive multiple sclerosis (SPMS), and 17 patients with primary progressive multiple sclerosis (PPMS). The RRMS group included 20 patients in clinical remission and 5 patients whose blood was drawn at the time of an acute relapse.

Validation cohort

In order to replicate EZH2 findings, mRNA expression levels for EZH2 were also measured in PBMC from an independent validation cohort comprised of 12 HC and 13 treatment-naïve multiple sclerosis patients. Considering that EZH2 expression levels in the initial cohort were similar between different clinical forms of the disease, for the validation cohort, only patients with RRMS were included.

Treated cohort

EZH2 and TLN1 mRNA expression levels were determined in an additional cohort of 59 RRMS patients treated for at least 1 year with interferon-beta (n = 17), glatiramer acetate (n = 15), fingolimod (n = 16), or natalizumab (n = 11). Expression levels for these genes were compared with those observed in a subgroup of 14 untreated RRMS patients included in the initial cohort.

The study was approved by the local Ethics Committee [EPA(AG)57/2013(3834)], and participants gave written informed consent. Tables 1 and 2 summarize demographic and baseline clinical characteristics of multiple sclerosis patients from the initial, validation, and treated cohorts and the HC included in the study.

Sample collection and determination of mRNA expression levels of EZH2, TLN1, and VAV1 by real-time PCR

PBMC from multiple sclerosis patients and HC were isolated by Ficoll-Isopaque density gradient centrifugation (Gibco BRL, Life Technologies LTD, UK) and stored in liquid nitrogen until used. Total RNA was extracted from PBMC using an RNeasy kit (Quiagen, Santa Clarita, USA) and cDNA synthesized using the High-Capacity cDNA Archive kit (Applied Biosystems, Foster City, CA, USA). mRNA expression levels for EZH2, TLN1, and VAV1 were determined with TaqMan® probes specific for the gene (Applied Biosystems). The housekeeping gene glyceraldehyde-3-phosphate dehydrogenase (GAPDH) was used as an endogenous control (Applied Biosystems). Assays were run on the ABI PRISM® 7900HT system (Applied Biosystems), and data were analyzed with the $2^{-\Delta\Delta CT}$ method [4].

Determination of microRNA expression levels by real-time PCR

Expression levels for miR-124 and miR-155 were determined according to sample availability in PBMC from a subgroup of 18 HC and 21 untreated multiple sclerosis patients (15 RRMS and 6 SPMS patients) who were also included in the initial cohort. Additional file 1: Table S1 summarizes demographic and main clinical characteristics of individuals included for this part of the study. PBMC were collected and processed in the same conditions as described in the previous section. Expression levels for miR-124 and miR-155 were measured with Taq Man® probes specific for the microRNAs (Applied Biosystems) using RNU 6b as endogenous control. Analysis was performed as described above with the $2^{-\Delta\Delta CT}$ method [4].

EZH2 immunophenotyping

EZH2 protein expression was determined by flow cytometry according to sample availability in PBMC from 13 HC [9 females (69.2%); mean age (standard deviation), 35.8 years (10.9)] and 10 RRMS patients [5 females (50%); mean age, 32.1 years (13.5); mean disease duration, 4.5 (3.5)] at baseline and after 1 year of natalizumab treatment. Only one MS patient and one HC were also included in the initial cohort whereas the remaining individuals corresponded to new multiple sclerosis patients and HC. EZH2 expression was also determined in cerebrospinal fluid (CSF) cells from 3 untreated RRMS patients [2 females (66.7%); mean age, 34.3 years (11.9); mean disease duration, 0.4 (0.5)]. CSF samples were collected by lumbar puncture for clinical purposes and centrifuged at 1200g for 15 min. Supernatants were stored at − 80 °C until processed for clinical tests and CSF cells resuspended in PBS and labeled as described below.

Table 1 Demographic and baseline clinical characteristics of the MS patients and healthy controls

Baseline characteristics	HC	RRMS	SPMS	PPMS	Relapse
Initial cohort					
N	24	20	20	17	5
Age (years)	30.2 (7.2)	30.0 (7.8)	45.7 (8.7)	50.2 (7.3)	30.8 (8.7)
Female/male (% women)	18/6 (75.0)	10/10 (50.0)	11/9 (55.0)	11/6 (64.7)	2/3 (40.0)
Duration of disease (years)	–	4.8 (4.6)	11.5 (7.6)	12.2 (7.9)	2.2 (2.7)
EDSS[a]	–	1.7 (1.0–4.2)	4.0 (3.5–5.1)	6.0 (4.0–6.0)	3.0 (2.5–5.3)
Numbers of relapses[b]	–	2.2 (0.7)	0.8 (0.8)	–	2.6 (1.3)
Validation cohort					
N	12	13			
Age (years)	28.2 (6.0)	37.6 (9.3)			
Female/male (% women)	8/3 (72.7)	12/2 (85.7)			
Duration of disease (years)	–	3.8 (3.2)			
EDSS[a]	–	2.5 (1.0–3.5)			
Numbers of relapses[b]	–	2.5 (0.8)			

Data are expressed as mean (standard deviation) unless otherwise stated

RRMS relapsing-remitting multiple sclerosis, *SPMS* secondary progressive multiple sclerosis, *PPMS* primary progressive multiple sclerosis, *Relapse* RRMS patients whose blood was collected at the time of an acute exacerbation

[a]Data are expressed as mean (interquartile range)

[b]The number of relapses in the 2 years before blood collection

Monoclonal antibodies

The following monoclonal antibodies were used in the study: EZH2-Alexa Fluor 488, CD197-PE (CCR7-PE), CD3-PE, granulocyte/macrophage colony-stimulating factor (GM-CSF)-PE, CD16-PE-Cy5, tumor necrosis factor (TNF)-α-PercP-Cy5.5, CD19-PE-Cy7, CD45RO-APC, CD56-APC, CD8-APC-H7, CD14-APC-H7, CD3-BV421, CD45-V450, CD45-V500 (all from BD Biosciences, San Diego, CA), and IL-17-APC (R&D Systems, Minneapolis, MN).

Characterization of EZH2 expression by CSF cells

CSF cells were stained for 30 min at 4 °C in the dark with the appropriate amounts of monoclonal antibodies recognizing the surface antigens. Subsequently, cells were washed with PBS, fixed and permeabilized for 20 min at 4 °C in the dark with Cytofix/Cytoperm Kit (BD Biosciences), washed twice with Perm/Wash solution

(BD Biosciences) and stained intracellularly for 30 min at 4 °C in the dark with a monoclonal antibody recognizing EZH2, and washed and analyzed in a FACSCanto II flow cytometer (BD Biosciences).

Intracellular cytokine staining

Aliquots of 10^6 PBMC were resuspended in 1 ml of complete medium with 50 ng/ml phorbol 12-myristate 13-acetate (PMA) (Sigma-Aldrich, St. Louis, MO) and 750 ng/ml ionomycin (Sigma-Aldrich), in the presence of 2 μg/ml brefeldin A (GolgiPlug, BD Biosciences) and 2.1 μM monensin (Golgi Stop, BD Biosciences) in poly-propylene tubes, and incubated for 4 h at 37 °C in 5% CO_2. Cells were washed in PBS and surface stained as indicated above. Afterward, cells were fixed and perme-abilized for 20 min at 4 °C in the dark with Cytofix/Cytoperm Kit (BD Biosciences), washed twice with Perm/Wash solution (BD Biosciences), and stained with

Table 2 Summary of demographic and baseline clinical characteristics of the treated MS cohort

Characteristics	UNT	IFN	GA	FG	NTZ
N	14	17	15	16	11
Age (years)	28.3 (6.3)	34.8 (7.5)	32.3 (7.9)	30.3 (7.8)	27.7 (14.5)
Female/male (% women)	8/6 (57.2)	9/8 (52.9)	8/7 (53.3)	11/5 (68.7)	7/4 (63.6)
Duration of disease (years)	3.3 (2.7)	5.0 (10.7)	6.7 (5.8)	3.0 (3.8)	6.1 (7.0)
EDSS[a]	1.8 (1.4–2.5)	1.6 (1.0–2.0)	2.2 (1.5–3.0)	1.6 (1.0–2.0)	2.5 (1.6–3.5)
Numbers of relapses[b]	2.0 (0.8)	1.5 (0.8)	2.3 (1.5)	2.2 (0.7)	1.9 (0.6)

Data are expressed as mean (standard deviation) unless otherwise stated

UNT untreated relapsing-remitting MS patients, *IFN* interferon-beta, *GA* glatiramer acetate, *FG* fingolimod, *NTZ* natalizumab

[a]Data are expressed as mean (interquartile range) and refers to EDSS at the time of treatment onset

[b]The number of relapses in the 2 years before treatment onset

monoclonal antibodies recognizing GM-CSF, TNF-α, and IL-17.

Flow cytometry analysis

Cells were always analyzed within 1 h of staining. Mean autofluorescence values were set using appropriate negative isotype controls. Data analysis was performed using FACSDiva Software V.8.0 (BD Biosciences). A gate including lymphocytes and monocytes and excluding debris and apoptotic cells was established; a minimum amount of 30,000 events for PBMC samples and 500 events for CSF cells were analyzed.

EZH2 expression in EAE mice

Anesthetized C57BL/6 mice were immunized by subcutaneous injections of PBS containing 50 μg of MOG$_{35-55}$ (Proteomics Section, Universitat Pompeu Fabra, Barcelona, Spain) or PBS, emulsified in complete Freund's adjuvant (Sigma Chemical, St. Louis, MO, USA), and supplemented with 2 mg/ml *Mycobacterium tuberculosis* H37RA (Difco Laboratories, Detroit, MI, USA). The animals received an additional intravenous injection of 150 ng pertussis toxin in 100 μl PBS on the day of immunization and again 48 h later. Four animals per group (EAE or controls—PBS) were sacrificed at 8, 16, 22, 29, 36, and 50 days post-immunization, and spinal cord tissue was subsequently obtained. mRNA expression levels of EZH2 and CD3e were determined by real-time PCR as previously described. Changes in gene expression were always compared with animals treated with PBS at the respective days.

EZH2 expression in human brain tissue
Samples

Paraffin-embedded brain samples from RRMS patients and non-neurological controls were provided by the UK Multiple Sclerosis Tissue Bank. Tissue sections were stained with hematoxylin and eosin (HE) and Klüver-Barrera (KB) for inflammation and demyelination assessment. Ten samples from multiple sclerosis patients with chronic active lesions and four control samples were selected for the study (demographic and clinical information was not available for these patients).

Immunohistochemistries

Immunostainings were developed with the automated Benchmark XT platform from Ventana Medical System. Briefly, 4-μm-thick, paraffin-embedded serial sections were deparaffinized with EZ prepTM (Ventana Medical System). Antigen retrieval was performed with Cell Conditioning 1 pH = 8 (Ventana Medical System) for 30 min. Endogenous peroxidase activity was blocked with hydrogen peroxide 3%. Samples were incubated with rabbit anti-EZH2 (clone EPR9307(2), Abcam) for 36 min and visualized with ultraView Universal DAB (Ventana Medical

Systems). Subsequently, samples were kept at 95 °C for 8 min and incubated with rabbit anti-CD4 (clone SP35, Ventana Medical System) or rabbit anti-CD8 (clone SP57, Ventana Medical System) for 40 min and visualized with ultraView Universal Alkaline Phosphatase Red Detection (Ventana Medical Systems). All samples were counterstained with hematoxylin.

Immunostaining assessment

A range between 5 and 20 pictures were taken for each multiple sclerosis sample. Total CD4+ and CD8+ T cells and double-positive EZH2 and CD4 or CD8 cells were counted. The percentages of double-positive cells were calculated with respect to the total of CD4+ or CD8+ T cells.

EZH2 blocking and gene expression microarrays

PBMC from 7 untreated RRMS patients [5 females (71.4%); mean age, 39.0 years (8.0); mean disease duration, 7.0 years (5.1)] were plated into 24-well plates for 24 h in the presence or absence of an EZH2 inhibitor (histone deacetylase inhibitor suberoylanilide hydroxamic acid—SAHA) at 1 μg/μl concentration. After 24 h, cells were harvested and total RNA isolated using the RNeasy kit (Quiagen) and hybridized to Affymetrix Human Transcriptome Arrays (HTA 2.0) (Affymetrix, Santa Clara, CA, USA) according to the manufacturer's protocol (GeneChip WT Pico Reagent Kit (Affymetrix)).

Statistical analysis

Statistical analysis was performed by using the SPSS 17.0 package (SPSS Inc., Chicago, IL) for MS Windows. Comparisons of mRNA expression levels for EZH2, TLN1, and VAV1; expression levels for miR-124 and miR-155; and the percentage of EZH2-positive cells between the different study groups were performed by parametric and non-parametric tests depending on the applicability conditions. Real-time PCR data were expressed as fold change in gene expression in controls relative to the whole group of multiple sclerosis patients and patients stratified according to the different clinical forms, in RRMS patients in clinical remission relative to patients in relapse, and in treated RRMS relative to untreated patients. For microarray analysis, images were processed with AGCC, Affymetrix GeneChip Command Console, to generate .CEL files. Raw expression values obtained directly from .CEL files were pre-processed using the RMA method [5]. These normalized values were the basis for all the subsequent analyses. Previous to any analysis data were submitted to non-specific filtering to remove low-signal genes (those genes whose mean signal in each group did not exceed a minimum threshold) and low-variability genes (those genes whose standard deviation between all samples did not exceed a minimum threshold). The selection of differentially expressed genes between the untreated and the EZH2 blocking conditions was based on a linear model analysis with empirical Bayes moderation of the variance estimates following the methodology developed by Smyth [6]. In order to deal with the multiple testing issues derived from the fact that many tests (one per gene) were performed simultaneously, p values were adjusted to obtain strong control over the false discovery rate using the Benjamini and Hochberg method [7].

Results

EZH2 expression is decreased in multiple sclerosis patients

In order to investigate the role of EZH2 in multiple sclerosis, we first measured the mRNA expression levels of EZH2 and EZH2-associated genes in PBMC from an initial cohort of 62 untreated multiple sclerosis patients and 24 HC. As shown in Fig. 1a, expression levels for EZH2, TLN1, and VAV1 were significantly decreased in PBMC from the whole multiple sclerosis group compared to controls. Further stratification of the multiple sclerosis group into the different clinical forms revealed significantly decreased gene expression levels of EZH2, TLN1, and VAV1 in PBMC from RRMS, SPMS, and PPMS patients compared to HC (Fig. 1b). As depicted in Fig. 1c, mRNA expression levels for EZH2, TLN1, and VAV1 were not changed in RRMS patients at the time of acute exacerbations, and expression levels for these genes were similar between RRMS patients in clinical remission and RRMS patients during relapse.

EZH2 findings were validated in an independent cohort of 13 untreated multiple sclerosis patients and 12 HC, and mRNA expression levels for EZH2 were again found to be significantly decreased in PBMC from the multiple sclerosis group compared to the HC group ($p = 0.01$; Fig. 1d).

Expression levels of miR-124 are increased in multiple sclerosis patients

We next investigated the expression levels of miR-124 and miR-155, two microRNAs that are known on the one hand to target EZH2 [8, 9] and on the other hand to be involved in multiple sclerosis [10, 11]. Following the determination of microRNA expression levels in 21 untreated multiple sclerosis patients and 18 HC, miR-124 expression was found to be significantly upregulated in PBMC from multiple sclerosis patients compared to controls ($p = 0.03$), whereas miR-155 expression levels were similar between patients and HC (Fig. 2). These results may suggest a potential and inverse relationship between EZH2 and miR-124 expression levels in multiple sclerosis patients.

EZH2 expression is increased in treated multiple sclerosis patients

As a next step, we investigated whether EZH2 and TLN1 expression was modulated by commonly used multiple sclerosis therapies. For this, mRNA expression levels for EZH2 and TLN1 were determined in PBMC from 59 treated patients. Compared to untreated patients, EZH2 and TLN1 expression was significantly upregulated in PBMC by the effect of interferon-beta, Copaxone, and natalizumab treatments (Fig. 3). In contrast, whereas fingolimod significantly increased TLN1 expression, this treatment had no effect on EZH2 expression (Fig. 3). Overall, the increased EZH2 and TLN1 expression in PBMC from treated MS patients may indicate a reduced leukocyte trafficking into the CNS by the effect of treatment.

EZH2 is expressed by circulating CD4+ and CD8+ T cells with effector memory and central memory phenotypes respectively

In order to characterize the PBMC populations that express EZH2, immunophenotyping for EZH2 and flow cytometry analysis was performed in T cells (CD3+, CD4+, and CD8+), B cells, monocytes, and NK cells from 10 multiple sclerosis patients and 13 HC. EZH2 expression was restricted to CD3+ (both CD4+ and CD8+) T cells and CD56dim NK cells (Fig. 4a), whereas it was absent in B cells and monocytes. Similar to the mRNA expression findings observed in the whole PBMC population, the percentage of EZH2-positive cells in CD4+ and CD8+ T cells was significantly reduced in untreated multiple sclerosis patients compared to controls (Fig. 4a). Although treatment with natalizumab, which was selected as control therapy, increased EZH2 expression by T cells, differences did not reach statistical significance (Fig. 4a). In contrast, EZH2 expression by CD56dim NK cells was similar across the different groups (Fig. 4a).

Further, EZH2 immunophenotyping in naïve and different memory T cell populations revealed that CD4+ T cells expressing EZH2 had a clear effector memory phenotype with low contribution of naïve T cells compared to CD4+ T cells negative for EZH2 expression (Fig. 4b). In contrast, CD8+ T cells expressing EZH2 exhibited a predominant central memory phenotype compared to EZH2-negative CD8+ T cells (Fig. 4c). A trend towards decreased expression of EZH2 ($p = 0.07$) was observed in terminally differentiated effector CD4+ T cells from untreated multiple sclerosis patients compared to HC, and EZH2 expression was significantly upregulated in patients by the effect of natalizumab treatment ($p = 0.03$) (Fig. 4b). However, a similar pattern was also observed in terminally differentiated effector CD4+ T cells negative for EZH2 ($p = 0.05$ and $p = 0.003$ in untreated patients versus controls and patients receiving treatment respectively) (Fig. 4b).

Finally, in order to evaluate the pathogenic potential of EZH2-positive cells, staining for proinflammatory cytokines such as TNF-α, GM-CSF, and IL-17 was also included in CD4+ and CD8+ T cells from a subgroup of untreated ($N = 4$) and treated ($N = 4$) patients and HC

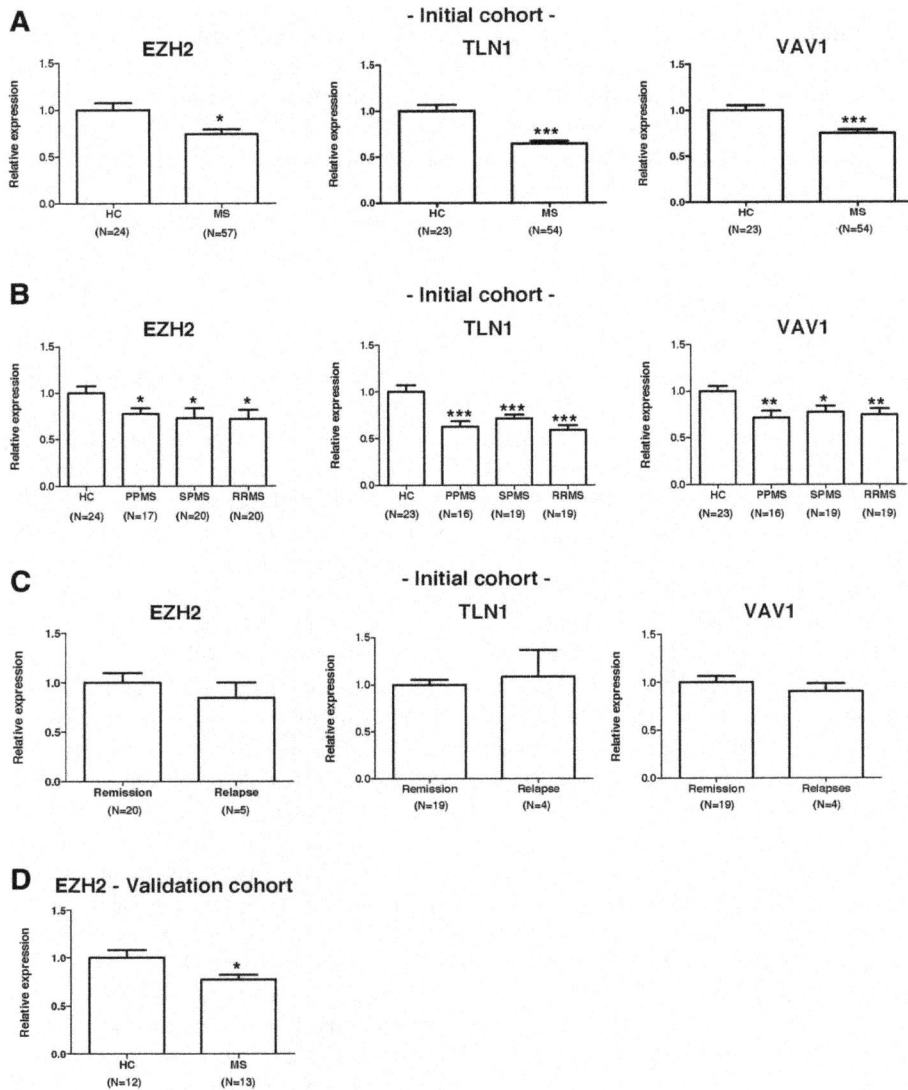

Fig. 1 Expression levels of EZH2 and EZH2-associated molecules in multiple sclerosis patients and controls. mRNA expression levels for EZH2, TLN1, and VAV1 were determined in PBMC from untreated multiple sclerosis patients and healthy controls by real-time PCR relative quantification, as described in the "Methods" section. Graphs showing expression levels for EZH2, TLN1, and VAV1 **a–c** in the initial discovery cohort and **d** in an independent cohort of patients and controls. Results are expressed as fold change (standard error of the mean) in gene expression in multiple sclerosis patients relative to controls and in patients in relapse relative to patients in remission. Statistics: unpaired Student's *t* test. *p values < 0.05; **p values < 0.01; ***p values < 0.001. HC healthy controls, MS whole group of multiple sclerosis patients, RRMS relapsing-remitting multiple sclerosis, SPMS secondary progressive multiple sclerosis, PPMS primary progressive multiple sclerosis, Remission RRMS patients in clinical remission, Relapse RRMS patients whose blood was collected at the time of an acute exacerbation, EZH2 enhancer of zeste 2 polycomb repressive complex 2 subunit, TLN1 talin 1, VAV1 vav guanine nucleotide exchange factor 1

($N = 7$). EZH2-positive cells expressed TNF-α though were negative for GM-CSF and IL-17 expression. Interestingly, trends towards decreased percentage of TNF-α-positive cells were observed in CD4+ and CD8+ T cells expressing EZH2 from untreated patients compared to HC ($p = 0.08$ and $p = 0.07$ respectively), whereas no similar findings were seen in their EZH2-negative counterparts (Fig. 4d). Furthermore, natalizumab treatment was associated with significant increases in the percentage of TNF-α-positive cells in CD4+ and CD8+ T cells expressing EZH2 ($p = 0.02$ and $p = 0.04$ respectively), while treatment had no effect in the percentage of TNF-α-positive cells by EZH2-negative CD4+ and CD8+ T cells (Fig. 4d).

Altogether, these data point to a different expression of EZH2 depending on the differentiation stages of the CD4+ and CD8+ T cells and suggest a common pathogenic potential of EZH2-positive cells in MS via TNF-α production.

Expression levels of microRNAs

miR-124

miR-155

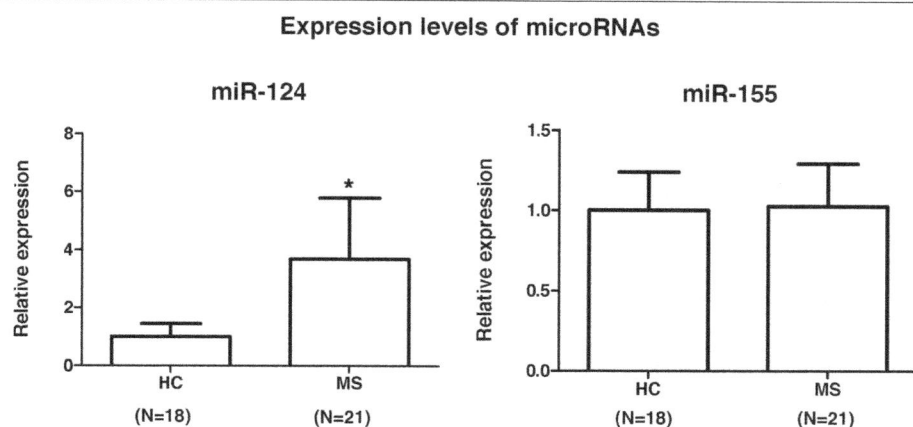

Fig. 2 Expression levels of miR-124 and miR-155 in multiple sclerosis patients and controls. Expression levels for miR-124 and miR-155 were determined in PBMC from untreated multiple sclerosis patients and controls by real-time PCR relative quantification. Results are expressed as fold change (standard error of the mean) in gene expression in patients relative to controls. Statistics: unpaired Student's t test. *p value = 0.03. HC healthy controls, MS whole group of untreated multiple sclerosis patients, which included 15 RRMS and 6 SPMS patients

EZH2-positive T cells migrate to the CNS during EAE and multiple sclerosis

Based on the gene and protein expression findings, we hypothesized that the decrease of circulating EZH2-positive T cells in untreated multiple patients compared to controls was secondary to the migration of EZH2-positive T cells into the CNS. To evaluate this hypothesis, we first investigated EZH2 expression in the CNS of EAE mice and observed that EZH2 was expressed in spinal cord tissue during EAE, and EZH2 expression levels peaked at the inflammatory phase of the disease (day 16 post-immunization) (Fig. 5a). Interestingly, EZH2 followed a similar temporal pattern of CNS expression to Cd3 in EAE mice, and expression levels for these two genes correlated with each other (Spearman correlation coefficient =

0.63, $p = 0.002$), suggesting a relationship between EZH2 expression and the inflammatory cell infiltrate during EAE (Fig. 5a). We next aimed to extrapolate these findings to patients with multiple sclerosis by determining EZH2 expression in CSF cells from three untreated patients. As shown in Fig. 5b, EZH2-positive T cells were enriched in the CSF compartment, and the percentage of CD3+ T cells expressing EZH2 was significantly increased in the CSF compared to peripheral blood ($p = 0.007$). In contrast, in CD56dim NK cells, a cell subset that also expressed EZH2 (Fig. 4a), the percentage of EZH2-positive cells did not differ between the CSF and blood compartments, indicating a preferential capacity for EZH2-positive T cells to migrate into the CNS. In this line, we finally investigated EZH2 expression in chronic active lesions from 10 multiple sclerosis

Effect of treatment in EZH2 and TLN1 expression

EZH2

TLN1

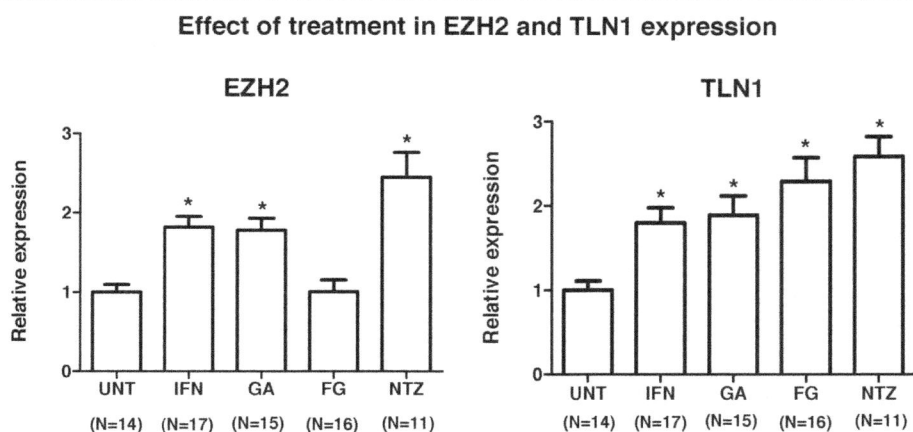

Fig. 3 Expression levels of EZH2 and TLN1 in treated multiple sclerosis patients. mRNA expression levels for EZH2 and TLN1 were determined by real-time PCR relative quantification in PBMC from untreated multiple sclerosis patients and patients receiving disease-modifying therapies for at least 1 year. Results are expressed as fold change (standard error of the mean) in gene expression in patients relative to controls. Statistics: Mann-Whitney U test. *p values < 0.001. UNT untreated patients, IFN interferon-beta, GA glatiramer acetate, FG fingolimod, NTZ natalizumab, EZH2 enhancer of zeste 2 polycomb repressive complex 2 subunit, TLN1 talin 1

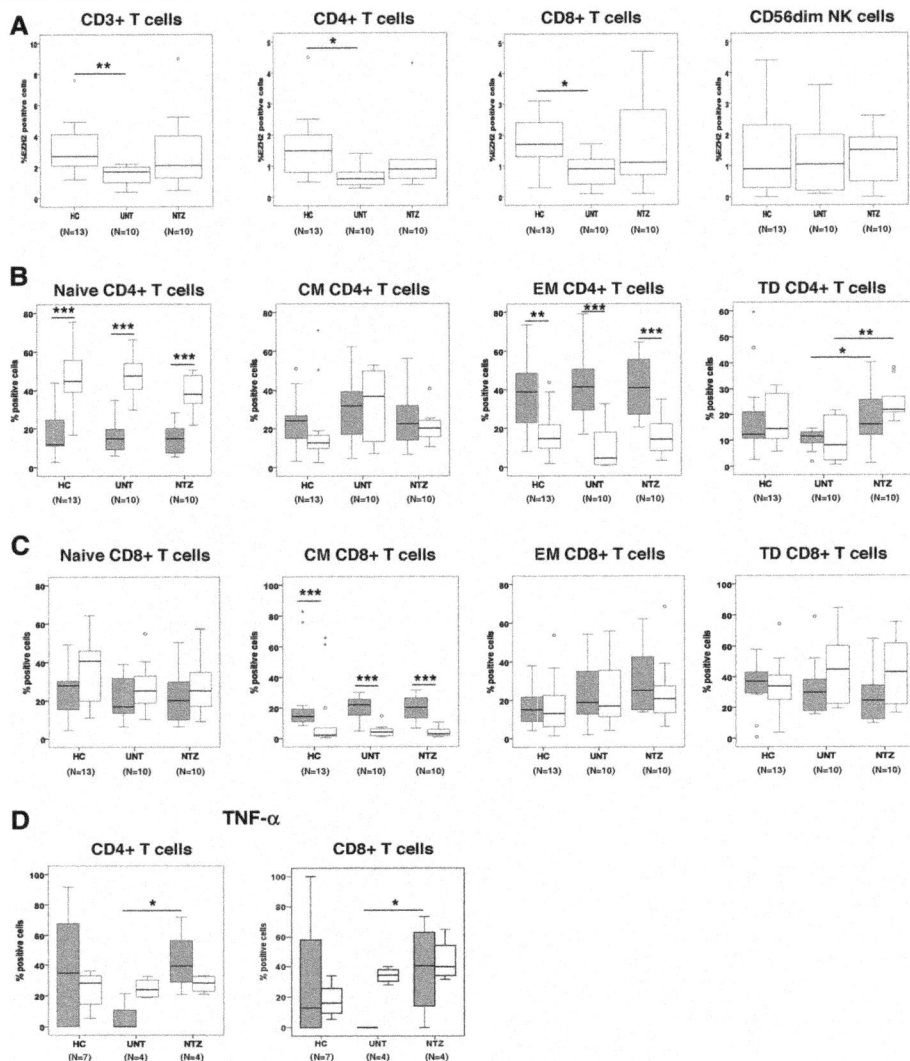

Fig. 4 EZH2 immunophenotyping in PBMC from multiple sclerosis patients and controls. **a** Graphs showing the percentage of EZH2-positive cells in T cells and CD56dim NK cells from healthy controls (HC; $n = 13$), untreated multiple sclerosis patients (UNT; $n = 10$), and the same cohort of patients after 1 year of natalizumab treatment (NTZ; $n = 10$). **b, c** Graphs showing EZH2 expression in different CD4+ and CD8+ T cell subsets (HC, $n = 13$; UNT, $n = 10$; NTZ, $n = 10$). Naïve T cells were defined as CD45RO−/CCR7+. Central memory (CM) T cells were defined as CD45RO+/CCR7+. Effector memory (EM) T cells were defined as CD45RO+/CCR7−. Terminally differentiated (TD) effector T cells were defined as CD45RO−/CCR7+. Gray boxes, EZH2-positive cells; open boxes, EZH2-negative cells. **d** Graphs showing the percentage of tumor necrosis factor (TNF)-α-positive cells in CD4+ and CD8+ T cells expressing EZH2 (HC, $n = 7$; UNT, $n = 4$; NTZ, $n = 4$). Gray boxes, EZH2-positive cells; open boxes, EZH2-negative cells. Statistics: **a, b** unpaired Student's t test; **c, d** Mann-Whitney U test. *p values < 0.05; **p values < 0.01; ***p values < 0.001. EZH2 enhancer of zeste 2 polycomb repressive complex 2 subunit

patients and observed that 8.5% (mean percentage) and 10.9% of the total CD4+ and CD8+ T cells were expressing EZH2 respectively (Fig. 5c). Occasionally, EZH2 expression was also observed in the nuclei of few glial cells, and brain tissues from non-neurological controls were negative for EZH2 expression (data not shown).

EZH2 blocking downregulates T cell adhesion molecules
As a last step, we incubated in vitro PBMC from seven untreated multiple sclerosis patients with an EZH2

inhibitor in order to investigate the genes modulated by EZH2 and aiming to better understand the role of EZH2 in disease pathophysiology. A total of 6763 genes were significantly up- or downregulated by the effect of the EZH2 inhibitor (with p values < 0.05; data not shown). Interestingly, among the top 1% of differentially expressed genes between the untreated and treated conditions, we identified key T cell adhesion molecules that were strikingly downregulated by the EZH2 inhibitor such as selectin L (SELL, also known as CD62L; adjusted p value versus the

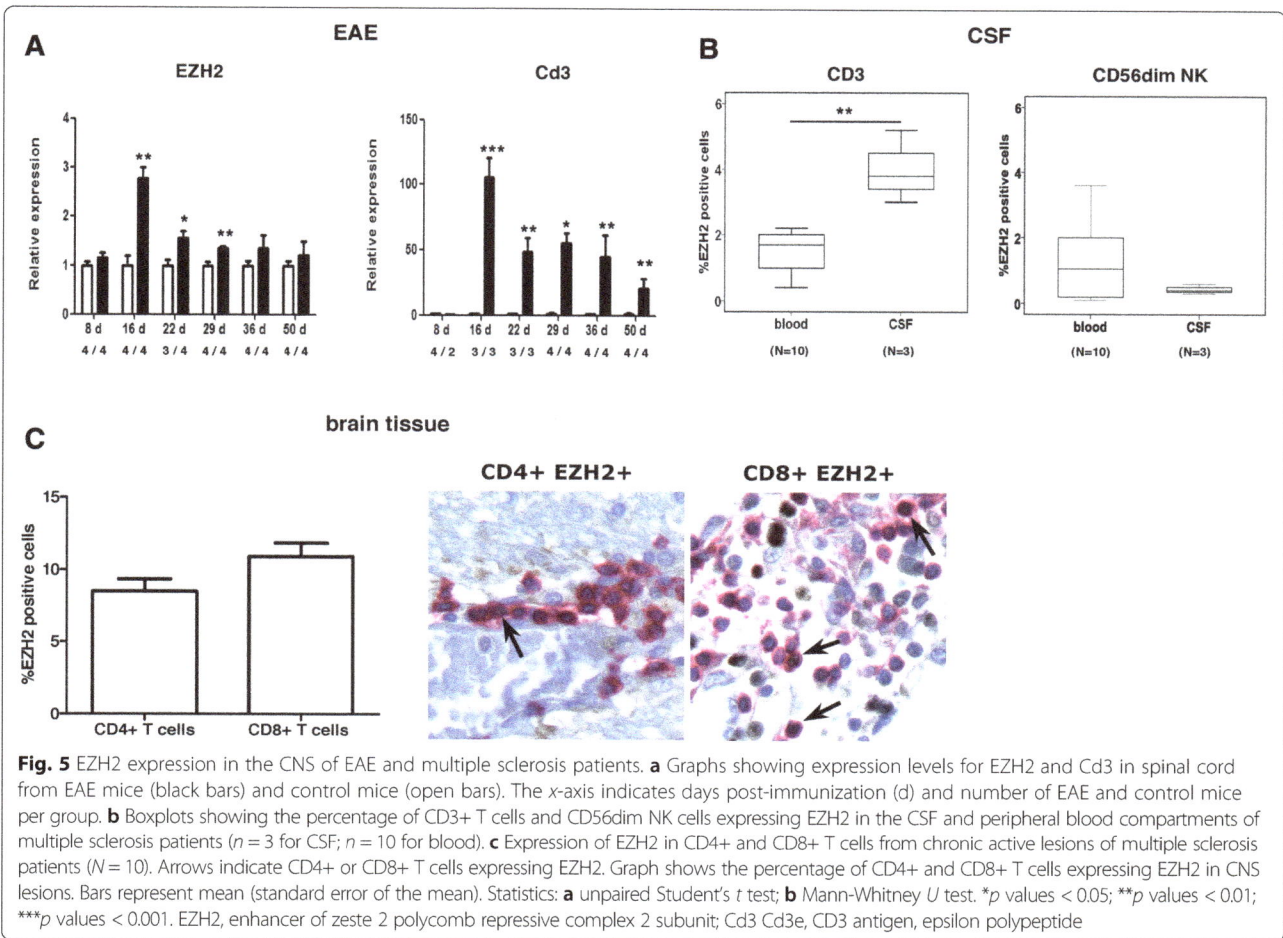

Fig. 5 EZH2 expression in the CNS of EAE and multiple sclerosis patients. **a** Graphs showing expression levels for EZH2 and Cd3 in spinal cord from EAE mice (black bars) and control mice (open bars). The x-axis indicates days post-immunization (d) and number of EAE and control mice per group. **b** Boxplots showing the percentage of CD3+ T cells and CD56dim NK cells expressing EZH2 in the CSF and peripheral blood compartments of multiple sclerosis patients (n = 3 for CSF; n = 10 for blood). **c** Expression of EZH2 in CD4+ and CD8+ T cells from chronic active lesions of multiple sclerosis patients (N = 10). Arrows indicate CD4+ or CD8+ T cells expressing EZH2. Graph shows the percentage of CD4+ and CD8+ T cells expressing EZH2 in CNS lesions. Bars represent mean (standard error of the mean). Statistics: **a** unpaired Student's t test; **b** Mann-Whitney U test. *p values < 0.05; **p values < 0.01; ***p values < 0.001. EZH2, enhancer of zeste 2 polycomb repressive complex 2 subunit; Cd3 Cd3e, CD3 antigen, epsilon polypeptide

untreated condition = 6.4×10^{-20}), integrin subunit alpha 4 (ITGA4, also known as CD49D; $p = 3.6 \times 10^{-16}$), integrin subunit alpha L (ITGAL, also known as CD11A; $p = 1.1 \times 10^{-13}$), and platelet and endothelial cell adhesion molecule 1 (PECAM1; $p = 5.2 \times 10^{-14}$) (Fig. 6). These data support a role of EZH2 in the adhesion of circulating T cells.

Discussion

Extensive literature exists about the role of EZH2 as histone methyltransferase and, particularly, about EZH2 involvement in a wide range of malignant tumors [8, 12, 13] due to its function as epigenetic silencer [14]. The identification of a cytosolic methyltransferase complex containing EZH2 suggested that, in addition to its nuclear role, EZH2 could also be involved in other important cellular processes such as cell adhesion and migration [2]. In an attempt to characterize more in depth the cytosolic role of EZH2, Gunawan et al. [2] recently reported that EZH2 was critical for regulating leukocyte migration to sites of inflammation in EAE mice, findings that opened a potential and attractive link between EZH2 and auto-immune disorders such as multiple sclerosis in which

cell adhesion and migration are critical pathogenic mechanisms [15]. Despite this initial publication in the animal model of multiple sclerosis [3], to date, there are no studies of EZH2 in patients with multiple sclerosis. Aiming to explore the role of EZH2 in multiple sclerosis, we first determined mRNA expression levels in PBMC from untreated patients and healthy individuals and observed that EZH2, together with molecules reported to be associated with cytosolic EZH2 such as TLN1 and VAV1 [3], were all downregulated in multiple sclerosis patients regardless of whether they were having relapse-onset or progressive clinical forms, or whether they were in clinical remission or in acute relapse. The decreased expression of EZH2 in PBMC from patients with multiple sclerosis was replicated in an independent validation cohort of patients and controls. These initial observations at the gene expression level suggested an involvement of EZH2 in the disease, which was explored in additional experiments.

We first explored microRNAs, which are known to exert regulatory functions at the posttranscriptional level via binding to the 3′ untranslated region of target mRNAs

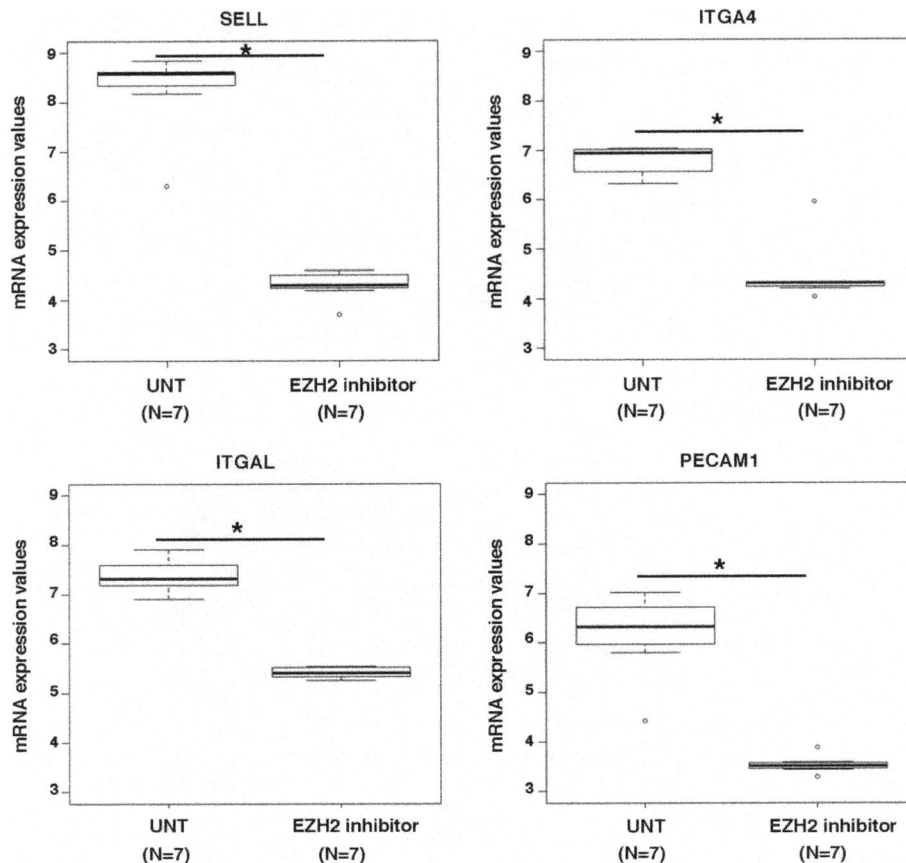

Fig. 6 Expression of cell adhesion molecules in PBMC following EZH2 blocking. Boxplots showing expression levels obtained with microarrays for adhesion molecules before and after incubation of PBMC from multiple sclerosis patients with an EZH2 inhibitor for 24 h. The asterisk symbol refers to adjusted p values < 0.001. UNT untreated condition, SELL selectin L, ITGA4 integrin subunit alpha 4, ITGAL integrin subunit alpha L, PECAM1 platelet and endothelial cell adhesion molecule 1

[16]. In the search for potential microRNAs that on the one hand regulated EZH2 expression and on the other hand were involved in multiple sclerosis, the microRNAs miR-124 and miR-155 emerged as attractive candidates [8, 9]. In this context, expression levels for miR-124 were found increased in demyelinated hippocampi from postmortem brains of multiple sclerosis patients [10]. miR-155 expression was upregulated in peripheral blood monocytes and active lesions from patients [11]. In our study, when expression levels for these two microRNAs were determined in PBMC from a subgroup of untreated multiple sclerosis patients and controls, miR-124 but not miR-155 was significantly upregulated in patients, suggesting a potential functional relationship between decreased EZH2 mRNA expression levels and miR-124 upregulation in patients with multiple sclerosis. These findings warrant future studies to investigate the cell types that contribute to miR-124 upregulation.

In order to explore whether the expression of EZH2 and associated molecules was modulated by commonly used disease-modifying therapies in patients with multiple sclerosis, a cohort of patients treated with interferon-beta, glatiramer acetate, fingolimod, and natalizumab was also included in the study. Treatment with interferon-beta, glatiramer acetate, and natalizumab was associated with increased expression levels of EZH2 and TLN1. By contrast, fingolimod treatment was only associated with upregulated expression of TLN1. Although based on a small number of samples and in spite of the descriptive nature of the experiments, it is tempting to speculate that this finding may be due to the different mechanisms by which these drugs regulate leukocyte migration to the CNS, being the mechanism of action of fingolimod not exerted in peripheral blood but in the lymph nodes where it retains naïve and central memory lymphocytes [17–20]. In view of these data, we hypothesize that the reduction in EZH2 expression observed in untreated patients with subsequent upregulation after treatment may indicate a migration capacity of PBMC expressing EZH2 to the CNS that is inhibited by the effect of treatment. These findings also open a new research avenue to investigate whether the increase in EZH2 expression observed after treatment is associated with the response to therapies and hence may differ between responders and non-responders to each particular therapeutic strategy.

Immunophenotyping of the major PBMC populations revealed restricted EZH2 expression in CD4+ and CD8+ T cells as well as CD56dim NK cells. Similar to the gene expression findings, the percentage of EZH2-positive T cells was reduced in untreated multiple sclerosis patients compared to controls, pointing to a role of EZH2 in this particular cell subset rather than in CD56dim NK cells, which showed similar percentages of EZH2-positive cells in patients and controls. It is worth highlighting that except for one patient and one control, the immunophenotyping cohort included new individuals, and hence, the decrease of EZH2-positive T cells observed in patients can also be considered as a new validation of the EZH2 expression findings at the protein level. Natalizumab, which was selected as control therapy because of its known effects reducing T cell trafficking into the CNS, increased the percentage of EZH2-positive T cells, but, contrary to gene expression results, differences did not reach statistical significance. Interestingly, further T cell immunophenotyping showed heterogeneity in the T cell subsets positive for EZH2 expression. In this context, most CD4+ T cells expressing EZH2 were effector memory T cells, a population that per se has the capacity to migrate to non-lymphoid tissues including the CNS [21]. In contrast, CD8+ T cells positive for EZH2 had a predominant central memory phenotype, suggesting that this particular subset can migrate to the CNS in MS and may later differentiate into effector memory populations in the sites of inflammation. Of note, EZH2-positive cells both in CD4+ and CD8+ T cells may have pathogenic potential through the secretion of TNF-α, a pro-inflammatory cytokine involved in the pathogenesis of multiple sclerosis [22]. Although caution should be taken when considering these data owing to the small sample size and high variability, these findings altogether warrant additional studies to deepen into the pathogenic capacity of T cells expressing EZH2 and explore whether EZH2 may become a therapeutic target in MS patients to reduce disease activity.

The potential for EZH2-positive T cells to migrate to the CNS was first suggested in the EAE study, which showed EZH2 expression in spinal cord tissue from EAE mice following a similar pattern to Cd3 expression over time. Confirmation of the migratory capacity of EZH2-positive T cells was provided by their detection in the CSF and brain lesions from multiple sclerosis patients. Noteworthy, the enrichment for CD4+ and CD8+ T cells expressing EZH2 in the CSF and chronic active lesions compared to the blood compartment suggested that the decrease of EZH2-positive T cells observed in untreated multiple sclerosis patients compared to healthy individuals was secondary to their migration into the CNS. This notion was further supported by the observation that other EZH2-expressing blood cell populations such as CD56dim NK cells, which did not depict differences between patients and controls in blood, were not enriched in the CSF. Although EZH2 expression in brain lesions from multiple sclerosis patients seemed restricted to CD4+ and CD8+ T cells, additional sources of EZH2 expression within the CNS cannot be totally ruled out, as evidenced by EZH2 immunohistochemistry. In contrast, EZH2 expression was not observed in brain tissue from non-neurological controls, a finding that confers specificity for EZH2 expression in the CNS of multiple sclerosis patients.

Conclusions

Finally, the implication of EZH2 in T cell adhesion, an important step for cell migration, was supported by the microarray findings conducted after EZH2 blocking with a histone deacetylase inhibitor that regulates EZH2 expression [23], which showed striking downregulation of cell adhesion molecules expressed in T cells such as SELL [24], ITGA4 [25], ITGAL [26], and PECAM1 [27]. The aggregate results from the study suggest a role for EZH2 in the migration of T cells into the CNS in patients with multiple sclerosis and also suggest a potential pathogenic capacity of EZH2-positive T cells that will need to be explored more in depth in future studies.

Additional file

Additional file 1: Table S1. Demographic and clinical characteristics of the multiple sclerosis patients and HC included for the determination of microRNA expression levels. (DOC 36 kb)

Abbreviations

EAE: Experimental autoimmune encephalomyelitis; EZH2: Enhancer of zeste 2 polycomb repressive complex 2 subunit; GM-CSF: Granulocyte/macrophage colony-stimulating factor; H3K27: Histone H3 at lysine 27; HC: Healthy controls; ITGA4: Integrin subunit alpha 4; ITGAL: Integrin subunit alpha L; KB: Klüver-Barrera; mRNA: Messenger RNA; MS: Multiple sclerosis; PBMC: Peripheral blood mononuclear cells; PECAM1: Platelet and endothelial cell adhesion molecule 1; PMA: Phorbol 12-myristate 13-acetate; PPMS: Patients with primary progressive multiple sclerosis; RRMS: Relapsing-remitting multiple sclerosis; SAHA: Suberoylanilide hydroxamic acid; SELL: Selectin L; TLN1: Talin 1; TNF: Tumor necrosis factor

Acknowledgements

The authors would like to thank the nurses, laboratory technicians, and patients for their participation in sample collection.

Funding

The authors thank the "Red Española de Esclerosis Múltiple (REEM)" sponsored by the FEDER-FIS and the "Ajuts per donar Suport als Grups de Recerca de Catalunya," sponsored by the "Agència de Gestió d'Ajuts Universitaris i de Recerca" (AGAUR), Generalitat de Catalunya, Spain.

Authors' contributions

SM, LMV, XM, and MC contributed to the conception and study design. CC, LM, MCu SMe, NF, JR, JC, JCA-C, and AS contributed to the data acquisition and analysis. SM, LMV, and MC contributed to the drafting of the manuscript and figures. All authors read and approved the final manuscript.

Competing interests

The authors declare that they have no competing interests.

Author details

[1]Servei de Neurologia-Neuroimmunologia, Centre d'Esclerosi Múltiple de Catalunya (Cemcat), Institut de Recerca Vall d'Hebron (VHIR), Hospital Universitari Vall d'Hebron, Universitat Autònoma de Barcelona, Barcelona, Spain. [2]Departments of Neurology and Immunology, Hospital Universitario Ramón y Cajal, Instituto Ramón y Cajal de Investigacion Sanitaria, Madrid, Spain. [3]Departament d'Estadística, Facultat de Biologia, Universitat de Barcelona, Barcelona, Spain. [4]Unitat d'Estadística i Bioinformàtica, Institut de Recerca, HUVH, Barcelona, Spain. [5]Genetics, Microbiology and Statistics Department, Universitat de Barcelona, Barcelona, Spain.

References

1. Cao R, Wang L, Wang H, Xia L, Erdjument-Bromage H, Tempst P, et al. Role of histone H3 lysine 27 methylation in polycomb-group silencing. Science. 2002;298:1039–43.
2. Su IH, Dobenecker MW, Dickinson E, Oser M, Basavaraj A, Marqueron R, et al. Polycomb group protein ezh2 controls actin polymerization and cell signaling. Cell. 2005;121:425–36.
3. Gunawan M, Venkatesan N, Loh JT, Wong JF, Berger H, Neo WH, et al. The methyltransferase Ezh2 controls cell adhesion and migration through direct methylation of the extranuclear regulatory protein talin. Nat Immunol. 2015. 2015;16:505–16.
4. Livak KJ, Schmittgen TD. Analysis of relative gene expression data using real-time quantitative PCR and the 2(-Delta Delta C(T)). Methods. 2001;25: 402–8.
5. Irizarry RA, Hobbs B, Collin F, Beazer-Barclay YD, Antonellis KJ, Scherf U, et al. Exploration, normalization, and summaries of high density oligonucleotide array probe level data. Biostatistics. 2003;4:249–64.
6. Smyth GK. Linear models and empirical Bayes methods for assessing differential expression in microarray experiments. Stat Appl Genet Mol Biol. 2004;3:Article3.
7. Benjamin Y, Hochberg Y. Controlling the false discovery rate: a practical and powerful approach to multiple testing. J Roy Stat Soc B. 1995;57:289–30.
8. Zheng F, Liao YJ, Cai MY, Liu YH, Liu TH, et al. The putative tumour suppressor microRNA-124 modulates hepatocellular carcinoma cell aggressiveness by repressing ROCK2 and EZH2. Gut. 2012;61:278–89.
9. Mei S, Liu Y, Bao Y, Zhang Y, Min S, Liu Y, et al. Dendritic cell-associated miRNAs are modulated via chromatin remodeling in response to different environments. PLoS One. 2014;9:e90231.
10. Dutta R, Chomyk AM, Chang A, Ribaudo MV, Deckard SA, Doud MK, et al. Hippocampal demyelination and memory dysfunction are associated with increased levels of the neuronal microRNA miR-124 and reduced AMPA receptors. Ann Neurol. 2013;73:637–45.
11. Moore CS, Rao VT, Durafourt BA, Bedell BJ, Ludwin SK, Bar-Or A, et al. miR-155 as a multiple sclerosis-relevant regulator of myeloid cell polarization. Ann Neurol. 2013;74:709–20.
12. Lee SR, Roh YG, Kim SK, Lee JS, Seol SY, Lee HH, et al. Activation of EZH2 and SUZ12 regulated by E2F1 predicts the disease progression and aggressive characteristics of bladder cancer. Clin Cancer Res. 2015;21:5391–403.
13. Zingg D, Debbache J, Schaefer SM, Tuncer E, Frommel SC, Cheng P, et al. The epigenetic modifier EZH2 controls melanoma growth and metastasis through silencing of distinct tumour suppressors. Nat Commun. 2015;6:6051.
14. Sun S, Yu F, Zhang L, Zhou X. EZH2, an on–off valve in signal network of tumor cells. Cell Signal. 2016;28:481–7.
15. Sospedra M, Martin R. Immunology of multiple sclerosis. Annu Rev Immunol. 2015;23:683–747.
16. Macfarlane LA, Murphy PR. MicroRNA: biogenesis, function and role in cancer. Curr Genom. 2010;11:537–61.
17. Niino M, Bodner C, Simard ML, Alatab S, Gano D, Kim HJ, et al. Natalizumab effects on immune cell responses in multiple sclerosis. Ann Neurol. 2006;59: 748–54.
18. Dhib-Jalbut S, Marks S. Interferon-beta mechanisms of action in multiple sclerosis. Neurology. 2010;74:S17–24.
19. Griffith JW, Luster AD. Targeting cells in motion: migrating toward improved therapies. Eur J Immunol. 2013;43:1430–5.
20. Sellner J, Koczi W, Harrer A, Oppermann K, Obregon-Castrillo E, Pilz G, et al. Glatiramer acetate attenuates the pro-migratory profile of adhesion molecules on various immune cell subsets in multiple sclerosis. Clin Exp Immunol. 2013;173:381–9.
21. Mueller SN, Gebhardt T, Carbone FR, Heath WR. Memory T cell subsets, migration patterns, and tissue residence. Annu Rev Immunol. 2013;31:137–61.
22. Caminero A, Comabella M, Montalban X. Tumor necrosis factor alpha (TNF-α), anti-TNF-α and demyelination revisited: an ongoing story. J Neuroimmunol. 2011;234:1–6.
23. Yamaguchi J, Sasaki M, Sato Y, Itatsu K, Harada K, Zen Y, et al. Histone deacetylase inhibitor (SAHA) and repression of EZH2 synergistically inhibit proliferation of gallbladder carcinoma. Cancer Sci. 2010;101:355–62.
24. Wedepohl S, Beceren-Braun F, Riese S, Buscher K, Enders S, Bernhard G, et al. L-selectin--a dynamic regulator of leukocyte migration. Eur J Cell Biol. 2012;91:257–64.
25. Cobo-Calvo Á, Figueras A, Bau L, Matas E, Mañé Martínez MA, León I, et al. Leukocyte adhesion molecule dynamics after natalizumab withdrawal in multiple sclerosis. Clin Immunol. 2016;171:18–24.
26. Jilek S, Mathias A, Canales M, Lysandropoulos A, Pantaleo G, Schluep M, et al. Natalizumab treatment alters the expression of T-cell trafficking marker LFA-1 α-chain (CD11a) in MS patients. Mult Scler. 2014;20:837–42.
27. Qing Z, Sandor M, Radvany Z, Sewell D, Falus A, Potthoff D, et al. Inhibition of antigen-specific T cell trafficking into the central nervous system via blocking PECAM1/CD31 molecule. J Neuropathol Exp Neurol. 2001;60:798–807.

4

TLR4 inhibitor TAK-242 attenuates the adverse neural effects of diet-induced obesity

V. Alexandra Moser[1], Mariana F. Uchoa[1] and Christian J. Pike[1,2]*

Abstract

Background: Obesity exerts negative effects on brain health, including decreased neurogenesis, impaired learning and memory, and increased risk for Alzheimer's disease and related dementias. Because obesity promotes glial activation, chronic neuroinflammation, and neural injury, microglia are implicated in the deleterious effects of obesity. One pathway that is particularly important in mediating the effects of obesity in peripheral tissues is toll-like receptor 4 (TLR4) signaling. The potential contribution of TLR4 pathways in mediating adverse neural outcomes of obesity has not been well addressed. To investigate this possibility, we examined how pharmacological inhibition of TLR4 affects the peripheral and neural outcomes of diet-induced obesity.

Methods: Male C57BL6/J mice were maintained on either a control or high-fat diet for 12 weeks in the presence or absence of the specific TLR4 signaling inhibitor TAK-242. Outcomes examined included metabolic indices, a range of behavioral assessments, microglial activation, systemic and neuroinflammation, and neural health endpoints.

Results: Peripherally, TAK-242 treatment was associated with partial inhibition of inflammation in the adipose tissue but exerted no significant effects on body weight, adiposity, and a range of metabolic measures. In the brain, obese mice treated with TAK-242 exhibited a significant reduction in microglial activation, improved levels of neurogenesis, and inhibition of Alzheimer-related amyloidogenic pathways. High-fat diet and TAK-242 were associated with only very modest effects on a range of behavioral measures.

Conclusions: These results demonstrate a significant protective effect of TLR4 inhibition on neural consequences of obesity, findings that further define the role of microglia in obesity-mediated outcomes and identify a strategy for improving brain health in obese individuals.

Keywords: Adiposity, Alzheimer's disease, Inflammation, Obesity, Toll-like receptor 4, Microglia

Background

The high prevalence of obesity presents a major public health concern since obesity is strongly linked with increased risk for several diseases including type 2 diabetes, cardiovascular disease, and cancer [1]. Importantly, obesity is also associated with adverse effects on the brain and neural function. In humans, obesity is linked with decreases in hippocampal volume and white matter integrity [2–4] as well as with functional consequences that lead to accelerated cognitive decline [5, 6] and increased risk of dementia [7]. In rodent models, diet-induced obesity (DIO) has been demonstrated to impair neurogenesis [8, 9], synaptic plasticity [10, 11], and neural function [12], as well as promote Alzheimer's disease (AD)-related pathology [13, 14].

Although the mechanisms by which obesity impairs neural health have yet to be fully elucidated, pathways associated with microglial activation are compelling candidates. Obesity is characterized by chronic activation of macrophages in peripheral tissues [15–17] and both microglia and astrocytes in the brain [18–21]. Activated macrophages yield unresolved inflammation in peripheral organs including the adipose tissue [15, 22] and liver

* Correspondence: cjpike@usc.edu
[1]Neuroscience Graduate Program, University of Southern California, 3641 Watt Way, HNB 120, Los Angeles, CA 90089, USA
[2]Leonard Davis School of Gerontology, University of Southern California, 3715 McClintock Avenue, Los Angeles, CA 90089-0191, USA

[23], whereas activated microglia can drive neuroinflammation in the brain [24, 25]. Neuroinflammation is associated with numerous deleterious effects including reductions in neurogenesis [26] and synaptic plasticity [27] and acceleration of AD [28]. In addition to promoting pro-inflammatory pathways, activated microglia exhibit diverse phenotypes that are characterized by a range of morphological and gene expression signatures [29, 30] and presumed to underlie both beneficial and adverse effects [31, 32]. The pathways that may contribute to the neural effects of obesity remain to be fully defined.

The pattern recognition receptor Toll-like receptor 4 (TLR4) activates signaling pathways that may be particularly important in mediating obesity-associated microglial activation and its consequences. TLR4 stimulation results in downstream activation of at least two key transcription factors: NFκB, which increases expression of pro-inflammatory cytokines [33], and interferon regulatory factor 3, which promotes activated microglial phenotypes that are relatively anti-inflammatory [34, 35]. Thus, TLR4 activation may be expected to yield a range of activated microglial phenotypes. Interestingly, TLR4 binds to and is activated by saturated fatty acids, which are abundant in obesogenic diets and may contribute to obesity-induced increases in inflammation [36–40] and impaired insulin signaling [37, 41]. Prior work has implicated TLR4 signaling as an important regulator of DIO effects on peripheral tissues. For example, mice with either nonfunctional or deleted TLR4 exhibit significant protection against high-fat diet (HFD)-induced glucose dysregulation [42, 43], insulin resistance [44, 45], and peripheral inflammation [46–48], though other studies indicate these mice are not protected against the entire range of metabolic and inflammatory effects of HFD [48, 49]. Pharmacological inhibition of TLR4 also protects mice against HFD-associated adipose inflammation and fibrosis [50] and insulin resistance [51]. Disruption of TLR4 signaling appears to have only modest effects on increases in body weight and adiposity that result from HFD [45, 46, 52, 53].

The potential role of TLR4 signaling in mediating obesity-induced microglial activation and associated neural impairment is unclear. Prior work has implicated TLR4 in pro-inflammatory effects of saturated fatty acids and HFD in hypothalamus, which in turn may regulate diet-induced changes in metabolic function [54–56]. Given that TLR4 is highly expressed in microglia [57, 58], TLR4 signaling pathways are implicated in activated microglial phenotypes, and activated microglia are thought to drive many of the adverse effects of obesity and HFD in hippocampus and other brain regions [10, 59], TLR4 may mediate HFD-induced microglial activation and dysfunction in hippocampus. To address this possibility, we evaluated HFD-induced effects on metabolic, inflammatory, microglial, and neural outcomes in the presence and absence of a pharmacological inhibitor of TLR4 signaling. We report that treatment with a specific TLR4 inhibitor reduced peripheral inflammation and largely prevented both microglia activation and impaired neurogenesis in hippocampus independently of the effects on weight gain and metabolic dysregulation associated with HFD.

Methods
Animal procedures
Ten-week-old male C57BL6/J mice were purchased from Jackson Labs (Bar Harbor, ME, USA) and allowed to acclimate to our vivarium facility at the University of Southern California for 2 weeks. Animals were housed under a 12-h light/dark cycle with lights on at 6 AM and ad libitum access to food and water. At 12 weeks of age, mice were randomized to a total of four dietary and drug treatments groups ($N = 10–14$/group). Dietary treatments were either control (CTL; 10% fat; #D12450J, Research Diets, New Brunswick, NJ, USA) or high-fat diet (HFD; 60% fat; #D12492, Research Diets). Drug treatments were either vehicle (0.09% sterile saline) or the TLR4 inhibitor TAK-242 (3 mg/kg in saline; #614316, EMD Millipore, Billerica, MA, USA). Drugs were administered via intraperitoneal (IP) injection 6 days/week. Dosage was based upon a previous study in which TAK-242 delivered at 3 mg/kg via IP injection yielded significant brain levels of the drug that were sufficiently maintained for at least 24 h after administration [60]. Treatments were maintained over a 12-week experimental period, during which body weights were recorded daily and food consumption was measured weekly.

At the conclusion of the experimental period, mice were euthanized with inhalant carbon dioxide and the brains were rapidly removed. One hemi-brain was immersion fixed for 48 h in 4% paraformaldehyde/0.1 M PBS, then stored at 4 °C in 0.1 M PBS/0.03% NaN_3 until processed for immunohistochemistry. Hippocampus was dissected and snap frozen for subsequent use in RNA extraction, while the remainder of the hemi-brain was snap frozen for subsequent use in protein extraction to examine soluble β-amyloid (Aβ) levels. Blood was collected via cardiac puncture into EDTA-coated tubes and centrifuged to separate plasma, which was stored in aliquots at – 80 °C. Gonadal and retroperitoneal (RP) fat pads were dissected and weighed as measures of adiposity. Both fat pads were snap frozen for subsequent RNA extraction. All animal procedures were conducted under protocols approved by the University of Southern California Institutional Animal Care and Use Committee and in accordance with National Institute of Health standards.

Body composition

Body composition was determined 1 day prior to euthanization using the Bruker LF90 Minispec (Bruker Optics, Billerica, MA, USA). Mice were placed and loosely restrained inside an acrylic cylinder. The cylinder was placed inside the bore of the magnet, and measurements of fat, lean, and fluid mass percentages were recorded. Animals were returned to their home cages in less than 2 min.

Glucose, cholesterol, and triglyceride measurements

At weeks 0, 4, 8, and 11, blood glucose readings were measured after overnight fasting (16 h). Blood was collected from the lateral tail vein and immediately assessed for glucose levels using the Precision Xtra Blood Glucose and Ketone Monitoring System (Abbott Diabetes Care, Alameda, CA, USA).

At week 11, glucose tolerance testing (GTT) was performed. First, baseline fasting glucose levels were taken. Mice were then administered a glucose bolus (2 g/kg body weight) via IP injection. Blood glucose levels were recorded from lateral tail vein 15, 30, 60, and 120 min after the glucose bolus. Area under the curve (AUC) was calculated.

Plasma cholesterol and triglyceride levels were measured enzymatically at the conclusion of the experimental period. Commercially available kits for both cholesterol (Total Cholesterol Colorimetric Assay kit, #K603, BioVision, Milpitas, CA, USA) and triglycerides (LabAssay Triglycerides, #290-63701, Wako Chemicals, Richmond, VA, USA) were used following the manufacturers' protocols.

Behavioral analyses

All behavioral testing was conducted between the hours of 6 AM and 1 PM. For all behavioral assays, mice were brought into the behavior room and allowed to acclimate for 30 min prior to testing. After each trial, animals were returned to their home cages and the testing arenas were disinfected with 70% ethanol.

Open field and forced swim testing were video recorded and analyzed by a rater blind to experimental treatment groups. Elevated plus maze and spontaneous alternation behavior were scored live. Fear conditioning was recorded using Noldus Ethovision XT software (Leesburg, VA, USA) and the Ugo Basille Fear Conditioning System NG (Gemonia, Varese, Italy).

Anxiety and exploratory activity: open field and elevated plus maze (EPM)

Open field test was performed during week 8 of treatments. Briefly, animals were placed into a 40-cm^2 plexiglass arena and allowed to move freely for 5 min. The arena floor was lightly marked off into 9 squares, with 3 squares along each wall and 1 center square. The following behaviors were recorded: (1) center crossings: the number of times the animal crossed into the center square with both front paws; (2) center time: the amount of time the animal spent with both front paws in the center square; and (3) crossings: the total number of times the animal crossed a line entering a different square.

EPM testing was performed on the day immediately following the open field assay. After being habituated to the room, mice were placed in the center of the EPM, facing a closed arm, and allowed to move freely on the maze for 5 min. The following behaviors were recorded: (1) open arm entries: the number of times the mouse placed both front paws into the open arm; (2) open arm time: the amount of time the animal spent with both front paws in the open arm; and (3) latency to enter the open arm for the first time.

Learning and memory: spontaneous alternation behavior (SAB) and fear conditioning

At week 10, SAB was tested in the Y-maze as previously described [61, 62]. Briefly, animals were placed into the long arm and allowed to explore the maze for 5 min. Arm choices were recorded, and behavior was scored as the number of alternations divided by the total number of arm entries.

Fear conditioning was performed over 3 consecutive days beginning 48 h after SAB. On day 1, animals were placed in the conditioning chamber, a box (17 cm × 17 cm × 25 cm) with an electrified grid floor, placed inside a sound attenuated chest (Ugo Basile). White noise was used to block out external sounds. After a 3 min habituation, mice were exposed to 5 tone-and-foot shock pairings that were each placed 3 min apart (20 s tone at 85 dB and 2 kHz, followed by a 20 s trace period, and a 1 sec 1 mA foot shock). Animals were returned to their home cages 1 min after the final tone-shock pairing. Twenty-four hours after training, cued fear conditioning was tested by placing animals back into the chamber but changing the context by altering the pattern of the walls, placing a floor board over the grid floor, and adding a cotton ball with vanilla extract to change the scent of the chamber. After a 3-min baseline period, the tone was played 3 times, but was not followed by the foot shock. Freezing behavior (defined as the absence of all movement except breathing) to the tone and during the 20 s after the tone was recorded. On day 3, 24 h after cued testing, contextual fear conditioning was assessed by placing animals back into the chamber that had the same appearance and odor as it did during training on day 1. Freezing behavior was measured over 8 min. Behavior in the fear conditioning chamber was recorded using Noldus Ethovision XT software.

Depression-like behavior: forced swim test (FST)

FST was conducted 1 week after fear conditioning, during week 11, and was the last behavioral assessment. As previously described [61], the animals were placed into a 2-L cylindrical tank (20 cm height × 13 cm diameter) filled with 15 cm of water heated to 23–25 °C. At this depth, neither the feet nor tails of animals reached the floor of the cylinder. Mice remained in the cylinder for 5 min, during which behavior was videotaped from the side of the cylinder. Animals were scored as being immobile if they were making only the movements necessary to keep their head above water. The number of immobile bouts, the total time spent immobile, and the duration of the longest bout of immobility were recorded.

Immunohistochemistry and quantification

Fixed hemi-brains were completely sectioned at 40 μm in the horizontal plane, using a vibratome (Leica Biosystems, Buffalo Grove, IL, USA). A standard avidin/biotin peroxidase approach using ABC Vector Elite kits (Vector Laboratories, Burlingame, CA, USA) was used to perform immunohistochemistry, as previously described [63]. Every eighth section was processed for ionized calcium binding adaptor molecule 1 (IBA-1), doublecortin (DCX), and bromodeoxyuridine (BrdU). A different initial antigen retrieval step was performed for each antibody, after which the same protocol was followed. For IBA-1 staining, sections were boiled in 10 mM EDTA, pH 6.0 for 10 min, then rinsed in water three times for 5 min each. For DCX staining, tissue was pretreated with 95% formic acid for 5 min, followed by rinsing in TBS. Finally, for BrdU staining, sections were placed in 1% NP40 detergent for 20 min, rinsed in TBS, then incubated in 2 N HCl at 37 °C for 30 min, followed by 10 min in 0.1 M boric acid and rinsing in TBS. Following the various antigen retrieval steps, sections were treated with an endogenous blocking solution for 10 min, then rinsed with 0.2% Triton-X in TBS, 3 times for 10 min each. Tissue was then incubated for 1 h in a blocking solution consisting of 2% bovine serum albumin and 0.2% Triton-X in TBS for IBA-1, plus 2% normal goat serum for BrdU. For DCX, the blocking solution was made up of 3% normal horse serum and 0.2% Triton-X in TBS. Blocked sections were incubated overnight at 4 °C in primary antibody directed against IBA-1 (#019-19741, 1:500 dilution, Wako Chemicals); DCX (#sc-271390, 1:1000 dilution, Santa Cruz Biotechnology, Dallas, TX, USA); or BrdU (#MCA2483, 1:200 dilution, Bio-Rad, Hercules, CA, USA). All primary antibodies were diluted in the respective blocking solution used. On the following day, sections were rinsed and incubated in

biotinylated secondary antibody diluted in blocking solution. Finally, immunoreactivity was visualized using 3,3′-diaminobenzidine (Vector Laboratories).

Density and activation states of microglia were determined using live imaging under bright-field microscopy with a × 40 objective (Olympus, BX50, CASTGrid software, Olympus, Tokyo, Japan). As previously described [63, 64], each cell was scored as having either a resting or reactive phenotype. Specifically, resting or type 1 microglia were defined as having spherical cell bodies with numerous thin, branched processes. Both type 2 and 3 microglia were considered reactive: type 2 cells had enlarged, rod-shaped cell bodies with fewer and thicker processes, while type 3 cells were enlarged and had either very few or no processes, or several filopodia. Microglia were quantified in the entorhinal cortex (4 fields/section), subiculum (4 fields/section), CA1 (5 fields/section), and CA2/3 (3 fields/section) across 4 tissue sections for a total of 64 fields and an average of ∼ 450 cells per brain. Because increased soma size is a robust indicator of microglial activation [65], we also examined microglial soma size. Images of IBA-1 immunostaining in the CA1 subregion of the hippocampus were digitally captured using an Olympus BX50 microscope and DP74 camera paired with a computer running CellSens software (Olympus). Microglial cell bodies were outlined, and their area was determined using NIH ImageJ 1.50i (US National Institutes of Health, Bethesda, MD, USA).

DCX- and BrdU-immunoreactive cells were also quantified using live imaging under bright-field microscopy with a × 100 oil immersion lens (Olympus). Cells were counted in non-overlapping fields of the subgranular zone and granule cell layer of the dentate gyrus, across 8 sections per animal. Additionally, to examine the relative maturity of DCX-expressing cells, the morphology of their dendritic processes was assessed as previously described [66–68]. Briefly, immature or type 1 cells were defined as having very short or no processes, intermediate or type 2 cells as having processes that extended only within the granule cell layer and do not extend into the molecular layer, and post-mitotic or type 3 cells as having dendrites that extend and branch into the molecular layer or having multiple branches within the granule cell layer. Morphology of DCX-positive cells was assayed across 4 sections per animal, and the relative proportions of type 1, 2, and 3 cells were calculated.

RNA isolation and quantitative PCR

RNA was extracted from the gonadal fat pads and the hippocampus using TRIzol reagent (Invitrogen Corporation, Carlsbad, CA, USA), following the manufacturer's protocol. To remove any remaining DNA contamination, the RNA pellet was treated with RNase-free DNase I (Epicentre, Madison, WI, USA) for 30 min at 37 °C after which a phenol-chloroform extraction was performed to isolate RNA. cDNA was reverse transcribed from 1 μg of purified RNA using the iScript cDNA synthesis system (Bio-Rad). The resulting cDNA was used to run real-time quantitative PCR using SsoAdvanced Universal SYBR Green Supermix (Bio-Rad) and a Bio-Rad CFX Connect Thermocycler, as previously described [63]. Both hippocampus and adipose tissue were analyzed for expression levels of cluster of differentiation 68 (CD68), EGF-like module-containing mucin-like hormone receptor-like 1 (F4/80), major histocompatibility complex class II (MHC II), cluster of differentiation 74 (CD74) transcript variant 1, interleukin-6 (IL-6), and interleukin-1β (IL-1β). Additionally, hippocampal tissue was assessed for lipoprotein lipase (LPL) and CD36, as well as for the Aβ clearance and production factors neprilysin, insulin-degrading enzyme (IDE), and β-site APP cleaving enzyme (BACE1). Finally, levels of the cytokine tumor necrosis factor α (TNFα) transcript variant 1 were examined in adipose tissue. Primer pair sequences for target genes are shown in Table 1. All samples were run in duplicate, and PCR products were normalized with corresponding expression levels of β-actin and/or phosphoglycerate kinase 1 (Pgk1) in the brain and succinate dehydrogenase complex, subunit A, flavoprotein (SDHA) in the adipose tissue. The $\Delta\Delta$-CT method was used to determine relative mRNA levels. For hippocampal samples, the Ct value of each reference gene (β-actin and/or Pgk1) was subtracted separately from the target genes and the resulting values were averaged and used to calculate fold changes relative to the control-diet, vehicle-treated group. CD68, F4/80, MHCII, CD74, IL6, IL1β, LPL, and CD36 were run with both reference genes and neprilysin, IDE, and BACE1 only with β-actin.

β-Amyloid enzyme-linked immunosorbent assay

Levels of soluble Aβ42 peptides were determined by enzyme-linked immunosorbent assay (ELISA) as described previously [69], with noted modifications. Briefly, the remaining hemi-brain portions were homogenized in buffer (0.2% diethylamine, 50 mM NaCl, 1 mL/200 mg tissue) using a polytron on ice. Resulting homogenates were centrifuged at 4 °C for 1 h at 15,000 g. Supernatants

Table 1 Target genes for the PCR analyses are listed with their corresponding GeneID number and oligonucleotide sequences for the forward and reverse primers

Target gene	Primer sequence
β-actin *Gene ID: 11461*	Forward: 5'-AGCCATGTACGTAGCCATCC-3' Reverse: 5'-CTCTCAGCTGTGGTGGTGAA-3'
β-site APP cleaving enzyme (BACE1) *GeneID: 23821*	Forward: 5'-TCGCTGTCTCACAGTCATCC-3' Reverse: 5'-AACAAACGGACCTTCCACTG-3'
Cluster of differentiation factor 36 (CD36) *GeneID: 12491*	Forward: 5'-TATTGGTGCAGTCCTGGCTG-3' Reverse: 5'-CTGCTGTTCTTTGCCACGTC-3'
Cluster of differentiation factor 68 (CD68) *GeneID: 12514*	Forward: 5'-TTCTGCTGTGGAAATGCAAG-3' Reverse: 5'-AGAGGGGCTGGTAGGTTGAT-3'
Cluster of differentiation factor 74 (CD74), transcript variant 1 *GeneID: 16149*	Forward: 5'-CAAGTACGGCAACATGACCC-3' Reverse: 5'-GCACTTGGTCAGTACTTTAGGTG-3'
EGF-like module-containing mucin-like hormone receptor-like 1 (F4/80) *GeneID: 13733*	Forward: 5'-TGCATCTAGCAATGGACAGC-3' Reverse: 5'-GCCTTCTGGATCCATTTGAA-3'
Insulin-degrading enzyme (IDE) *GeneID: 15925*	Forward: 5'-TGTTTCCACACACAGGCAAT-3' Reverse: 5'-ACCTGTGAAAAGCCGAGAGA-3'
Interleukin-1β (IL1β) *GeneID: 16176*	Forward: 5'-GCAACTGTTCCTGAACTCAACT-3' Reverse: 5'-ATCTTTTGGGGTCCGTCAACT-3'
Interleukin-6 (IL6) *GeneID:16193*	Forward: 5'-CTCTGGGAAATCGTGGAAAT-3' Reverse: 5'-CCAGTTTGGTAGCATCCATC-3'
Lipoprotein lipase (LPL) *GeneID: 16956*	Forward: 5'-GGGCCCAGCAACATTATCCA-3' Reverse: 5'-GGGGGCTTCTGCATACTCAA-3'
Major histocompatibility complex class II (MHC II) *GeneID: 14961*	Forward: 5'-CAGACGCCGAGTACTGGAAC-3' Reverse: 5'-CAGCGCACTTTGATCTTGGC-3'
Neprilysin *GeneID: 17380*	Forward: 5'-GAGAAAAGCCCACTTGCTTG-3' Reverse: 5'-GAAAGACAAAATGGGGCAGA-3'
Phosphoglycerate kinase 1 (Pgk1) *GeneID: 18655*	Forward: 5'-GCCTGTTGACTTTGTCACTGC-3' Reverse: 5'-GAGTGACTTGGTTCCCCTGG-3'
Succinate dehydrogenase complex, subunit A, flavoprotein (SDHA) *Gene ID: 66945*	Forward: 5'-ACACAGACCTGGTGGAGACC-3' Reverse: 5'-GGATGGGCTTGGAGTAATCA-3'
Tumor necrosis factor α (TNFα), transcript variant 1 *GeneID: 21926*	Forward: 5'-CCCTCACACTCAGATCATCTTCT-3' Reverse: 5'-GCTACGACGTGGGCTACAG-5'

were collected and neutralized with 1/10th volume of 0.5 M Tris-HCl, pH 6.8. Samples were then analyzed using a commercially available Aβ42 ELISA (Human/Rat β Amyloid 42 ELISA Kit High Sensitive; 292-64501; Wako Chemicals) according to manufacturer's directions.

Statistical analyses

All data were analyzed using Prism software (version 7, GraphPad Software, La Jolla, CA, USA). Two-way repeated measures ANOVAs were performed for the analyses of body weight and glucose tolerance. All other data were analyzed by two-way ANOVAs. In the case of significant main effects, planned comparisons between groups were made using the Bonferroni correction. All data are represented as the mean ± the standard error of the mean (SEM). Significance was set at a threshold of $p < 0.05$.

Results

Effects of HFD and TAK-242 on body weight and adiposity

We first examined measures of DIO in vehicle-treated and TAK-242-treated animals to assess whether drug treatment altered the obesogenic effects of HFD. The control diet was associated with a ~ 5% weight gain in both vehicle-treated and TAK-242-treated mice, whereas HFD was associated with a 39.6 ± 4.2% increase in body weight in vehicle-treated mice and a 34.4 ± 3.0% increase in TAK-242-treated mice (Fig. 1a). Two-way repeated measures ANOVA showed that HFD significantly increased body weight ($F = 38.9$, $p < 0.0001$). There was no significant effect of drug treatment on body weight. Between-group comparisons revealed that mice fed HFD weighed more than those fed CTL diets at the 4-, 8-, and 12-week time points ($p < 0.05$); this was true for both vehicle-treated and TAK-242-treated groups. When examining final body weight, we found a main effect of diet ($F = 63.88$, $p < 0.0001$; Fig. 1b), which was significant across both drug treatments ($p < 0.0001$). There were no significant interactions between diet and drug on measures of body weight.

Next, we examined adiposity by both body composition analysis and weights of gonadal and RP fat pads. We found that HFD was associated with a significant decrease in percent lean body mass ($F = 103.0$, $p < 0.0001$; Fig. 1c) and a corresponding significant increase in percent body fat ($F = 98.7$, $p < 0.0001$; Fig. 1d) in both vehicle-treated and TAK-242-treated mice ($p < 0.0001$). There was no interaction effect between diet and drug, nor were there significant main effects of drug on lean mass or body fat. The same pattern was found with fat depot weight, such that HFD significantly increased weights of both RP ($F = 117.1$, $p < 0.0001$; Fig. 1e) and gonadal ($F = 108.4$, $p < 0.0001$; Fig. 1f) fat pads. There were neither significant main

effects of drug nor interaction effects between diet and drug.

We also examined food intake and found that HFD feeding was associated with a significant increase in the average daily kilocalorie consumption ($F = 52.5$, $p < 0.0001$; Fig. 1g), as would be expected given the higher caloric density of HFD relative to control diet. Importantly, drug treatment did not significantly affect caloric intake, and there were no significant interactions between diet and drug.

Effects of HFD and TAK-242 on metabolic outcomes

Another established outcome of DIO is dysregulation of glucose homeostasis [70, 71]. We first examined changes in fasting glucose levels over the treatment period. We found that HFD was associated with a significant increase in glucose levels ($F = 23.78$, $p < 0.0001$; Fig. 2a) at the 4-, 8-, and 11-week time points ($p < 0.05$). Additionally, there was a significant main effect of diet on percent change in glucose levels from baseline to the end of the treatment period ($F = 13.7$, $p < 0.001$; Fig. 2b). However, between-group comparisons revealed that the effect of HFD on increasing fasting glucose was only significant in vehicle-treated ($p < 0.01$), not in TAK-242-treated animals. There were neither significant interaction effects nor main effects of drug treatment on these measures of glucose homeostasis.

In addition to fasting glucose levels, we examined responses to a glucose bolus. There was a main effect of diet on glucose clearance in GTT ($F = 49.95$, $p < 0.0001$; Fig. 2c) that was significant in both vehicle-treated and TAK-242-treated mice ($p < 0.05$). We also calculated the AUC for GTT and again found a significant effect of diet ($F = 55.11$, $p < 0.0001$; Fig. 2d) such that HFD increased AUC regardless of drug treatment. There were no significant interactions or main effects of drug treatment on GTT measures.

Finally, we examined the effects of diet and drug treatments on levels of plasma triglycerides and cholesterol. HFD was associated with significantly increased triglyceride levels ($F = 15.64$, $p < 0.001$; Fig. 2e) in both drug treatment groups ($p < 0.05$). There was a non-significant trend towards increased cholesterol levels by HFD ($F = 3.41$, $p = 0.07$; Fig. 2f). There were no main effects of drug nor were there interactions between diet and drug on levels of either triglycerides or cholesterol.

Effects of HFD and TAK-242 on peripheral inflammation

DIO is known to increase inflammation in a number of organs, including adipose tissue [72]. To assess effects of HFD on peripheral tissue inflammation, we examined gene expression of markers of macrophage activation and inflammatory cytokines in gonadal fat (Fig. 3). We

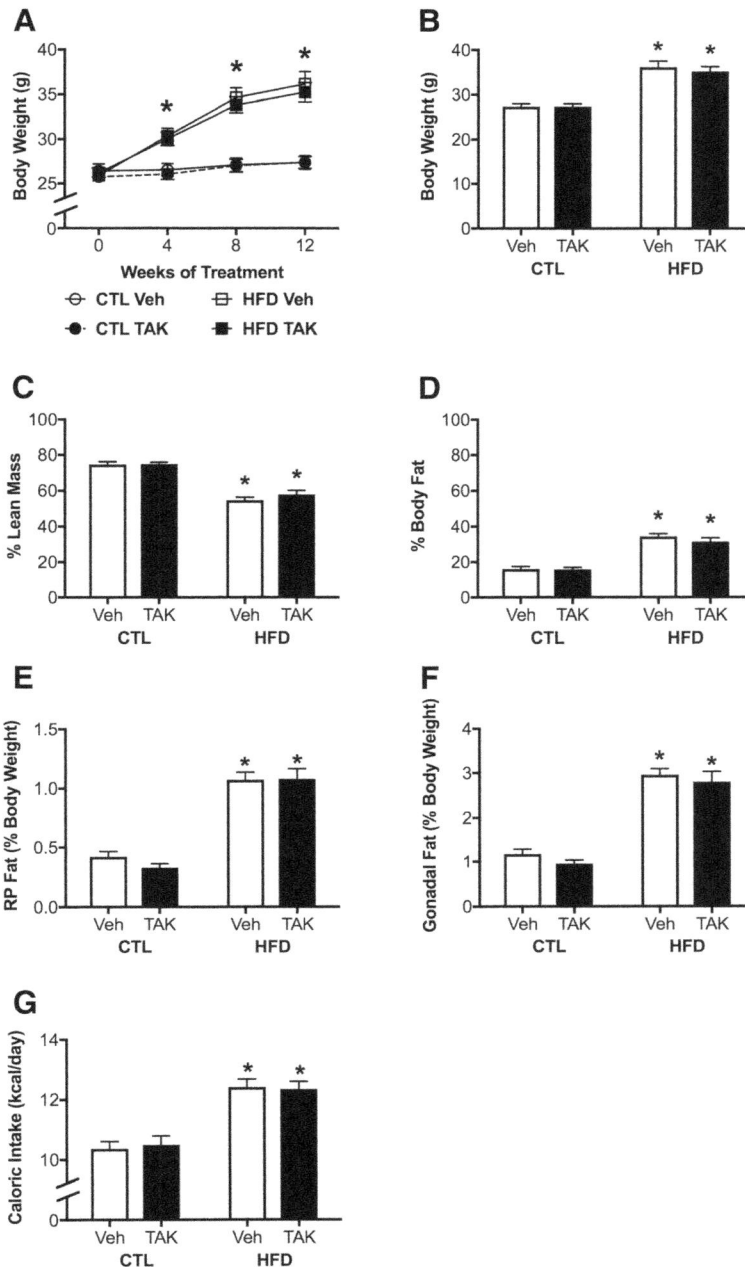

Fig. 1 Metabolic outcomes associated with diet-induced obesity in mice treated with vehicle (Veh) or the TLR4 inhibitor TAK-242 (TAK). **a** Body weights in male C57BL6/J mice maintained on control (CTL) and high-fat (HFD) diets and vehicle (Veh) and TAK-242 (TAK) treatments taken at baseline (week 0) and 4-week intervals across the 12-week experimental period, and **b** body weights at the end of the treatment period. **c** Lean mass and **d** percent body fat via NMR scan. **e, f** Adiposity as measured by **e** retroperitoneal (RP) fat pad and **f** gonadal fat pad weights. **g** Average daily caloric intake across the experimental period. Data are presented as mean (±SEM) values; $n = 10$–14/group. For data presented across time, control diet-fed mice are shown as circles, high-fat diet-fed mice are shown as squares; vehicle-treated are open symbols, TAK-242-treated are filled symbols; for all other panels, vehicle-treated animals are shown in white bars and TAK-242-treated are shown in black bars. Statistical significance is based on ANOVA followed by Bonferroni correction. * $p < 0.05$ relative to drug treatment-matched mice in control diet condition

found a significant effect of diet on adipose tissue levels of CD68 ($F = 17.14$, $p < 0.001$; Fig. 3a), F4/80 ($F = 10.06$, $p < 0.01$; Fig. 3b), MHCII ($F = 16.42$, $p < 0.001$; Fig. 3c), CD74 ($F = 7.42$, $p < 0.05$; Fig. 3d), IL-6 ($F = 6.52$, $p < 0.05$;

Fig. 3e), IL-1β ($F = 9.99$, $p < 0.01$; Fig. 3f), and TNFα ($F = 10.85$, $p < 0.01$; Fig. 3g). However, for the markers of CD68, F4/80, MHC II, IL6, and TNFα, this effect was only statistically significant in vehicle-treated HFD-fed

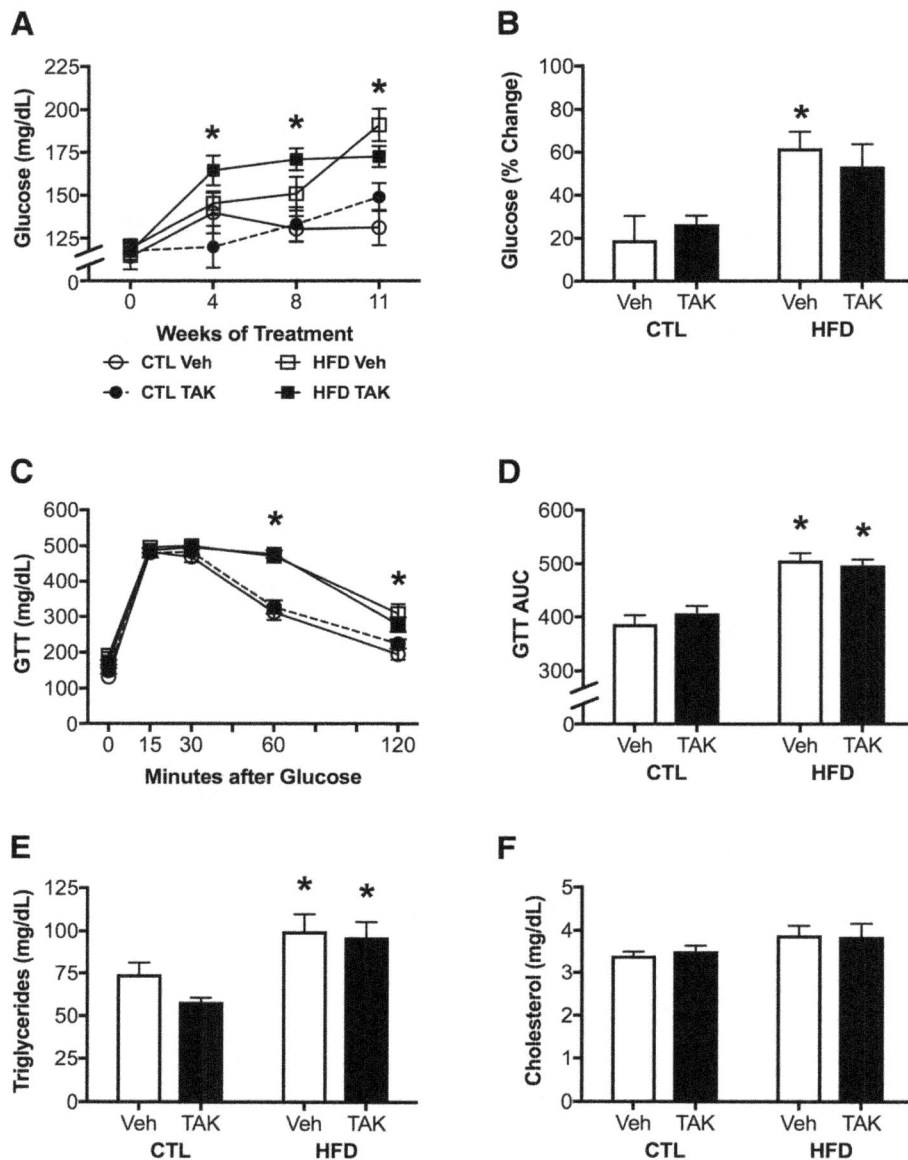

Fig. 2 Peripheral effects of diet-induced obesity in mice treated with vehicle (Veh) or the TLR4 inhibitor, TAK-242 (TAK). **a** Baseline fasting glucose levels in male C57BL6/J mice maintained on control (CTL) and high-fat diets (HFD) and drug treatments taken at baseline (week 0) and weeks 4, 8, and 11. **b** Percent change in fasting blood glucose levels relative to baseline after 12 weeks of control or high-fat diet. **c** Glucose tolerance test showing blood glucose levels over time after administration of a glucose bolus and **d** area under the curve (AUC) for the glucose tolerance test. **e** Plasma triglyceride levels and **f** plasma cholesterol levels at the end of the experimental period. Data are presented as mean (±SEM) values; $n = 10$–14/group. For data presented across time, control diet-fed mice are shown as circles, high-fat diet-fed mice are shown as squares; vehicle-treated are open symbols, TAK-242-treated are filled symbols; for all other panels, vehicle-treated animals are shown in white bars and TAK-242-treated are shown in black bars. Statistical significance is based on ANOVA followed by Bonferroni correction. * $p < 0.05$ relative to drug treatment-matched mice in control diet condition

mice and did not reach statistical significance in TAK-242-treated HFD-fed mice. For CD74 and IL-1β the main effect of diet failed to reach statistical significance in either of the HFD-fed groups. There was neither a main effect of drug, nor an interaction effect between diet and drug on expression of any probed genes.

Effects of HFD and TAK-242 on hippocampal microgliosis
In addition to causing macrophage activation and inflammation in peripheral tissues, HFD is associated with increased glial activation and inflammation in the brain [73, 74]. Because microglia express high levels of TLR4 [57, 58] and have been shown to adopt activated phenotypes in response to HFD [40, 75, 76], we examined

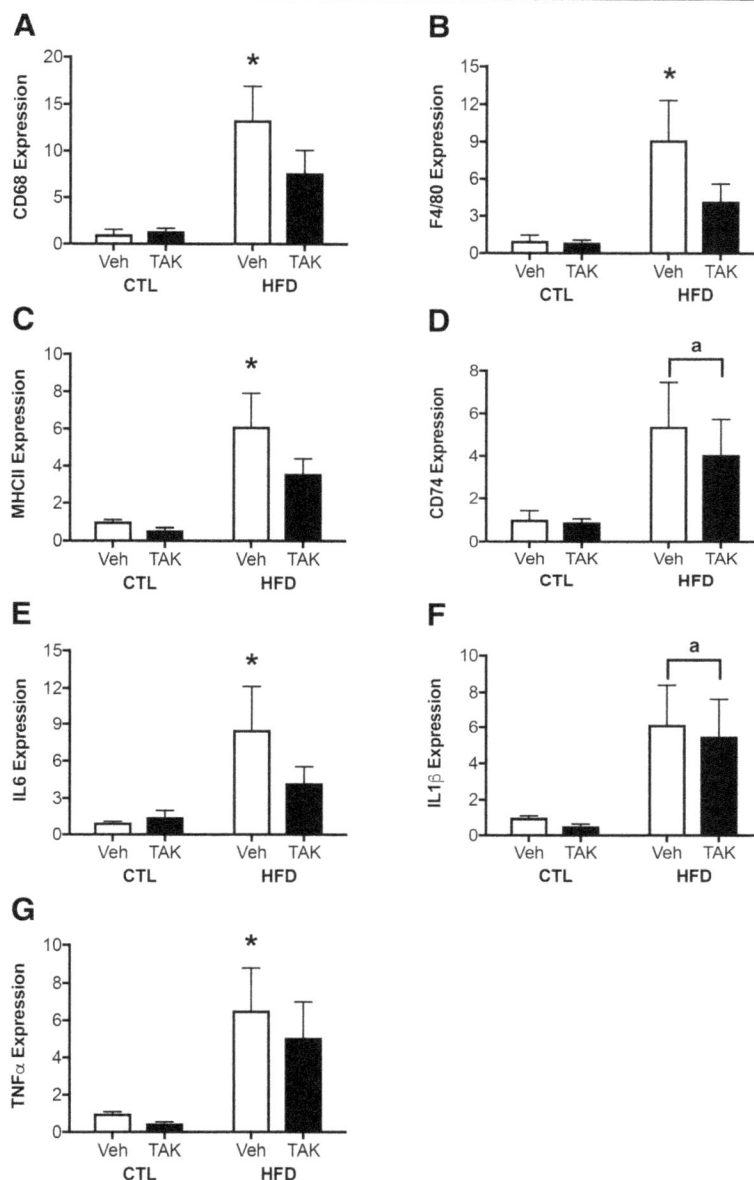

Fig. 3 Expression of mRNA levels of genes associated with macrophage activation and inflammation in adipose tissue from vehicle (Veh) and TAK-242 (TAK)-treated mice fed a control (CTL) or high-fat diet (HFD). mRNA from gonadal fat pads was probed for levels of the macrophage markers **a** CD68 and **b** F4/80, as well as for the antigen presenting molecules **c** MHC II and **d** CD74. Pro-inflammatory cytokine expression was examined by probing for levels of **e** IL-6, **f** IL-1β, and **g** TNFα. Data show fold difference means and standard error of the means (SEM) relative to vehicle-treated mice fed a control diet $n = 10$/group. Vehicle-treated animals are shown in white bars and TAK-242-treated are shown in black bars. Statistical significance is based on ANOVA followed by Bonferroni correction. *$p < 0.05$ relative to drug treatment-matched mice in control diet condition. [a]$p < 0.05$ for main effect of diet that does not reach statistical significance in between-group comparisons

microgliosis in brain sections. We analyzed both cell density and morphology of labeled cells following immunostaining for IBA-1 in entorhinal cortex and in the subiculum, CA1, and CA2/3 regions of the hippocampus. Figure 4a–c illustrates morphological phenotype characteristic of resting (type 1; Fig. 4a) microglia, with multiple, thin processes, and activated microglia with fewer, thicker processes (type 2; Fig. 4b), or amoeboid

appearance (type 3; Fig. 4c). When examining microglial density, we found neither significant effects of diet or drug treatment, nor an interaction between these factors in entorhinal cortex (Fig. 4d), subiculum (Fig. 4f), CA1 (Fig. 4h), or CA2/3 (Fig. 4j). However, we found significant interactions between diet and drug treatment on microglial activation in entorhinal cortex ($F = 36.27$, $p < 0.0001$; Fig. 4e), subiculum ($F = 38.93$, $p < 0.0001$; Fig. 4g),

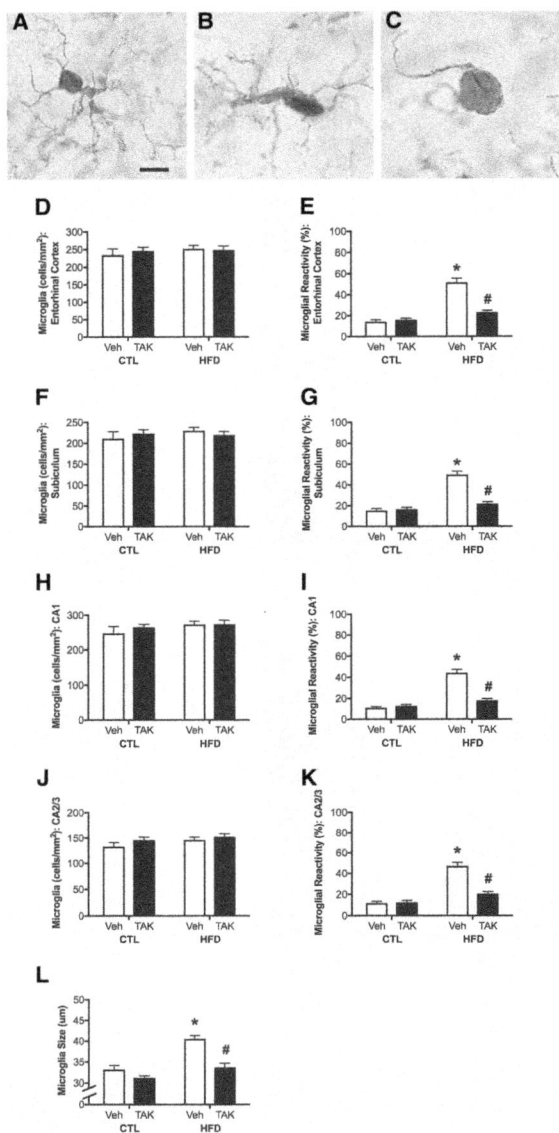

Fig. 4 Microglial number, morphological status, and soma size as assessed by IBA-1 immunohistochemistry in control (CTL) and high-fat diet (HFD)-fed mice treated with vehicle (Veh) or the TLR4 inhibitor, TAK-242 (TAK). **a–c** Representative images of microglial morphology. Scale bar = 10 μm. **a** Resting (type 1) microglial cells are characterized by small cell bodies with numerous branching processes. Reactive microglia are either **b** type 2 cells with rod-shaped cell bodies and fewer, thicker projections, or **c** amoeboid cells with no processes or with filopodia. Densities of IBA-1 immunoreactive cells were quantified in **d** entorhinal cortex and in the **f** subiculum, **h** CA1, and **j** CA2/3 of the hippocampus. Percentages of reactive microglia (type 2 and 3 cells) were quantified in **e** entorhinal cortex and in the hippocampal subregions **g** subiculum, **i** CA1, and **k** CA2/3. **l** Microglial soma size was assessed specifically in CA1 of the hippocampus. Data are presented as mean (±SEM) values; $n = 10$/group. Vehicle-treated animals are shown in white bars, and TAK-242-treated are shown in black bars. Statistical significance is based on ANOVA followed by Bonferroni correction. *$p < 0.05$ relative to drug treatment-matched mice in control diet condition. #$p < 0.05$ relative to vehicle-treated mice in the same diet condition

CA1 ($F = 47.16$, $p < 0.0001$; Fig. 4i), and CA2/3 ($F = 31.7$, $p < 0.0001$; Fig. 4k). Between-group comparisons revealed that across all brain regions, HFD increased microglial reactivity exclusively in vehicle-treated animals, and TAK-242 was associated with significantly reduced microglial reactivity specifically in HFD-fed animals.

Activation phenotypes of microglia are also associated with increased soma size [65]. We measured microglial soma size as a complementary measure of microgliosis, specifically in the CA1 region of the hippocampus. Our data show similar results to findings on microglial morphology. That is, there is a significant interaction effect between diet and drug treatment ($F = 8.62$, $p < 0.01$; Fig. 4l), such that diet significantly increased soma size only in vehicle-treated animals ($p < 0.0001$), and TAK-242 treatment was associated with significantly decreased soma size compared to the vehicle group only in HFD-fed animals ($p < 0.0001$).

Effects of HFD and TAK-242 on hippocampal gene expression

One frequent consequence of microgliosis is the increased expression of various microglia/macrophage markers and pro-inflammatory cytokines [77, 78]. We examined gene expression levels of several such factors in hippocampus (Fig. 5), including CD68 and F4/80 as general microglia/macrophage markers [79], with CD68 being characteristic of a more activated cell phenotype [80–82]. We found a significant interaction between diet and drug ($F = 7.06$, $p < 0.05$; Fig. 5a) on expression levels of CD68. Between-group comparisons revealed that HFD increased CD68 expression only in vehicle-treated but not in TAK-242-treated animals ($p < 0.01$), and TAK-242 significantly decreased CD68 only in HFD-fed mice ($p < 0.05$). There were neither significant effects of diet or drug treatment, nor an interaction between these factors on hippocampal gene expression of F4/80 (Fig. 5b).

We next examined levels of MHC II, which is expressed specifically in microglia in the brain [83, 84], enhances TLR4 signaling [85], and is increased in microglia by HFD [10], and of CD74, which is also expressed specifically by microglia and macrophages [86], and is involved in the formation and transport of MHC II [87]. Additionally, CD74 expression has been shown to correlate with obesity-induced increases in body weight and metabolic changes in adipose tissue [88], and is increased in hippocampus of HFD-fed mice [89]. There was a statistically non-significant trend of increased MHC II in the HFD-vehicle group (Fig. 5c), and no significant diet or drug effects on CD74 expression (Fig. 5d).

Increased production of pro-inflammatory cytokines is a one potential outcome of increased microglial

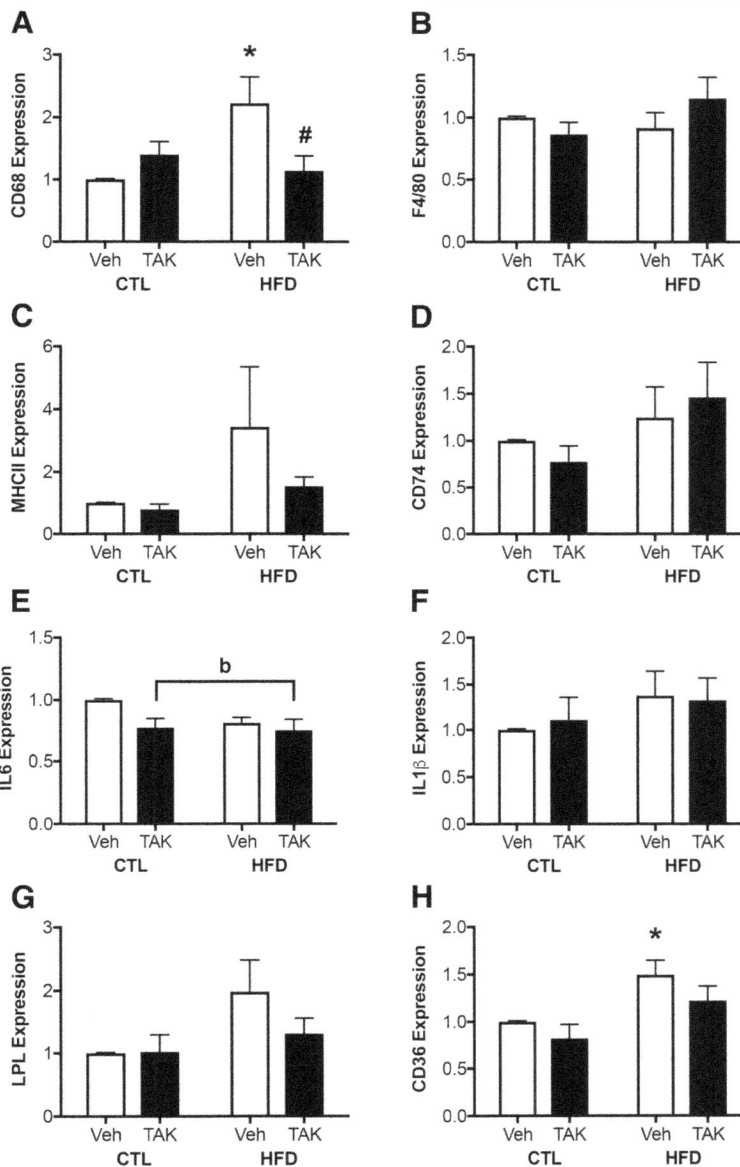

Fig. 5 Hippocampal mRNA expression of genes associated with activated microglial phenotypes and neuroinflammation in mice fed a control (CTL) or high-fat diet (HFD) and treated with vehicle (Veh) or the TLR4 inhibitor, TAK-242 (TAK). Hippocampal mRNA was probed for levels of the microglia/macrophage markers **a** CD68 and **b** F4/80, and for the innate immune antigen presentation markers **c** MHC II and **d** CD74. Pro-inflammatory cytokine expression was examined using **e** IL-6 and **f** IL-1β. Gene expression of two factors involved in microglial phenotype, lipid transport, and uptake **g** LPL and **h** CD36 were also assayed in hippocampus. Data show fold difference means and standard error of the means (SEM) relative to vehicle-treated mice fed a control diet $n = 10$/group. Vehicle-treated animals are shown in white bars and TAK-242-treated are shown in black bars. Statistical significance is based on ANOVA followed by Bonferroni correction. *$p < 0.05$ relative to drug treatment-matched mice in control diet condition. #$p < 0.05$ relative to vehicle-treated mice in same diet condition. b$p < 0.05$ for main effect of drug treatment that does not reach statistical significance in between-group comparisons

activation [78] as well as of obesity [21]. Thus, we probed for two pro-inflammatory cytokines: IL-6 (Fig. 5e) and IL-1β (Fig. 5f). Though diet did not significantly affect gene expression of either cytokine, we found a significant main effect of drug on levels of IL-6 ($F = 4.73$, $p < 0.05$); however, this did not reach statistical significance in either CTL-fed or HFD-fed mice.

Finally, we examined mRNA levels of two factors involved in fatty acid transport and uptake as well as regulation of activated microglial phenotypes: LPL [90, 91] and CD36 [92, 93]. Results demonstrated a statistically non-significant trend of a main effect of diet on LPL levels ($F = 3.03$, $p = 0.08$; Fig. 5g), as well as a statistically significant effect of diet on CD36 expression ($F = 10.99$; $p < 0.01$;

Fig. 5h). Between-group comparisons showed that HFD significantly increased CD36 only in vehicle-treated but not in TAK-242-treated mice ($p < 0.05$).

Effects of HFD and TAK-242 on neurogenesis

An established negative consequence of DIO is impaired neurogenesis [8, 9]. We examined neurogenesis across groups using techniques to quantify both neural stem cells committed to a neuronal phenotype (DCX-labeling) and proliferation of neural stem cells (BrdU labeling) in the dentate gyrus region of the hippocampus. Figure 6 shows representative images of DCX immunohistochemistry, which qualitatively show a decrease in labeled cells with HFD that is prevented by TAK-242 treatment (Fig. 6a–d). Quantification of DCX-labeled cell density showed a significant main effect of drug ($F = 5.01$, $p < 0.05$; Fig. 6e). Between-group comparisons revealed that this effect of drug treatment was significant only in HFD-fed mice ($p < 0.05$). In addition, there was a non-significant trend towards an interaction between diet and drug ($F = 3.05$, $p = 0.08$; Fig. 6e). There was no significant effect of diet on DCX-labeled cells. We also determined the relative maturity of DCX-positive cells by examining their dendritic morphology and arborization [66, 67]. Diet and drug treatments did not significantly affect maturation states of new neurons, as the proportion of subtypes was roughly equivalent

between treatment groups (Fig. 6f). Parallel assessment of BrdU-labeled cells revealed neither significant main effects of diet or drug, nor an interaction between these factors (Fig. 6g).

Effects of HFD and TAK-242 on amyloidogenic pathways

DIO has been shown to promote Alzheimer-related amyloidogenic pathways in rodent models, in part by regulating neural expression of factors involved in Aβ production and clearance [94–98]. We measured hippocampal expression levels of three key genes to investigate if HFD and TAK-242 treatments affect Aβ homeostasis pathways. We found no significant effects of diet or drug treatment, nor an interaction between these factors, on expression levels of the Aβ-degrading enzymes neprilysin (Fig. 7a) and IDE (Fig. 7b). However, we found a significant interaction between diet and drug treatment ($F = 4.90$, $p < 0.05$; Fig. 7c) on levels of the pro-amyloidogenic Aβ enzyme BACE1. Between-group comparisons revealed that HFD significantly increased BACE1 in vehicle-treated animals ($p < 0.05$) but not in TAK-242-treated mice. Finally, we determined levels of soluble Aβ42 peptides by ELISA. There were no statistically significant effects of diet or drug treatment and no interaction between these factors, though there were non-significant trends consistent with the BACE1 data (Fig. 7d).

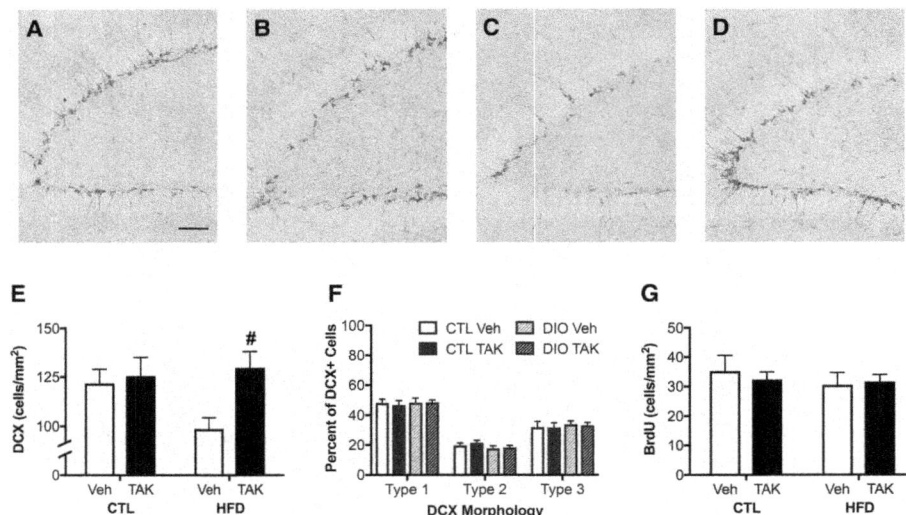

Fig. 6 Neurogenesis and cell proliferation as assessed by DCX and BrdU immunohistochemistry in mice maintained on control (CTL) or high-fat diets (HFD) and treated with vehicle (Veh) or the TLR4 inhibitor, TAK-242 (TAK). a–d Representative images of DCX immunohistochemistry in mice treated with a control diet (CTL) and vehicle (Veh), b control diet and TAK-242 (TAK), c high-fat diet (HFD) and vehicle, and d high-fat diet and TAK-242. Scale bar = 50 µm. e Densities of DCX immunoreactive cells were quantified in the dentate gyrus. f The maturation state of DCX-positive cells was assessed, and cells were categorized as type 1, type 2, or type 3 based on their dendritic morphology. g BrdU-positive cells were quantified in the dentate gyrus. Data are presented as mean (±SEM) values; n = 10/group. Vehicle-treated animals are shown in white bars, and TAK-242-treated are shown in black bars; for DCX morphology, CTL diet-fed animals are shown in solid bars and HFD-fed animals are shown in striped bars. Statistical significance is based on ANOVA followed by Bonferroni correction. #p < 0.05 relative to vehicle-treated mice in the same diet condition

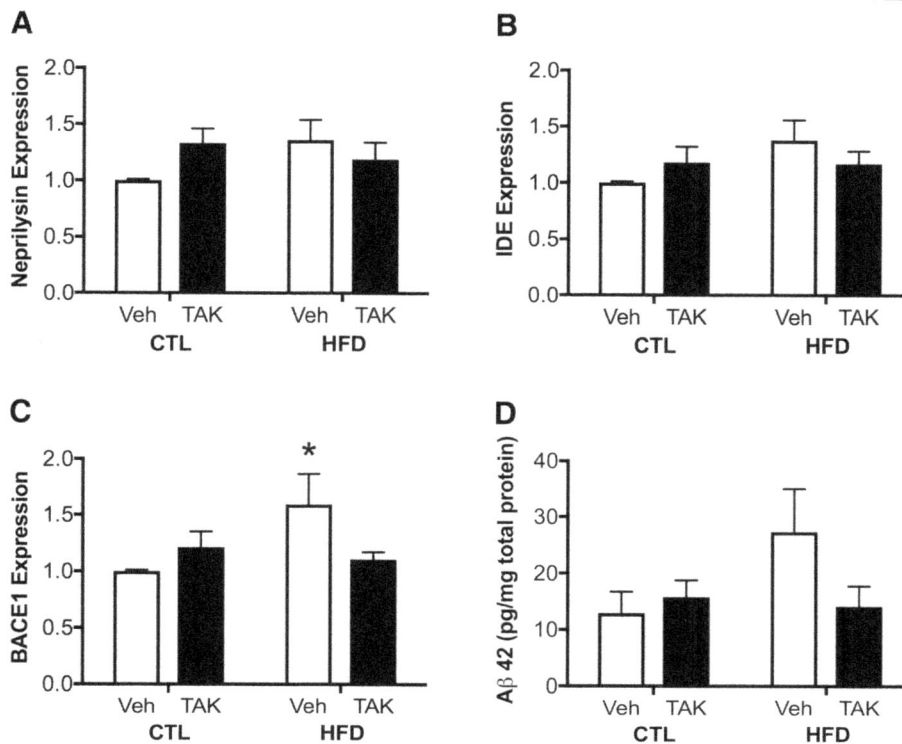

Fig. 7 Expression of Aβ production and degrading factors and soluble Aβ42 in mice fed a control (CTL) or high-fat diet (HFD) and treated with vehicle (Veh) or the TLR4 inhibitor TAK-242 (TAK). **a–c** Hippocampal gene expression of the Aβ clearance factors **a** neprilysin, and **b** insulin-degrading enzyme, and the Aβ production factor **c** BACE1, as assessed by qPCR. Data show fold differences relative to vehicle-treated mice fed a control diet. **d** Protein levels of soluble Aβ42 as measured by ELISA (expressed as pg Aβ42 per to mg total protein). Data are presented as mean (±SEM) values; $n = 10$/group. Vehicle-treated animals are shown in white bars, and TAK-242-treated are shown in black bars. Statistical significance is based on ANOVA followed by Bonferroni correction. *$p < 0.05$ relative to drug treatment-matched mice in control diet condition

Effects of HFD and TAK-242 on exploration, anxiety-like, and depressive-like behaviors

To determine whether the drug treatment affected general behavioral performance, we compared animals on measures of activity, anxiety, and depression, using the behavioral assays of open field, elevated plus maze, and forced swim test, respectively. We found no statistically significant main effects of drug treatment on any of these three behavioral tasks (Additional file 1: Figure S1). There were only two statistically significant effects on any of the outcome measures in these assays, and both of these were in exploratory activity in the open field. First, there was a significant interaction between diet and drug treatment on the number of times the animals crossed into the center field ($F = 4.91$, $p < 0.05$; Additional file 1: Figure S1A), such that HFD increased center crossings only in TAK-242-treated mice ($p < 0.05$). Second, there was a significant main effect of diet on time spent in the center field ($F = 4.23$, $p < 0.05$; Additional file 1: Figure S1B), such that HFD again increased this measure specifically in TAK-242-treated animals ($p < 0.05$). There were no statistically significant effects on any measures of anxiety-like or depressive-like behaviors.

Effects of HFD and TAK-242 on behavioral performance in cognitive tasks

Finally, we examined cognitive performance in two behavioral assays. The spontaneous alternation behavior (SAB) task assays short-term working memory and visual attention. Total arm entries did not vary by either diet or drug treatment (Fig. 8a). However, there was a main effect of diet on alternation behavior ($F = 7.86$, $p < 0.01$; Fig. 8b), which was significantly only in TAK-242-treated mice ($p < 0.05$), though performance of the TAK-242-treated HFD mice (49%) is not significantly different from that observed in vehicle-treated HFD mice (50%).

As a measure of hippocampal-dependent and hippocampal-independent memory, we tested animals using the fear-conditioning paradigm. When examining freezing during the day 1 training trials, we found no significant differences between groups in initial freezing before the tone/shock pairing or in freezing during the tone/shock pairings and inter-trial periods. Figure 8c shows time spent freezing during the trace period between the tone and shock during the final presentation of the tone/shock pairing on day 1.

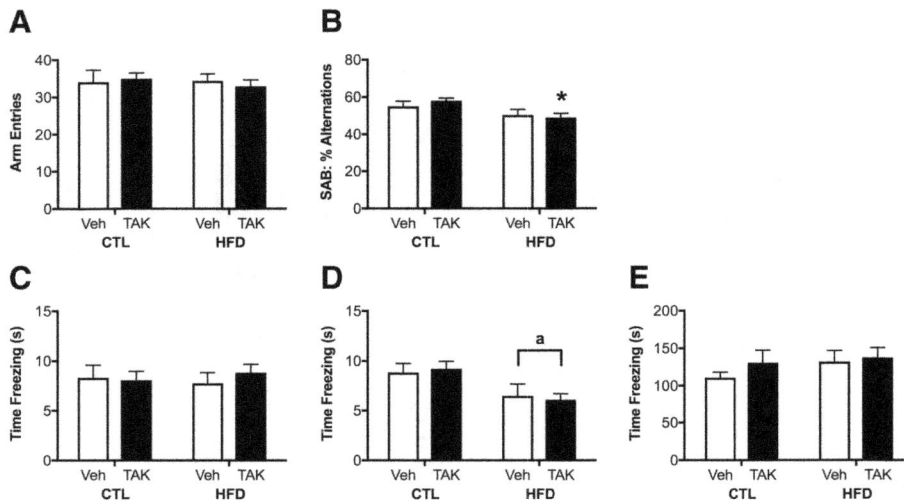

Fig. 8 Working memory and cued and contextual memory performance in mice maintained on control (CTL) or high-fat diet (HFD) and given vehicle (Veh) or the TLR4 inhibitor, TAK-242 (TAK). **a, b** Short-term working memory was assessed by spontaneous alternation behavior. **a** Total arm entries in the Y maze. **b** Spontaneous alternation behavior (SAB) in the Y maze. **c–e** Cued and contextual memory was tested in the fear conditioning paradigm. **c** Learning was assessed by examining freezing behavior during the trace period between the tone and shock on the 5th trial of the training day. **d** Cued memory was tested 24 h later in a different context. **e** Contextual memory was assessed 24 h after the cued test. Data are presented as mean (±SEM) values; $n = 10$–14/group. Vehicle-treated animals are shown in white bars, and TAK-242-treated are shown in black bars. Statistical significance is based on ANOVA followed by Bonferroni correction. *$p < 0.05$ relative to drug treatment-matched mice in control diet condition

Cued memory was assessed on day 2 by changing the appearance and odor of the chamber and examining freezing to the tone, without presenting the shock. There were no group differences in freezing during the baseline period before presentation of the tone (data not shown). There was a main effect of diet on freezing during the trace period immediately after the first presentation of the tone ($F = 4.76$, $p < 0.05$; Fig. 8d), but this did not reach statistical significance across the different drug treatments. There were no significant group differences on freezing during the following 2 tone presentations (data not shown).

Contextual memory was examined on day 3 by placing animals back into the chamber with the same appearance and odor as during day 1 and examining freezing to this context. There were no significant effects of either diet or drug treatment, nor was there an interaction between these factors, on freezing in response to the context (Fig. 8e).

Discussion

The goal of this study is to examine the role of TLR4 signaling in mediating the effects of obesity on microglial activation and adverse neural outcomes. Comparing animals fed control versus HFD in the presence or absence of the TLR4 inhibitor TAK-242, we demonstrate that TAK-242 treatment was associated with attenuation of HFD-induced adipose tissue inflammation, microgliosis, and reduction in neurogenesis in the hippocampus.

However, TAK-242 treatment did not improve the metabolic dysregulation induced by HFD feeding. The finding that TLR4 inhibition did not protect against effects of HFD on weight gain and adiposity is consistent with numerous other studies [42, 44–46, 49, 52, 53]. In contrast to our findings, however, many of these studies show that obesity-associated dysregulation of insulin and glucose signaling was improved in the absence of TLR4 signaling [42–47, 53]. One possible reason for this discordance is that several studies used mice with either knockout or dysfunctional TLR4, whereas we used a pharmacological approach to inhibit TLR4. Constitutive absence of TLR4 signaling may result in metabolic changes even in the absence of HFD and is likely to result in more complete inhibition of TLR4 and different outcomes than pharmacological approaches.

Our findings support the conclusion that TLR4 contributes to obesity-induced activation of peripheral macrophages and brain microglia. First, our observations in adipose tissue of partial reductions in both markers of macrophage activation (CD68, F4/80, MHCII) and pro-inflammatory cytokines (IL-6, TNFα) in HFD-fed mice treated with TAK-242 is consistent with previous findings [42, 44, 46, 48, 53]. Second, we demonstrate that the TLR4 inhibitor attenuates HFD-induced microgliosis in hippocampus, as evidenced by changes in microglial morphology and soma size and mRNA levels of the activated microglia markers CD68 and, to a lesser extent, CD36 or fatty acid translocase. CD36 is a pattern recognition receptor that exhibits increased expression in obesity [93] as well as in AD [99, 100], where it mediates recruitment of microglia to Aβ deposits [101, 102]. Interestingly, CD36 has been found to form a complex with TLR4 and TLR6 through which both Aβ and lipids can induce inflammation [103]. Collectively, these findings support and extend prior work by Milanski and colleagues that implicated TLR4 in obesity-induced glial activation in hypothalamus, which may contribute to systemic metabolic disturbances [54, 55].

Although we observed an increase in activated microglia in response to HFD, it is noteworthy that hippocampal expression of the pro-inflammatory cytokines IL-6 and IL1-β was not increased by obesogenic diet. Though HFD is often associated with both microglial activation and increased cytokine expression [104], others show changes only in some brain regions [105], or no changes in pro-inflammatory cytokines [106]. Here, we find DIO-associated changes in specific markers of activated microglia but not in cytokines, which is consistent with previous work by Setti and colleagues [89]. Although it is reasonable to predict that a more chronic exposure to HFD may be required for increased neural cytokine expression, cytokine expression in hypothalamus is significantly increased by high-fat diet exposures as brief as 1 day [107]. We posit that the observed microglial activation in the absence of significantly increased expression of pro-inflammatory cytokines is consistent with the known heterogeneity in activated microglial phenotypes [29, 30]. Indeed, accumulating evidence indicates that deleterious effects of microglia are mediated by numerous factors rather than simply increased levels of pro-inflammatory cytokines [32, 108]. The extent to which various activated microglial phenotypes differentially affect neural outcomes is an important topic that remains to be fully elucidated.

One deleterious neural consequence common to both diet-induced obesity and activated microglia is promotion of amyloidogenesis. HFD is known to increase gene expression and/or enzyme activity of the pro-amyloidogenic BACE1 [95] and decrease levels of the Aβ-degrading enzymes neprilysin [94] and insulin-degrading enzyme [97]. These effects on Aβ homeostasis likely contribute to observations that experimental obesity drives Aβ accumulation in transgenic mouse models of AD [13, 14]. Additionally, it has been shown that inflammation can increase levels of BACE1 [109] and decrease levels of neprilysin [110]. Thus, microglial activation and associated neuroinflammation are likely significant mediators of the obesity-induced increase in Aβ. We found that HFD significantly increased levels of BACE1 in vehicle-treated, but not in TAK-242-treated mice. This suggests that HFD caused a shift towards more pro-amyloidogenic processing via TLR4 signaling. Although not statistically significant, our analyses of soluble brain Aβ42 showed trends towards increased levels in HFD mice in the absence but not the presence of TLR4 inhibitor.

Another negative effect of obesity is attenuation of neurogenesis. We found that treatment with TAK-242 significantly increased the number of new neurons in dentate gyrus specifically in HFD-fed mice, indicating a protective effect of TLR4 inhibition on obesity-related impairment in neurogenesis. Because BrdU labeling, a marker of cell proliferation, was not affected by diet or drug treatments, the protective effect of TAK-242 appears to involve the survival and or differentiation of newborn neurons rather than stem cell proliferation. The possibility that TLR4 inhibition yielded a generalized increase in new neuron survival is consistent with our finding that the relative proportion of subtypes of newly formed neurons was not significantly altered by either diet or TLR4 inhibition. The reported effects of HFD on neurogenesis and cell proliferation are somewhat mixed in the literature, with some studies finding decreases in both [111, 112] and others finding changes in only one [9, 113] or neither [114] marker of neurogenesis. Differences in experimental parameters including the composition of the diet may affect the extent to which cell proliferation and/or survival of newborn neurons are affected by HFD. Our observed effects were likely mediated by microglia, which have previously been shown to attenuate neurogenesis during states of activation such as after LPS [115, 116] or seizure [26]. Further, our finding of increased neurogenesis with TAK-242 treatment in HFD-fed mice is consistent with prior data showing that TLR4 signaling regulates neurogenesis in response to neural injury and microgliosis [117, 118]. Importantly, adult neurogenesis is regulated both positively and negatively by a range of activated microglial phenotypes [32, 119], reinforcing the emerging complexity of the associations between microglial functions and their activation states.

One limitation of this study is that we were not able to fully determine the effects of TLR4 inhibition on HFD-induced behavioral changes. Although behavioral impairment is often associated with obesity, we found very subtle effects of diet and drug treatments on overall behavioral outcomes. Specifically, mice fed HFD and treated with TAK-242 showed small but significantly increased exploratory behavior/decreased anxiety-like behavior in the open field test, and worse spontaneous alternation in the Y-maze, and HFD was associated with decreased cued memory in fear conditioning. There were no significant effects of our diet or drug manipulations on anxiety-like behavior in EPM, depressive-like behavior in forced swim, or on contextual fear conditioning. Though a number of studies demonstrated cognitive impairments after HFD exposure [120–124], others did not [125–128]. The age at which rodents are exposed to diet-induced obesity may be a factor. For example, one study found significant effects of HFD on behavior in mice started on diet at 5 weeks of age, but not in animals started at 8 weeks [129], whereas another found behavioral impairments in response to HFD in aged but not young adult rats [130]. These studies suggest that the age at which exposure to HFD occurs may be important in determining whether behavioral deficits are observed. As with the induction of neuroinflammation, it is unlikely that the length of HFD exposure is the key variable in whether or not behavioral impairment occurs. Previous studies of HFD outcomes in rodents have showed changes in both neuroinflammation [107, 130] and behavioral outcomes [130, 131] within 3 days of HFD feeding. Moreover, deficits in cognitive performance have also been observed after 9 days [132], 1 month [133], and 3 months [131] of diet exposure.

Though complete elucidation of the mechanisms underlying the effects of obesity on the brain remains to be established, our findings suggest a stronger role for microglial activation than for metabolic dysregulation. That is, despite having similar weight gain and metabolic outcomes in response to HFD, mice treated with a TLR4 inhibitor showed significant reductions in microglial activation and increased neurogenesis in comparison to vehicle-treated mice. This position is consistent with findings in the human literature that the effects of obesity on cognitive impairment are mediated largely by glial/inflammatory rather than metabolic factors [134–136]. Because TAK-242 has systemic effects and we observed partial attenuation of inflammation in adipose tissue, peripheral effects of TLR4 inhibition may have contributed to the observed neural benefits. The role of other mechanisms like vascular and microbiota changes in the effects of obesity on the brain cannot be ruled out and should be addressed in future studies, especially given that inflammation may be important in these systems as well [137, 138].

Conclusions

To our knowledge, this study provides the first evidence that TLR4 signaling significantly contributes to the adverse effects of obesity on the hippocampus. Though TLR4 is well established as mediating the effects of saturated fatty acids on adverse outcomes in metabolic measures [42–47, 53] and inflammation [42, 44–48, 50, 53], its regulation of obesity-related changes in brain have not been thoroughly investigated. Our data demonstrate that treatment with an inhibitor of TLR4 signaling in the

context of obesogenic diet attenuates microgliosis, increases neurogenesis, and trends towards reductions in pro-amyloidogenic pathways. These findings implicate a significant role for microglial function as a key mediator of the neural effects of obesity. Additionally, these findings point to TLR4 as a therapeutic target for obesity, which has important health implications for a range of systemic and neural disorders including type 2 diabetes, cardiovascular disease, and dementia.

Additional file

> **Additional file 1: Figure S1.** Effects of diet and TLR4 inhibition on exploration, anxiety-like, and depressive-like behaviors. Exploration, anxiety-like, and depressive-like behaviors in control (CTL) and high-fat diet (HFD)-fed mice treated with vehicle (Veh) or the TLR4 inhibitor, TAK-242 (TAK). A-C) Explorative and anxiety-like behaviors were examined in the open field. A) The number of times animals entered the center square of the open field and B) the amount of time they spent in the center field. C) General locomotor activity as assessed by the total number of square crossings. D-F) Anxiety-like behavior was assessed in the elevated plus maze. D) The amount of time spent in the open arm of the maze, and E) the number of times the animals crossed into the open arm. F) The latency to enter the open arm for the first time. G-I) Depressive-like behaviors were examined in the forced swim test. G) The total amount of time the animals spent immobile and H) the number of times the animals were immobile. I) The length of the single longest time spent immobile. Vehicle-treated animals are shown in white bars and TAK-242-treated are shown in black bars. *p < 0.05 relative to drug treatment-matched mice in control diet condition. (TIFF 681 kb)

Abbreviations

AD: Alzheimer's disease; ANOVA: Analysis of variance; AUC: Area under the curve; Aβ: β-Amyloid; BACE1: β-Site APP cleaving enzyme; BrdU: Bromodeoxyuridine; CD36: Cluster of differentiation 36; CD68: Cluster of differentiation 68; CD74: Cluster of differentiation 74; CTL: Control; DCX: Doublecortin; DIO: Diet-induced obesity; ELISA: Enzyme-linked immunosorbent assay; EPM: Elevated plus maze; F4/80: EGF-like module-containing mucin-like hormone receptor-like 1; FST: Forced swim test; GTT: Glucose tolerance testing; HFD: High-fat diet; IBA-1: Ionized calcium binding adaptor molecule 1; IDE: Insulin-degrading enzyme; IL-1β: Interleukin-1β; IL-6: Interleukin-6; IP: Intraperitoneal; LPL: Lipoprotein lipase; MHCII: Major histocompatibility complex class II; Pgk1: Phosphoglycerate kinase 1; RP: Retroperitoneal; SAB: Spontaneous alternation behavior; SDHA: Succinate dehydrogenase complex, subunit A, flavoprotein; SEM: Standard error of the mean; TLR4: Toll-like receptor 4; TNFα: Tumor necrosis factor α; Veh: Vehicle

Acknowledgements

The authors thank Dr. Sean Curran for helpful discussions and Ms. Wenjie Qian for assistance with immunohistochemical analyses.

Funding

This work was supported by NIH grants AG051521 and AG26572 and by the Alzheimer's Association (SAGA-17-419-408).

Authors' contributions

VAM, MFU, and CJP conceptualized and designed this study. VAM and MFU coordinated execution of the studies and performed animal procedures and sample collection. VAM performed PCR, ELISAs, immunohistochemistry, histological analyses, and statistical analyses. VAM and CJP wrote the manuscript. All authors have read and approved the final manuscript.

Competing interests

The authors declare that they have no competing interests.

References

1. Zheng Y, Manson JE, Yuan C, Liang MH, Grodstein F, Stampfer MJ, et al. Associations of weight gain from early to middle adulthood with major health outcomes later in life. JAMA. 2017;318:255–69. https://doi.org/10.1001/jama.2017.7092.
2. Jagust W, Harvey D, Mungas D, Haan M. Central obesity and the aging brain. Arch Neurol. 2005;62:1545–8. https://doi.org/10.1001/archneur.62.10.1545.
3. Ho AJ, Raji CA, Becker JT, Lopez OL, Kuller LH, Hua X, et al. Obesity is linked with lower brain volume in 700 AD and MCI patients. Neurobiol Aging. 2010;31:1326–39. https://doi.org/10.1016/j.neurobiolaging.2010.04.006.
4. Stanek KM, Grieve SM, Brickman AM, Korgaonkar MS, Paul RH, Cohen RA, et al. Obesity is associated with reduced white matter integrity in otherwise healthy adults. Obesity (Silver Spring). 2011;19:500–4. https://doi.org/10.1038/oby.2010.312.
5. Elias MF, Elias PK, Sullivan LM, Wolf PA, D'Agostino RB. Obesity, diabetes and cognitive deficit: the Framingham heart study. Neurobiol Aging. 2005;26(Suppl 1):11–6. https://doi.org/10.1016/j.neurobiolaging.2005.08.019.
6. Cournot M, Marquié JC, Ansiau D, Martinaud C, Fonds H, Ferrières J, et al. Relation between body mass index and cognitive function in healthy middle-aged men and women. Neurology. 2006;67:1208–14. https://doi.org/10.1212/01.wnl.0000238082.13860.50.
7. Whitmer RA, Gustafson DR, Barrett-Connor E, Haan MN, Gunderson EP, Yaffe K. Central obesity and increased risk of dementia more than three decades later. Neurology. 2008;71:1057–64. https://doi.org/10.1212/01.wnl.0000306313.89165.ef.
8. Lindqvist A, Mohapel P, Bouter B, Frielingsdorf H, Pizzo D, Brundin P, et al. High-fat diet impairs hippocampal neurogenesis in male rats. Eur J Neurol. 2006;13:1385–8. https://doi.org/10.1111/j.1468-1331.2006.01500.x.
9. Park HR, Park M, Choi J, Park K-Y, Chung HY, Lee J. A high-fat diet impairs neurogenesis: involvement of lipid peroxidation and brain-derived neurotrophic factor. Neurosci Lett. 2010;482:235–9. https://doi.org/10.1016/j.neulet.2010.07.046.
10. Hao S, Dey A, Yu X, Stranahan AM. Dietary obesity reversibly induces synaptic stripping by microglia and impairs hippocampal plasticity. Brain Behav Immun. 2016;51:230–9. https://doi.org/10.1016/j.bbi.2015.08.023.
11. Stranahan AM, Norman ED, Lee K, Cutler RG, Telljohann RS, Egan JM, et al. Diet-induced insulin resistance impairs hippocampal synaptic plasticity and cognition in middle-aged rats. Hippocampus. 2008;18:1085–8. https://doi.org/10.1002/hipo.20470.
12. Jayaraman A, Lent-Schochet D, Pike CJ. Diet-induced obesity and low testosterone increase neuroinflammation and impair neural function. J Neuroinflammation. 2014;11:162. https://doi.org/10.1186/s12974-014-0162-y.
13. Julien C, Tremblay C, Phivilay A, Berthiaume L, Emond V, Julien P, et al. High-fat diet aggravates amyloid-beta and tau pathologies in the 3xTg-AD mouse model. Neurobiol Aging. 2010;31:1516–31. https://doi.org/10.1016/j.neurobiolaging.2008.08.022.
14. Barron AM, Rosario ER, Elteriefi R, Pike CJ. Sex-specific effects of high fat diet on indices of metabolic syndrome in 3xTg-AD mice: implications for Alzheimer's disease. PLoS One. 2013;8:e78554. https://doi.org/10.1371/journal.pone.0078554.
15. Weisberg SP, McCann D, Desai M, Rosenbaum M, Leibel RL, Ferrante AW. Obesity is associated with macrophage accumulation in adipose tissue. J Clin Invest. 2003;112:1796–808. https://doi.org/10.1172/JCI19246.
16. Cancello R, Tordjman J, Poitou C, Guilhem G, Bouillot JL, Hugol D, et al. Increased infiltration of macrophages in omental adipose tissue is associated with marked hepatic lesions in morbid human obesity. Diabetes. 2006;55:1554–61. https://doi.org/10.2337/db06-0133.
17. Lumeng CN, Deyoung SM, Bodzin JL, Saltiel AR. Increased inflammatory properties of adipose tissue macrophages recruited during diet-induced obesity. Diabetes. 2007;56:16–23. https://doi.org/10.2337/db06-1076.
18. García-Cáceres C, Yi C-X, Tschöp MH. Hypothalamic astrocytes in obesity. Endocrinol Metab Clin N Am. 2013;42:57–66. https://doi.org/10.1016/j.ecl.2012.11.003.
19. Buckman LB, Hasty AH, Flaherty DK, Buckman CT, Thompson MM, Matlock BK, et al. Obesity induced by a high-fat diet is associated with increased immune cell entry into the central nervous system. Brain Behav Immun. 2014;35:33–42. https://doi.org/10.1016/j.bbi.2013.06.007.
20. Lee EB, Mattson MP. The neuropathology of obesity: insights from human disease. Acta Neuropathol. 2014;127:3–28. https://doi.org/10.1007/s00401-013-1190-x.
21. Maldonado-Ruiz R, Montalvo-Martínez L, Fuentes-Mera L, Camacho A. Microglia activation due to obesity programs metabolic failure leading to type two diabetes. Nutr Diabetes. 2017;7:e254. https://doi.org/10.1038/nutd.2017.10.
22. Zeyda M, Stulnig TM. Obesity, inflammation, and insulin resistance--a mini-review. Gerontology. 2009;55:379–86. https://doi.org/10.1159/000212758.
23. Park EJ, Lee JH, Yu G-Y, He G, Ali SR, Holzer RG, et al. Dietary and genetic obesity promote liver inflammation and tumorigenesis by enhancing IL-6 and TNF expression. Cell. 2010;140:197–208. https://doi.org/10.1016/j.cell.2009.12.052.
24. Koga S, Kojima A, Kuwabara S, Yoshiyama Y. Immunohistochemical analysis of tau phosphorylation and astroglial activation with enhanced leptin receptor expression in diet-induced obesity mouse hippocampus. Neurosci Lett. 2014;571:11–6. https://doi.org/10.1016/j.neulet.2014.04.028.
25. Dorfman MD, Thaler JP. Hypothalamic inflammation and gliosis in obesity. Curr Opin Endocrinol Diabetes Obes. 2015;22:325–30. https://doi.org/10.1097/MED.0000000000000182.
26. Ekdahl CT, Claasen J-H, Bonde S, Kokaia Z, Lindvall O. Inflammation is detrimental for neurogenesis in adult brain. Proc Natl Acad Sci U S A. 2003;100:13632–7. https://doi.org/10.1073/pnas.2234031100.
27. Di Filippo M, Chiasserini D, Gardoni F, Viviani B, Tozzi A, Giampà C, et al. Effects of central and peripheral inflammation on hippocampal synaptic plasticity. Neurobiol Dis. 2013;52:229–36. https://doi.org/10.1016/j.nbd.2012.12.009.
28. Heneka MT, Carson MJ, El Khoury J, Landreth GE, Brosseron F, Feinstein DL, et al. Neuroinflammation in Alzheimer's disease. Lancet Neurol. 2015;14:388–405. https://doi.org/10.1016/S1474-4422(15)70016-5.
29. Dubbelaar ML, Kracht L, Eggen BJL, Boddeke EWGM. The kaleidoscope of microglial phenotypes. Front Immunol. 2018;9:1753. https://doi.org/10.3389/fimmu.2018.01753.
30. Olah M, Biber K, Vinet J, Boddeke HWGM. Microglia phenotype diversity. CNS Neurol Disord Drug Targets. 2011;10:108–18.
31. Cherry JD, Olschowka JA, O'Banion MK. Neuroinflammation and M2 microglia: the good, the bad, and the inflamed. J Neuroinflammation. 2014;11:98. https://doi.org/10.1186/1742-2094-11-98.
32. Ekdahl CT, Kokaia Z, Lindvall O. Brain inflammation and adult neurogenesis: the dual role of microglia. Neuroscience. 2009;158:1021–9. https://doi.org/10.1016/j.neuroscience.2008.06.052.
33. Chow JC, Young DW, Golenbock DT, Christ WJ, Gusovsky F. Toll-like receptor-4 mediates lipopolysaccharide-induced signal transduction. J Biol Chem. 1999;274:10689–92. https://doi.org/10.1074/jbc.274.16.10689.
34. Tarassishin L, Suh H-S, Lee SC. Interferon regulatory factor 3 plays an anti-inflammatory role in microglia by activating the PI3K/Akt pathway. J Neuroinflammation. 2011;8:187. https://doi.org/10.1186/1742-2094-8-187.
35. Mathur V, Burai R, Vest RT, Bonanno LN, Lehallier B, Zardeneta ME, et al. Activation of the STING-dependent type I interferon response reduces microglial reactivity and neuroinflammation. Neuron. 2017;96:1290–1302.e6. https://doi.org/10.1016/j.neuron.2017.11.032.
36. Lee JY, Sohn KH, Rhee SH, Hwang D. Saturated fatty acids, but not unsaturated fatty acids, induce the expression of cyclooxygenase-2 mediated through Toll-like receptor 4. J Biol Chem. 2001;276:16683–9. https://doi.org/10.1074/jbc.M011695200.
37. Shi H, Kokoeva MV, Inouye K, Tzameli I, Yin H, Flier JS. TLR4 links innate immunity and fatty acid-induced insulin resistance. J Clin Invest. 2006;116:3015–25. https://doi.org/10.1172/JCI28898.
38. Reyna SM, Ghosh S, Tantiwong P, Meka CSR, Eagan P, Jenkinson CP, et al. Elevated Toll-like receptor 4 expression and signaling in muscle from insulin-resistant subjects. Diabetes. 2008;57:2595–602. https://doi.org/10.2337/db08-0038.
39. Schaeffler A, Gross P, Buettner R, Bollheimer C, Buechler C, Neumeier M, et al. Fatty acid-induced induction of Toll-like receptor-4/nuclear factor-kappaB pathway in adipocytes links nutritional signalling with innate immunity. Immunology. 2009;126:233–45. https://doi.org/10.1111/j.1365-2567.2008.02892.x.
40. Wang Z, Liu D, Wang F, Liu S, Zhao S, Ling E-A, et al. Saturated fatty acids activate microglia via Toll-like receptor 4/NF-κB signalling. Br J Nutr. 2012;107:229–41. https://doi.org/10.1017/S0007114511002868.
41. Song MJ, Kim KH, Yoon JM, Kim JB. Activation of Toll-like receptor 4 is associated with insulin resistance in adipocytes. Biochem Biophys Res Commun. 2006;346:739–45. https://doi.org/10.1016/j.bbrc.2006.05.170.

42. Poggi M, Bastelica D, Gual P, Iglesias MA, Gremeaux T, Knauf C, et al. C3H/HeJ mice carrying a Toll-like receptor 4 mutation are protected against the development of insulin resistance in white adipose tissue in response to a high-fat diet. Diabetologia. 2007;50:1267–76. https://doi.org/10.1007/s00125-007-0654-8.

43. Liang C-F, Liu JT, Wang Y, Xu A, Vanhoutte PM. Toll-like receptor 4 mutation protects obese mice against endothelial dysfunction by decreasing NADPH oxidase isoforms 1 and 4. Arterioscler Thromb Vasc Biol. 2013;33:777–84. https://doi.org/10.1161/ATVBAHA.112.301087.

44. Suganami T, Mieda T, Itoh M, Shimoda Y, Kamei Y, Ogawa Y. Attenuation of obesity-induced adipose tissue inflammation in C3H/HeJ mice carrying a Toll-like receptor 4 mutation. Biochem Biophys Res Commun. 2007;354:45–9. https://doi.org/10.1016/j.bbrc.2006.12.190.

45. Kim F, Pham M, Luttrell I, Bannerman DD, Tupper J, Thaler J, et al. Toll-like receptor-4 mediates vascular inflammation and insulin resistance in diet-induced obesity. Circ Res. 2007;100:1589–96. https://doi.org/10.1161/CIRCRESAHA.106.142851.

46. Jia L, Vianna CR, Fukuda M, Berglund ED, Liu C, Tao C, et al. Hepatocyte Toll-like receptor 4 regulates obesity-induced inflammation and insulin resistance. Nat Commun. 2014;5:3878. https://doi.org/10.1038/ncomms4878.

47. Li J, Chen S, Qiang J, Wang X, Chen L, Zou D. Diet-induced obesity mediates a proinflammatory response in pancreatic β cell via Toll-like receptor 4. Cent Eur J Immunol. 2014;39:306–15. https://doi.org/10.5114/ceji.2014.45940.

48. Kim JI, Huh JY, Sohn JH, Choe SS, Lee YS, Lim CY, et al. Lipid-overloaded enlarged adipocytes provoke insulin resistance independent of inflammation. Mol Cell Biol. 2015;35:1686–99. https://doi.org/10.1128/MCB.01321-14.

49. Ding Y, Subramanian S, Montes VN, Goodspeed L, Wang S, Han C, et al. Toll-like receptor 4 deficiency decreases atherosclerosis but does not protect against inflammation in obese low-density lipoprotein receptor-deficient mice. Arterioscler Thromb Vasc Biol. 2012;32:1596–604. https://doi.org/10.1161/ATVBAHA.112.249847.

50. Vila IK, Badin P-M, Marques M-A, Monbrun L, Lefort C, Mir L, et al. Immune cell Toll-like receptor 4 mediates the development of obesity- and endotoxemia-associated adipose tissue fibrosis. Cell Rep. 2014;7:1116–29. https://doi.org/10.1016/j.celrep.2014.03.062.

51. Zhang N, Liang H, Farese RV, Li J, Musi N, Hussey SE. Pharmacological TLR4 inhibition protects against acute and chronic fat-induced insulin resistance in rats. PLoS One. 2015;10:e0132575. https://doi.org/10.1371/journal.pone.0132575.

52. Coenen KR, Gruen ML, Lee-Young RS, Puglisi MJ, Wasserman DH, Hasty AH. Impact of macrophage Toll-like receptor 4 deficiency on macrophage infiltration into adipose tissue and the artery wall in mice. Diabetologia. 2009;52:318–28. https://doi.org/10.1007/s00125-008-1221-7.

53. Saberi M, Woods N-B, de Luca C, Schenk S, Lu JC, Bandyopadhyay G, et al. Hematopoietic cell-specific deletion of Toll-like receptor 4 ameliorates hepatic and adipose tissue insulin resistance in high-fat-fed mice. Cell Metab. 2009;10:419–29. https://doi.org/10.1016/j.cmet.2009.09.006.

54. Milanski M, Degasperi G, Coope A, Morari J, Denis R, Cintra DE, et al. Saturated fatty acids produce an inflammatory response predominantly through the activation of TLR4 signaling in hypothalamus: implications for the pathogenesis of obesity. J Neurosci. 2009;29:359–70. https://doi.org/10.1523/JNEUROSCI.2760-08.2009.

55. Milanski M, Arruda AP, Coope A, Ignacio-Souza LM, Nunez CE, Roman EA, et al. Inhibition of hypothalamic inflammation reverses diet-induced insulin resistance in the liver. Diabetes. 2012;61:1455–62. https://doi.org/10.2337/db11-0390.

56. Morari J, Anhe GF, Nascimento LF, de Moura RF, Razolli D, Solon C, et al. Fractalkine (CX3CL1) is involved in the early activation of hypothalamic inflammation in experimental obesity. Diabetes. 2014;63:3770–84. https://doi.org/10.2337/db13-1495.

57. Rehli M. Of mice and men: species variations of Toll-like receptor expression. Trends Immunol. 2002;23:375–8. https://doi.org/10.1016/S1471-4906(02)02259-7.

58. Vaure C, Liu Y. A comparative review of Toll-like receptor 4 expression and functionality in different animal species. Front Immunol. 2014;5:316. https://doi.org/10.3389/fimmu.2014.00316.

59. De Luca SN, Ziko I, Sominsky L, Nguyen JCD, Dinan T, Miller AA, et al. Early life overfeeding impairs spatial memory performance by reducing microglial sensitivity to learning. J Neuroinflammation. 2016;13:112. https://doi.org/10.1186/s12974-016-0578-7.

60. Hua F, Tang H, Wang J, Prunty MC, Hua X, Sayeed I, et al. TAK-242, an antagonist for Toll-like receptor 4, protects against acute cerebral ischemia/reperfusion injury in mice. J Cereb Blood Flow Metab. 2015;35:536–42. https://doi.org/10.1038/jcbfm.2014.240.

61. Carroll JC, Rosario ER, Villamagna A, Pike CJ. Continuous and cyclic progesterone differentially interact with estradiol in the regulation of Alzheimer-like pathology in female 3xTransgenic-Alzheimer's disease mice. Endocrinology. 2010;151:2713–22. https://doi.org/10.1210/en.2009-1487.

62. Christensen A, Pike CJ. Age-dependent regulation of obesity and Alzheimer-related outcomes by hormone therapy in female 3xTg-AD mice. PLoS One. 2017;12:e0178490. https://doi.org/10.1371/journal.pone.0178490.

63. Moser VA, Pike CJ. Obesity accelerates Alzheimer-related pathology in APOE4 but not APOE3 mice. Eneuro. 2017;4. https://doi.org/10.1523/ENEURO.0077-17.2017.

64. Ayoub AE, Salm AK. Increased morphological diversity of microglia in the activated hypothalamic supraoptic nucleus. J Neurosci. 2003;23:7759–66.

65. Kozlowski C, Weimer RM. An automated method to quantify microglia morphology and application to monitor activation state longitudinally in vivo. PLoS One. 2012;7:e31814. https://doi.org/10.1371/journal.pone.0031814.

66. Plümpe T, Ehninger D, Steiner B, Klempin F, Jessberger S, Brandt M, et al. Variability of doublecortin-associated dendrite maturation in adult hippocampal neurogenesis is independent of the regulation of precursor cell proliferation. BMC Neurosci. 2006;7:77. https://doi.org/10.1186/1471-2202-7-77.

67. Hamson DK, Wainwright SR, Taylor JR, Jones BA, Watson NV, Galea LAM. Androgens increase survival of adult-born neurons in the dentate gyrus by an androgen receptor-dependent mechanism in male rats. Endocrinology. 2013;154:3294–304. https://doi.org/10.1210/en.2013-1129.

68. Breunig JJ, Silbereis J, Vaccarino FM, Sestan N, Rakic P. Notch regulates cell fate and dendrite morphology of newborn neurons in the postnatal dentate gyrus. Proc Natl Acad Sci U S A. 2007;104:20558–63. https://doi.org/10.1073/pnas.0710156104.

69. Rosario ER, Chang L, Beckett TL, Carroll JC, Paul Murphy M, Stanczyk FZ, et al. Age-related changes in serum and brain levels of androgens in male Brown Norway rats. Neuroreport. 2009;20:1534–7. https://doi.org/10.1097/WNR.0b013e328331f968.

70. van den Top M, Zhao FY, Viriyapong R, Michael NJ, Munder AC, Pryor JT, et al. The impact of ageing, fasting and high-fat diet on central and peripheral glucose tolerance and glucose-sensing neural networks in the arcuate nucleus. J Neuroendocrinol. 2017;29. https://doi.org/10.1111/jne.12528.

71. Soltis AR, Kennedy NJ, Xin X, Zhou F, Ficarro SB, Yap YS, et al. Hepatic dysfunction caused by consumption of a high-fat diet. Cell Rep. 2017;21:3317–28. https://doi.org/10.1016/j.celrep.2017.11.059.

72. Lee B-C, Lee J. Cellular and molecular players in adipose tissue inflammation in the development of obesity-induced insulin resistance. Biochim Biophys Acta. 2014;1842:446–62. https://doi.org/10.1016/j.bbadis.2013.05.017.

73. Carlsen H, Haugen F, Zadelaar S, Kleemann R, Kooistra T, Drevon CA, et al. Diet-induced obesity increases NF-kappaB signaling in reporter mice. Genes Nutr. 2009;4:215–22. https://doi.org/10.1007/s12263-009-0133-6.

74. Valdearcos M, Douglass JD, Robblee MM, Dorfman MD, Stifler DR, Bennett ML, et al. Microglial inflammatory signaling orchestrates the hypothalamic immune response to dietary excess and mediates obesity susceptibility. Cell Metab. 2017;26:185–197.e3. https://doi.org/10.1016/j.cmet.2017.05.015.

75. Gzielo K, Kielbinski M, Ploszaj J, Janeczko K, Gazdzinski SP, Setkowicz Z. Long-term consumption of high-fat diet in rats: effects on microglial and astrocytic morphology and neuronal nitric oxide synthase expression. Cell Mol Neurobiol. 2017;37:783–9. https://doi.org/10.1007/s10571-016-0417-5.

76. Bocarsly ME, Fasolino M, Kane GA, LaMarca EA, Kirschen GW, Karatsoreos IN, et al. Obesity diminishes synaptic markers, alters microglial morphology, and impairs cognitive function. Proc Natl Acad Sci U S A. 2015;112:15731–6. https://doi.org/10.1073/pnas.1511593112.

77. Chhor V, Le Charpentier T, Lebon S, Oré M-V, Celador IL, Josserand J, et al. Characterization of phenotype markers and neuronotoxic potential of polarised primary microglia in vitro. Brain Behav Immun. 2013;32:70–85. https://doi.org/10.1016/j.bbi.2013.02.005.

78. Hanisch U-K. Microglia as a source and target of cytokines. Glia. 2002;40:140–55. https://doi.org/10.1002/glia.10161.

79. Korzhevskii DE, Kirik OV. Brain microglia and microglial markers. Neurosci Behav Physiol. 2016;46:284–90. https://doi.org/10.1007/s11055-016-0231-z.

80. Bodea L-G, Wang Y, Linnartz-Gerlach B, Kopatz J, Sinkkonen L, Musgrove R, et al. Neurodegeneration by activation of the microglial complement-phagosome pathway. J Neurosci. 2014;34:8546–56. https://doi.org/10.1523/JNEUROSCI.5002-13.2014.

81. Perego C, Fumagalli S, De Simoni M-G. Temporal pattern of expression and colocalization of microglia/macrophage phenotype markers following brain ischemic injury in mice. J Neuroinflammation. 2011;8:174. https://doi.org/10.1186/1742-2094-8-174.

82. Graeber MB, Streit WJ, Kiefer R, Schoen SW, Kreutzberg GW. New expression of myelomonocytic antigens by microglia and perivascular cells following lethal motor neuron injury. J Neuroimmunol. 1990;27:121–32.

83. Hayes GM, Woodroofe MN, Cuzner ML. Microglia are the major cell type expressing MHC class II in human white matter. J Neurol Sci. 1987;80:25–37. https://doi.org/10.1016/0022-510X(87)90218-8.

84. Bö L, Mörk S, Kong PA, Nyland H, Pardo CA, Trapp BD. Detection of MHC class II-antigens on macrophages and microglia, but not on astrocytes and endothelia in active multiple sclerosis lesions. J Neuroimmunol. 1994;51:135–46.

85. Frei R, Steinle J, Birchler T, Loeliger S, Roduit C, Steinhoff D, et al. MHC class II molecules enhance Toll-like receptor mediated innate immune responses. PLoS One. 2010;5:e8808. https://doi.org/10.1371/journal.pone.0008808.

86. Zeiner PS, Preusse C, Blank A-E, Zachskorn C, Baumgarten P, Caspary L, et al. MIF receptor CD74 is restricted to microglia/macrophages, associated with a M1-polarized immune milieu and prolonged patient survival in gliomas. Brain Pathol. 2015;25:491–504. https://doi.org/10.1111/bpa.12194.

87. Cresswell P. Assembly, transport, and function of MHC class II molecules. Annu Rev Immunol. 1994;12:259–93. https://doi.org/10.1146/annurev.iy.12.040194.001355.

88. Chan P-C, Wu T-N, Chen Y-C, Lu C-H, Wabitsch M, Tian Y-F, et al. Targetted inhibition of CD74 attenuates adipose COX-2-MIF-mediated M1 macrophage polarization and retards obesity-related adipose tissue inflammation and insulin resistance. Clin Sci. 2018;132:1581–96. https://doi.org/10.1042/CS20180041.

89. Setti SE, Littlefield AM, Johnson SW, Kohman RA. Diet-induced obesity attenuates endotoxin-induced cognitive deficits. Physiol Behav. 2015;141:1–8. https://doi.org/10.1016/j.physbeh.2014.12.036.

90. Bruce KD, Gorkhali S, Given K, Coates AM, Boyle KE, Macklin WB, et al. Lipoprotein lipase is a feature of alternatively-activated microglia and may facilitate lipid uptake in the CNS during demyelination. Front Mol Neurosci. 2018;11:57. https://doi.org/10.3389/fnmol.2018.00057.

91. Gao Y, Vidal-Itriago A, Kalsbeek MJ, Layritz C, García-Cáceres C, Tom RZ, et al. Lipoprotein lipase maintains microglial innate immunity in obesity. Cell Rep. 2017;20:3034–42. https://doi.org/10.1016/j.celrep.2017.09.008.

92. Goudriaan JR, den Boer MAM, Rensen PCN, Febbraio M, Kuipers F, Romijn JA, et al. CD36 deficiency in mice impairs lipoprotein lipase-mediated triglyceride clearance. J Lipid Res. 2005;46:2175–81. https://doi.org/10.1194/jlr.M500112-JLR200.

93. Bonen A, Tandon NN, Glatz JFC, Luiken JJFP, Heigenhauser GJF. The fatty acid transporter FAT/CD36 is upregulated in subcutaneous and visceral adipose tissues in human obesity and type 2 diabetes. Int J Obes. 2006;30:877–83. https://doi.org/10.1038/sj.ijo.0803212.

94. Standeven KF, Hess K, Carter AM, Rice GI, Cordell PA, Balmforth AJ, et al. Neprilysin, obesity and the metabolic syndrome. Int J Obes. 2011;35:1031–40. https://doi.org/10.1038/ijo.2010.227.

95. Maesako M, Uemura M, Tashiro Y, Sasaki K, Watanabe K, Noda Y, et al. High fat diet enhances β-site cleavage of amyloid precursor protein (APP) via promoting β-site APP cleaving enzyme 1/adaptor protein 2/clathrin complex formation. PLoS One. 2015;10:e0131199. https://doi.org/10.1371/journal.pone.0131199.

96. Maesako M, Uemura K, Kubota M, Kuzuya A, Sasaki K, Hayashida N, et al. Exercise is more effective than diet control in preventing high fat diet-induced β-amyloid deposition and memory deficit in amyloid precursor protein transgenic mice. J Biol Chem. 2012;287:23024–33. https://doi.org/10.1074/jbcM112.367011.

97. Brandimarti P, Costa-Júnior JM, Ferreira SM, Protzek AO, Santos GJ, Carneiro EM, et al. Cafeteria diet inhibits insulin clearance by reduced insulin-degrading enzyme expression and mRNA splicing. J Endocrinol. 2013;219:173–82. https://doi.org/10.1530/JOE-13-0177.

98. Wei X, Ke B, Zhao Z, Ye X, Gao Z, Ye J. Regulation of insulin degrading enzyme activity by obesity-associated factors and pioglitazone in liver of diet-induced obese mice. PLoS One. 2014;9:e95399. https://doi.org/10.1371/journal.pone.0095399.

99. Martin E, Boucher C, Fontaine B, Delarasse C. Distinct inflammatory phenotypes of microglia and monocyte-derived macrophages in Alzheimer's disease models: effects of aging and amyloid pathology. Aging Cell. 2017;16:27–38. https://doi.org/10.1111/acel.12522.

100. Ricciarelli R, D'Abramo C, Zingg J-M, Giliberto L, Markesbery W, Azzi A, et al. CD36 overexpression in human brain correlates with beta-amyloid deposition but not with Alzheimer's disease. Free Radic Biol Med. 2004;36:1018–24. https://doi.org/10.1016/j.freeradbiomed.2004.01.007.

101. El Khoury JB, Moore KJ, Means TK, Leung J, Terada K, Toft M, et al. CD36 mediates the innate host response to beta-amyloid. J Exp Med. 2003;197:1657–66. https://doi.org/10.1084/jem.20021546.

102. Moore KJ, El Khoury J, Medeiros LA, Terada K, Geula C, Luster AD, et al. A CD36-initiated signaling cascade mediates inflammatory effects of beta-amyloid. J Biol Chem. 2002;277:47373–9. https://doi.org/10.1074/jbc.M208788200.

103. Stewart CR, Stuart LM, Wilkinson K, van Gils JM, Deng J, Halle A, et al. CD36 ligands promote sterile inflammation through assembly of a Toll-like receptor 4 and 6 heterodimer. Nat Immunol. 2010;11:155–61. https://doi.org/10.1038/ni.1836.

104. Pistell PJ, Morrison CD, Gupta S, Knight AG, Keller JN, Ingram DK, et al. Cognitive impairment following high fat diet consumption is associated with brain inflammation. J Neuroimmunol. 2010;219:25–32. https://doi.org/10.1016/j.jneuroim.2009.11.010.

105. Guillemot-Legris O, Masquelier J, Everard A, Cani PD, Alhouayek M, Muccioli GG. High-fat diet feeding differentially affects the development of inflammation in the central nervous system. J Neuroinflammation. 2016;13:206. https://doi.org/10.1186/s12974-016-0666-8.

106. Baumgarner KM, Setti S, Diaz C, Littlefield A, Jones A, Kohman RA. Diet-induced obesity attenuates cytokine production following an immune challenge. Behav Brain Res. 2014;267:33–41. https://doi.org/10.1016/j.bbr.2014.03.017.

107. Thaler JP, Yi C-X, Schur EA, Guyenet SJ, Hwang BH, Dietrich MO, et al. Obesity is associated with hypothalamic injury in rodents and humans. J Clin Invest. 2012;122:153–62. https://doi.org/10.1172/JCI59660.

108. Singhal G, Baune BT. Microglia: an interface between the loss of neuroplasticity and depression. Front Cell Neurosci. 2017;11:270. https://doi.org/10.3389/fncel.2017.00270.

109. Sastre M, Walter J, Gentleman SM. Interactions between APP secretases and inflammatory mediators. J Neuroinflammation. 2008;5:25. https://doi.org/10.1186/1742-2094-5-25.

110. Wong SS, Sun NN, Fastje CD, Witten ML, Lantz RC, Lu B, et al. Role of neprilysin in airway inflammation induced by diesel exhaust emissions. Res Rep Health Eff Inst. 2011;159:3–40.

111. Yoo DY, Kim W, Nam SM, Yoo K-Y, Lee CH, Choi JH, et al. Reduced cell proliferation and neuroblast differentiation in the dentate gyrus of high fat diet-fed mice are ameliorated by metformin and glimepiride treatment. Neurochem Res. 2011;36:2401–8. https://doi.org/10.1007/s11064-011-0566-3.

112. Kim IY, Hwang IK, Choi JW, Yoo K-Y, Kim YN, Yi SS, et al. Effects of high cholesterol diet on newly generated cells in the dentate gyrus of C57BL/6N and C3H/HeN mice. J Vet Med Sci. 2009;71:753–8.

113. Tozuka Y, Wada E, Wada K. Diet-induced obesity in female mice leads to peroxidized lipid accumulations and impairment of hippocampal neurogenesis during the early life of their offspring. FASEB J. 2009;23:1920–34. https://doi.org/10.1096/fj.08-124784.

114. Rivera P, Romero-Zerbo Y, Pavón FJ, Serrano A, López-Ávalos M-D, Cifuentes M, et al. Obesity-dependent cannabinoid modulation of proliferation in adult neurogenic regions. Eur J Neurosci. 2011;33:1577–86. https://doi.org/10.1111/j.1460-9568.2011.07650.x.

115. Cacci E, Ajmone-Cat MA, Anelli T, Biagioni S, Minghetti L. In vitro neuronal and glial differentiation from embryonic or adult neural precursor cells are differently affected by chronic or acute activation of microglia. Glia. 2008;56:412–25. https://doi.org/10.1002/glia.20616.

116. Monje ML, Toda H, Palmer TD. Inflammatory blockade restores adult hippocampal neurogenesis. Science. 2003;302:1760–5. https://doi.org/10.1126/science.1088417.

117. Moraga A, Pradillo JM, Cuartero MI, Hernández-Jiménez M, Oses M, Moro MA, et al. Toll-like receptor 4 modulates cell migration and cortical neurogenesis after focal cerebral ischemia. FASEB J. 2014;28:4710–8. https://doi.org/10.1096/fj.14-252452.

118. Mouihate A. TLR4-mediated brain inflammation halts neurogenesis: impact of hormonal replacement therapy. Front Cell Neurosci. 2014;8:146. https://doi.org/10.3389/fncel.2014.00146.

119. Kohman RA, Rhodes JS. Neurogenesis, inflammation and behavior. Brain Behav Immun. 2013;27:22–32. https://doi.org/10.1016/j.bbi.2012.09.003.

120. Hwang L-L, Wang C-H, Li T-L, Chang S-D, Lin L-C, Chen C-P, et al. Sex differences in high-fat diet-induced obesity, metabolic alterations and learning, and synaptic plasticity deficits in mice. Obesity (Silver Spring). 2010;18:463–9. https://doi.org/10.1038/oby.2009.273.

121. Jurdak N, Lichtenstein AH, Kanarek RB. Diet-induced obesity and spatial cognition in young male rats. Nutr Neurosci. 2008;11:48–54. https://doi.org/10.1179/147683008X301333.

122. Arnold SE, Lucki I, Brookshire BR, Carlson GC, Browne CA, Kazi H, et al. High fat diet produces brain insulin resistance, synaptodendritic abnormalities and altered behavior in mice. Neurobiol Dis. 2014;67:79–87. https://doi.org/10.1016/j.nbd.2014.03.011.

123. Kosari S, Badoer E, Nguyen JCD, Killcross AS, Jenkins TA. Effect of western and high fat diets on memory and cholinergic measures in the rat. Behav Brain Res. 2012;235:98–103. https://doi.org/10.1016/j.bbr.2012.07.017.

124. Kaczmarczyk MM, Machaj AS, Chiu GS, Lawson MA, Gainey SJ, York JM, et al. Methylphenidate prevents high-fat diet (HFD)-induced learning/memory impairment in juvenile mice. Psychoneuroendocrinology. 2013;38:1553–64. https://doi.org/10.1016/j.psyneuen.2013.01.004.

125. Lavin DN, Joesting JJ, Chiu GS, Moon ML, Meng J, Dilger RN, et al. Fasting induces an anti-inflammatory effect on the neuroimmune system which a high-fat diet prevents. Obesity (Silver Spring). 2011;19:1586–94. https://doi.org/10.1038/oby.2011.73.

126. Mielke JG, Nicolitch K, Avellaneda V, Earlam K, Ahuja T, Mealing G, et al. Longitudinal study of the effects of a high-fat diet on glucose regulation, hippocampal function, and cerebral insulin sensitivity in C57BL/6 mice. Behav Brain Res. 2006;175:374–82. https://doi.org/10.1016/j.bbr.2006.09.010.

127. Li L, Wang Z, Zuo Z. Chronic intermittent fasting improves cognitive functions and brain structures in mice. PLoS One. 2013;8:e66069. https://doi.org/10.1371/journal.pone.0066069.

128. Tucker KR, Godbey SJ, Thiebaud N, Fadool DA. Olfactory ability and object memory in three mouse models of varying body weight, metabolic hormones, and adiposity. Physiol Behav. 2012;107:424–32. https://doi.org/10.1016/j.physbeh.2012.09.007.

129. Valladolid-Acebes I, Fole A, Martín M, Morales L, Cano MV, Ruiz-Gayo M, et al. Spatial memory impairment and changes in hippocampal morphology are triggered by high-fat diets in adolescent mice. Is there a role of leptin? Neurobiol Learn Mem. 2013;106:18–25. https://doi.org/10.1016/j.nlm.2013.06.012.

130. Spencer SJ, D'Angelo H, Soch A, Watkins LR, Maier SF, Barrientos RM. High-fat diet and aging interact to produce neuroinflammation and impair hippocampal- and amygdalar-dependent memory. Neurobiol Aging. 2017;58:88–101. https://doi.org/10.1016/j.neurobiolaging.2017.06.014.

131. Kanoski SE, Davidson TL. Different patterns of memory impairments accompany short- and longer-term maintenance on a high-energy diet. J Exp Psychol Anim Behav Process. 2010;36:313–9. https://doi.org/10.1037/a0017228.

132. Murray AJ, Knight NS, Cochlin LE, McAleese S, Deacon RMJ, Rawlins JNP, et al. Deterioration of physical performance and cognitive function in rats with short-term high-fat feeding. FASEB J. 2009;23:4353–60. https://doi.org/10.1096/fj.09-139691.

133. Hsu TM, Konanur VR, Taing L, Usui R, Kayser BD, Goran MI, et al. Effects of sucrose and high fructose corn syrup consumption on spatial memory function and hippocampal neuroinflammation in adolescent rats. Hippocampus. 2015;25:227–39. https://doi.org/10.1002/hipo.22368.

134. Dik MG, Jonker C, Comijs HC, Deeg DJH, Kok A, Yaffe K, et al. Contribution of metabolic syndrome components to cognition in older individuals. Diabetes Care. 2007;30:2655–60. https://doi.org/10.2337/dc06-1190.

135. Yaffe K, Haan M, Blackwell T, Cherkasova E, Whitmer RA, West N. Metabolic syndrome and cognitive decline in elderly Latinos: findings from the Sacramento Area Latino Study of Aging study. J Am Geriatr Soc. 2007;55:758–62. https://doi.org/10.1111/j.1532-5415.2007.01139.x.

136. Spyridaki EC, Simos P, Avgoustinaki PD, Dermitzaki E, Venihaki M, Bardos AN, et al. The association between obesity and fluid intelligence impairment is mediated by chronic low-grade inflammation. Br J Nutr. 2014;112:1724–34. https://doi.org/10.1017/S0007114514002207.

137. Bell RD, Winkler EA, Singh I, Sagare AP, Deane R, Wu Z, et al. Apolipoprotein E controls cerebrovascular integrity via cyclophilin A. Nature. 2012;485:512–6. https://doi.org/10.1038/nature11087.

138. Zhao Y, Lukiw WJ. Microbiome-generated amyloid and potential impact on amyloidogenesis in Alzheimer's disease (AD). J Nat Sci. 2015;1(7):e138.

5

Hashimoto's thyroiditis induces neuroinflammation and emotional alterations in euthyroid mice

Yao-Jun Cai[1], Fen Wang[1], Zhang-Xiang Chen[1], Li Li[1], Hua Fan[1], Zhang-Bi Wu[1], Jin-Fang Ge[2], Wen Hu[3], Qu-Nan Wang[4*] and De-Fa Zhu[1*] (iD)

Abstract

Background: Although studies have reported an increased risk for mood disorders in Hashimoto's thyroiditis (HT) patients even in the euthyroid state, the mechanisms involved remain unclear. Neuroinflammation may play a key role in the etiology of mood disorders in humans and behavioral disturbances in rodents. Therefore, this study established a euthyroid HT model in mice and investigated whether HT itself was capable of triggering neuroinflammation accompanied by emotional alterations.

Methods: Experimental HT was induced by immunizing NOD mice with thyroglobulin and adjuvant twice. Four weeks after the last challenge, mice were tested for anxiety-like behavior in the open field and elevated plus maze tests and depression-like behavior in the forced swimming and tail suspension tests. Then, animals were sacrificed for thyroid-related parameter measure as well as detection of cellular and molecular events associated with neuroinflammation. The changes in components of central serotonin signaling were also investigated.

Results: HT mice showed intrathyroidal monocyte infiltration and rising serum thyroid autoantibody levels accompanied by normal thyroid function, which defines euthyroid HT in humans. These mice displayed more anxiety- and depressive-like behaviors than controls. HT mice further showed microglia and astrocyte activation in the frontal cortex detected by immunohistochemistry, real-time RT-PCR, and transmission electron microscopy (TEM). These observations were also accompanied by enhanced gene expression of proinflammatory cytokines *IL-1β* and *TNF-α* in the frontal cortex. Despite this inflammatory response, no signs of neuronal apoptosis were visible by the TUNEL staining and TEM in the frontal cortex of HT mice. Additionally, IDO1 and SERT, key serotonin-system-related genes activated by proinflammatory cytokines, were upregulated in HT mice, accompanied by reduced frontal cortex serotonin levels.

Conclusions: Our results are the first to suggest that HT induces neuroinflammation and alters related serotonin signaling in the euthyroid state, which may underlie the deleterious effects of HT itself on emotional function.

Keywords: Hashimoto's thyroiditis, Neuroinflammation, Anxiety, Depression, Serotonin

Background

Hashimoto's thyroiditis (HT) is a frequent autoimmune thyroid disease, affecting approximately 5% of the general population, especially women [1]. HT is characterized by intrathyroidal monocyte infiltration along with rising serum autoantibodies, such as anti-thyroglobulin antibody (anti-Tg) and anti-thyroid peroxidase antibody (anti-TPO), and is the leading cause of hypothyroidism worldwide [2]. However, most patients (approximately 79.3%) show normal thyroid function at diagnosis [3] and may be euthyroid for many years [2]. Hypothyroidism may lead to neuropsychological deficits, including depression and anxiety [4]. Only in recent years, a high prevalence of psychiatric involvement in HT patients has been increasingly recognized, independent of thyroid function [5–9]. Symptoms of depression and anxiety are more common in euthyroid HT patients than in the general population,

* Correspondence: wqn@ahmu.edu.cn; zdfa0168@sina.com
[4]Department of Toxicology, School of Public Health, Anhui Medical University, Hefei 230032, China
[1]Department of Endocrinology, Anhui Geriatric Institute, the First Affiliated Hospital of Anhui Medical University, Hefei 230032, China
Full list of author information is available at the end of the article

with up to 52.9% demonstrating affective illness [7]. Neuroimaging data of euthyroid HT patients, even those without psychiatric symptoms, reveals cerebral perfusion impairments, particularly in the frontal cortex [10], a key brain region for the control of emotional behaviors [11]. In line with this, another imaging study showed decreased gray matter density in the left inferior frontal gyrus in these patients [12]. In addition, a severe neuropsychiatric disorder independent of thyroid status has been described to exceptionally target patients suffering with HT [13, 14]. Taken together, these data strongly suggest a primary brain-specific mechanism that is independent of thyroid hormone level. However, the mechanisms of brain injury responsible for the psychological impairments in the context of euthyroid HT remain unclear.

HT is the most prevalent autoimmune disease, frequently co-occurring with other autoimmunological diseases [15], including rheumatoid arthritis and systemic lupus erythematosus. These illness have also been found to present a high comorbidity with depression and anxiety [16, 17], the mechanism of which has been reported to be associated with significant neuroinflammation [17, 18]. Neuroinflammation is an essential innate response against brain injury. However, uncontrolled neuroinflammation can result in a series of deleterious consequences involving brain cells, immune cells, and signaling molecules [19]. Glial cells, including microglia and astroglia, are the immune cells of the central nervous system and the main cellular regulators of neuroinflammation [20]. Normally, glial cells exist in the resting state, but under pathological conditions, they become over-activated and release a plethora of neurotoxic species, such as proinflammatory cytokine interleukin-1β (IL-1β), tumor necrosis factor-α (TNF-α), and interleukin-6 (IL-6) [20]. These events appear to negatively impact the synthesis and reuptake of neurotransmitters relevant to mood regulation, especially serotonin (5-HT) [21]. As such, neuroinflammation, characterized by neuroglia activation and the related generation of pro-inflammatory cytokines, has been acknowledged as a triggering factor for psychiatric conditions [22, 23]. Given the significant role of neuroinflammation in mental pathology, we hypothesize that neuroinflammation may provide a mechanism for the pathogenesis of psychological impairments in the context of euthyroid HT.

To test this hypothesis, this study built a classical model for the human disease HT in which female NOD mice were immunized with thyroglobulin [24] and investigated whether HT itself was capable of triggering neuroinflammation accompanied by anxiety/depressive-like behaviors in mice. As the frontal cortex is reported to be predominantly affected in euthyroid patients with HT [10, 12] and play a substantial role in mood regulation [11], we focused on the frontal cortex and set out to examine the cellular

and molecular events associated with neuroinflammation, such as the activation status of microglia and astrocytes as well as the expression of proinflammatory cytokines IL-1β, TNF-α, and IL-6. The consequences of such inflammation on the neurons and the components of serotonin signaling were also examined.

Methods

Animals

Female NOD mice (8–9 weeks old; 22~25 g) were obtained from Beijing HFK Bioscience Co., Ltd. (Beijing, China) and randomly assigned into two groups: the control group (Con group, $n = 10$) and Hashimoto's thyroiditis group (HT group, $n = 10$). These mice were housed in cohorts of three to four under standard laboratory conditions (23 ± 2 °C, a 12-h light/12-h dark cycle, $55 \pm 5\%$ humidity) and had ad libitum access to tap water and rodent chow. The NOD mouse strain is a common model of autoimmune diseases. The animals spontaneously develop autoimmune diabetes with aging. Considerable evidence has confirmed that diabetes in NOD mice can be inhibited by a single injection of complete Freund's adjuvant [25–27], so this condition may not be a major issue when NOD mice, following immunization with thyroglobulin in complete Freund's adjuvant, are used for HT in this study [24].

Immunization and experimental design

After 7 days of acclimatizing, mice in the HT group were challenged with 25 μg porcine thyroglobulin (Tg; Sigma-Aldrich, USA) emulsified in complete Freund's adjuvant (CFA; Sigma-Aldrich, USA) injected subcutaneously at the base of the tail, and with a booster injection of an equal dose of Tg in incomplete Freund's adjuvant (IFA; Sigma-Aldrich, USA) performed 14 days later. Mice treated with phosphate buffered saline (PBS) instead of Tg at the same time served as controls. Four weeks after the second challenge, the behavioral and biochemical parameters of all mice were evaluated (please see Fig. 1).

Behavioral tests

Behavioral tests were performed to examine the anxiety/depression-like states in animals. Mice were taken to the test room 60 min before the test. Behavioral procedures were conducted between 0830 and 1200 h in a dim and quiet room. The observers were blind to the experimental design. During the test, all animals were tracked and recorded by ANY-Maze™ Video Tracking Software (Stoelting Co., Illinois, USA) with a digital camera.

Open field test (OFT)

The OFT is widely applied to test motor and anxiety-like behavior of rodents in a novel environment [28, 29]. The equipment consisted of a black square arena (40 × 40 cm)

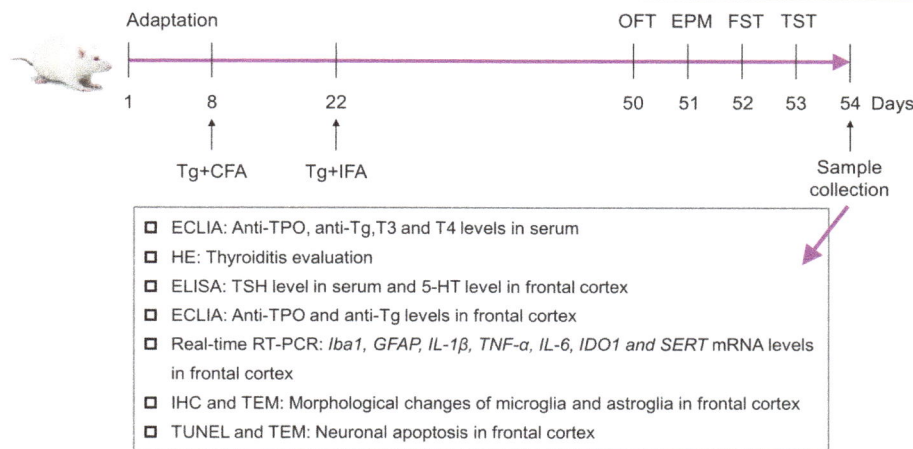

Fig. 1 Experiment schedule. Annotations: Tg, thyroglobulin; CFA, complete Freund's adjuvant; IFA, incomplete Freund's adjuvant; OFT, open field test; EPM, elevated plus maze; FST, forced swimming test; TST, tail suspension test; Anti-TPO: anti-thyroid peroxidase antibody; Anti-Tg: anti-thyroglobulin antibody; T3: triiodothyronine; T4: thyroxin; TSH: thyroid-stimulating hormone; 5-HT: serotonin; Iba1: ionized calcium-binding adapter molecule 1; GFAP: glial fibrillary acidic protein; IL-1β: interleukin-1β; TNF-α: tumor necrosis factor-α; IL-6: interleukin-6; IDO1: indoleamine-2,3-dioxygenase; SERT: serotonin transporter

with walls of 40 cm in height. The computer defined the grid lines dividing the box floor into 16 equal-sized squares, with the central four squares regarded as the center. Each mouse was gently placed at one corner of the arena facing the wall and videotaped for 5 min. Time in the center, entries into the center, total moving distance, mean speed, rearing number, and grooming number were analyzed. After each test, the equipment was wiped down with ethanol.

Elevated plus maze (EPM)
The EPM is a well-validated instrument used to analyze anxiety-like traits in rodents [28]. The maze (80 cm in height from the ground) is made up of two opposite open arms (30 cm × 5 cm, without edges), two opposite closed arms (30 cm × 5 cm × 15 cm), and a central zone (5 cm × 5 cm). Each animal was gently mildly placed in the central area facing an open arm and left to move freely for 5 min. Open-arm entries, open-arm time, the percentage of open/total-arm entries, and the percentage of open/total-arm time were recorded and analyzed. After each test, the equipment was wiped down with ethanol.

Forced swimming test (FST)
The FST was applied to measure depressive-like behavior based on previously described methods [30]. Each mouse was gently placed into a plexiglass cylinder (30 cm in height, 11 cm in diameter) filled with 25 cm of tap water (24 ± 1 °C) for a 6-min test. The trial was videotaped for later manual summation of immobility time during the final 4 min by using a stopwatch. Immobility, defined as floating with only the small movements required to keep the head above water, was evaluated by

two observers blind to experimental design and averaged. After each trial, animals were towel-dried, placed under a heat lamp, and returned to the housing cage. The water was replaced in between mice.

Tail suspension test (TST)
The TST was applied to measure depressive-like behavior as described by Ge et al [29]. In brief, each animal was hung by adhesive tape and suspended from a fixed hook (50 cm in height from the floor) for 6 min. The trial was videotaped for later manual summation of immobility time during the final 4 min by using a stopwatch. Immobility, defined as no active movements except for respiration and whisker movement, was evaluated by two observers blind to experimental design and averaged. After each test, the apparatus was cleaned.

Tissue preparation
On the last day following the TST, mice were deeply anesthetized and randomly sacrificed in the morning (09:00–11:30 am). Blood, the thyroid, and the brain were collected immediately. Blood samples were centrifuged for measuring serological parameters. The thyroids were collected for histopathology. The brains was carefully dissected on ice and randomly assigned for later assay: right frontal lobes for electrochemiluminescence immunoassay, enzyme-linked immunosorbent assay, and transmission electron microscopy and left frontal lobes for immunohistochemistry, TUNEL staining, and real-time RT-PCR.

Electrochemiluminescence immunoassay (ECLIA)
Serum samples were kept at − 80 °C until use. The levels of serum triiodothyronine (T3), thyroxin (T4), anti-TPO, and

anti-Tg were quantified through ECLIA on Cobas e411 immunoassay analyzer (Roche, Mannheim, Germany). The procedures for ECLIA were as described in detail elsewhere [31]. In addition, the frontal cortex tissues were homogenized in PBS at a ratio of 1:9 (weight to volume) and then centrifuged at 12,000g for 20 min at 4 °C. The supernatants were collected for an analysis of protein content using the BCA method and then for 5-HT content measure as well as detection of thyroid autoantibody levels. Frontal cortex anti-TPO and anti-Tg levels in mice were measured with ECLIA and modified by the corresponding protein concentration. Data were expressed as international units per milligram protein of brain issue.

Enzyme-linked immunosorbent assay (ELISA)

The levels of thyroid-stimulating hormone (TSH) in serum and 5-HT in the frontal cortex were analyzed utilizing ELISA kits (TSH: USCN Life Science Inc., Wuhan, China; 5-HT: Enzo Life Science, NY, USA) [32, 33], in accordance with the manufacturer's guidelines. Data were expressed as picograms per milliliter of serum or picograms per milligram protein of brain issue.

Hematoxylin and eosin (HE)

For histopathology, fresh thyroid tissues were fixed and processed for HE. From each animal, five noncontiguous coronal sections were used to examine thyroid histopathology. The thyroiditis classification standard was based on the percentage of thyroid infiltrated, as previously described [24]: 0 = absence of infiltrate; 1 = interstitial accumulation of inflammatory cells around one or two follicles; 2 = one or two foci of inflammatory cells reaching the size of a follicle; 3 = 10–40% inflammatory cells infiltration; 4 = greater than 40% inflammatory cells infiltration. The histological scores were evaluated and averaged by two investigators blind to experimental design.

Immunohistochemistry (IHC)

The fixed left hemispheres were processed for paraffin embedding. Serial coronal sections (5 μm thick) were cut at the levels of the frontal cortex following a mouse brain atlas [34]. Histological sections were used to immunostain ionized calcium-binding adapter molecule 1 (Iba1, Wako) and glial fibrillary acidic protein (GFAP, Abcam). Iba1 immunolabeling was able to identify activated microglia characterized by enlarged, darkened soma and thickened processes [35]. GFAP immunolabeling allowed for identification of activated astrocytes as demonstrated by hypertrophy of the cell body and stem processes [36]. For immunohistochemical analysis, five sections (1/5 serial sections) per antibody were used. Sections were dewaxed in xylene and rehydrated through gradient ethanol. After optimum antigen retrieval and quenching endogenous peroxidase, sections were incubated overnight at 4 °C with different primary antibodies, such as rabbit anti-Iba1 (1:500) or rabbit anti-GFAP (1:2000). Subsequently, appropriate secondary antibodies were used, followed by incubation with avidin-biotin complex (Zsgb-bio, Beijing, China). Finally, chromogen was added to each section and counterstained with hematoxylin.

For histopathological analysis, slides were photographed with a Nikon 80i microscope (Nikon, Tokyo, Japan). In each section, three nonoverlapping fields were randomly selected in the frontal cortex at magnification × 100. The numbers of activated microglia and astroglia in the frontal cortex were calculated [37, 38] . In addition to cell counting, Iba1 and GFAP immunoreactivity was analyzed by determining the percentage of Iba1 or GFAP-stained area, respectively, as described previously [38, 39]. All images were analyzed by two blinded observers using the public domain NIH ImageJ Program.

Transmission electron microscopy (TEM)

For ultrastructure studies of microglia, astrocytes, and neurons, the frontal cortex in HT mice and the equivalent area in Con mice were obtained according to the mouse brain atlas. The entire TEM procedure was well described in our previous study [40]. Observations of neuroglia and neurons were made using magnifications ranging from 8000 to 12,000×.

Terminal deoxynucleotidyl transferase-mediated dUTP-biotin nick end labeling (TUNEL) staining

Apoptotic neurons in the frontal cortex were visualized using a TUNEL kit (Roche, Basel, Switzerland) following the manufacturer's protocol. Briefly, serial coronal sections from the left frontal cortex were dewaxed in xylene and rehydrated through gradient ethanol. After rinsing with PBS, the sections were incubated with proteinase K solution at 37 °C for 20 min. Then they were incubated at 37 °C for 2 h with TUNEL reaction mixture in a dark, humidified chamber. Following five PBS washes, the nuclei were stained with DAPI (Servicebio, Wuhan, China) at room temperature for 10 min and slides were coverslipped. TUNEL-positive signals in the frontal cortex were examined using a fluorescent microscope (Nikon Eclipse C1).

RNA purification and real-time RT-PCR

Total RNA was extracted from the frontal cortex using TRI reagent (Invitrogen, Carlsbad, CA) and treated with RNase-free DNase followed by reverse transcription with AMV (Promega, Wisconsin, USA) according to the manufacturer's guidelines. The primers used for PCR are listed as follows: *Iba1*: Forward Primer (FP) - CTT GAA GCG AAT GCT GGA GAA, Reverse Primer (RP) - GGC AGC TCG GAG ATA GCT TT; *GFAP*: FP - CGG AGA CGC ATC ACC TCTG, RP - TGG AGG AGT CAT TCG AGA

CAA; *IL-1β*: FP - GAA ATG CCC CTT TTG ACA GTG, RP - TGG ATG CTC TCA TCA GGA CAG; *TNF-α*: FP - CAG GCG GTG CCT ATG TCTC, RP - CGA TCA CCC CGA AGT TCA GTAG; *IL-6*: FP - CTG CAA GAG ACT TCC ATC CAG, RP - AGT GGT ATA GAC AGG TCT GTT GG; *IDO1*: FP - TGG CGT ATG TGT GGA ACCG, RP - CTC GCA GTA GGG AAC AGC AA; *SERT*: FP - CTC CGC AGT TCC CAG TAC AAG, RP - CAC GGC ATA GCC AAT GAC AGA; *18S*: FP - GTA ACC CGT TGA ACC CCA TT, RP - CCA TCC AAT CGG TAG TAG CG. The PCR was conducted on a Light Cycler® 480 Instrument (Roche, Mannheim, Germany) with an initial hold step (95 °C for 5 min) and 50 cycles of 15 s at 95 °C, 15 s at 60 °C, and 30 s at 72 °C. Relative mRNA expression was analyzed using the $2^{-\Delta\Delta Ct}$ method and normalized to the 18s rRNA levels.

Statistical analysis

All statistical analyses were performed using GraphPad Prism 5.0 (San Diego, CA, USA). Values are presented as the mean ± standard error (SEM). Mann-Whitney U test was used to analyze the severity of thyroiditis. The other data were compared by unpaired two-tailed Student's t test. The significance criterion was set at p value < 0.05.

Results

Building a euthyroid HT model in mice

As depicted in Fig. 2a, histological examination showed that control mice had intact thyroid follicles with an even distribution, and monocyte infiltration was hardly found in thyroid tissues. In contrast, HT mice displayed significant thyroid enlargement with disorderly and destroyed thyroid follicles, and monocyte infiltration was found more or less in thyroid tissues. Further quantitative analysis revealed that the severity of thyroiditis in HT mice was significantly higher than that in controls (Fig. 2b). On the other hand, as seen in Fig. 2c–g, serum concentrations of thyroid autoantibodies (anti-TPO and anti-Tg) in the HT group were apparently higher than those in the Con group (Fig. 2c, d), while no differences in serum T3, T4, or TSH levels (Fig. 2e–g) was detected between groups. Moreover, frontal cortex levels of anti-Tg were significantly higher in HT mice than those in controls (Fig. 3a). As well, there was a similar, albeit not significant, tendency for frontal cortex anti-TPO levels between groups (p = 0.09, Fig. 3b). Taken together, these findings indicated that a euthyroid HT model was successfully established in mice. Since NOD mice spontaneously develop autoimmune diabetes, we examined serum glucose levels in all mice using a glucose analyzer (Roche, Indianapolis, IN), and no significant difference was detected in serum glucose levels between Con mice and HT mice (5.50 ± 0.55 vs. 6.31 ± 0.52 mmol/L, p = 0.30, n = 10), in line with previous studies [24, 25].

Euthyroid HT induces anxiety-like behavior in mice

As depicted in Fig. 4, anxiety-like behavior was tested in animals by the OFT and EPM. When exposed to the OFT,

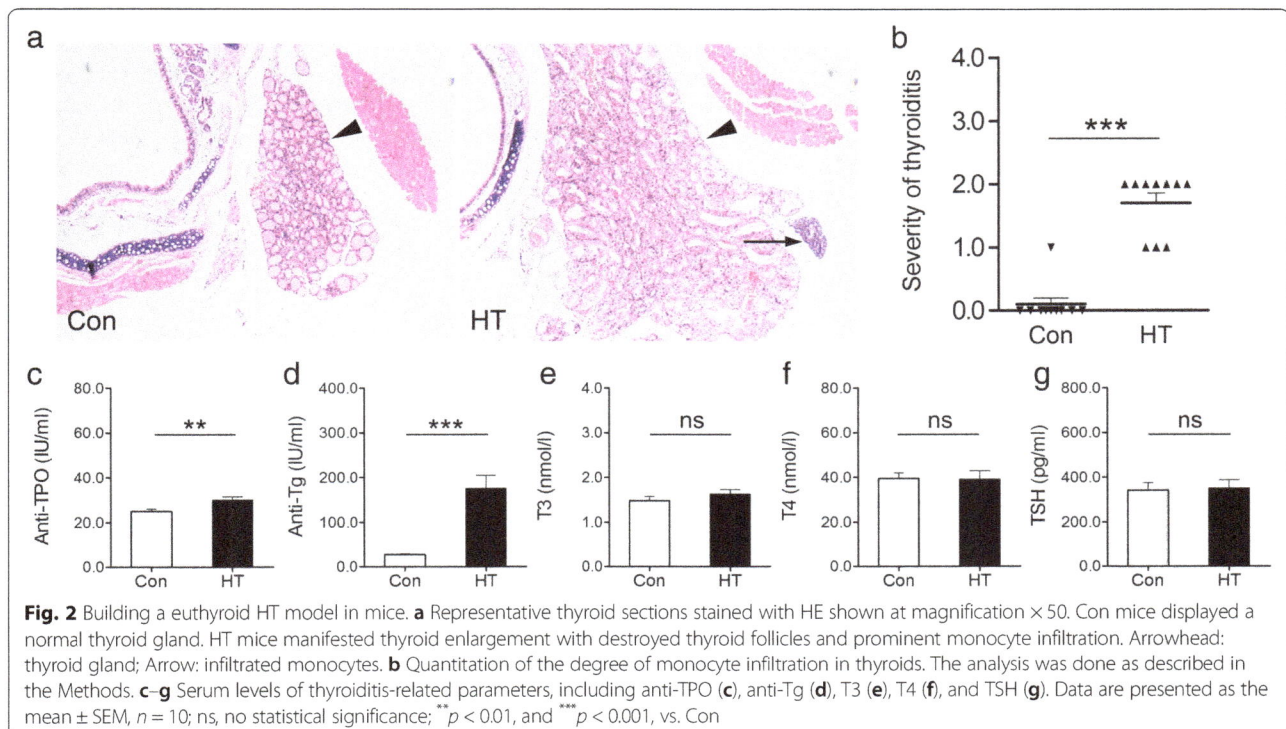

Fig. 2 Building a euthyroid HT model in mice. **a** Representative thyroid sections stained with HE shown at magnification × 50. Con mice displayed a normal thyroid gland. HT mice manifested thyroid enlargement with destroyed thyroid follicles and prominent monocyte infiltration. Arrowhead: thyroid gland; Arrow: infiltrated monocytes. **b** Quantitation of the degree of monocyte infiltration in thyroids. The analysis was done as described in the Methods. **c–g** Serum levels of thyroiditis-related parameters, including anti-TPO (**c**), anti-Tg (**d**), T3 (**e**), T4 (**f**), and TSH (**g**). Data are presented as the mean ± SEM, n = 10; ns, no statistical significance; **p < 0.01, and ***p < 0.001, vs. Con

HT mice made significantly fewer entries into and spent less time in the central zone than did control mice (Fig. 4b, c), while motor function examined by total distance and mean speed did not differ between groups (Fig. 4d, e). In the EPM, HT mice tended to spend less time in and made fewer entries into the open arms relative to control animals (Fig. 4i, j). Additionally, HT mice exhibited a significant decrement in the percentage of open-arm time and number of open-arm entries (Fig. 4k, l).

Euthyroid HT induces depressive-like behavior in mice

As depicted in Fig. 5, depressive-like behavior was evaluated in animals by the FST and TST. In the FST, HT mice showed a significant elevation in immobility time compared to control mice (Fig. 5a). This behavioral pattern was also detected in the TST, with HT mice spending more time in immobility state (Fig. 5b). Consistent with these results, rearing and grooming actions as assessed during the OFT were markedly reduced in HT mice compared to those in control mice (Fig. 4f, g), suggestive of a depressive-like state.

Euthyroid HT induces microglia and astroglia activation in the frontal cortex

Microglia and astroglia are the main executors in the process of neuroinflammation [20]. Therefore, we examined the activation status of microglia and astrocytes in the frontal cortex of mice from both groups by using immunohistochemistry, real-time RT-PCR, and TEM. Representative images of Iba-1 (for microglia) and GFAP (for astrocytes) staining are shown in Fig. 6a, b. We noted that there was an apparent increase in microglial activation in HT mice compared to that in controls, as demonstrated by the greater numbers of activated microglia and higher percentages of Iba1-stained areas in the captured photographs (Fig. 6c). Similarly, the

astrocytes also showed intense activation, identified by more activated cells and greater areas of GFAP expression in HT mice than in controls (Fig. 6d). These immunohistochemical results demonstrated that euthyroid HT induced microglia and astroglia activation in the frontal cortex. A quantitative analysis of Iba1 and GFAP mRNA levels in the frontal cortex (Fig. 6e) confirmed these results.

We also observed the ultrastructural features of glial cells by using TEM (Fig. 7). In HT mice, an intense microglial reaction was observed in the frontal cortex. The activated microglia displayed an enlarged nucleus with large, dense clumps of heterochromatin beneath the nuclear envelope. The cytoplasm of glial cells from HT mice contained more lysosomes, including primary lysosomes and secondary lysosomes, than that of control mice (Fig. 7b). These pathological features were associated with phagocytic cells [41]. In addition, the astrocytes, identified by their classical appearance of a narrow rim of chromatin beneath the nuclear membrane, also showed signs of activation in HT mice. These cells tended to show the features involved in active proteosynthesis [42], such as a well-developed Golgi apparatus, some endoplasmic reticulum, and many mitochondria, in HT mice (Fig. 7d).

Euthyroid HT promotes proinflammatory cytokine expression in the frontal cortex

Activated neuroglia are widely accepted to be able to produce classical proinflammatory cytokines, such as IL-1β, TNF-α, and IL-6 [19]. Accordingly, we probed expression of the cytokines by real-time RT-PCR. Here, frontal cortex expression of $IL-1\beta$ and $TNF-\alpha$ was significantly upregulated in HT mice compared to the expression in controls (Fig. 8a, b). In line with this, there was a tendency (albeit not significant) for higher $IL-6$ expression in the frontal

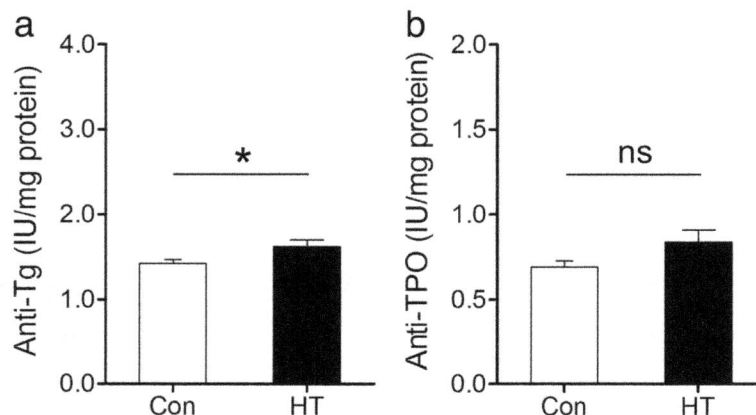

Fig. 3 Frontal cortex levels of anti-Tg and anti-TPO in mice. ECLIA was performed to detect thyroid autoantibody levels in mouse brain homogenate supernatant. **a** Frontal cortex anti-Tg levels. **b** Frontal cortex anti-TPO levels. Data are presented as the mean ± SEM, $n = 7$; ns, no statistical significance; $^*p < 0.05$, vs. Con

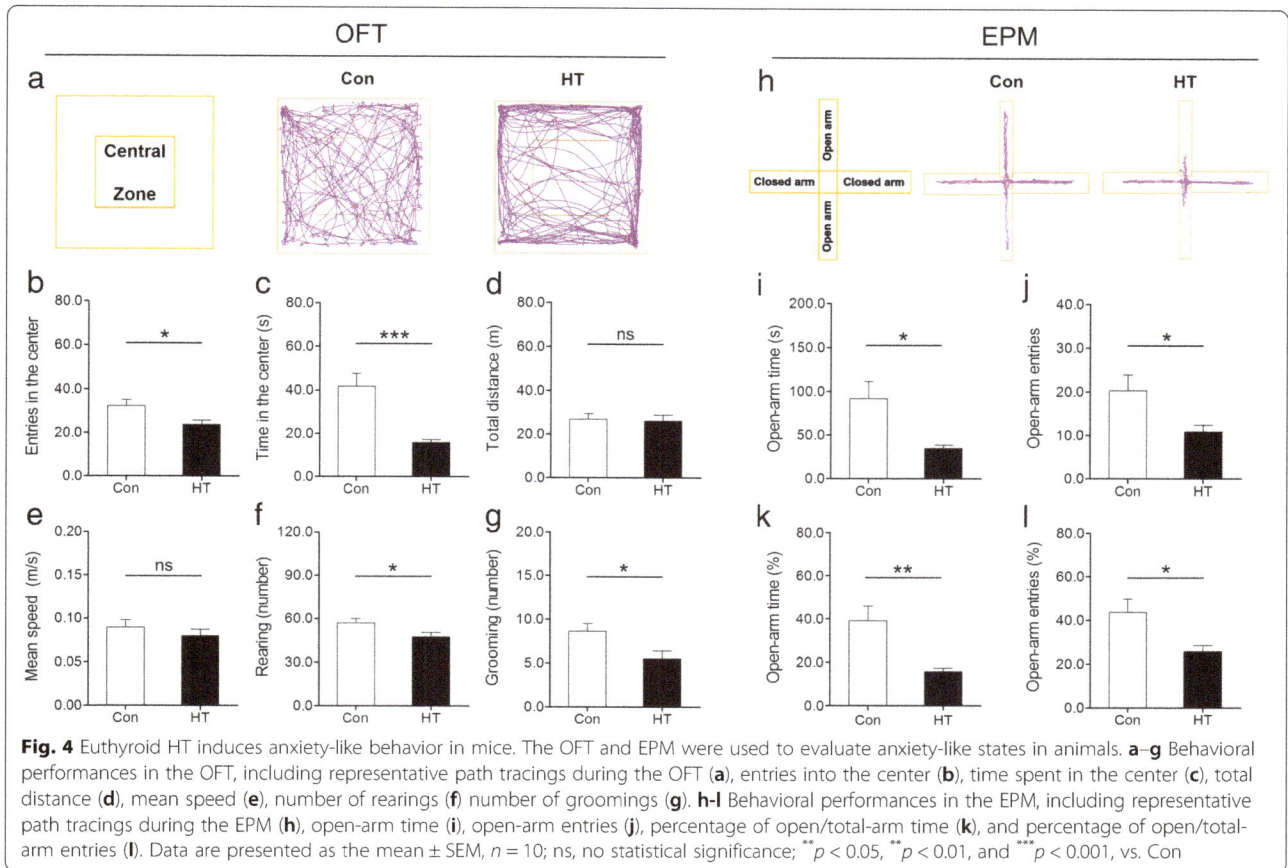

Fig. 4 Euthyroid HT induces anxiety-like behavior in mice. The OFT and EPM were used to evaluate anxiety-like states in animals. **a–g** Behavioral performances in the OFT, including representative path tracings during the OFT (**a**), entries into the center (**b**), time spent in the center (**c**), total distance (**d**), mean speed (**e**), number of rearings (**f**) number of groomings (**g**). **h-l** Behavioral performances in the EPM, including representative path tracings during the EPM (**h**), open-arm time (**i**), open-arm entries (**j**), percentage of open/total-arm time (**k**), and percentage of open/total-arm entries (**l**). Data are presented as the mean ± SEM, $n = 10$; ns, no statistical significance; $^{**}p < 0.05$, $^{**}p < 0.01$, and $^{***}p < 0.001$, vs. Con

cortex of HT mice than in that of controls ($p = 0.08$, Fig. 8c).

Euthyroid HT does not induce neuronal apoptosis in the frontal cortex

In this study, we performed TUNEL staining and TEM to identify neuronal apoptosis in the frontal cortex. As shown in Fig. 9a, we did not observe any changes in TUNEL-positive neurons in the frontal cortex between groups. In addition, ultrastructure of frontal cortex neurons in HT

mice was similar to Con mice with the nucleus with intact nuclear membranes and evenly distributed chromatin (Fig. 9b). There were no apoptotic features, such as chromatin margination or nuclear condensation [43], in the neurons examined.

Euthyroid HT alters 5-HT signaling in the frontal cortex

Since our data clearly showed inflammation induction in the frontal cortex of HT mice, we further extended the work to study key mediators involved in the central 5-HT

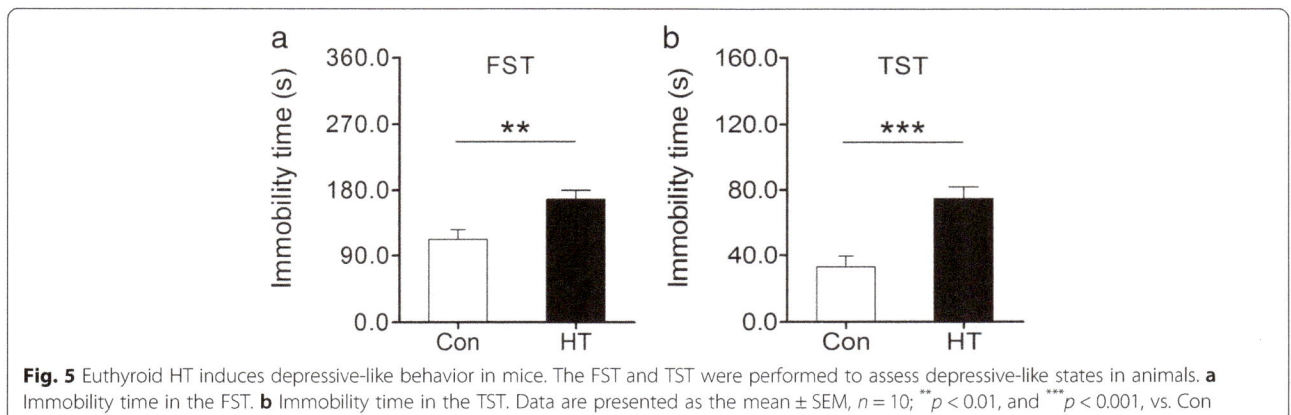

Fig. 5 Euthyroid HT induces depressive-like behavior in mice. The FST and TST were performed to assess depressive-like states in animals. **a** Immobility time in the FST. **b** Immobility time in the TST. Data are presented as the mean ± SEM, $n = 10$; $^{**}p < 0.01$, and $^{***}p < 0.001$, vs. Con

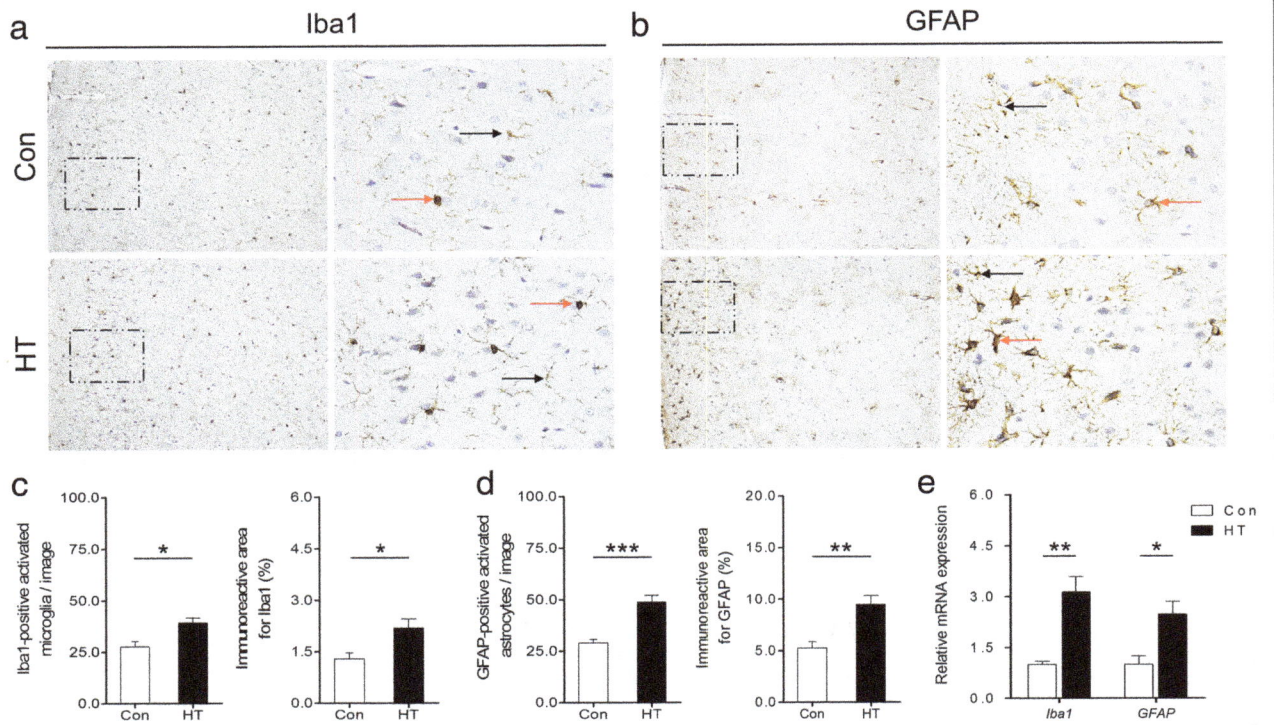

Fig. 6 Euthyroid HT induces microglia and astroglia activation in the frontal cortex. IHC and real-time RT-PCR were performed to assess the activation state of microglia and astrocytes in animals. **a, b** Representative images of Iba1 (microglia marker) and GFAP (astrocyte marker) staining in the frontal cortex. Each right-hand panel (× 400) depicts a magnified image of the boxed area of the corresponding image in the left panel (× 100). Black arrows indicate resting microglia or astroglia. Red arrows indicate activated microglia or astroglia. **c** Quantitative analysis of Iba1 immunoreactivity. **d** Quantitative analysis of GFAP immunoreactivity. **e** PCR analysis of *Iba1* and *GFAP*. Data are presented as the mean ± SEM, $n = 5$; *$p < 0.05$, **$p < 0.01$, and ***$p < 0.001$, vs. Con

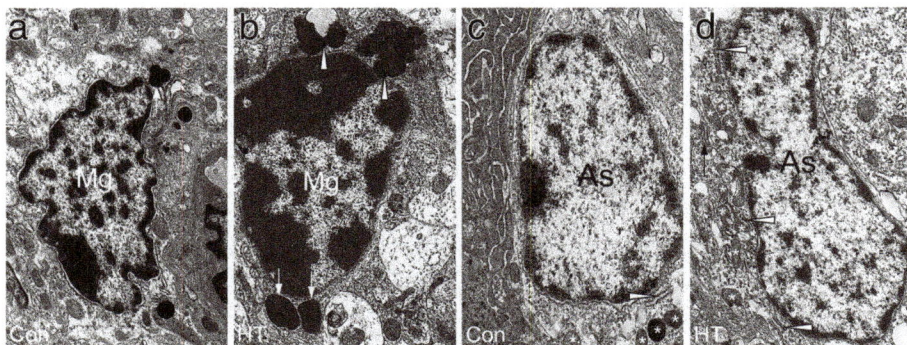

Fig. 7 Ultrastructural observations of microglia and astrocytes in the frontal cortex. **a, b** Representative TEM images of microglia. The control group (**a**) showed an irregular nucleolus with chromatin condensation beneath the nuclear membrane and a primary lysosome (arrow). In contrast, the HT group (**b**) showed an enlarged nucleolus with increased lysosomes including primary lysosomes (arrows) and secondary lysosomes (arrowheads). Mg, microglia. Magnification × 12,000. **c, d** Representative TEM images of astrocytes. The control group (**c**) showed the classical appearance of astrocyte with a narrow rim of chromatin beneath the nuclear membrane. The cytoplasm was pale, contained an endoplasmic reticulum (arrowheads) and a few mitochondria (asterisk). In contrast, the astroglia in the HT group (**d**) had an organelle-rich cytoplasm that included a well-developed Golgi apparatus (arrow), some endoplasmic reticulum (arrowheads), and many mitochondria (asterisks). As, astroglia. Magnification × 10,000

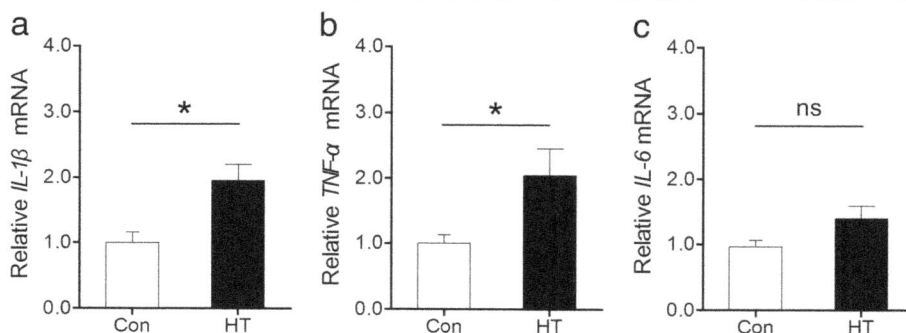

Fig. 8 Euthyroid HT promotes proinflammatory cytokine expression in the frontal cortex. Proinflammatory cytokine expression was probed by real-time RT-PCR. **a–c** Expression of *IL-1β* (**a**), *TNF-α* (**b**), and *IL-6* (**c**) mRNA. Data are presented as the mean ± SEM, $n = 5$; ns, no statistical significance; *$p < 0.05$, vs. Con

signaling that were sensitive to inflammatory cytokines [23]. We found that mRNA expression of tryptophan-degrading enzyme indoleamine-2,3-dioxygenase (IDO1) and 5-HT transporter (SERT) was significantly higher in HT mice than in control mice (Fig. 10a, b). As expected, the levels of 5-HT measured by ELISA showed a significant reduction in the frontal cortex of HT mice compared to that in controls (Fig. 10c).

Discussion

Tg is a well-known thyroid auto-antigen associated with the development of thyroiditis in both rodents and humans. Tg-induced thyroiditis is a classic model for studying HT [24] and can be established in susceptible mice, such as NOD mice, leading to the development of HT-like illness characterized by monocyte infiltration into the thyroid gland and presence of autoantibodies against Tg and TPO, which are serological hallmarks of HT [2]. Thus, this model has been widely used to explore the pathogenesis of HT and test therapeutics [24, 44, 45]. In our study, mice immunized with Tg showed intrathyroidal monocyte infiltration and rising serum thyroid autoantibody (TA) levels accompanied by normal T3, T4, and TSH levels, which defines euthyroid HT in humans. To our knowledge, our study is the first to use this model to investigate the effect of HT itself on emotional function in mice, focusing on the possible contribution of neuroinflammation in mediating such an effect.

Thyroid diseases resulting in thyroid dysfunctions are well known to be able to induce psychological deficits, including anxiety and depression [4]. However, the literature on the emotional effects of euthyroid HT are limited and controversial. An early epidemiological study indicated that no association was found between thyroid autoantibodies and anxiety or depression, neither crude nor adjusted for T4 and TSH [46]. On the other hand, other researchers reported impairments of mental well-being in patients with HT that were shown to be independent of

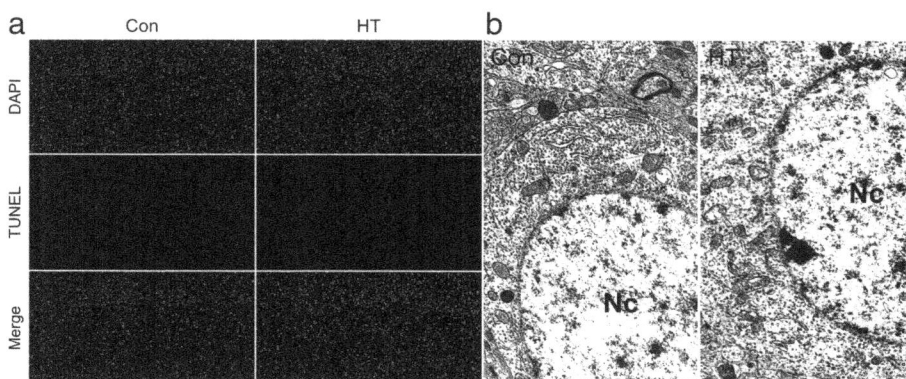

Fig. 9 Euthyroid HT does not induce neuronal apoptosis in the frontal cortex. Neuronal apoptosis was identified by the TUNEL staining and TEM. **a** Representative fluorescent images showing TUNEL-labeled (green) apoptotic cells counterstained with DAPI (blue) in the frontal cortex of control mice and HT mice ($n = 5$/group). Magnification × 100. **b** Representative TEM images of frontal cortex neurons in Con mice and HT mice ($n = 3$/group). The neuronal nuclei (Nc) had no signs of apoptosis, such as chromatin margination or nuclear condensation, in the neurons examined. Magnification × 8000

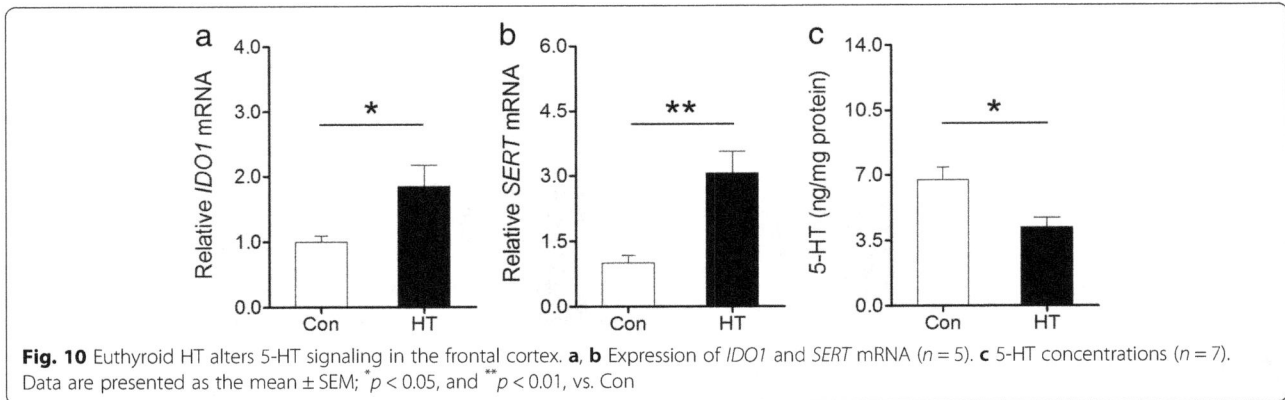

Fig. 10 Euthyroid HT alters 5-HT signaling in the frontal cortex. **a, b** Expression of *IDO1* and *SERT* mRNA ($n = 5$). **c** 5-HT concentrations ($n = 7$). Data are presented as the mean ± SEM; $^*p < 0.05$, and $^{**}p < 0.01$, vs. Con

thyroid function [5–8]. In this study, we first investigated whether HT affected emotional performance regardless of thyroid dysfunctions in mice. Here, HT mice displayed more anxiety-like behavior during the OFT and EPM than control mice despite a similar thyroid functional state between groups. These mice also displayed prolonged immobility time in the FST and TST, suggestive of depressive-like behavior. These results indicated that HT itself induced behaviors relevant to mood disorders in mice, providing preliminary evidence to support the clinical literature linking euthyroid HT to increased emotional reactivity.

Recently, the crucial role of neuroinflammation in the development of psychological disorders including depression and anxiety has received more attention. Characteristic features of neuroinflammation include the activation of microglia and astroglia and generation of proinflammatory cytokines [19]. An increasing number of human studies have reported microglia activation in the CNS of patients with psychiatric disorders, such as depression, schizophrenia, and anxiety [47, 48]. Results from animal models have shown that neuroinflammation is closely associated with abnormal emotional behavior, which could be improved after antiinflammatory treatment [49–51]. Notably, studies on brain biopsy revealed activated microglia and reactive astrocytes in patients with Hashimoto's encephalopathy [13, 14], a severe form of a deterioration of the CNS in patients suffering with HT. In the present study, the effects of HT itself on neuroinflammation were examined. Using immunohistochemistry, we found that microglia and astrocytes were activated in the frontal cortex of HT mice. Ultrastructural observations further confirmed glia activation in HT mice, with microglia showing phagocytic function and astrocytes tending to show features involved in active proteosynthesis. Moreover, these observations were accompanied by an increase in the expression of glial marker *Iba1* and *GFAP* as well as pro-inflammatory cytokines *IL-1β* and *TNF-α*. These results demonstrated that HT induced neuroinflammation in the euthyroid

state. Thus, HT-induced emotional alterations may be, at least partially, attributed to neuroinflammation.

The mechanisms by which HT induces neuroinflammation in the euthyroid state are still unknown. A recent study showed experimental hyperthyroidism promoted activation of microglia and astrocytes in the cerebral cortex of young mice [52]. In another animal model, hypothyroidism was associated with an increased number of astrocyte cells in the brain [53]. In our study, neuroinflammatory reactions, such as glia activation, were unlikely to be due to thyroid dysfunctions, because serum T3 and T4, as well as TSH, were within the normal range. On the other hand, increased TA themselves may also be pathogenic, given that anti-TPO specifically binds to astrocytes in vitro [54]. Moreover, different studies described the presence of antigenic sites for TA on neural tissues [55, 56], and most recently, anti-Tg has been shown to immunolocalize to vascular smooth muscle of all limbic regions, including frontal cortex [57]. The present study described the increased presence of TA in the frontal cortex of HT mice. It appears reasonable to then propose that TA may cross-react with auto-antigens expressed in the brain and modulate local immune responses. Further studies are needed to explore the detailed mechanisms underlying neuroinflammation in the context of euthyroid HT.

Interestingly, despite this inflammatory response, no signs of neuronal apoptosis were visible by the TUNEL staining and TEM in the frontal cortex of HT mice. This result was in line with previous studies showing that increased brain inflammatory response was not functionally associated to neuronal apoptosis or neuronal damage [58–61]. It is interesting to speculate that HT could not induce neuronal damage. This may explain the very consistent finding of normal neural activity on resting-state functional magnetic resonance imaging in patients with euthyroid HT [62]. Utilization of other markers to assess neurodegeneration or neurogenesis would have been useful but it was beyond the scope of the study. Despite no evident structural alterations of neurons, emotional dysfunction can occur due to functional impairments, for example, of the serotonergic signaling system, which are important mechanisms in the regulation of mood [63].

Recent studies have revealed that the serotonergic signaling system may be a major target for immune mediators, such as proinflammatory cytokines. In vitro results have shown that treatment with proinflammatory cytokines, such as IL-1β and TNF-α, directly induce IDO1 and SERT expression in neuroglia and/or neurons [64–67]. In vivo studies have suggested that central inflammatory signaling activation significantly upregulates IDO1 and/or SERT, resulting in depressive-like behavior in animals [68–70]. Indeed, IDO-1 and SERT are crucial regulators of central 5-HT signaling, which plays vital roles in the development of psychiatric symptoms in humans and animals [63]. In this study, frontal cortex expression of *IDO-1* and *SERT* was sharply increased in HT mice. Moreover, the 5-HT concentration in the frontal cortex was lower in HT mice than in controls. These results demonstrated that elevated expression of IL-1β and TNF-α paralleled by glial activation provoked by HT may impact 5-HT signaling and thereby contribute to the emotional disturbance. Different studies have revealed that antiinflammatory drugs such as celecoxib have an inhibitory effect on the neuroinflammatory response [38, 71, 72] and that celecoxib therapy exerts a beneficial effect on psychiatric symptoms in some cases [73, 74]. Detailed data on the effects of antiinflammatory therapy upon psychiatric symptoms related with euthyroid HT is of interest for future studies.

There are some deficiencies in the present study. First, all behavioral tests were conducted on the same group of mice. The stress associated with exposure of the mice to behavioral tests may consequently affect performance in the subsequent behavioral tests; therefore, we are unable to entirely exclude an interactive effect among the behavioral tests. However, the mice in control group underwent the same behavioral tests in this study. Second, although IL-1β, TNF-α, and IL-6 are the most common cytokines involved in process of neuroinflammation, they do not represent the entire range of inflammatory molecules. Therefore, other inflammatory cytokines related to neuroinflammation remain to be considered. Third, this study focused on the frontal cortex because this brain area is involved in mood control and is the primary region affected in euthyroid HT patients. Other brain regions relevant to mood regulation, such as the hippocampus, should be examined in further studies.

Conclusions

In summary, emerging clinical studies have shown that HT renders individuals vulnerable to psychopathology in the euthyroid state. Using an animal model, this study provides further evidence for such arguments, showing for the first time that euthyroid HT induced emotional alterations in mice, at least partially, through induction of neuroinflammation and alterations in 5-HT signaling in the frontal cortex. These findings provide preliminary leads to further explore the potential role of neuroinflammation in mediating these psychological consequences of euthyroid HT and to develop effective approaches to combat them.

Abbreviations
5-HT: Serotonin; Anti-Tg: Anti-thyroglobulin antibody; Anti-TPO: Anti-thyroid peroxidase antibody; CFA: Complete Freund's adjuvant; ECLIA: Electrochemiluminescence immunoassay; ELISA: Enzyme-linked immunosorbent assay; EPM: Elevated plus maze; FST: Forced swimming test; GFAP: Glial fibrillary acidic protein; HE: Hematoxylin and eosin; HT: Hashimoto's thyroiditis; Iba1: Ionized calcium-binding adapter molecule 1; IDO1: Indoleamine-2,3-dioxygenase; IFA: Incomplete Freund's adjuvant; IL-1β: Interleukin-1β; IL-6: Interleukin-6; OFT: Open field test; SERT: Serotonin transporter; T3: Triiodothyronine; T4: Thyroxin; TEM: Transmission electron microscopy; Tg: Thyroglobulin; TNF-α: Tumor necrosis factor-α; TSH: Thyroid-stimulating hormone; TST: Tail suspension test; TUNEL: Terminal deoxynucleotidyl transferase-mediated dUTP-biotin nick end labeling

Acknowledgements
The authors wish to thank PhD student Zhen Yu of Department of Maternal, Child and Adolescent Health, School of Public Health, Anhui Medical University, for his excellent technical assistance.

Funding
This study was supported by the National Natural Science Foundation of China (No. 81272152) and Natural Science Foundation of Anhui province (No. 1708085MH221).

Authors' contributions
DFZ, QNW, and YJC designed the study. YJC, ZXC, LL, HF, ZBW, and WH performed the experiment and collected the data. FW and JFG conducted the statistical analysis and participated in data interpretation. YJC contributed to writing the manuscript, with the help of FW. DFZ and QNW proofread the final version of the manuscript. All authors read and approved the final manuscript.

Competing interests
The authors declare that they have no competing interests.

Author details
[1]Department of Endocrinology, Anhui Geriatric Institute, the First Affiliated Hospital of Anhui Medical University, Hefei 230032, China. [2]Anhui Key Laboratory of Bioactivity of Natural Products, School of Pharmacy, Anhui Medical University, Hefei 230032, China. [3]Department of Pathology, Anhui Provincial Hospital Affiliated to Anhui Medical University, Hefei 230032, China. [4]Department of Toxicology, School of Public Health, Anhui Medical University, Hefei 230032, China.

References
1. Siriweera EH, Ratnatunga NV. Profile of Hashimoto's thyroiditis in Sri Lankans: is there an increased risk of ancillary pathologies in Hashimoto's thyroiditis? J Thyroid Res. 2010. https://doi.org/10.4061/2010/124264.
2. Pearce EN, Farwell AP, Braverman LE. Thyroiditis. N Engl J Med. 2003;348: 2646–55.

3. Kapila K, Sathar SA, Al-Rabah NA, Prahash A, Seshadri MS. Chronic lymphocytic (Hashimoto's) thyroiditis in Kuwait diagnosed by fine needle aspirates. Ann Saudi Med. 1995;15:363–6.

4. Bauer M, Goetz T, Glenn T, Whybrow PC. The thyroid-brain interaction in thyroid disorders and mood disorders. J Neuroendocrinol. 2008;20:1101–14.

5. Carta MG, Hardoy MC, Carpiniello B, Murru A, Marci AR, Carbone F, Deiana L, Cadeddu M, Mariotti S. A case control study on psychiatric disorders in Hashimoto disease and Euthyroid goitre: not only depressive but also anxiety disorders are associated with thyroid autoimmunity. Clin Pract Epidemiol Ment Health. 2005;1:23.

6. Kirim S, Keskek SO, Koksal F, Haydardedeoglu FE, Bozkirli E, Toledano Y. Depression in patients with euthyroid chronic autoimmune thyroiditis. Endocr J. 2012;59:705–8.

7. Giynas Ayhan M, Uguz F, Askin R, Gonen MS. The prevalence of depression and anxiety disorders in patients with euthyroid Hashimoto's thyroiditis: a comparative study. Gen Hosp Psychiatry. 2014;36:95–8.

8. Yalcin MM, Altinova AE, Cavnar B, Bolayir B, Akturk M, Arslan E, Ozkan C, Cakir N, Balos Toruner F. Is thyroid autoimmunity itself associated with psychological well-being in euthyroid Hashimoto's thyroiditis? Endocr J. 2017;64:425–9.

9. Mussig K, Kunle A, Sauberlich AL, Weinert C, Ethofer T, Saur R, Klein R, Haring HU, Klingberg S, Gallwitz B, Leyhe T. Thyroid peroxidase antibody positivity is associated with symptomatic distress in patients with Hashimoto's thyroiditis. Brain Behav Immun. 2012;26:559–63.

10. Piga M, Serra A, Deiana L, Loi GL, Satta L, Di Liberto M, Mariotti S. Brain perfusion abnormalities in patients with euthyroid autoimmune thyroiditis. Eur J Nucl Med Mol Imaging. 2004;31:1639–44.

11. Millan MJ, Rivet JM, Gobert A. The frontal cortex as a network hub controlling mood and cognition: probing its neurochemical substrates for improved therapy of psychiatric and neurological disorders. J Psychopharmacol. 2016;30:1099–128.

12. Leyhe T, Ethofer T, Bretscher J, Kunle A, Sauberlich AL, Klein R, Gallwitz B, Haring HU, Fallgatter A, Klingberg S, et al. Low performance in attention testing is associated with reduced grey matter density of the left inferior frontal gyrus in euthyroid patients with Hashimoto's thyroiditis. Brain Behav Immun. 2013;27:33–7.

13. Doherty CP, Schlossmacher M, Torres N, Bromfield E, Samuels MA, Folkerth R. Hashimoto's encephalopathy mimicking Creutzfeldt-Jakob disease: brain biopsy findings. J Neurol Neurosurg Psychiatry. 2002;73:601–2.

14. Zhao W, Li J, Wang J, Guo Y, Tuo H, Kang Z, Jiang B, Wang R, Wang D. A case of Hashimoto encephalopathy: clinical manifestation, imaging, pathology, treatment, and prognosis. Neurologist. 2011;17:141–3.

15. Cardenas-Roldan J, Rojas-Villarraga A, Anaya JM. How do autoimmune diseases cluster in families? A systematic review and meta-analysis. BMC Med. 2013;11:73.

16. Bruce TO. Comorbid depression in rheumatoid arthritis: pathophysiology and clinical implications. Curr Psychiatry Rep. 2008;10:258–64.

17. Jeltsch-David H, Muller S. Autoimmunity, neuroinflammation, pathogen load: a decisive crosstalk in neuropsychiatric SLE. J Autoimmun. 2016;74:13–26.

18. Fuggle NR, Howe FA, Allen RL, Sofat N. New insights into the impact of neuro-inflammation in rheumatoid arthritis. Front Neurosci. 2014;8:357.

19. Kempuraj D, Thangavel R, Selvakumar GP, Zaheer S, Ahmed ME, Raikwar SP, Zahoor H, Saeed D, Natteru PA, Iyer S, Zaheer A. Brain and peripheral atypical inflammatory mediators potentiate Neuroinflammation and neurodegeneration. Front Cell Neurosci. 2017;11:216.

20. Hendriksen E, van Bergeijk D, Oosting RS, Redegeld FA. Mast cells in neuroinflammation and brain disorders. Neurosci Biobehav Rev. 2017;79:119–33.

21. Capuron L, Miller AH. Immune system to brain signaling: neuropsychopharmacological implications. Pharmacol Ther. 2011;130:226–38.

22. Najjar S, Pearlman DM, Alper K, Najjar A, Devinsky O. Neuroinflammation and psychiatric illness. J Neuroinflammation. 2013;10:43.

23. Rosenblat JD, Cha DS, Mansur RB, McIntyre RS. Inflamed moods: a review of the interactions between inflammation and mood disorders. Prog Neuro-Psychopharmacol Biol Psychiatry. 2014;53:23–34.

24. Damotte D, Colomb E, Cailleau C, Brousse N, Charreire J, Carnaud C. Analysis of susceptibility of NOD mice to spontaneous and experimentally induced thyroiditis. Eur J Immunol. 1997;27:2854–62.

25. Sadelain MW, Qin HY, Lauzon J, Singh B. Prevention of type I diabetes in NOD mice by adjuvant immunotherapy. Diabetes. 1990;39:583–9.

26. Qin HY, Sadelain MW, Hitchon C, Lauzon J, Singh B. Complete Freund's adjuvant-induced T cells prevent the development and adoptive transfer of diabetes in nonobese diabetic mice. J Immunol. 1993;150:2072–80.

27. Lee IF, Qin H, Trudeau J, Dutz J, Tan R. Regulation of autoimmune diabetes by complete Freund's adjuvant is mediated by NK cells. J Immunol. 2004; 172:937–42.

28. Chen Z, Xu YY, Wu R, Han YX, Yu Y, Ge JF, Chen FH. Impaired learning and memory in rats induced by a high-fat diet: involvement with the imbalance of nesfatin-1 abundance and copine 6 expression. J Neuroendocrinol. 2017. https://doi.org/10.1111/jne.12462.

29. Ge JF, Gao WC, Cheng WM, Lu WL, Tang J, Peng L, Li N, Chen FH. Orcinol glucoside produces antidepressant effects by blocking the behavioural and neuronal deficits caused by chronic stress. Eur Neuropsychopharmacol. 2014;24:172–80.

30. Li M, Li C, Yu H, Cai X, Shen X, Sun X, Wang J, Zhang Y, Wang C. Lentivirus-mediated interleukin-1beta (IL-1beta) knock-down in the hippocampus alleviates lipopolysaccharide (LPS)-induced memory deficits and anxiety- and depression-like behaviors in mice. J Neuroinflammation. 2017;14:190.

31. Yu Z, Han Y, Shen R, Huang K, Xu YY, Wang QN, Zhou SS, Xu DX, Tao FB. Gestational di-(2-ethylhexyl) phthalate exposure causes fetal intrauterine growth restriction through disturbing placental thyroid hormone receptor signaling. Toxicol Lett. 2018;294:1–10.

32. Wang X, Liu H, Zhang Y, Li J, Teng X, Liu A, Yu X, Shan Z, Teng W. Effects of isolated positive maternal thyroglobulin antibodies on brain development of offspring in an experimental autoimmune thyroiditis model. Thyroid. 2015;25:551–8.

33. Houlden A, Goldrick M, Brough D, Vizi ES, Lenart N, Martinecz B, Roberts IS, Denes A. Brain injury induces specific changes in the caecal microbiota of mice via altered autonomic activity and mucoprotein production. Brain Behav Immun. 2016;57:10–20.

34. Paxinos G, Franklin K. Paxinos and Franklin's the mouse brain in stereotaxic coordinates. 4th ed. Amsterdam: Elsevier/Academic Press; 2013.

35. Kreutzberg GW. Microglia: a sensor for pathological events in the CNS. Trends Neurosci. 1996;19:312–8.

36. Sofroniew MV, Vinters HV. Astrocytes: biology and pathology. Acta Neuropathol. 2010;119:7–35.

37. Wixey JA, Reinebrant HE, Spencer SJ, Buller KM. Efficacy of post-insult minocycline administration to alter long-term hypoxia-ischemia-induced damage to the serotonergic system in the immature rat brain. Neuroscience. 2011;182:184–92.

38. Kaizaki A, Tien LT, Pang Y, Cai Z, Tanaka S, Numazawa S, Bhatt AJ, Fan LW. Celecoxib reduces brain dopaminergic neuronal dysfunction, and improves sensorimotor behavioral performance in neonatal rats exposed to systemic lipopolysaccharide. J Neuroinflammation. 2013;10:45.

39. Yanguas-Casas N, Barreda-Manso MA, Nieto-Sampedro M, Romero-Ramirez L. Tauroursodeoxycholic acid reduces glial cell activation in an animal model of acute neuroinflammation. J Neuroinflammation. 2014;11:50.

40. Wang F, Wu Z, Zha X, Cai Y, Wu B, Jia X, Zhu D. Concurrent administration of thyroxine and donepezil induces plastic changes in the prefrontal cortex of adult hypothyroid rats. Mol Med Rep. 2017;16:3233–41.

41. Dahlke C, Saberi D, Ott B, Brand-Saberi B, Schmitt-John T, Theiss C. Inflammation and neuronal death in the motor cortex of the wobbler mouse, an ALS animal model. J Neuroinflammation. 2015;12:215.

42. Casamenti F, Prosperi C, Scali C, Giovannelli L, Colivicchi MA, Faussone-Pellegrini MS, Pepeu G. Interleukin-1beta activates forebrain glial cells and increases nitric oxide production and cortical glutamate and GABA release in vivo: implications for Alzheimer's disease. Neuroscience. 1999;91:831–42.

43. Cheng C, Zochodne DW. Sensory neurons with activated caspase-3 survive long-term experimental diabetes. Diabetes. 2003;52:2363–71.

44. Jin Z, Mori K, Fujimori K, Hoshikawa S, Tani J, Satoh J, Ito S, Satomi S, Yoshida K. Experimental autoimmune thyroiditis in nonobese diabetic mice lacking interferon regulatory factor-1. Clin Immunol. 2004;113:187–92.

45. Mori K, Yoshida K, Tani J, Nakagawa Y, Hoshikawa S, Ozaki H, Ito S. Effects of angiotensin II blockade on the development of autoimmune thyroiditis in nonobese diabetic mice. Clin Immunol. 2008;126:97–103.

46. Engum A, Bjoro T, Mykletun A, Dahl AA. Thyroid autoimmunity, depression and anxiety; are there any connections? An epidemiological study of a large population. J Psychosom Res. 2005;59:263–8.

47. van der Doef TF, Doorduin J, van Berckel BNM, Cervenka S. Assessing brain immune activation in psychiatric disorders: clinical and preclinical PET imaging studies of the 18-kDa translocator protein. Clin Transl Imaging. 2015;3:449–60.

48. Setiawan E, Wilson AA, Mizrahi R, Rusjan PM, Miler L, Rajkowska G, Suridjan I, Kennedy JL, Rekkas PV, Houle S, Meyer JH. Role of translocator protein density, a marker of neuroinflammation, in the brain during major depressive episodes. JAMA Psychiatry. 2015;72:268–75.

49. Wang YL, Han QQ, Gong WQ, Pan DH, Wang LZ, Hu W, Yang M, Li B, Yu J, Liu Q. Microglial activation mediates chronic mild stress-induced depressive- and anxiety-like behavior in adult rats. J Neuroinflammation. 2018;15:21.

50. da Silva Dias IC, Carabelli B, Ishii DK, de Morais H, de Carvalho MC, Rizzo de Souza LE, Zanata SM, Brandao ML, Cunha TM, Ferraz AC, et al. Indoleamine-2,3-dioxygenase/kynurenine pathway as a potential pharmacological target to treat depression associated with diabetes. Mol Neurobiol. 2016;53:6997–7009.

51. Haile M, Boutajangout A, Chung K, Chan J, Stolper T, Vincent N, Batchan M, D'Urso J, Lin Y, Kline R, et al. The Cox-2 Inhibitor Meloxicam Ameliorates Neuroinflammation and Depressive Behavior in Adult Mice after Splenectomy. J Neurophysiol Neurol Disord. 2016;3:1–9.

52. Noda M. Thyroid hormone in the CNS: contribution of neuron-glia interaction. Vitam Horm. 2018;106:313–31.

53. Cortes C, Eugenin E, Aliaga E, Carreno LJ, Bueno SM, Gonzalez PA, Gayol S, Naranjo D, Noches V, Marassi MP, et al. Hypothyroidism in the adult rat causes incremental changes in brain-derived neurotrophic factor, neuronal and astrocyte apoptosis, gliosis, and deterioration of postsynaptic density. Thyroid. 2012;22:951–63.

54. Blanchin S, Coffin C, Viader F, Ruf J, Carayon P, Potier F, Portier E, Comby E, Allouche S, Ollivier Y, et al. Anti-thyroperoxidase antibodies from patients with Hashimoto's encephalopathy bind to cerebellar astrocytes. J Neuroimmunol. 2007;192:13–20.

55. Ota K, Matsui M, Milford EL, Mackin GA, Weiner HL, Hafler DA. T-cell recognition of an immunodominant myelin basic protein epitope in multiple sclerosis. Nature. 1990;346:183–7.

56. Moodley K, Botha J, Raidoo DM, Naidoo S. Immuno-localisation of anti-thyroid antibodies in adult human cerebral cortex. J Neurol Sci. 2011;302:114–7.

57. Naicker M, Naidoo S. Expression of thyroid-stimulating hormone receptors and thyroglobulin in limbic regions in the adult human brain. Metab Brain Dis. 2018;33:481–9.

58. Mouihate A, Pittman QJ. Lipopolysaccharide-induced fever is dissociated from apoptotic cell death in the rat brain. Brain Res. 1998;805:95–103.

59. Aid S, Langenbach R, Bosetti F. Neuroinflammatory response to lipopolysaccharide is exacerbated in mice genetically deficient in cyclooxygenase-2. J Neuroinflammation. 2008;5:17.

60. Francois A, Terro F, Quellard N, Fernandez B, Chassaing D, Janet T, Rioux Bilan A, Paccalin M, Page G. Impairment of autophagy in the central nervous system during lipopolysaccharide-induced inflammatory stress in mice. Mol Brain. 2014;7:56.

61. Sapin E, Peyron C, Roche F, Gay N, Carcenac C, Savasta M, Levy P, Dematteis M. Chronic intermittent hypoxia induces chronic low-grade neuroinflammation in the dorsal hippocampus of mice. Sleep. 2015;38:1537–46.

62. Quinque EM, Karger S, Arelin K, Schroeter ML, Kratzsch J, Villringer A. Structural and functional MRI study of the brain, cognition and mood in long-term adequately treated Hashimoto's thyroiditis. Psychoneuroendocrinology. 2014;42:188–98.

63. Cowen PJ. Serotonin and depression: pathophysiological mechanism or marketing myth? Trends Pharmacol Sci. 2008;29:433–6.

64. Hochstrasser T, Ullrich C, Sperner-Unterweger B, Humpel C. Inflammatory stimuli reduce survival of serotonergic neurons and induce neuronal expression of indoleamine 2,3-dioxygenase in rat dorsal raphe nucleus organotypic brain slices. Neuroscience. 2011;184:128–38.

65. Zunszain PA, Anacker C, Cattaneo A, Choudhury S, Musaelyan K, Myint AM, Thuret S, Price J, Pariante CM. Interleukin-1beta: a new regulator of the kynurenine pathway affecting human hippocampal neurogenesis. Neuropsychopharmacology. 2012;37:939–49.

66. Zhu CB, Blakely RD, Hewlett WA. The proinflammatory cytokines interleukin-1beta and tumor necrosis factor-alpha activate serotonin transporters. Neuropsychopharmacology. 2006. https://doi.org/10.1038/sj.npp.1301029.

67. Malynn S, Campos-Torres A, Moynagh P, Haase J. The pro-inflammatory cytokine TNF-alpha regulates the activity and expression of the serotonin transporter (SERT) in astrocytes. Neurochem Res. 2013;38:694–704.

68. Fu X, Zunich SM, O'Connor JC, Kavelaars A, Dantzer R, Kelley KW. Central administration of lipopolysaccharide induces depressive-like behavior in vivo and activates brain indoleamine 2,3 dioxygenase in murine organotypic hippocampal slice cultures. J Neuroinflammation. 2010;7:43.

69. Zhu CB, Lindler KM, Owens AW, Daws LC, Blakely RD, Hewlett WA. Interleukin-1 receptor activation by systemic lipopolysaccharide induces behavioral despair linked to MAPK regulation of CNS serotonin transporters. Neuropsychopharmacology. 2010;35:2510–20.

70. Dobos N, de Vries EF, Kema IP, Patas K, Prins M, Nijholt IM, Dierckx RA, Korf J, den Boer JA, Luiten PG, Eisel UL. The role of indoleamine 2,3-dioxygenase in a mouse model of neuroinflammation-induced depression. J Alzheimers Dis. 2012;28:905–15.

71. Villa V, Thellung S, Corsaro A, Novelli F, Tasso B, Colucci-D'Amato L, Gatta E, Tonelli M, Florio T. Celecoxib inhibits prion protein 90-231-mediated pro-inflammatory responses in microglial cells. Mol Neurobiol. 2016;53:57–72.

72. Mhillaj E, Morgese MG, Tucci P, Furiano A, Luongo L, Bove M, Maione S, Cuomo V, Schiavone S, Trabace L. Celecoxib prevents cognitive impairment and neuroinflammation in soluble amyloid beta-treated rats. Neuroscience. 2018;372:58–73.

73. Muller N, Schwarz MJ, Dehning S, Douhe A, Cerovecki A, Goldstein-Muller B, Spellmann I, Hetzel G, Maino K, Kleindienst N, et al. The cyclooxygenase-2 inhibitor celecoxib has therapeutic effects in major depression: results of a double-blind, randomized, placebo controlled, add-on pilot study to reboxetine. Mol Psychiatry. 2006;11:680–4.

74. Kohler O, Benros ME, Nordentoft M, Farkouh ME, Iyengar RL, Mors O, Krogh J. Effect of anti-inflammatory treatment on depression, depressive symptoms, and adverse effects: a systematic review and meta-analysis of randomized clinical trials. JAMA Psychiatry. 2014;71:1381–91.

6

Protein kinase C-delta inhibition protects blood-brain barrier from sepsis-induced vascular damage

Yuan Tang[1], Fariborz Soroush[1], Shuang Sun[2], Elisabetta Liverani[3], Jordan C. Langston[1], Qingliang Yang[1], Laurie E. Kilpatrick[2] and Mohammad F. Kiani[1,4*]

Abstract

Background: Neuroinflammation often develops in sepsis leading to activation of cerebral endothelium, increased permeability of the blood-brain barrier (BBB), and neutrophil infiltration. We have identified protein kinase C-delta (PKCδ) as a critical regulator of the inflammatory response and demonstrated that pharmacologic inhibition of PKCδ by a peptide inhibitor (PKCδ-i) protected endothelial cells, decreased sepsis-mediated neutrophil influx into the lung, and prevented tissue damage. The objective of this study was to elucidate the regulation and relative contribution of PKCδ in the control of individual steps in neuroinflammation during sepsis.

Methods: The role of PKCδ in mediating human brain microvascular endothelial (HBMVEC) permeability, junctional protein expression, and leukocyte adhesion and migration was investigated in vitro using our novel BBB on-a-chip (B³C) microfluidic assay and in vivo in a rat model of sepsis induced by cecal ligation and puncture (CLP). HBMVEC were cultured under flow in the vascular channels of B³C. Confocal imaging and staining were used to confirm tight junction and lumen formation. Confluent HBMVEC were pretreated with TNF-α (10 U/ml) for 4 h in the absence or presence of PKCδ-i (5 μM) to quantify neutrophil adhesion and migration in the B³C. Permeability was measured using a 40-kDa fluorescent dextran in vitro and Evans blue dye in vivo.

Results: During sepsis, PKCδ is activated in the rat brain resulting in membrane translocation, a step that is attenuated by treatment with PKCδ-i. Similarly, TNF-α-mediated activation of PKCδ and its translocation in HBMVEC are attenuated by PKCδ-i in vitro. PKCδ inhibition significantly reduced TNF-α-mediated hyperpermeability and TEER decrease in vitro in activated HBMVEC and rat brain in vivo 24 h after CLP induced sepsis. TNF-α-treated HBMVEC showed interrupted tight junction expression, whereas continuous expression of tight junction protein was observed in non-treated or PKCδ-i-treated cells. PKCδ inhibition also reduced TNF-α-mediated neutrophil adhesion and migration across HBMVEC in B³C. Interestingly, while PKCδ inhibition decreased the number of adherent neutrophils to baseline (no-treatment group), it significantly reduced the number of migrated neutrophils below the baseline, suggesting a critical role of PKCδ in regulating neutrophil transmigration.

Conclusions: The BBB on-a-chip (B³C) in vitro assay is suitable for the study of BBB function as well as screening of novel therapeutics in real-time. PKCδ activation is a key signaling event that alters the structural and functional integrity of BBB leading to vascular damage and inflammation-induced tissue damage. PKCδ-TAT peptide inhibitor has therapeutic potential for the prevention or reduction of cerebrovascular injury in sepsis-induced vascular damage.

Keywords: Blood-brain barrier, Protein kinase C-delta, Microvascular endothelial cells, Microfluidic assay, Sepsis, Neuroinflammation

* Correspondence: mkiani@temple.edu
[1]Department of Mechanical Engineering, College of Engineering, Temple University, Philadelphia, PA 19122, USA
[4]Department of Radiation Oncology, Lewis Katz School of Medicine, Temple University, Philadelphia, PA 19140, USA
Full list of author information is available at the end of the article

Background

Sepsis is a life-threatening organ dysfunction caused by a dysregulated host response to infection [1]. It is one of the leading causes of death in ICUs causing more than 200,000 deaths/year in the USA [2, 3]. Patients who recover from sepsis suffer from impaired quality of life and rapid degradation in cognition and functional capacity which is more pronounced in middle-aged and older survivors [4].

During sepsis, the endothelium is an active participant in the recruitment and activation of neutrophils through the production of chemokines/cytokines and expression of adhesion molecules [5–7]. Sepsis induces activation of cerebral endothelial cell (EC) which initiates a cascade of proinflammatory events by releasing various mediators into the brain [8], resulting in alterations in the blood-brain barrier (BBB), leukocyte dysregulation, and subsequent brain tissue damage [9]. A key step in neutrophil-mediated brain damage is the migration of neutrophils across the damaged BBB. BBB properties are primarily determined by tight and adherens junctions between the cerebral EC [10]. Normally, junctional complexes prevent the transmigration of blood cells. However, in sepsis, BBB disruption leads to the influx of neutrophils into brain tissue. To date, there are no specific pharmacological therapies available that protect brain from neutrophil-mediated tissue damage [2, 11].

Our group has identified protein kinase C-delta (PKCδ) as a critical regulator of the inflammatory response and an important regulator of endothelial proinflammatory signaling [12–18]. PKCδ inhibition had an anti-inflammatory and lung protective effect indicating that targeting PKCδ may offer a unique therapeutic strategy for the protection of EC and control of neutrophil-induced tissue damage [16, 18]. PKCδ is a member of the protein kinase C (PKC) superfamily. While PKCδ has been identified as an important regulator of inflammation, the mechanisms by which PKCδ regulates BBB permeability, EC adhesion molecule/junctional protein expression, and neutrophil migration in sepsis are incompletely understood and further studies are needed to elucidate the regulation and relative contribution of PKCδ in the control of individual steps in this process.

Given the complexity of existing in vivo models of the inflammatory process, several in vitro models have been developed. While 2D flow chambers can be used to examine adhesion molecule/junctional protein expression, as well as neutrophil rolling/adhesion phenomena, they lack the appropriate geometry to model EC permeability/TEER changes and neutrophil transmigration. Boyden/transwell chambers can be used for migration studies, however do not account for in vivo fluid shear and size/topology of microvessels which is essential for the expression of junctional proteins or

provide real-time visualization of the above-mentioned events. As there are no models that can monitor all these critical parameters and events in a single assay, the understanding of the inflammation cascade and the development of anti-inflammatory drugs has been hindered. In this study, we have modified our previously developed novel blood-brain barrier on-a-chip (B^{3}C) microfluidic assay [19] so that it resolves and facilitates real-time assessment of the characteristics of the BBB as well as individual steps including rolling, firm arrest, spreading, and migration of neutrophils into the extravascular tissue space in a single system. This integrated microfluidic assay was then used to study the role of PKCδ in the modulation of each individual steps involved in inflammation of the brain during sepsis in a realistic microvasculature geometry with physiological shear conditions which allows direct observation and quantification of permeability, protein expression, leukocytes rolling, adhesion, and migration over time.

The objective of this study is to test the hypothesis that inhibition of PKCδ prevents activation of EC, protects BBB structural integrity, prevents neutrophil migration, and attenuates the development of brain inflammation. This study will provide important insight into the molecular mechanisms and functional role of PKCδ in the underlying pathophysiology of brain inflammation during sepsis and will ascertain whether targeting PKCδ offers a unique therapeutic strategy for the control of BBB damage in sepsis.

Materials and methods
Materials, equipment, and reagents

A rabbit polyclonal anti-rat PKCδ (Ser643/676) antibody was purchased from Cell Signaling Technology (Beverly, MA). A rabbit polyclonal anti-human TJP1/Tight Junction Protein 1 antibody was purchased from Boster Biological Technology (Pleasanton, CA); Alexa Fluor® 568 goat anti-rabbit polyclonal antibody and Alexa Fluor® 488 Phalloindin were purchased from Life Technologies Corporation (Carlsbad, CA). Human fibronectin was obtained from BD Biosciences (San Jose, CA). Human brain microvascular endothelial cell (HBMVEC), human astrocytes, endothelial cell media (ECM), and astrocyte media were purchased from ScienCell (Carlsbad, CA). Subcellular Protein Fractionation Kit, bovine serum albumin (BSA), phosphate buffered saline (PBS), Hanks' Balanced Salt solution (HBSS), Trypsin/EDTA, formalin, Triton X-100, Draq5, 40 kDa Texas Red-conjugated dextran, and Hoechst 33342 were purchased from Thermofisher Scientific (Rockford, IL). Formamide was purchased from MilliporeSigma (Burlington, MA). B^{3}C microfluidic assay platform was manufactured at the Synvivo, Inc. (Huntsville, AL).

A Nikon TE200 fluorescence microscope equipped with an automated stage was used for performing experiments. Images were acquired using an ORCA Flash 4 camera (Hamamatsu Corp., USA). An Olympus FluoView FV1000 confocal microscope equipped with a fully automated stage was used for capturing confocal image stacks. PhD Ultra Syringe pump (Harvard Apparatus, USA) was used for injecting growth media, permeability dye, or neutrophil/microparticle suspension to the B³C with high precision. A stage warmer was used to keep the B³C at 37 °C. NIS Elements software (Nikon Instruments Inc., Melville, NY) was used to control the microscope stage and the camera.

Synthesis of PKCδ-TAT inhibitor peptide

A peptide antagonist (PKCδ-TAT) was synthesized to selectively inhibit PKCδ activity. The peptide, derived from the first unique region (V1) of PKCδ (SFNSYELGSL: amino acids 8–17), was coupled to a membrane-permeant peptide sequence in the HIV TAT gene product (YGRKKRRQRRR: amino acids 47–57 of TAT) via an N-terminal Cys-Cys bond [20]. The resulting PKCδ-TAT peptide produces a unique dominant-negative phenotype that effectively inhibits activation of PKCδ but not other PKC isotypes. The PKCδ-TAT inhibitory peptide was synthesized by Mimotopes (Melbourne, Australia) and purified to > 95% by HPLC.

In vivo sepsis model

Animal procedures and handling were conducted in accordance with the NIH standards and were approved by the Institutional Animal Care and Use Committee at Temple University. Male Sprague-Dawley rats (300–350 g) (Charles River, Boston, MA) were used in all experiments. Rats were acclimated for at least 1 week in a climate-controlled facility and given free access to food and water. Sepsis was induced by the cecal ligation and puncture (CLP) method as described previously [21, 22]. Briefly, a midline laparotomy was performed and the cecum identified, the mesentery trimmed, and the stalk joining the cecum to the large intestine was ligated. The cecum was punctured with a 21-gauge needle, stool expressed and the cecum returned to the abdomen, and the incision closed in two layers. Sham controls underwent a laparotomy without cecal ligation or puncture. Following CLP or sham surgery, the abdominal incision was closed, and the animals were orally intubated with a 16-gauge intravenous cannula and randomized to receive either the PKCδ-TAT inhibitory peptide (200 μg/kg in 200 μl of PBS) or a like volume of PBS (vehicle).

PKCδ phosphorylation and translocation in rats

At 24 h post-surgery, animals were euthanized and the brains were harvested. Cell membrane and cytoplasm fractions of brain tissue were isolated using a Subcellular Protein Fractionation Kit for Tissues. For Western blot analysis, isolated tissue samples were mixed with 2X sample buffer to a final concentration of 30 μg/lane and heated for 5 min at 95 °C. Purity of membrane and cytosolic fractions were routinely monitored by probing cell membrane marker VE-cadherin. Proteins were separated on 4–12% SDS-PAGE gels and transferred to nitrocellulose membranes for blotting. The presence of phosphorylated PKCδ in membrane and cytoplasm fractions was determined by a phospho-specific PKCδ (Ser643/676) antibody [23–25]. PKCδ membrane translocation was then quantified by densitometry analysis to Western blot films in ImageJ software, and the values were expressed as a ratio of membrane fraction density to cytosolic fraction density.

Permeability measurements in vivo

Twenty-four hours post-sham or CLP surgery, animals were anesthetized, and Evans blue dye (4% in saline) was given at 2 ml/kg via tail vein. Thirty minutes post-dye injection, each rat was perfused with 50 ml of saline by direct injection through left ventricle into the ascending aorta. Brain samples were then collected, weighed, and homogenized in PBS. Evans blue was extracted from tissue homogenates by incubating samples in formamide at 60 °C for 14–18 h. The concentration of Evans blue in brain homogenate supernatants was quantified by a dual wavelength spectrophotometric method at absorptions of 620 and 740 nm that allows for correction of contaminating heme pigments using the following formula:

$$E620(\text{corrected}) = E620 - (1.426 \times E740 + 0.030)$$

$$(1)$$

Data are expressed as micrograms per milligram brain weight.

Design and fabrication of the B³C microfluidic assay

The blood-brain barrier on a chip (B³C) microfluidic assay used in this study (Fig. 1) is based on a modification of our previous design [19]. Vascular channels as well as tissue compartment were reproduced on a glass slide using soft-lithography processes as reported previously [19, 26]. This B³C microfluidic assay consists of vascular channels, which were covered with human brain microvascular endothelial cells (HBMVEC), in connection with a tissue compartment via a porous barrier. Microfabricated pillars (10 μm diameter) were used to fabricate the 3 μm × 100 μm pores resulting in vascular channels connected to a tissue compartment via 3 μm porous barrier, which is the optimum size for neutrophil migration.

Culturing of endothelial cells in B³C

HBMVEC and human astrocytes were cultured in their corresponding culture media and used between passages 1 and 2. The astrocyte-conditioned media (ACM) was prepared by culturing 10^7 astrocytes in 75 cm² culture flask with 12 ml of growth media for 48 h, after which the media were collected and filtered as reported previously [27]. The collected ACM was mixed with fresh ECM at 50/50 ratio and was used as the culture media for EC in B³C. Before EC seeding, the B³C was first degassed, washed with sterile deionized water, and then coated with human fibronectin at 37 °C for 30 min to facilitate cell attachment. HBMVEC suspended in ECM at a concentration of 5×10^6 cells/ml were seeded into the B³C using a programmable syringe pump and incubated at 37 °C for 4 h prior to shear flow (0.1 µl/min at the entry of the network) for 48 h. HBMVEC in B³C formed a confluent lumen and aligned in the direction of flow (Fig. 1). Formation of the 3D lumen in vascular channels under physiological conditions was confirmed using confocal microscopy [19, 28]. Assays in which neutrophils freely entered the tissue compartment without attachment were discarded.

Permeability and transendothelial electrical resistance measurements in B³C

HBMVEC integrity in the vascular channels was quantified by measuring the flux of a 40-kDa Texas Red fluorescent dextran (25 µM in ECM) from the vascular to the tissue compartment. The vascular channels were connected to a Hamilton gas-tight syringe filled with dextran solution maintained at 37 °C mounted on a programmable syringe pump. The B³C was then mounted on a Nikon TE200 fluorescence microscope equipped with a temperature controllable automated stage. Permeability was measured by imaging the B³C every minute for 2 h while the dextran solution flowed through the vascular channel (flow rate 0.1 µl/min). Using our previously published method [19, 27], the following equation was used to calculate permeability (P) of dextran across the endothelium in B³C:

$$P = \frac{1}{I_{v_0}} \frac{V}{S} \frac{dI_t}{dt} \tag{2}$$

where I_t is the average intensity in the tissue compartment, I_{v_0} is the maximum fluorescence intensity of the vascular channel, and $\frac{V}{S}$ is the ratio of vascular channel volume to its surface area.

Transendothelial electrical resistance (TEER) was measured following our established method [19] using an electrode compartment outside the vascular channels. Ag/AgCl electrodes were placed on either side of the HBMVEC in the vascular and tissue compartments and connected to SynVivo Cell Resistance Analyzer (SynVivo Inc., Huntsville, AL). Impedance measurements were acquired at 10 kHz with a voltage of 10 mV. Baseline TEER of the confluent EC monolayer

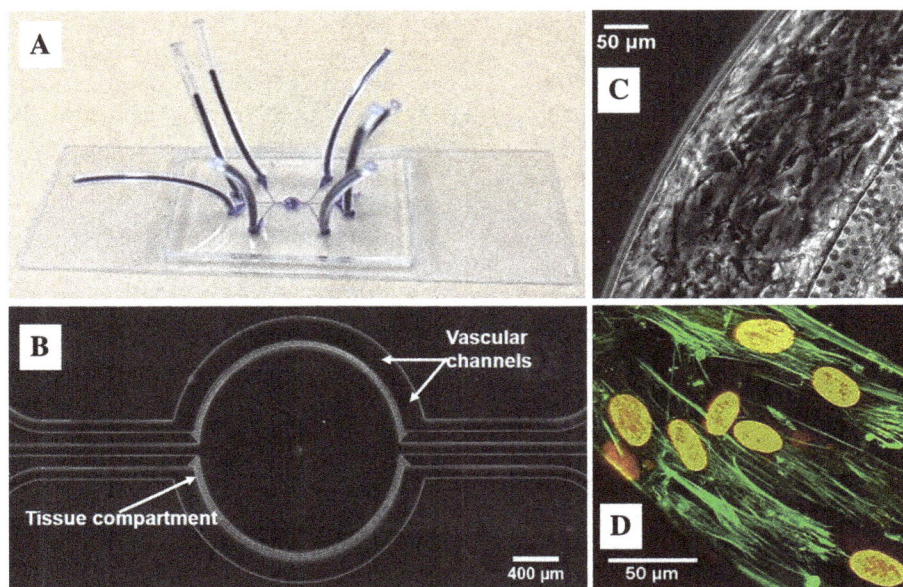

Fig. 1 HBMVEC cultured under flow in the vascular channel of B³C form a complete lumen. The B³C is assembled on a microscope glass slide (**a**) with plastic tubes (dark blue) allowing access to individual vascular channels and the tissue compartment (**b**). Magnified (**c**) view shows HBMVEC were cultured to confluence in the vascular channels. 3D reconstruction of confocal images (**d**) of HBMVEC stained with f-actin (green) and Draq5 (red) after 72 h of flow culture (0.1 µl/min)

was determined and then at 0, 24, and 48 h following the addition of TNF-α.

Neutrophil adhesion and migration in B³C

Following informed consent, human heparinized blood was obtained from healthy male or female adult donors. Human neutrophils were isolated by ficoll-hypaque separation, dextran sedimentation, and hypotonic lysis to remove erythrocytes [21, 23]. Isolated neutrophils were suspended in HBSS (5×10^6 cells/ml) and labeled using CFDA/SE probe for 10 min at room temperature. All procedures were approved by the Temple University Institutional Review Board (Philadelphia, PA, USA).

Neutrophils were introduced into the vascular channels of the B³C at a flow rate of 0.1 μl/min. Neutrophils in contact with EC that did not move for 30 s were considered adherent. Adhesion level of neutrophils to the endothelium reached steady state after 10 min of flow and was quantified by scanning the entire network [28]. The number of migrated neutrophils was quantified using time-lapse imaging every 3 min for 60 min.

Immunofluorescence staining of the EC in B³C

To study morphological changes in cells, actin filaments were stained with phalloidin and cell nucleus was stained with Hoechst 33342. To examine EC barrier function after sepsis with or without PKCδ-i treatment, the formation of endothelial cell-to-cell tight junction was characterized using immunostaining against zonula occludens-1 (ZO-1). Briefly, the B³C was perfused with 4% neutral buffered formalin to fix the cells followed by 10-min treatment with 0.1% Triton X-100 to expose ZO-1 protein. After blocking with 5% goat serum in PBS for 1 h at 37 °C, the vascular channel of the B³C was incubated with mouse monoclonal primary antibody against ZO-1 (1:100) overnight at 4 °C. On the second day, the B³C was then incubated with fluorophore-conjugated secondary antibodies Alexa fluor 594 goat anti-mouse IgG for 1 h at 37 °C. Cells in B³C were washed with PBS containing 5% serum between each step using a syringe. Images were taken using the same microscope and camera system as described before. The background noise was removed from the image by thresholding, and the ZO-1 staining was enhanced in the ImageJ software using the "Find Edges" function.

PKCδ phosphorylation and translocation in HBMVEC

The presence and subcellular distribution of phosphorylated PKCδ in HBMVEC was determined by immunostaining followed by fluorescence imaging. PKCδ phosphorylation was quantified by intensity analysis in ImageJ software, and the values were expressed as a ratio of cell nucleus intensity to cytosolic intensity. HBMVEC cultured in chamber slides were fixed with 4% neutral buffered formalin followed by 0.1% Triton X-100 permeabilization. After blocking with 5% goat serum in PBS for 1 h at 37 °C, HBMVEC were incubated with phospho-specific PKCδ (Ser643/676) antibody (1:100) overnight at 4 °C. On the second day, the cells were washed and then incubated with Alexa fluor 594 fluorescent goat anti-rabbit secondary antibody for 1 h at 37 °C. Cells were washed with PBS containing 5% serum between each step. Images were taken using the same microscope and camera system as described before.

Data analysis

Nikon Elements and Fiji software were used to collect and analyze the data [29]. Data are presented as mean ± SEM. Statistical significance was determined by one-way or two-way analysis of variance (ANOVA) with Tukey-Kramer post hoc using SigmaPlot software. Differences were considered statistically significant if $p < 0.05$.

Results

Brain EC form a complete lumen in B³C

The schematic of the B³C microfluidic assay is shown in Fig. 1a. Two independent vascular channels with dimensions of 200 μm (width) × 100 μm (height) × 2762 μm (length) were placed around the tissue compartment. The dimensions of the vascular channels which closely approximate the size and morphology of microvessels in vivo permit the B³C to maintain physiologically relevant shear flow conditions for HBMVEC growth (Fig. 1c). Simultaneous real-time visualization of the vascular and tissue compartments was achieved by the side-by-side placement of optically clear polydimethylsiloxane (PDMS) onto a glass slide. The vascular channels and tissue compartment were separated by a porous interface which was constructed by a tightly packed cylindrical micro-pillar array to allow for biochemical and cellular communications. Previously, we have reported that brain EC barrier function was dependent on the presence of astrocytes or ACM [19]. Moreover, no significant differences were detected in EC permeability, TEER, or ZO-1 expression when comparing EC treated with ACM vs. EC co-cultured with astrocytes [19]. Therefore, in this study, HBMVEC was cultured with ACM in the vascular channels without astrocytes in the tissue compartment. To allow for real-time monitoring of EC barrier function as well as neutrophil-endothelial interaction, the B³C is constructed from optically clear PDMS assembled on a microscope slide (Fig. 1b). HBMVEC cultured with ACM under flow formed a complete 3D lumen in the vascular channels (Fig. 1d), which mimics the normal EC lining observed in vivo.

Sepsis-induced PKCδ activation and BBB barrier damage in rats are attenuated by treatment with a PKCδ peptide inhibitor

PKCδ activation requires phosphorylation on key serine/threonine sites, and translocation of PKCδ from the cell cytosol to membrane sites is a critical step in the activation of PKCδ in brain inflammation [23, 30]. To demonstrate that sepsis leads to PKCδ activation in the rat brain, we performed Western blot analysis on the subcellular fractionation of brain homogenates. As shown in Fig. 2a, in sham-operated rats, the majority of phosphorylated PKCδ was located in the cytosolic fraction as compared to the membrane fraction. In contrast, at 24 h post-CLP surgery, there was a significant increase in translocation of PKCδ from the cytosolic site to the membrane site. The PKCδ translocation pattern in CLP rats treated with the PKCδ-*i* was similar to that of sham-operated animals, indicating that the PKCδ activity was inhibited in treated animals. Densitometric analysis (Fig. 2b) of the Western blot images demonstrated that PKCδ translocation in septic rat brains was significantly increased and that treatment of septic animals with PKCδ-*i* inhibited this translocation. This pattern of PKCδ phosphorylation is consistent with our in vivo observations where PKCδ inhibition significantly reduced sepsis-induced Evans blue extravasation into the brain tissue at 24 h post-CLP surgery (Fig. 2c).

Inflammation-mediated activation of PKCδ in HBMVEC is inhibited by treatment with a PKCδ peptide inhibitor

To examine the effect of inflammation on PKCδ activation in brain endothelial cells, we determined PKCδ phosphorylation by immunostaining of HBMVEC in culture. As shown in Fig. 3a, in response to TNF treatment, there was a significant increase in PKCδ phosphorylation and enzyme translocation as compared to cells treated with buffer alone (no treatment). The addition of the PKCδ peptide inhibitor (TNF-α + PKCδ-*i*) attenuated TNF-mediated phosphorylation and translocation of PKCδ. This observation was confirmed by fluorescence intensity analysis as shown in Fig. 3b.

PKCδ inhibition modulates increased permeability in activated HBMVEC in B³C

In vitro, the HBMVEC permeability was quantified in the B³C with no treatment or 4 h after TNF-α with or without PKCδ-*i* treatment. As shown in Fig. 4a, a threefold increase was observed in dextran permeability from vascular channels to the tissue compartment in TNF-α-treated HBMVEC ($3.7 \pm 1.0 \times 10^{-7}$ to $12.8 \pm 0.7 \times 10^{-7}$ cm/s). Significant reduction in dextran permeability was observed when TNF-α-activated HBMVEC ($5.3 \pm 0.8 \times 10^{-7}$ cm/s) were treated with the PKCδ-*i*.

PKCδ inhibition modulates TEER decrease in activated HBMVEC in B³C

Our microfluidic system has electrodes in the two compartments for TEER measurements. Under static conditions, TEER of HBMVEC remained relatively constant over 96 h at 50 kΩ (data not shown). Under shear flow conditions, tight junctional endothelial integrity was significantly enhanced and TEER values increased by more than twofold (108.6 ± 4.0 kΩ). Addition of TNF-α produced a significant decrease in TEER indicating decreased EC barrier, whereas treatment with PKCδ-*i* of TNF-α-activated HBMVEC modulated this decrease to the control level (116.7 ± 5.4 kΩ) (Fig. 4b).

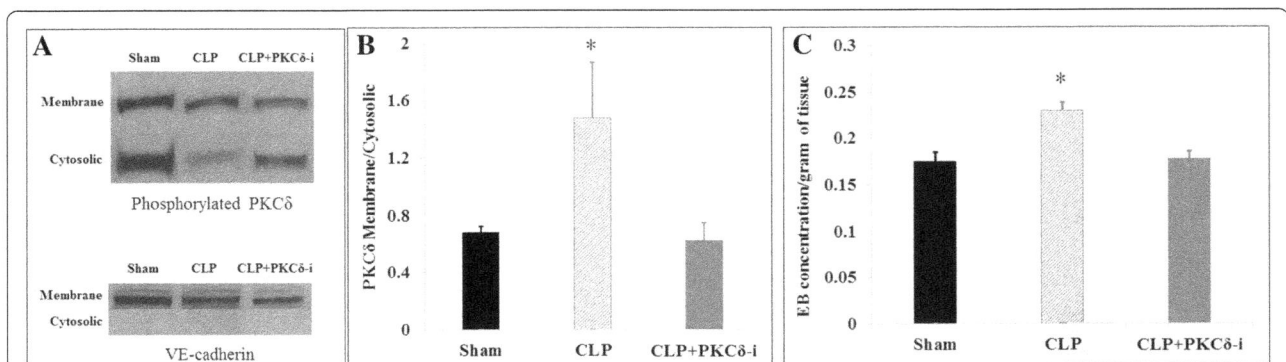

Fig. 2 Sepsis-induced PKCδ activation and BBB barrier damage in rats are attenuated by PKCδ inhibition. **a** Representative Western blot images of phosphor-PKCδ membrane and cytosolic fractions in the brain samples of sham-operated, septic (CLP), or treated septic (CLP+PKCδ-*i*) rats. VE-cadherin was used as a marker for the membrane fraction. **b** Densitometry analysis of phosphorylated PKCδ (Ser643) translocation. Values are expressed as the density ratio of the membrane to the cytosolic fraction. **c** PKCδ inhibition (PKCδ-*i*) also attenuates sepsis (CLP) induced Evans blue (EB) dye extravasation in rat brain. Data are presented as mean ± SEM (*n* = 3). *$p < 0.05$ compared to sham and CLP+PKCδ-*i* by ANOVA with Tukey-Kramer post hoc

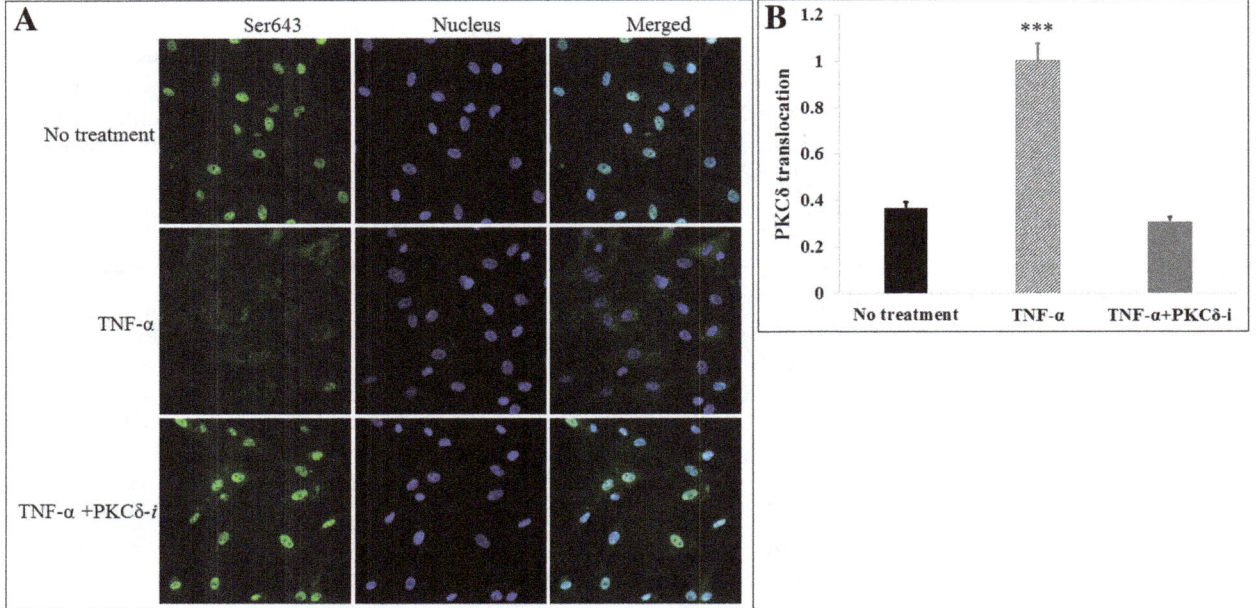

Fig. 3 Cytokine-induced PKCδ phosphorylation in vitro is attenuated by PKCδ inhibition. **a** Representative immunostaining images of phosphor-PKCδ distribution in non-treated, TNF-α-activated, or TNF-α + PKCδ-i-treated HBMVEC in static culture. **b** Fluorescence intensity analysis of phosphorylated PKCδ (Ser643) translocation. Values are expressed as the intensity ratio of the cell nucleus to the cytosol. Data are presented as mean ± SEM ($n = 3$). ***$p < 0.0001$ compared to no treatment and TNF-α + PKCδ-i by ANOVA with Tukey-Kramer post hoc

PKCδ inhibition attenuates neutrophil adhesion and migration in B³C

To further explore the effect of PKCδ inhibition on neutrophil-endothelial cell interaction during sepsis, neutrophil adhesion to and migration across HBMVEC under shear flow was investigated. Cytokine activation (4 h TNF-α treatment) significantly increased the number of adhering neutrophils to ECs as compared to controls ($77 ± 7$ vs. $199 ± 10$). PKCδ inhibition significantly reduced the total number of

adhered neutrophils by 54%, a level which is not statistically different from control levels ($77 ± 7$ vs. $91 ± 16$) (Fig. 5a).

Neutrophil migration across HBMVEC into the tissue compartment was used to further assess endothelial barrier function after cytokine activation with or without PKCδ inhibition. In B³C, the number of migrated neutrophils across TNF-α-activated endothelium in response to the chemoattractant (fMLP) significantly increased over 60 min. Neutrophil migration across cytokine-activated

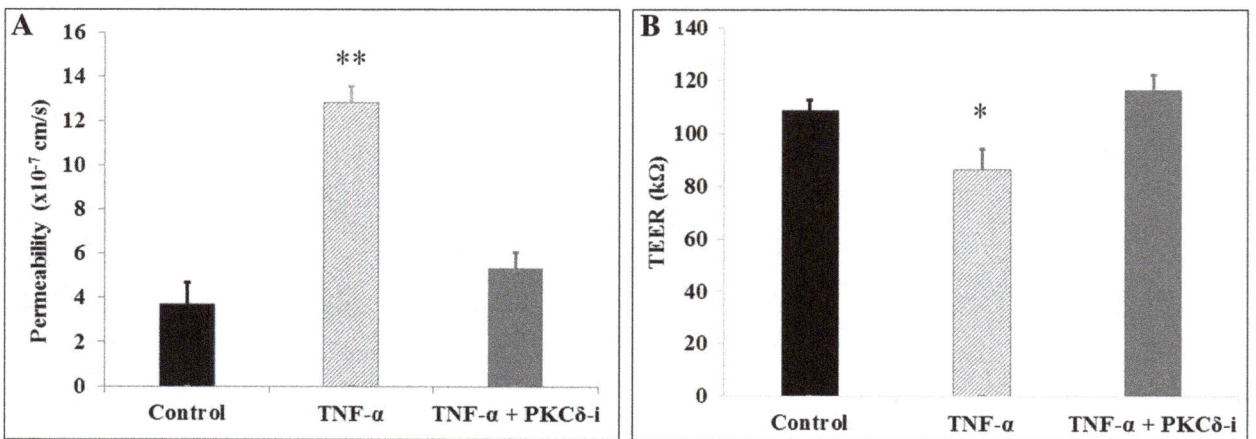

Fig. 4 PKCδ inhibition (PKCδ-i) attenuates TNF-α-induced permeability increase (**a**) and TEER decrease (**b**) in vitro in B³C after 4 h of TNF-α activation. Data are presented as mean ± SEM ($n = 3$). **$p < 0.01$, *$p < 0.05$, compared to control and TNF-α + PCKδ-i treatment group by ANOVA with Tukey-Kramer post hoc

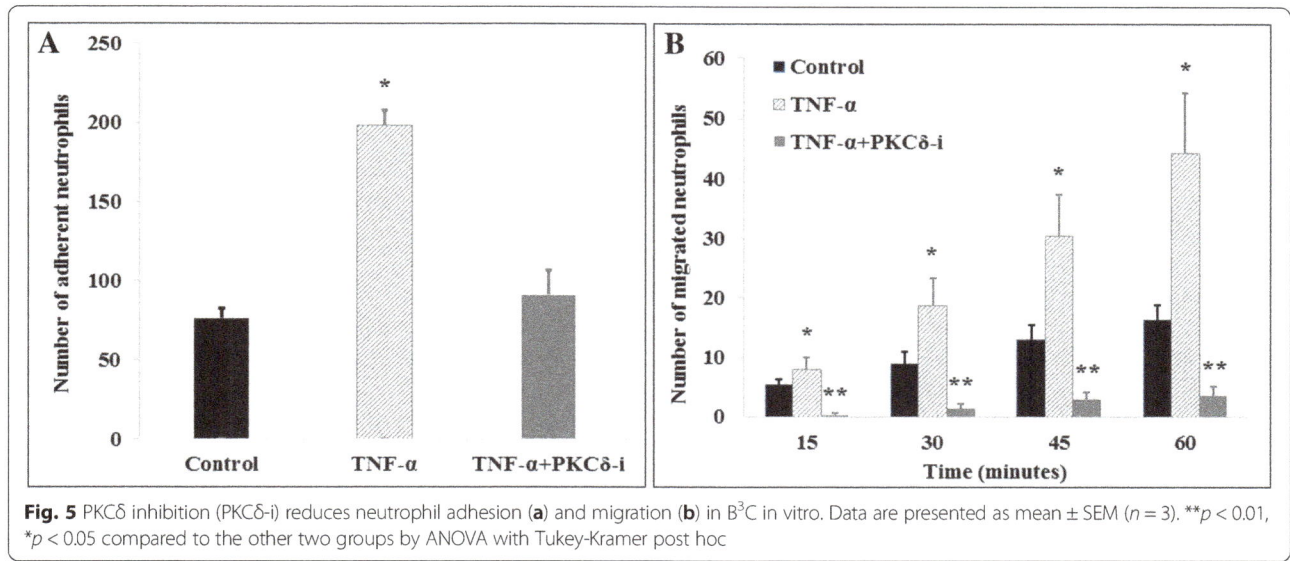

Fig. 5 PKCδ inhibition (PKCδ-i) reduces neutrophil adhesion (**a**) and migration (**b**) in B³C in vitro. Data are presented as mean ± SEM ($n = 3$). **$p < 0.01$, *$p < 0.05$ compared to the other two groups by ANOVA with Tukey-Kramer post hoc

HBMVEC was almost completely inhibited after PKCδ-TAT treatment (Fig. 5b), making it significantly lower than the control level of neutrophil migration.

PKCδ inhibition attenuates cytokine-induced tight junction damage in B³C

Tight junctions are important for regulating the barrier properties of BBB. Immunofluorescence staining for ZO-1 was used to highlight HBMVEC tight junction molecule expression under control conditions, after treatment with TNF-α, or treatment with TNF-α and PKCδ-TAT inhibitor (Fig. 6). Under control conditions, HBMVEC continuously expressed tight junctions when cultured using HA-conditioned media under shear flow in B³C as indicated by strong continuous ZO-1 staining in the vascular compartment (Fig. 6q). This shows that our B³C assay not

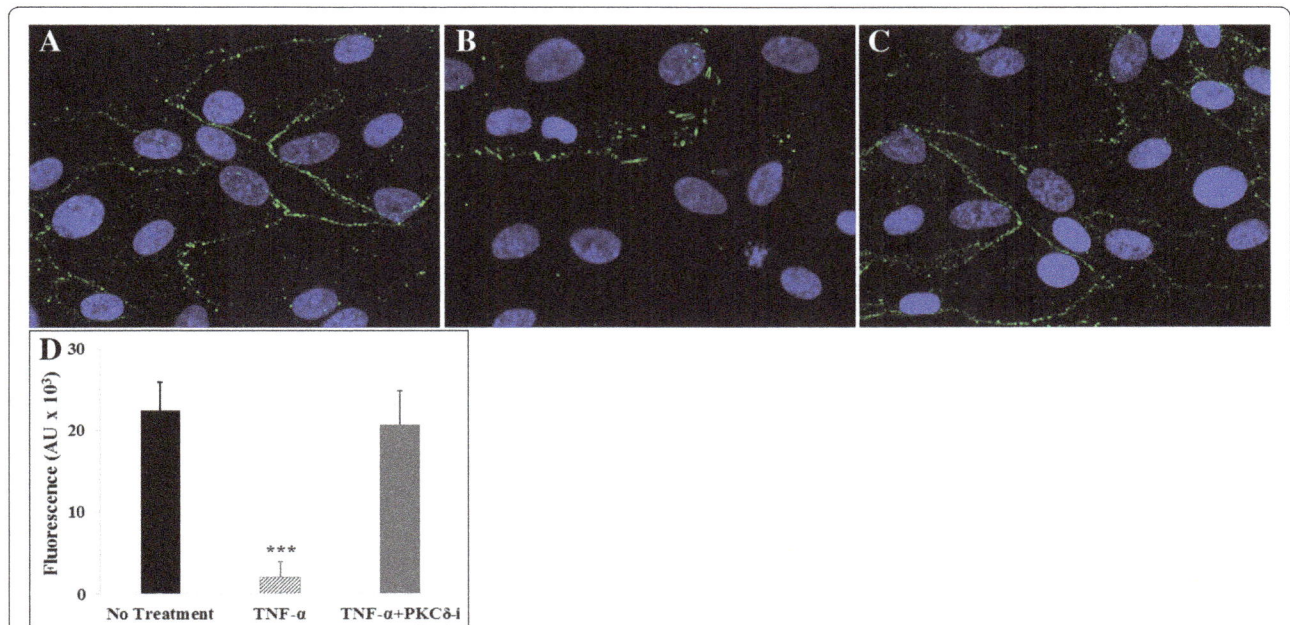

Fig. 6 Tight junction formation by HBMVEC under flow conditions as indicated by immunofluorescence staining of ZO-1. PKCδ inhibition (PKCδ-i) attenuates TNF-α-induced tight junction damage in vitro in B³C. When cultured with normal media, tight junctions were fully established between adjacent cells (**a**). Tight junction expression was disrupted after 4 h of TNF-α activation (**b**), while PKCδ inhibition (TNF-α + PKCδ-i) restored tight junction expression (**c**). HBMVEC cultured for 72 h under flow (0.1 μl/min) were stained with ZO-1 (red) and Hoechst 33342 (blue). **d** Quantitative analysis to the total tight junction fluorescence intensity confirmed our observation. Data are presented as mean ± SEM ($n = 3$). *** $p < 0.001$ compared to no treatment and TNF-α + PKCδ-i by ANOVA with Tukey-Kramer post hoc

only provides an in vivo-like shear flow environment, but also permits junction formation in ECs cultured in the vascular compartment. TNF-α activation significantly downregulated tight junction expression as indicated by a lack of ZO-1 in some cells as well as intermittent ZO-1 expression along the edges of the remaining cells (Fig. 6b). The expression of ZO-1 in PKCδ-TAT-treated, TNF-α-activated HBMVEC (Fig. 6c) was similar to those observed in control ECs (Fig. 6a), indicating that PKCδ inhibition attenuates cytokine activation-induced tight junction damage. This observation was confirmed by quantitative analysis to the total tight junction fluorescence intensity (Fig. 6d).

Discussion

The inflammatory response is composed of multiple overlapping and redundant mechanisms, and recent research has shifted the focus to developing therapeutics that can regulate common control signaling points which are activated by diverse signals. In vitro studies using our bioinspired microfluidic assay (bMFA) demonstrated a role for pulmonary endothelial PKCδ in mediating neutrophil-endothelial interaction [28]. Studies also suggest that PKCδ may be a major mediator and/or modulator of inflammatory responses in brain [31, 32], suggesting a critical role of PKCδ in mediating BBB damage during sepsis. In this study, we demonstrate that activation of PKCδ results in alterations in tight junction protein expression and functional integrity of the BBB after cytokine activation or CLP-induced sepsis. In vitro, inhibition of PKCδ prevented activation of ECs, protected BBB structure integrity, and prevented neutrophil migration across the brain EC. Treatment of septic animals with the PKCδ inhibitor prevented activation of PKCδ and restored BBB permeability to control levels. Our findings support the hypothesis that PKCδ inhibition can attenuate the disruption of ZO-1 tight junction protein, resulting in a decrease in permeability and an increase in electrical resistance across the endothelial cell barrier.

Maintenance of normal brain function is very much dependent on the integrity of BBB that is highly selective to the passage of molecules and cells from the blood to the brain tissue. Extravasation of dyes and changes in transendothelial electrical resistance are often used to measure permeability of the BBB barrier in vivo and in vitro. For example, Evans blue is widely regarded as the standard measurement of BBB permeability and its extravasation has been used by numerous studies to quantify BBB breakdown in vivo [33–37], despite some reported limitations [38–40]. Transport of macromolecules larger than 5 nm, such as the 40-kDa dextran, occurs through the transcellular pathway (through the cell body regulated by the cell membrane lipid bilayer) [41–44] that is regulated in part by cytoskeleton proteins

such as actin and is altered by TNF-α activation [45]. Under pathological conditions such as cytokine stimulations, the distribution of junctions between endothelial cells, as well as cytoskeleton proteins such as actin, can be downregulated resulting in paracellular transport of macromolecules. TNF-α stimulation has been shown to induce alterations in cell-cell and cell-matrix interaction [45]. Components of adherens (cadherin) and tight junctions (occludins) were found to be downregulated in TNF-α stimulated cells and the contacts between neighboring cells were breached [46–50]. TEER on the other hand is an index of current flow via the paracellular route (through the junctions between cells and regulated by junctional proteins) and via the transcellular route [51]. These different regulatory mechanisms may become more prominent depending on the phenomenon being studied. In this study, TNF-α activation had a larger impact on BBB permeability to a 40-kDa dextran (threefold increase) as compared to TEER (23% reduction) indicating a shift from transcellular to paracellular transport.

The role of PKC in the regulation of BBB has been studied in several disease conditions in vivo [52–55]. However, the relative contribution of each of the different PKC isoforms is still not clear. To date, there are at least 12 different PKC isoforms discovered [56]. Conflicting data on the critical role of PKCδ in these diseases have been described. For example, three PKC family isotypes (PKCα, PKCδ, and PKCε) were found to be co-localized with EC after blast exposure [52]. However, high levels of PKCθ, PKCζ, and PKCγ isozyme expression were seen in cortical endothelial cells in a rat hypoxia and post-hypoxic reoxygenation model [54]. In a rat hypertension model, sustained pharmacological inhibition of PKCδ prevented the development of hypertensive encephalopathy through prevention of BBB breakdown [55]. Utilizing an in vitro transwell co-culture model of the BBB of mouse bEnd.3 cells, Kim et al. demonstrated that both PKCβII and PKCδ were activated during aglycemic hypoxia and while PKCδ activation was found to be protective of BBB integrity, PKCβII activation was detrimental to BBB integrity [53]. Thus, whereas these studies have shown the potential role of PKC in barrier permeability, there is still some uncertainty about the specific role of the δ isoform. The differential regulation of BBB by PKCδ in diverse cell systems is not surprising as specific regulatory roles for PKCδ are context specific and dependent on mechanisms of PKCδ activation, phosphorylation patterns, and input from other signaling pathways [23, 57, 58]. To our knowledge, the present study is the first to provide direct evidence of BBB disruption caused by PKCδ activation in sepsis. Meanwhile, no studies have examined the effects of PKCδ inhibition as a therapeutic approach for treatment of sepsis-induced brain damage.

Previous studies from our group demonstrated a key role for PKCδ in the regulation of proinflammatory signaling controlling the activation and recruitment of neutrophils [14, 16, 18, 28, 59, 60]. Our recent study using a PKCδ Knock-in mouse model of sepsis and an in vitro biomimetic microfluidic assay further demonstrated that PKCδ activation (tyrosine 155 phosphorylation) is required for neutrophil activation, adherence, and transmigration through pulmonary endothelium [61]. Consistent with these findings, in the current study, we show that PKCδ not only plays a significant role in regulating EC permeability, TEER, and tight junction protein expression in activated HBMVEC in the absence of neutrophils, but also inhibits neutrophil-endothelial cell interaction.

A novel aspect of this study is assessment of vascular integrity using a biomimetic blood-brain barrier microfluidic platform (B³C) where EC permeability and TEER as well as neutrophil transmigration can be directly evaluated. Compared to traditional transwell-based BBB models, the permeability of our B³C model was significantly lower and more closely mimic reported in vivo values [19]. More importantly, B³C allowed for real-time monitoring of neutrophil-endothelial interaction under physiologically relevant flow conditions.

Conclusions

We developed a first dynamic in vitro BBB on-a-chip (B³C) that offers the flexibility of real-time analysis and is suitable for studies of BBB function as well as screening of novel therapeutics. Our findings suggest that PKCδ activation is a key signaling event that dysregulates the structural and functional integrity of BBB, which leads to vascular damage and inflammation-induced tissue damage due to neutrophil transmigration. Our data suggest that PKCδ-TAT has therapeutic potential for the prevention or reduction of cerebrovascular injury in sepsis-induced vascular damage. Utilizing both in vivo (rat CLP model) and in vitro (B³C) tools, our findings support a novel therapeutic paradigm that targets PKCδ and neutrophil-endothelial interactions to protect BBB integrity and attenuate sepsis-induced brain tissue damage. These findings highlight an important control point of the proinflammatory signaling cascade and potential therapeutic targets for the treatment of sepsis-induced brain vascular damage.

Abbreviations

ACM: Astrocyte-conditioned media; ANOVA: Analysis of variance; B³C: Blood-brain barrier on-a-chip; BBB: Blood-brain barrier; bMFA: Bioinspired microfluidic assay; BSA: Bovine serum albumin; CFDA/SE: Carboxyfluorescein diacetate succinimidyl ester; CLP: Cecal ligation and puncture; EC: Endothelial cell; ECM: Endothelial cell media; fMLP: N-Formylmethionyl-leucyl-phenylalanine; HBMVEC: Human brain microvascular endothelial cell; HBSS: Hanks' Balanced Salt solution; PBS: Phosphate buffered saline; PDMS: Polydimethylsiloxane; PKC: Protein kinase C; PKCδ: Protein kinase C-delta; PKCδ-i: Protein kinase C-delta TAT peptide inhibitor; TEER: Transendothelial electrical resistance; TNF-α: Tumor necrosis factor α; ZO-1: Zonula occludens-1

Acknowledgements
Not applicable.

Funding
This work was supported by the American Heart Association (16GRNT29980001) and National Institutes of Health (GM114359 and HL111552).

Authors' contributions
YT and FS performed the research, analyzed the data, and wrote the manuscript and were also responsible for the statistical analyses. SS and EL performed the CLP surgery and Western blot. JCL and QY performed, edited, and analyzed the imaging and analysis tools. YT, LEK, and MFK designed the study, organized the experiments, analyzed the data, and wrote the manuscript. All authors read and approved the final manuscript.

Competing interests
L.E.K. is listed as an inventor on US Patent #8,470,766, entitled "Novel Protein Kinase C Therapy for the Treatment of Acute Lung Injury," which is assigned to the Children's Hospital of Philadelphia and the University of Pennsylvania.

Author details
[1]Department of Mechanical Engineering, College of Engineering, Temple University, Philadelphia, PA 19122, USA. [2]Center for Inflammation, Clinical and Translational Lung Research, Lewis Katz School of Medicine, Temple University, Philadelphia, PA 19140, USA. [3]Sol Sherry Thrombosis Research Center, Lewis Katz School of Medicine, Temple University, Philadelphia, PA 19140, USA. [4]Department of Radiation Oncology, Lewis Katz School of Medicine, Temple University, Philadelphia, PA 19140, USA.

References
1. Singer M, Deutschman CS, Seymour C, et al. The third international consensus definitions for sepsis and septic shock (sepsis-3). JAMA. 2016;315:801–10.
2. Deutschman Clifford S, Tracey Kevin J. Sepsis: current dogma and new perspectives. Immunity. 2014;40:463–75.
3. Angus DC, van der Poll T. Severe sepsis and septic shock. N Engl J Med. 2013;369:840–51.
4. Leibovici L. Long-term consequences of severe infections. Clin Microbiol Infect. 2013;19:510–2.
5. Goldenberg NM, Steinberg BE, Slutsky AS, Lee WL. Broken barriers: a new take on sepsis pathogenesis. Sci Transl Med. 2011;3:88ps25.
6. Maniatis NA, Orfanos SE. The endothelium in acute lung injury/acute respiratory distress syndrome. Curr Opin Crit Care. 2008;14:22–30. https://doi.org/10.1097/MCC.1090b1013e3282f1269b1099.
7. Danese S, Dejana E, Fiocchi C. Immune regulation by microvascular endothelial cells: directing innate and adaptive immunity, coagulation, and inflammation. J Immunol. 2007;178:6017–22.
8. Handa O, Stephen J, Cepinskas G. Role of endothelial nitric oxide synthase-derived nitric oxide in activation and dysfunction of cerebrovascular endothelial cells during early onsets of sepsis. Am J Physiol Heart Circ Physiol. 2008;295:H1712–9.
9. Sonneville R, Verdonk F, Rauturier C, Klein IF, Wolff M, Annane D, Chretien F, Sharshar T. Understanding brain dysfunction in sepsis. Ann Intensive Care. 2013;3:15.
10. Stamatovic SM, Keep RF, Andjelkovic AV. Brain endothelial cell-cell junctions: how to "open" the blood brain barrier. Curr Neuropharmacol. 2008;6:179–92.
11. Iskander KN, Osuchowski MF, Stearns-Kurosawa DJ, Kurosawa S, Stepien D, Valentine C, Remick DG. Sepsis: multiple abnormalities, heterogeneous responses, and evolving understanding. Physiol Rev. 2013;93:1247–88.
12. Kilpatrick LE, Lee JY, Haines KM, Campbell DE, Sullivan KE, Korchak HM. A role for PKC-delta and PI 3-kinase in TNF-alpha-mediated antiapoptotic signaling in the human neutrophil. Am J Physiol Cell Physiol. 2002;283:C48–57.

13. Kilpatrick LE, Sun S, Korchak HM. Selective regulation by delta-PKC and PI 3-kinase in the assembly of the antiapoptotic TNFR-1 signaling complex in neutrophils. Am J Physiol Cell Physiol. 2004;287:C633–42.

14. Kilpatrick LE, Sun S, Mackie D, Baik F, Li H, Korchak HM. Regulation of TNF mediated antiapoptotic signaling in human neutrophils: role of {delta}-PKC and ERK1/2. J Leuk Biol. 2006;80:1512–21.

15. Liverani E, Mondrinos MJ, Sun S, Kunapuli SP, Kilpatrick LE. Role of Protein Kinase C-delta in regulating platelet activation and platelet-leukocyte interaction during sepsis. PLoS One. 2018;13:e0195379.

16. Kilpatrick LE, Standage SW, Li H, Raj NR, Korchak HM, Wolfson MR, Deutschman CS. Protection against sepsis-induced lung injury by selective inhibition of protein kinase C-δ (δ-PKC). J Leukoc Biol. 2011;89:3–10.

17. Mondrinos MJ, Kennedy PA, Lyons M, Deutschman CS, Kilpatrick LE. Protein kinase C and acute respiratory distress syndrome. Shock. 2013;39:467–79.

18. Mondrinos MJ, Zhang T, Sun S, Kennedy PA, King DJ, Wolfson MR, Knight LC, Scalia R, Kilpatrick LE. Pulmonary endothelial protein kinase C-Delta (PKCδ) regulates neutrophil migration in acute lung inflammation. Am J Pathol. 2014;184:200–13.

19. Deosarkar SP, Prabhakarpandian B, Wang B, Sheffield JB, Krynska B, Kiani MF. A novel dynamic neonatal blood-brain barrier on a chip. PLoS One. 2015;10:e0142725.

20. Chen L, Hahn H, Wu G, Chen CH, Liron T, Schechtman D, Cavallaro G, Banci L, Guo Y, Bolli R, et al. Opposing cardioprotective actions and parallel hypertrophic effects of delta PKC and epsilon PKC. Proc Natl Acad Sci U S A. 2001;98:11114–9.

21. Mondrinos MJ, Zhang T, Sun S, Kennedy PA, King DJ, Wolfson MR, Knight LC, Scalia R, Kilpatrick LE. Pulmonary endothelial protein kinase C-delta (PKCdelta) regulates neutrophil migration in acute lung inflammation. Am J Pathol. 2014;184:200–13.

22. Mondrinos MJ, Knight LC, Kennedy PA, Wu J, Kauffman M, Baker ST, Wolfson MR, Kilpatrick LE. Biodistribution and efficacy of targeted pulmonary delivery of a protein kinase C-delta inhibitory peptide: impact on indirect lung injury. J Pharmacol Exp Ther. 2015;355:86–98.

23. Kilpatrick LE, Sun S, Li H, Vary TC, Korchak HM. Regulation of TNF-induced oxygen radical production in human neutrophils: role of delta-PKC. J Leukoc Biol. 2010;87:153–64.

24. Begley R, Liron T, Baryza J, Mochly-Rosen D. Biodistribution of intracellularly acting peptides conjugated reversibly to Tat. Biochem Biophys Res Commun. 2004;318:949–54.

25. Vary TC, Goodman S, Kilpatrick LE, Lynch CJ. Nutrient regulation of PKCepsilon is mediated by leucine, not insulin, in skeletal muscle. Am J Physiol Endocrinol Metab. 2005;289:E684–94.

26. Prabhakarpandian B, Shen M-C, Pant K, Kiani MF. Microfluidic devices for modeling cell-cell and particle-cell interactions in the microvasculature. Microvasc Res. 2011;82:210–20.

27. Tang Y, Soroush F, Sheffield JB, Wang B, Prabhakarpandian B, Kiani MF. A biomimetic microfluidic tumor microenvironment platform mimicking the EPR effect for rapid screening of drug delivery systems. Sci Rep. 2017;7:9359.

28. Soroush F, Zhang T, King DJ, Tang Y, Deosarkar S, Prabhakarpandian B, Kilpatrick LE, Kiani MF. A novel microfluidic assay reveals a key role for protein kinase C delta in regulating human neutrophil-endothelium interaction. J Leukoc Biol. 2016;100:1027–35.

29. Schindelin J, Arganda-Carreras I, Frise E, Kaynig V, Longair M, Pietzsch T, Preibisch S, Rueden C, Saalfeld S, Schmid B, et al. Fiji: an open-source platform for biological-image analysis. Nat Methods. 2012;9:676–82.

30. Salzer E, Santos-Valente E, Keller B, Warnatz K, Boztug K. Protein kinase C delta: a gatekeeper of immune homeostasis. J Clin Immunol. 2016;36:631–40.

31. Gordon R, Anantharam V, Kanthasamy AG, Kanthasamy A. Proteolytic activation of proapoptotic kinase protein kinase Cdelta by tumor necrosis factor alpha death receptor signaling in dopaminergic neurons during neuroinflammation. J Neuroinflammation. 2012;9:82.

32. Kaasinen SK, Goldsteins G, Alhonen L, Janne J, Koistinaho J. Induction and activation of protein kinase C delta in hippocampus and cortex after kainic acid treatment. Exp Neurol. 2002;176:203–12.

33. Wang Z, Li Y, Cai S, Li R, Cao G. Cannabinoid receptor 2 agonist attenuates blood-brain barrier damage in a rat model of intracerebral hemorrhage by activating the Rac1 pathway. Int J Mol Med. 2018;42:2914–22.

34. Li T, Xu W, Gao L, Guan G, Zhang Z, He P, Xu H, Fan L, Yan F, Chen G. Mesencephalic astrocyte-derived neurotrophic factor affords neuroprotection to early brain injury induced by subarachnoid hemorrhage

35. Kucuk M, Ugur Yilmaz C, Orhan N, Ahishali B, Arican N, Elmas I, Gurses C, Kaya M. The effects of lipopolysaccharide on the disrupted blood-brain barrier in a rat model of preeclampsia. J Stroke Cerebrovasc Dis. 2018.

36. Sarami Foroshani M, Sobhani ZS, Mohammadi MT, Aryafar M. Fullerenol nanoparticles decrease blood-brain barrier interruption and brain edema during cerebral ischemia-reperfusion injury probably by reduction of interleukin-6 and matrix metalloproteinase-9 transcription. J Stroke Cerebrovasc Dis. 2018;27:3053–65.

37. Faezi M, Nasseri Maleki S, Aboutaleb N, Nikougoftar M. The membrane mesenchymal stem cell derived conditioned medium exerts neuroprotection against focal cerebral ischemia by targeting apoptosis. J Chem Neuroanat. 2018;94:21–31.

38. Wang HL, Lai TW. Optimization of Evans blue quantitation in limited rat tissue samples. Sci Rep. 2014;4:6588.

39. Saunders NR, Dziegielewska KM, Mollgard K, Habgood MD. Markers for blood-brain barrier integrity: how appropriate is Evans blue in the twenty-first century and what are the alternatives? Front Neurosci. 2015;9:385.

40. Yao L, Xue X, Yu P, Ni Y, Chen F. Evans blue dye: a revisit of its applications in biomedicine. Contrast Media Mol Imaging. 2018;2018:7628037.

41. Sukriti S, Tauseef M, Yazbeck P, Mehta D. Mechanisms regulating endothelial permeability. Pulm Circ. 2014;4:535–51.

42. Vogel SM, Malik AB. Cytoskeletal dynamics and lung fluid balance. Compr Physiol. 2012;2:449–78.

43. Komarova Y, Malik AB. Regulation of endothelial permeability via paracellular and transcellular transport pathways. Annu Rev Physiol. 2010;72:463–93.

44. Predescu SA, Predescu DN, Palade GE. Endothelial transcytotic machinery involves supramolecular protein-lipid complexes. Mol Biol Cell. 2001; 12:1019–33.

45. Seynhaeve AL, Vermeulen CE, Eggermont AM, ten Hagen TL. Cytokines and vascular permeability: an in vitro study on human endothelial cells in relation to tumor necrosis factor-alpha-primed peripheral blood mononuclear cells. Cell Biochem Biophys. 2006;44:157–69.

46. Coyne CB, Vanhook MK, Gambling TM, Carson JL, Boucher RC, Johnson LG. Regulation of airway tight junctions by proinflammatory cytokines. Mol Biol Cell. 2002;13:3218–34.

47. Wachtel M, Bolliger MF, Ishihara H, Frei K, Bluethmann H, Gloor SM. Down-regulation of occludin expression in astrocytes by tumour necrosis factor (TNF) is mediated via TNF type-1 receptor and nuclear factor-kappaB activation. J Neurochem. 2001;78:155–62.

48. Mankertz J, Tavalali S, Schmitz H, Mankertz A, Riecken EO, Fromm M, Schulzke JD. Expression from the human occludin promoter is affected by tumor necrosis factor alpha and interferon gamma. J Cell Sci. 2000;113(Pt 11):2085–90.

49. Kniesel U, Wolburg H. Tight junctions of the blood-brain barrier. Cell Mol Neurobiol. 2000;20:57–76.

50. Wright TJ, Leach L, Shaw PE, Jones P. Dynamics of vascular endothelial-cadherin and beta-catenin localization by vascular endothelial growth factor-induced angiogenesis in human umbilical vein cells. Exp Cell Res. 2002;280:159–68.

51. Benson K, Cramer S, Galla HJ. Impedance-based cell monitoring: barrier properties and beyond. Fluids Barriers CNS. 2013;10:5.

52. Lucke-Wold BP, Logsdon AF, Smith KE, Turner RC, Alkon DL, Tan Z, Naser ZJ, Knotts CM, Huber JD, Rosen CL. Bryostatin-1 restores blood brain barrier integrity following blast-induced traumatic brain injury. Mol Neurobiol. 2015; 52:1119–34.

53. Kim YA, Park SL, Kim MY, Lee SH, Baik EJ, Moon CH, Jung YS. Role of PKCbetaII and PKCdelta in blood-brain barrier permeability during aglycemic hypoxia. Neurosci Lett. 2010;468:254–8.

54. Willis CL, Meske DS, Davis TP. Protein kinase C activation modulates reversible increase in cortical blood-brain barrier permeability and tight junction protein expression during hypoxia and posthypoxic reoxygenation. J Cereb Blood Flow Metab. 2010;30:1847–59.

55. Qi X, Inagaki K, Sobel RA, Mochly-Rosen D. Sustained pharmacological inhibition of deltaPKC protects against hypertensive encephalopathy through prevention of blood-brain barrier breakdown in rats. J Clin Invest. 2008;118:173–82.

56. Yuan SY. Protein kinase signaling in the modulation of microvascular permeability. Vasc Pharmacol. 2002;39:213–23.

via activating Akt-dependent prosurvival pathway and defending blood-brain barrier integrity. FASEB J. 0:fj.201800227RR.

57. Steinberg SF. Distinctive activation mechanisms and functions for protein kinase Cdelta. Biochem J. 2004;384:449–59.

58. Chari R, Getz T, Nagy B Jr, Bhavaraju K, Mao Y, Bynagari YS, Murugappan S, Nakayama K, Kunapuli SP. Protein kinase C[delta] differentially regulates platelet functional responses. Arterioscler Thromb Vasc Biol. 2009;29: 699–705.

59. Kilpatrick LE, Sun S, Li H, Vary TC, Korchak HM. Regulation of TNF-induced oxygen radical production in human neutrophils: role of δ-PKC. J Leukoc Biol. 2010;87:153–64.

60. Mondrinos MJ, Knight LC, Kennedy PA, Wu J, Kauffman M, Baker ST, Wolfson MR, Kilpatrick LE. Biodistribution and efficacy of targeted pulmonary delivery of a protein kinase C-δ inhibitory peptide: impact on indirect lung injury. J Pharmacol Exp Ther. 2015;355:86–98.

61. Soroush F, Tang Y, Guglielmo K, Engelmann A, Liverani E, Langston J, Sun S, Kunapuli S, Kiani MF, Kilpatrick LE. Protein kinase C-delta (PKCdelta) tyrosine phosphorylation is a critical regulator of neutrophil-endothelial cell interaction in inflammation. Shock 9000. Publish Ahead of Print.

7

Peripheral myeloid cells contribute to brain injury in male neonatal mice

Peter L. P. Smith[1†], Amin Mottahedin[1†], Pernilla Svedin[1], Carl-Johan Mohn[1], Henrik Hagberg[1,2], Joakim Ek[1] and Carina Mallard[1*] ◉

Abstract

Background: Neonatal brain injury is increasingly understood to be linked to inflammatory processes that involve specialised CNS and peripheral immune interactions. However, the role of peripheral myeloid cells in neonatal hypoxic-ischemic (HI) brain injury remains to be fully investigated.

Methods: We employed the *Lys*-EGFP-*ki* mouse that allows enhanced green fluorescent protein (EGFP)-positive mature myeloid cells of peripheral origin to be easily identified in the CNS. Using both flow cytometry and confocal microscopy, we investigated the accumulation of total EGFP+ myeloid cells and myeloid cell subtypes: inflammatory monocytes, resident monocytes and granulocytes, in the CNS for several weeks following induction of cerebral HI in postnatal day 9 mice. We used antibody treatment to curb brain infiltration of myeloid cells and subsequently evaluated HI-induced brain injury.

Results: We demonstrate a temporally biphasic pattern of inflammatory monocyte and granulocyte infiltration, characterised by peak infiltration at 1 day and 7 days after hypoxia-ischemia. This occurs against a backdrop of continuous low-level resident monocyte infiltration. Antibody-mediated depletion of circulating myeloid cells reduced immune cell accumulation in the brain and reduced neuronal loss in male but not female mice.

Conclusion: This study offers new insight into sex-dependent central-peripheral immune communication following neonatal brain injury and merits renewed interest in the roles of granulocytes and monocytes in lesion development.

Keywords: Neuroinflammation, Newborn, Immune cell trafficking

Background

Inflammation is widely recognised as an important component of perinatal brain injury [1, 2]. Persistent inflammation is thought to negatively impact ongoing developmental processes and potentially sensitise to later life pathologies [3, 4]. The central nervous system (CNS), with its developmentally distinct population of mononuclear phagocytes [5], immune-suppressive environment and highly regulated interactions with the innate and adaptive arms of the immune system [6], is viewed as an immune-specialised organ [7]. In response to pathological insult, the immature CNS actively upregulates numerous chemoattractant molecules including

the binding partners of CCR2 (CCL2 and CCL7), CCR1 and CCR5 (CCL3) and CXCR2 (CXCL1) [8], respectively known for their roles in emigration of Ly6C^{hi} monocytes from the bone marrow and recruitment of monocytes into inflamed tissue [9]. Indeed, accumulation of macrophages [10], neutrophils [11–13], mast cells [14] and NK cells [11] occurs in response to neonatal hypoxia-ischemia (HI). An important question yet to be satisfactorily addressed in neonatal injury models is the relative contribution of microglial-derived macrophages (MiDMs) vs that of monocyte-derived macrophages (MDMs) to the CNS macrophage pool: historically, discrimination between these cell types has proved difficult due to their assumed similar morphology and common expression of cell surface epitopes such as Fc and complement receptors, CD11b, F4/80 [15] and CD45 [16]. Despite such shared characteristics, MiDMs and MDMs are increasingly appreciated to

* Correspondence: carina.mallard@neuro.gu.se
†Peter L. P. Smith and Amin Mottahedin contributed equally to this work.
[1]Institute of Neuroscience and Physiology, Department of Physiology, Sahlgrenska Academy, University of Gothenburg, Box 432, SE-405 30 Gothenburg, Sweden
Full list of author information is available at the end of the article

play differing roles in the context of CNS insult [17]. Matters are further complicated by the non-homogenous nature of blood-borne monocytes; at least two distinct subsets have been identified and classified as inflammatory and resident monocytes [18]. Inflammatory monocytes represent a relatively short-lived population that is actively recruited to inflamed tissue [18, 19], whereas resident monocytes are physiologically recruited to non-inflamed tissue [18] and have the capacity to rapidly respond to tissue damage or infection [20]. These monocyte subsets display differential migratory dynamics in adult cerebral ischemia: inflammatory monocytes make a rapid but transient appearance, while resident monocytes display a delayed but progressive accumulation [21]. The inflammatory characteristics of each subset may underpin such dynamics: inflammatory monocytes upregulate inflammatory mediators including *TNFα* and *IL1*, while resident monocytes display a more reparative phenotype with elevated expression of genes involved in tissue remodelling such as *arg1* and *Fizz1* [20], drawing comparisons respective to M1 and M2 macrophage phenotypes [22].

Here, we employed immunohistochemistry and flow cytometry to investigate MDM and granulocyte infiltration in the post-ischemic neonatal brain. We performed experimental HI on postnatal day (P) 9 *Lys*-EGFP-*ki* mice, allowing identification of peripheral myeloid cells in the brain [23, 24]. For the first time, we describe the differential dynamics of resident and inflammatory monocytes in this model and that inhibition of myeloid cell accumulation in the brain protects against HI injury in male, but not female, neonatal mice.

Methods

Animals

Pregnant C57BL/6J dams were sourced from Janvier Laboratories (Le Genest-Saint-Isle, Fr). *Lys*-EGFP-*ki* mice were obtained from Dr. Tomas Graf, Autonomous University of Barcelona [22]. Animals were housed and bred at the University of Gothenburg's Laboratory for Experimental Biomedicine on a 12-h light-dark cycle (illuminated 07:00–19:00) at constant temperature (24 °C) and relative humidity (50–60%) with ad libitum access to food and water. All experimental procedures were approved by the Gothenburg Animal Research Ethics Committee (No. 337/2012, 139/2013, 18/2015).

Experimental hypoxia-ischemia

HI brain injury was induced in male and female mice on postnatal day (P) 9. Pups with body weight < 4 g at the time of HI were excluded from experiments. The mortality rate was < 5% throughout the study. A total of 306 animals were included in the study. Briefly, mice were anaesthetised with isoflurane in a 1:1 nitrous oxide to oxygen mix (4% induction, 2% maintenance) and

subjected to permanent occlusion of the left common carotid artery. Mice were then allowed a 1-h recovery period before being transferred to a temperature-controlled (36 °C) humidified incubator for 50 min of hypoxia (10% O_2). Sham animals were subjected to anaesthesia, and the carotid artery was exposed as above but without ligation of the artery and hypoxia.

EGFP, CD31, IBA1 and Ly6G immunohistochemistry

Mice were deeply anaesthetised and transcardially perfused with ice-cold 0.9% saline followed by 4% paraformaldehyde (PFA). Brains were rapidly removed, post-fixed in 4% PFA for 24 h at 4 °C and cryoprotected in 30% sucrose for a minimum of 3 days. Cryoprotected brains were snap-frozen on dry ice and sectioned serially at 40 μm on a Leica CM3050S cryostat (Leica, SE). Cut sections were transferred to a cryoprotectant solution (25% ethylene glycol, 25% glycerine, in 0.1 M phosphate buffer) and stored at − 20 °C. Sodium citrate antigen retrieval (10 mM sodium citrate, pH 6, 97 °C, 10 min) was performed prior to all staining procedures. Blocking of non-specific binding sites was achieved through a 30-min incubation in Tris-buffered saline (TBS) containing 3% donkey serum (hereafter referred to as blocking buffer). Sections were then incubated at 4 °C overnight with given combinations of primary antibodies which were later visualised via a 2-h room temperature incubation with relevant secondary antibodies (see Table 1).

Microscopy

Tile-scanned images of entire brain sections were captured on a Zeiss Axio Observer upright microscope equipped with an Apotome module and Zen blue software (Zeiss, Oberkochen, DE). From each experimental group ($n = 4$), 2−3 sections at hippocampus and striatum levels were analysed. Each z-stack consisted of 8–10 images with a z-plane distance of 3 μm. All other images were captured using a Zeiss LSM 700 inverted confocal (Zeiss, Oberkochen, DE). Z-projections were produced in ImageJ (NIH, Bethesda, http://rsbweb.nih.gov/ij/), and figures were compiled in Adobe CS6.

Tissue collection and preparation for flow cytometry

Brain samples were collected at 6 h, 1 day, 3 days, 7 days, 14 days and 28 days after HI. Mice were deeply anaesthetised and transcardially perfused with ice-cold 0.9% saline, brains were rapidly removed and dissected hemispheres were transferred to ice-cold Hanks' Balanced Salt Solution (HBSS) containing 0.5% bovine albumin serum (BSA) (hereafter referred to as FACS buffer) and kept on ice until dissociation. Single-cell suspensions were obtained through enzymatic dissociation (0.01% papain [Bionordika, Stockholm, SE], 0.1% dispase II [Bionordika, Stockholm, SE], 0.01% DNase I

Table 1 Antibodies for immunohistochemistry and flow cytometry

Application	Antigen	Host	Clone/target	Reactivity*	Conjugate	Company	Product number	Dilution**
Immunohistochemistry	GFP	Rabbit	Poly	Mouse	A488	Invitrogen	A21311	1:200
	CD31	Goat	Poly	Mouse	–	R&D systems	AF3628	1:200
	Iba1	Goat	Poly	Mouse	–	Abcam	Ab5076	1:500
	Ly6G	Rat	Mono (1A8)	Mouse	–	BioLegend	127602	1:250
	IgG	Donkey	Poly	Goat	CF555	VWR	89138-464	1:1000
	IgG	Goat	Poly	Rat	CF555	Sigma	SAB46000070	1:1000
Flow cytometry	CD11b	Rat	M1/70	Mouse	PE-Cy7	BioLegend	101216	0.25 µg
	CD45	Rat	30-F11	Mouse	APC-CY7	BD	557659	0.25 µg
	GR-1	Rat	RB6-8C5	Mouse	PerCp-Cy5.5	eBiosciences	45-5931	0.25 µg
	Ly6C	Rat	HK1.4	Mouse	APC	eBiosciences	17-5932	0.25 µg
	CD16/CD32	Rat	2.4G2	Mouse	–	BD	553142	0.1 µg

*Where antibody is reactive to multiple species, only relevant species are listed
**For flow cytometry, given values represent microgram antibody per 10^6 cells

[Roche, Bromma, SE], 12.4 mM $MgSO_4$ in Ca/Mg-free HBSS); briefly, samples underwent three rounds of enzymatic (10-min incubation at 37 °C) and mechanical (repetitive pipetting) dissociation. Resultant samples were passed over a 40-µm cell strainer, centrifuged (500g, 5 min), resuspended in FACS buffer and quantified on a BioRad TC10 automated cell counter (BioRad, Solna, SE). Samples were incubated for 15 min at 4 °C with Fc block (CD16/CD32) and then primary antibodies in relevant combinations (Table 1). Stained samples were centrifuged (500g, 5 min), re-suspended in FACS buffer and kept at 4 °C until analysis.

Flow cytometry
Cell viability was determined, in pilot experiments using 7AAD, to be 98.47 ± 0.39% (n = 12). Debris were excluded by gating on size and granularity (P1 gate; Fig. 1a). Myeloid cells were identified by CD11b expression; a mean (from all analyses presented herein) of 38,000 CD11b$^+$ cells per sample was analysed (Figs. 1a–c and 4a for gating strategies). CD11b$^+$EGFP$^+$Ly6C$^+$ cells were considered myeloid cells of peripheral origin and further categorised by differential Ly6C expression as inflammatory monocytes (CD11b$^+$EGFP$^+$Gr1$^{lo/-}$Ly6C$^{int/hi}$), resident monocytes (CD11b$^+$EGFP$^+$Gr1$^{lo/-}$Ly6C$^{lo/-}$) [25] or granulocytes (CD11b$^+$EGFP$^+$Gr1^{hi}Ly6C^{int}) [26]. All data was collected using a BD FACSCanto flow cytometer with BD FACS-Diva software v.6.1.3 (BD Biosciences, Stockholm, SE); analysis was performed with FlowJo v.10 (Tree Star Inc., Ashland, OR, USA).

Bio-plex cytokine analysis
Brain and plasma samples were collected at 6 h, 1 day, 3 days, 7 days and 14 days after HI. Briefly, mice were deeply anaesthetised, blood was collected from the heart's right ventricle and transferred to EDTA-coated tubes and set aside for further processing, animals were then transcardially perfused with ice-cold 0.9% saline and brains were rapidly removed and frozen on dry ice. Plasma samples were isolated via centrifugation (10 min, 1000×g, 4 °C) and frozen on dry ice prior to storage at − 80 °C.

Brain lysates were prepared through mechanical dissociation of tissue samples in 600 µl of lysis buffer (10 mM EDTA, 1% Triton-X-100, 1% Protein Inhibitor Cocktail [Sigma-Aldrich#8340] in RNase-free PBS) followed by sonication and centrifugation (4500×g, 5 min, 4 °C). Protein concentration was assessed using a Pierce BCA Protein Assay Kit (Thermo Fisher Scientific) as per manufacturer's protocol, and the final concentration of the samples was adjusted to 1 mg/ml using the lysis buffer. Preparations were carried out at 4 °C, and samples were stored at − 80 °C.

Cytokine concentration in brain lysates and plasma samples were assessed using a Bio-Plex Pro Mouse Cytokine Standard 23-Plex (Bio-Rad) kit in accordance with manufacturers' instructions on a Bio-Plex 200 analyser. For brain samples, the results were normalised to the brain protein concentration.

Antibody-based depletion of circulating monocytes and neutrophils
Circulating monocytes and neutrophils were depleted via intraperitoneal (i.p.) administration of GR-1 antibody (clone RB6-8C5, 17 mg/kg; Bio X Cell# BE0075). Administration commenced 1 h after removal of mice from the hypoxia chamber and was repeated every 48 h thereafter until sacrifice. The antibody dose was selected based on previous work with a similar concentration that demonstrated successful depletion of monocytes and neutrophils in 8–12-week-old mice [27].

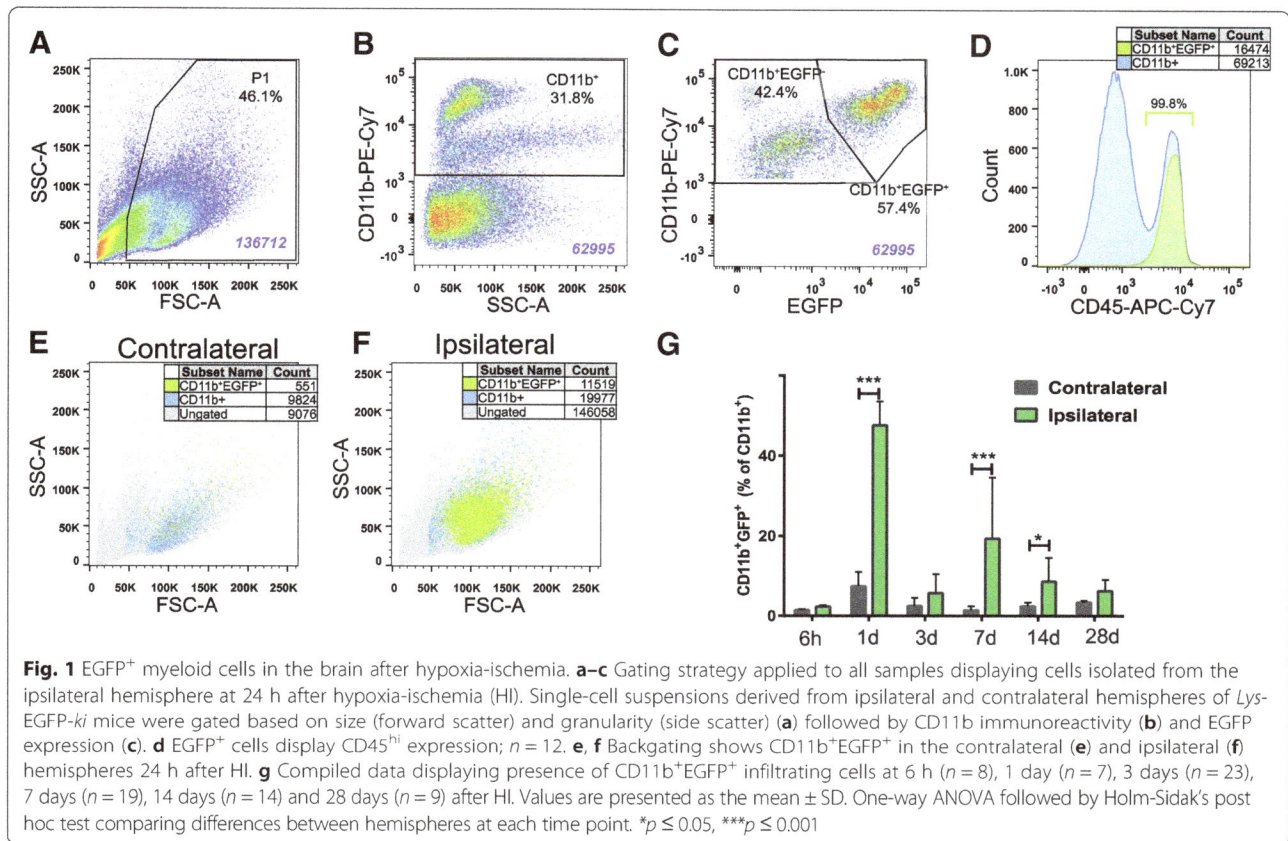

Fig. 1 EGFP$^+$ myeloid cells in the brain after hypoxia-ischemia. **a–c** Gating strategy applied to all samples displaying cells isolated from the ipsilateral hemisphere at 24 h after hypoxia-ischemia (HI). Single-cell suspensions derived from ipsilateral and contralateral hemispheres of *Lys-EGFP-ki* mice were gated based on size (forward scatter) and granularity (side scatter) (**a**) followed by CD11b immunoreactivity (**b**) and EGFP expression (**c**). **d** EGFP$^+$ cells display CD45^{hi} expression; $n = 12$. **e, f** Backgating shows CD11b$^+$EGFP$^+$ in the contralateral (**e**) and ipsilateral (**f**) hemispheres 24 h after HI. **g** Compiled data displaying presence of CD11b$^+$EGFP$^+$ infiltrating cells at 6 h ($n = 8$), 1 day ($n = 7$), 3 days ($n = 23$), 7 days ($n = 19$), 14 days ($n = 14$) and 28 days ($n = 9$) after HI. Values are presented as the mean ± SD. One-way ANOVA followed by Holm-Sidak's post hoc test comparing differences between hemispheres at each time point. *$p \leq 0.05$, ***$p \leq 0.001$

Brain injury analysis

Mice exposed to HI and treated with saline or RB6-8C5 antibody for 2 weeks, as described above, were deeply anaesthetised on P23 (i.e. 14 days after HI for assessing long-term outcome) and transcardially perfused with ice-cold 0.9% saline followed by 4% PFA. Brains were rapidly removed, post-fixed in 4% PFA for 24 h at 4 °C, dehydrated and embedded in paraffin. Brains were then serially cut at 10 μm (at 50-section intervals) on a Leica RM2165 microtome (Leica, SE). Three sections spanning the hippocampus (Fig. 7a) of each brain were analysed. Antigen retrieval was performed through boiling sections in sodium citrate buffer for 10 min, and non-specific binding was blocked by a 30-min incubation in PBS containing 1% horse serum, 3% BSA and 0.1% NaN$_3$. Sections were then incubated with antibodies against microtubule-associated protein-2 (MAP2) (clone HM.2, 1:1000; Sigma-Aldrich) or myelin basic protein (MBP) (clone SMI-94R, 1:10,000; Covance) overnight at 4 °C. Biotinylated secondary antibodies were applied for 1 h at room temperature and visualised using a Vectastatin ABC Elite followed by standard DAB staining. Brain images were captured using a Nikon Optiphot-2 microscope equipped with AVT dolphin F145B camera (Allied Vision Technologies). Percent loss of MAP2-positive tissue was calculated by subtracting the MAP2-positive area in the ipsilateral hemisphere from that measured in the contralateral hemisphere, then dividing the result by the MAP2-positive area of the contralateral hemisphere and converting to percent tissue loss. Percent loss of MBP-positive tissue was calculated in the same manner.

Statistics

Data are presented as group mean ± standard deviation (SD). Comparisons between ipsilateral and contralateral changes in number of infiltrating cells over time were assessed by one-way ANOVA followed by Holm-Sidak's multiple comparison tests. Differences were considered significant at *$p < 0.05$, **$p < 0.01$ and ***$p < 0.001$. Brain injury comparisons were performed using multiple unpaired Student's t tests at each brain level; p values were corrected for multiple comparisons using the Holm-Sidak method. Differences were considered significant at *$p < 0.05$. Analyses were performed using Prism (Graphpad, v.6.05).

Results

Peripheral immune cells are detected in the CNS for up to 14 days after experimental HI

To assess the potential influx of peripheral immune cells to the CNS following HI brain injury, we subjected P9 *lys-EGFP-ki* mice to experimental HI, collected tissue at

6 h, 1 day, 3 days, 7 days, 14 days and 28 days after HI and employed flow cytometry to quantitatively assess the presence of EGFP$^+$ infiltrating cells in injured vs uninjured cerebral hemispheres. Infiltrating myeloid cells were identified through a stepwise gating strategy: cells were first gated by size and granularity (Fig. 1a), followed by CD11b (Fig. 1b) and finally EGFP expression (Fig. 1c). We found that 99.80% ± 0.06% of cells identified as CD11b$^+$EGFP$^+$ were CD45^{hi}, confirming their peripheral origin (Fig. 1d). CD11b$^+$EGFP$^+$ infiltrating myeloid cells were significantly increased in the ipsilateral compared with the contralateral hemisphere at 1 day ($p < 0.001$), 7 days ($p < 0.001$) and 14 days ($p = 0.031$) after HI (Fig. 1e–g), with CD11b$^+$EGFP$^+$ cells respectively constituting 47.65 ± 2.40%, 19.41 ± 3.51% and 8.75 ± 1.56% of the injured hemisphere's total CD11b$^+$ cell population (Fig. 1g).

Different localisation patterns of infiltrating cells were determined at 1 day and 7 days after HI by immunohistochemical staining for EGFP. We further co-localised EGFP$^+$ staining with the endothelial cell marker CD31 at 1 day and 7 days after HI to assess parenchymal vs intraluminal localisation. At 1 day, EGFP$^+$ myeloid cells show a dispersed pattern of infiltration including invasion of the hippocampus, thalamus (Fig. 2a) and striatum (Additional file 1: Figure S1A). In contrast, at 7 days, invading cells showed a spatially distinct dense pattern of infiltration limited to the remaining parts of the hippocampus and hippocampal fimbriae as well as the white matter in the thalamus (Fig. 2b), with very little infiltration into the striatum (Additional file 1: Figure S1B). Cortical infiltration was also observed in cases with severe injury at both time points (Fig. 3a).

Invading EGFP$^+$ leukocytes include cell types of distinct morphologies

As *Lys*-EGFP-*ki* transgenic mice express EGFP in monocytes, MDMs and granulocytes [23], we employed confocal microscopy in conjunction with immunohistochemistry to investigate the morphological features and protein immunoreactivity of CNS-infiltrating cells 7 days after HI. In animals with severe injury, EGFP$^+$ infiltrating cells were present in the cortex and displayed low to negative immunoreactivity for microglial/monocyte marker Iba1$^+$ and were commonly round shaped (Fig. 3a). Similarly, in the injured hippocampus, EGFP$^+$ cells were commonly round and expressed the neutrophil marker Ly6G but were not associated with CD31$^+$ vessels (Fig. 3b).

CNS accumulation of inflammatory monocytes and granulocytes after HI follows a temporally biphasic pattern

In order to identify subpopulations of infiltrating CD11b$^+$EGFP$^+$ leukocytes, cells were gated based on their expression of Gr1 and Ly6C, allowing determination of inflammatory monocytes (CD11b$^+$EGFP$^+$Gr1$^{lo/-}$Ly6C$^{int/hi}$), resident monocytes (CD11b$^+$EGFP$^+$Gr1$^{lo/-}$Ly6C$^{lo/-}$) and granulocytes (CD11b$^+$EGFP$^+$Gr1^{hi}Ly6C^{int})

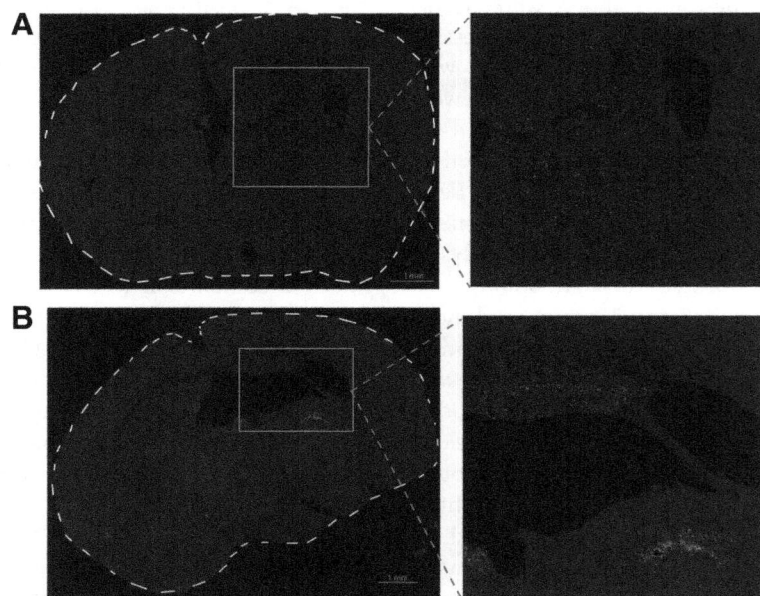

Fig. 2 EGFP$^+$ myeloid cell localisation in the brain after hypoxia-ischemia. **a** Representative tile-scanned confocal images of brain sections after hypoxia-ischemia (HI). **a** Dispersed pattern of EGFP$^+$ myeloid cell infiltration in the hippocampus and thalamus 1 day after HI. **b** EGFP$^+$ myeloid cells localised in the hippocampus and the white matter of the thalamus (medullary lamina of thalamus) in a spatially limited dense pattern 7 days after HI. $n = 4$/time point

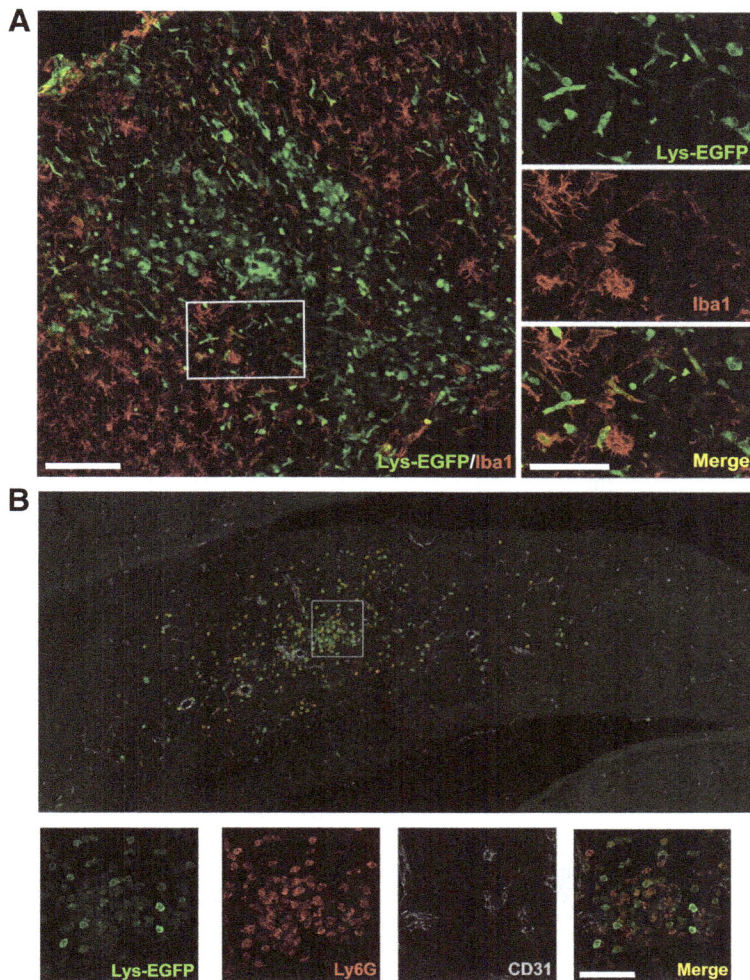

Fig. 3 EGFP$^+$ myeloid cells in the brain 7 days after hypoxia-ischemia are Iba-1$^-$ and Ly6G$^+$. **a** EGFP$^+$ cells are distinct from Iba-1-positive cells and display mostly round morphology in the ipsilateral cortex in animals with severe injury at 7 days after hypoxia-ischemia (HI). **b** Round-shaped EGFP$^+$ cells are largely Ly6G$^+$ and are not associated with CD31$^+$ vessels (example from the hippocampus). Scale bars = 100 μm (at low magnification) and 50 μm (at high magnification)

[26] (Fig. 4a). Backgating confirmed the relative lack of infiltrating cells in the contralateral hemisphere (Fig. 4b) and the distinct physical properties of each myeloid subpopulation in the ipsilateral hemisphere (Fig. 4c), with granulocytes and resident monocytes forming distinct populations based on size and granularity while inflammatory monocytes formed a less homogenous population.

CD11b$^+$EGFP$^+$Gr1$^{lo/-}$Ly6C$^{lo/-}$ resident monocytes could be detected at significantly greater levels in the ipsilateral hemisphere compared to contralateral levels at 3 days ($p < 0.001$), 7 days ($p < 0.01$) and 14 days ($p < 0.001$) after HI (Fig. 4d). Inflammatory monocytes were significantly increased in the ipsilateral compared to contralateral hemisphere at 1 day after HI and represented 31.9 ± 1.3% of the ipsilateral hemisphere's total CD11b$^+$ cell population (Fig. 4e; $p < 0.001$); by 3 days, however, they

were no longer detectable above control levels (Fig. 4e, $p > 0.05$). A second phase of infiltration occurred after 3 days with significantly more inflammatory monocytes detected at 7 days ($p < 0.001$) in the ipsilateral compared to the contralateral hemisphere. The infiltration of CD11b$^+$EGFP$^+$Gr1^{hi}Ly6C^{int} granulocytes (Fig. 4f) largely mirrored that of inflammatory monocytes with the increased number of granulocytes observed in the ipsilateral hemisphere at 1 day ($p < 0.001$) and 7 days ($p < 0.001$). Figure 4g displays an overview of the relative contribution of resident monocytes, inflammatory monocytes and granulocytes to the total population of peripherally derived myeloid cells in the ipsilateral hemisphere at each time point (expressed as percentage of total CD11b$^+$ cells). Overall, the temporal pattern of peripheral leukocyte influx was distinctly biphasic, characterised by peak accumulation

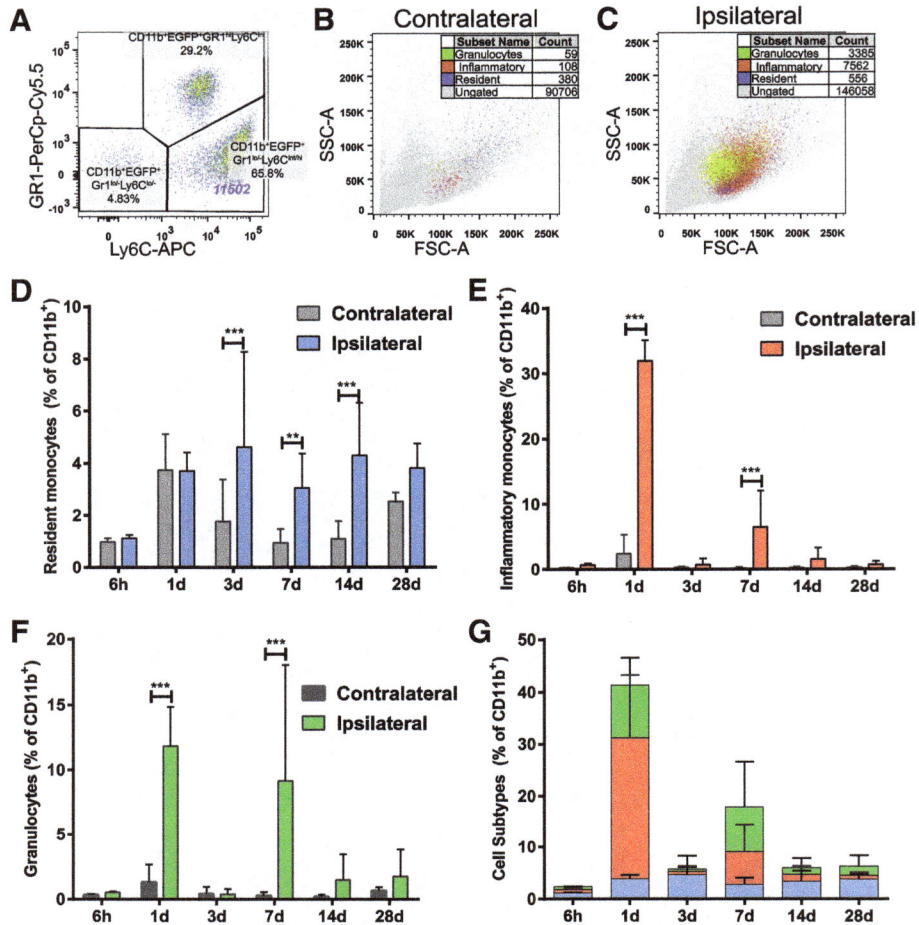

Fig. 4 Characterisation of EGFP$^+$ cells in the brain after hypoxia-ischemia. EGFP$^+$ myeloid cells were identified after hypoxia-ischemia (HI) through the gating strategy presented in Fig. 1a–c. **a** EGFP$^+$ were further characterised based on expression of Gr1 and Ly6C and defined as resident monocytes (CD11b$^+$EGFP$^+$Gr1$^{lo/-}$Ly6C$^{lo/-}$), inflammatory monocytes (CD11b$^+$EGFP$^+$Gr1$^{lo/-}$Ly6C$^{int/hi}$) and granulocytes (CD11b$^+$EGFP$^+$Gr1^{hi}Ly6C^{int}). **b**, **c** Backgating displays the presence of these cell populations in contralateral (**b**) and ipsilateral (**c**) hemispheres at 1 day after HI. **d–f** Compiled data demonstrate these cell subtypes in ipsilateral and contralateral hemispheres at 6 h ($n = 8$), 1 day ($n = 7$), 3 days ($n = 23$), 7 days ($n = 19$), 14 days ($n = 14$) and 28 days ($n = 9$) after HI. **g** Stacked bar graph showing the relative contribution of each cell population to the total EGFP$^+$ population at each time point. Values are presented as the mean ± SD. One-way ANOVA followed by Holm-Sidak's post hoc test comparing differences between hemispheres at each time point, **$p \leq 0.01$, ***$p \leq 0.001$

of inflammatory cells (inflammatory monocytes and granulocytes) at 1 day, relative quiescence at 3 days and renewed infiltration at 7 days.

Inflammatory cell accumulation in the brain is associated with elevated chemotactic and inflammatory cytokine levels

To assess whether the temporal pattern of leukocyte infiltration to the brain corresponded to a distinct cytokine profile, we performed a 23-plex multiplex cytokine assay covering the time points assessed in the flow cytometry experiment. At 6 h, before the peak of leukocyte accumulation, a marked increase was observed in several inflammatory cytokines (e.g. IL1a, IL1b and IL6) and

chemokines (e.g. KC, MCP1, MIP1a, MIP1b), as well as granulocyte and macrophage growth factors (e.g. G-CSF and GM-CSF), in the ipsilateral hemisphere compared to the contralateral hemisphere (Fig. 5, Additional file 2: Figure S2, Additional file 3 and Additional file 4: Table S1). Several cytokines (e.g. IL1a, IL1b and IL6; Fig. 5) were also increased in the contralateral hemisphere compared to that in the brains of sham-operated mice. Chemokine levels were similar in the contralateral hemisphere compared with that in the brains from sham-operated mice. Cytokine levels in the ipsilateral hemisphere remained elevated over time, except for the 7-day time point. Most chemokines were reduced to sham levels within 1–3 days and remained at levels similar to

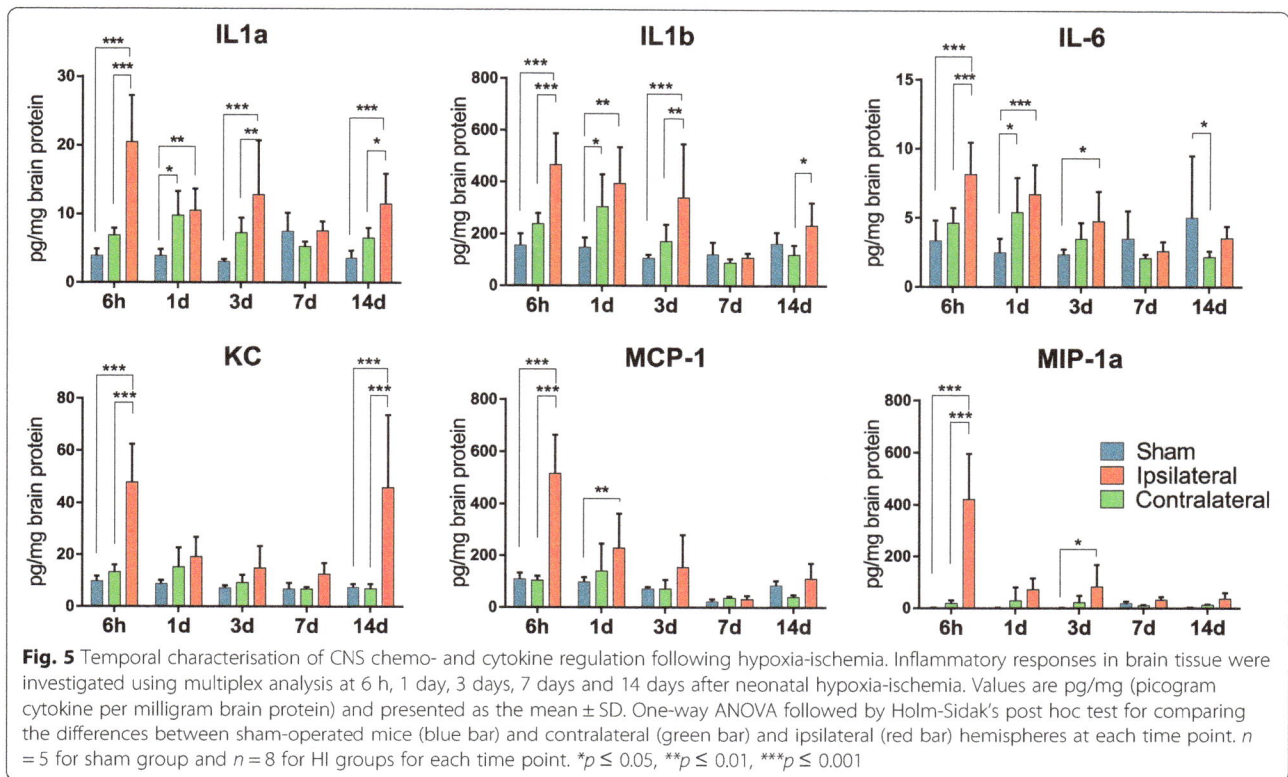

Fig. 5 Temporal characterisation of CNS chemo- and cytokine regulation following hypoxia-ischemia. Inflammatory responses in brain tissue were investigated using multiplex analysis at 6 h, 1 day, 3 days, 7 days and 14 days after neonatal hypoxia-ischemia. Values are pg/mg (picogram cytokine per milligram brain protein) and presented as the mean ± SD. One-way ANOVA followed by Holm-Sidak's post hoc test for comparing the differences between sham-operated mice (blue bar) and contralateral (green bar) and ipsilateral (red bar) hemispheres at each time point. n = 5 for sham group and n = 8 for HI groups for each time point. *$p \leq 0.05$, **$p \leq 0.01$, ***$p \leq 0.001$

those observed in sham-operated animals up to 2 weeks except for KC, which was markedly increased at 14 days after HI (Fig. 5).

Significant differences in plasma cytokine levels between HI mice and sham-operated mice were only detected for G-CSF at 1 day and four cytokines (IL1b, IL3, IL4 and eotaxin) which were elevated at the 14-day time point in HI mice (Additional file 3: Figure S3 and Additional file 5: Table S2).

Myeloid cell depletion protects the brain against hypoxic-ischemic injury in male mice

To investigate the role of the infiltrating myeloid cells, an antibody-based cell-depleting strategy was employed. Repeated systemic administration of RB6-8C5 blocked accumulation of myeloid cells in the brain after HI (Fig. 6b, c). At 1 day and 7 days after HI, the percentage of CD11b$^+$EGFP$^+$ infiltrating myeloid cells were significantly lower in the injured hemisphere of antibody-treated mice compared to that in the control mice (Fig. 6d). Likewise, antibody administration significantly reduced the percentage of inflammatory monocytes (CD11b$^+$EGFP$^+$Ly6C^{hi}) and granulocytes (CD11b$^+$EGFP$^+$Gr1$^+$Ly6C^{int}) in the injured hemisphere at both time points (Fig. 6f, g). Interestingly, the percentage of resident monocytes was also lower in antibody-treated mice at the 7-day time point (Fig. 6e).

Next, we asked whether inhibition of myeloid cell accumulation in the brain affects the HI injury. Treatment

with RB6-8C5 significantly reduced loss of MAP2-positive neuronal tissue in male mice ($p < 0.05$, Fig. 7a, b), but not in female mice (Fig. 7c). There was no significant change in loss of MBP-positive area (i.e. myelinated area) in either male (Fig. 7d, e) or female mice (Fig. 7f).

Discussion

In this study, we utilised the *Lys*-EGFP-*ki* mouse model, in which myeloid cells generated through definitive but not primitive haematopoiesis express EGFP [23, 28], to characterise the presence of peripherally derived myeloid cells in the injured CNS after neonatal HI. We show that EGFP-positive leukocytes home to the injured hemisphere and are morphologically distinct from CNS microglia and demonstrate a temporally biphasic pattern of inflammatory cell infiltration occurring over a background of stable resident monocyte infiltration. Further, we show that depletion of these cells reduces grey matter injury in male mice.

Myeloid cell accumulation has been demonstrated in numerous neonatal models of sterile brain injury [29] [10, 11, 30–32]. While identification of granulocytes in the CNS is relatively straightforward, discrimination of MDMs and MiDMs has presented a greater problem due to their similar characteristics and common expression of cell surface epitopes [15, 16]. *Lys*-EGFP-*ki* transgenic mice express EGFP in monocytes,

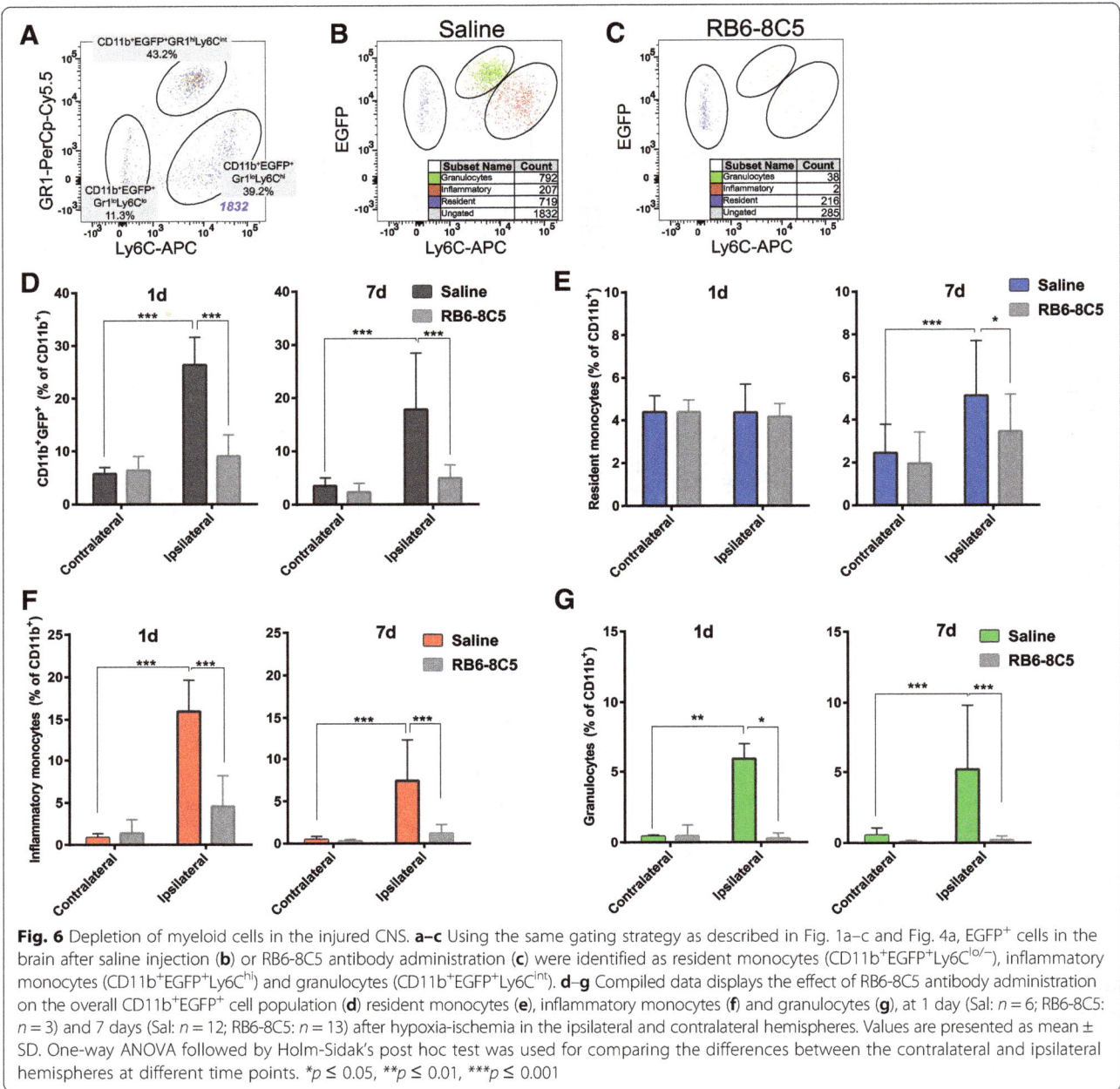

Fig. 6 Depletion of myeloid cells in the injured CNS. **a–c** Using the same gating strategy as described in Fig. 1a–c and Fig. 4a, EGFP$^+$ cells in the brain after saline injection (**b**) or RB6-8C5 antibody administration (**c**) were identified as resident monocytes (CD11b$^+$EGFP$^+$Ly6C$^{lo/-}$), inflammatory monocytes (CD11b$^+$EGFP$^+$Ly6C^{hi}) and granulocytes (CD11b$^+$EGFP$^+$Ly6C^{int}). **d–g** Compiled data displays the effect of RB6-8C5 antibody administration on the overall CD11b$^+$EGFP$^+$ cell population (**d**) resident monocytes (**e**), inflammatory monocytes (**f**) and granulocytes (**g**), at 1 day (Sal: $n = 6$; RB6-8C5: $n = 3$) and 7 days (Sal: $n = 12$; RB6-8C5: $n = 13$) after hypoxia-ischemia in the ipsilateral and contralateral hemispheres. Values are presented as mean ± SD. One-way ANOVA followed by Holm-Sidak's post hoc test was used for comparing the differences between the contralateral and ipsilateral hemispheres at different time points. *$p \leq 0.05$, **$p \leq 0.01$, ***$p \leq 0.001$

MDMs and granulocytes [23] allowing unambiguous identification of CNS-infiltrating cells and therefore discrimination of MDMs and MiDMs by flow cytometry and microscopy [28].

Our immunohistochemical investigation indicated extravasated EGFP$^+$ cells as early as 24 h after HI, with cells dispersed throughout the ipsilateral hemisphere. Later at the 7-day time point, there was a close correlation between peripheral myeloid cell accumulation and well-characterised areas of cerebral injury that has previously been described in the neonatal HI model [33]. Microscopic examination of EGFP$^+$ cells in the cortex at 7 days revealed distinct morphological characteristics of invading cells, which displayed few processes and low Iba1 immunoreactivity. Although qualitative in nature, this data reflects recent observations made following experimental autoimmune encephalomyelitis in CCR2-RFP/CX3CR1-GFP mice [17], where unlike the highly ramified microglia, MDMs were elongated or spindle shaped, smaller and rarely had processes. EGFP$^+$ cells often co-localised with Ly6G$^+$ cells but not with CD31$^+$ blood vessels (Fig. 3b), supporting that these cells were peripherally derived myeloid cells.

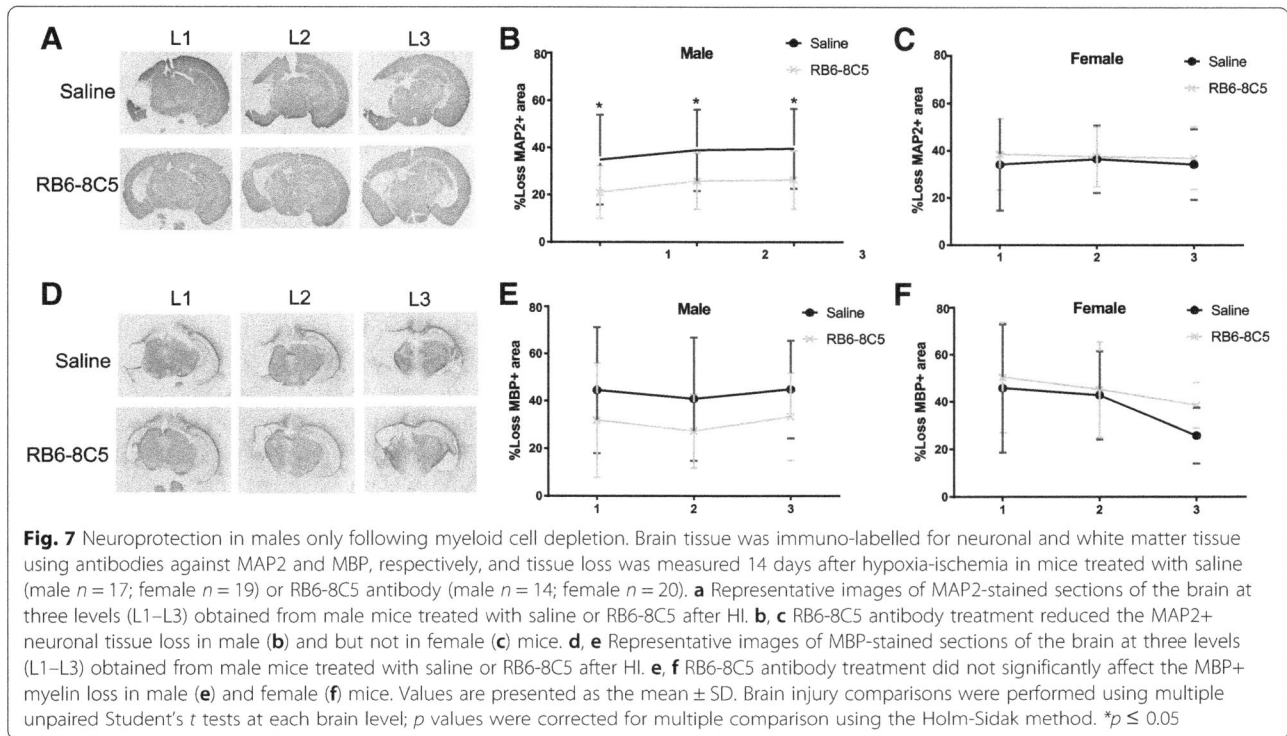

Fig. 7 Neuroprotection in males only following myeloid cell depletion. Brain tissue was immuno-labelled for neuronal and white matter tissue using antibodies against MAP2 and MBP, respectively, and tissue loss was measured 14 days after hypoxia-ischemia in mice treated with saline (male $n = 17$; female $n = 19$) or RB6-8C5 antibody (male $n = 14$; female $n = 20$). **a** Representative images of MAP2-stained sections of the brain at three levels (L1–L3) obtained from male mice treated with saline or RB6-8C5 after HI. **b**, **c** RB6-8C5 antibody treatment reduced the MAP2+ neuronal tissue loss in male (**b**) and but not in female (**c**) mice. **d**, **e** Representative images of MBP-stained sections of the brain at three levels (L1–L3) obtained from male mice treated with saline or RB6-8C5 after HI. **e**, **f** RB6-8C5 antibody treatment did not significantly affect the MBP+ myelin loss in male (**e**) and female (**f**) mice. Values are presented as the mean ± SD. Brain injury comparisons were performed using multiple unpaired Student's t tests at each brain level; p values were corrected for multiple comparison using the Holm-Sidak method. *$p \leq 0.05$

We have previously shown marked expansion of the CD11b+ cell population in the brain after neonatal HI [34]. Using quantitative flow cytometry-based analysis of CD11b+EGFP+ cells, our data indicates that a significant proportion of this CD11b+ cell population in the ipsilateral hemisphere consists of infiltrating myeloid cells, ranging from 28 to 48% of the total CD11b+ cells at 1 day after HI. The difference in percentage of infiltrating cells between experiments is likely due to the variability in the HI model. However, overall, our data indicates a larger response than that observed by Denker et al. in a neonatal stroke model where accumulation of 10% CD45^{hi}CD11b+ cells was observed at 1 day after MCAO [32]. The discrepancies in the different models may result from the utilisation of different strategies for the identification of infiltrating leukocytes, inherent differences of the rat neonatal stroke and mouse HI models, but also variability in respective models.

Further characterisation of the CD11b+EGFP+ cell populations based on differential expression of Ly6C and Gr1 facilitated discrimination of resident monocytes (CD11b+EGFP+Gr1$^{lo/-}$Ly6C$^{lo/-}$), inflammatory monocytes (CD11b+EGFP+Gr1$^{lo/-}$Ly6C$^{int/hi}$) [25] and granulocytes (CD11b+EGFP+Gr1^{hi}Ly6C^{int}) [26]. The two pro-inflammatory cell types identified, inflammatory monocytes and granulocytes, displayed temporally similar expression patterns with peak accumulation seen at 1 and 7 days after HI but with no significant increase at 3 days and a minimal but detectable

presence at 14 days, suggesting distinct phases of accumulation and clearance.

Previous studies examining neutrophil accumulation after neonatal HI reported varying results. Several studies demonstrated neuroprotective effects by depleting neutrophils before HI [12, 13, 35], suggesting an important role of neutrophils in injury development. One of these studies, however, was unable to show consistent hemispheric differences in myeloperoxidase (MPO) activity, number of MPO positive cells and number of anti-neutrophil serum-positive cells [12]. Nijboer et al. demonstrated increased MPO activity at 24 h and up to 48 h [13], and identification and quantification of neutrophils in H&E-stained sections revealed increased neutrophil counts at 12 h, but not at 24 h–35 days [11]. Our data complements the above described studies by displaying increased post-ischemia granulocyte accumulation as assessed in an unbiased and quantitative fashion.

The distinct peaks of inflammatory cell accumulation detected at 1 day and 7 days suggest distinct phases of infiltration and clearance, presumably by CNS resident macrophages. These observations are partially supported by previous studies: Winerdal et al. demonstrated peak CD11b+CD86+ macrophage presence at 1 day and 7 days, with reduced levels at 3 days after neonatal HI in mice [36], and in adult rats, distinct peaks of neutrophil engulfment by macrophages were observed 3 days and 15 days post-ischemia [37]. Speculatively, these studies suggest distinct phases of influx and phagocytic clearance of infiltrating inflammatory cells. Resident monocytes, by contrast, were detected at lower and more stable levels. This pattern of infiltration may be due to a slower accumulation of resident monocytes coupled with a lesser degree of phagocytic clearance: a fate that is in light of the proposed reparatory phenotype of these cells [20, 38].

Previous microarray data from our laboratory indicated peak expression of several chemokines in the brain, including CCL2, CCL7, CCL3 and CXCL1 at 8 h post-HI, with reduced levels at 3 days (the latest time point assessed), presumably produced by endogenous brain cells [8]. Thus, we now hypothesised that increased chemokine expression in the brain could attract peripheral immune cells. However, the multiplex analyses conducted in this study failed to demonstrate a correlation between elevated cytokine and chemokine levels and the temporal pattern of leukocyte accumulation. This was particularly apparent at the early time points where marked increases in chemokine levels were observed at 6 h, while peak leukocyte accumulation occurred at 24 h after HI. These data thus suggest that increased chemokine expression precedes cell accumulation. Hence, by the time significant cell accumulation can be detected, the chemokine gradient might have already started to fade away. In support, there was also no evidence of cytokine and chemokine changes in the brain at 7 days after HI, when the second phase of leukocyte accumulation was identified. However, we cannot exclude the possibility that a second wave of infiltration was due to cytokine/chemokine gradients between days 3 and 7. The lack of correlation between CNS inflammation and infiltrating cells could also be due to that we only investigated the overall response in the whole brain. It is possible that specific cell types/brain structures, for example the response in the vasculature, are more directly correlated to outcome. Further, interestingly, a number of cytokines/chemokines were increased in the brain even 14 days after HI. For example, KC showed a biphasic pattern of increase after HI, with the first and second phase at 6 h and 14 days after HI, respectively. It is unclear how this long-term CNS inflammation may have affected outcome. Previous studies using the neonatal HI model have shown a progressive cerebral atrophy which is only apparent from approximately 2 weeks after the initial injury [39]. Thus, it would be of interest to, in future experiments, investigate both inflammatory responses and immune cell infiltration over a more prolonged period of time and in specific brain/vascular structures.

In addition to chemokine gradients, the physiological status of the brain barriers may affect the magnitude of the leukocyte accumulation. However, we have previously shown an increase in blood-brain barrier permeability at 6 h and 24 h, but not at 7 days following neonatal HI [40]. These results suggest that other mechanisms are likely to be involved in the second wave of leukocyte accumulation. The choroid plexus has been shown to be the route of entry for T_H17 lymphocytes into the brain following inflammation-sensitised neonatal HI [38]. We recently showed that following systemic inflammation, induced by a toll-like receptor 2 agonist, marked leukocyte infiltration occurred through the choroid plexus [41]. Thus, it is possible that the trafficking across the choroid plexus may have contributed to the second wave of leukocyte accumulation.

Recruitment of peripheral neutrophils, monocytes or lymphocytes aggravates the damage in animal models of multiple sclerosis [42, 43], stroke [37, 44, 45] and epilepsy [46]. We have demonstrated that systemic activation of toll-like receptor 2 induces infiltration of leukocytes, mainly neutrophils and inflammatory monocytes, to the developing brain of mice and exacerbates HI brain injury [41, 47]. In contrast, a previous study in adult animals reported that a subtype population of monocytes homes to the injury site via the choroid plexus following spinal cord injury and contributes to the resolution of inflammation [48]. Therefore, current evidence suggests that invading leukocytes can play both detrimental and beneficial roles depending on their subtype, the nature of the injury and potentially age.

We found that the systemic depletion of neutrophil and monocyte populations inhibits their accumulation in the brain following HI and reduces the neuronal injury in males. The role of inflammatory cells in ischemic injury of the brain is controversial [49]. Recently, accumulation of neutrophils in the human brain after adult stroke has been documented [50], supported by similar observation in a mouse model of stroke [50]. Moreover, depletion of neutrophils has been shown to reduce the infarct size in a rat model of brain ischemic injury [51]. However, in a focal ischemic stroke rat model, depletion of neutrophils failed to reduce the brain injury [52]. Our results, particularly the gender-dependent aspect, corroborate the complex role leukocytes play in ischemic injuries. Accumulating evidence illustrates gender-related differences in immune responses to infection and injury in adults and newborns, which was attributed to effects of various sex hormones as well as of differences on the sex chromosome [53]. In adult mice, induction of certain cytokines in the brain was stronger in males in systemic inflammation models and in an experimental autoimmune encephalomyelitis model [54, 55]. In neonatal mice (P4), there are more microglia colonised in the brain of males than in females [56]. Very recently, it was discovered that microglial response to environmental challenges is sex-specific [57]. There are also differences between male and female in the quantity and function of neutrophils and monocytes [58–61]. Further, inflammatory responses and injury outcome after neonatal HI have been reported to diverge according to gender, with enhanced inflammation, microglia activation and monocyte infiltration in males compared to females [62, 63]. Therefore, it is not surprising that many neuroprotective agents for neonatal brain injury, such as the antibody treatment in the present study, act in a sex-specific manner [64–67].

In conclusion, we have assessed accumulation of peripherally derived myeloid cells in the immature CNS in response to experimental HI. We detected significant infiltration with highest levels of invading cells at 1 day after hypoxia-ischemia. Additionally, we demonstrate two distinct phases of inflammatory cell accumulation occurring over a background of stable resident monocyte accumulation. Moreover, inhibiting myeloid cell accumulation in the brain was shown to be neuroprotective in male mice. Our findings merit renewed interest in the roles of MDMs and polymorphonuclear leukocytes in the long-term aspects of neonatal brain injury.

Conclusion

By using *Lys*-EGFP-*ki* mice, allowing identification of peripheral myeloid cells in the brain, we demonstrate a temporally biphasic pattern of inflammatory monocyte and granulocyte infiltration after neonatal hypoxia-ischemia. Antibody-mediated depletion of circulating myeloid cells reduced immune cell accumulation in the brain and reduced neuronal loss in male but not female mice. This study offers new insights into sex-dependent central-peripheral immune communication following neonatal brain injury and merits renewed interest in the roles of granulocytes and monocytes in brain lesion development.

Additional files

Additional file 1: Figure S1. EGFP⁺ myeloid cell localisation in the brain after HI. Representative tile-scanned confocal images of brain sections after HI. EGFP⁺ myeloid cells markedly infiltrate the striatum 1 day (A) but not 7 days (B) after HI. $n = 4$. (PDF 7477 kb)

Additional file 2: Figure S2. Cytokine measurements in the brain after HI. Multiplex cytokine measurements in the brain at 6 h, 1 day, 3 days, 7 days and 14 days after neonatal hypoxia-ischemia (HI) or sham operation. Values are pg/mg protein and presented as the mean ± SD. The statistical results are presented in Additional file 4: Table S1. (PDF 172 kb)

Additional file 3: Figure S3. Cytokine measurements in plasma after HI. Multiplex cytokine measurement in plasma at 6 h, 1 day, 3 days, 7 days and 14 days after neonatal hypoxia-ischemia (HI) or sham operation. Values are pg/ml and presented as the mean ± SD. The statistical results are presented in Additional file 5: Table S2. (PDF 172 kb)

Additional file 4: Table S1. Statistical analysis of multiplex cytokine measurement in the brain after HI. One-way ANOVA followed by Holm-Sidak's post hoc test for comparing the differences between sham-operated mice and HI mice in the contralateral and ipsilateral hemispheres at each time point. $n = 5$ for sham group and $n = 8$ for

HI groups. ns: not significant, *$p < 0.05$, **$p < 0.01$, ***$p < 0.001$. (PDF 138 kb)

Additional file 5: Table S2. Statistical analysis of multiplex cytokine measurement in plasma after HI. Student's *t* test followed by Holm-Sidak's post hoc test to correct for multiple comparisons between sham-operated mice and HI mice at each time point. $n = 5$ for sham group and $n = 8$ for HI groups. ns: not significant, *$p < 0.05$. (PDF 164 kb)

Abbreviations
BSA: Bovine albumin serum; CNS: Central nervous system; EGFP: Enhanced green fluorescent protein; HBSS: Hanks' Balanced Salt Solution; HI: Hypoxia-ischemia; MAP 2: Microtubule-associated protein-2; MBP: Myelin basic protein; MDM: Monocyte-derived macrophages; MiDM: Microglial-derived macrophages; MPO: Myeloperoxidase; P: Postnatal day; PFA: Paraformaldehyde; TBS: Tris-buffered saline

Acknowledgements
We acknowledge the Centre for Cellular Imaging at the University of Gothenburg for use of their imaging equipment, instruction and support.

Funding
This research received financial assistance from the Swedish Medical Research Council (VR 2012-2992, 2015-02493), Government grant to a researcher in Public Health Service at the Sahlgrenska University Hospital (ALFGBG-142881; 137601; ALFGBG-426401), European Union grant FP7 (Neurobid, HEALTH-F2-2009-241778), ERA-net (EU;VR 529-2014-7551), Swedish Brain Foundation (FO 2017-0063; FO2015-0004), the Leducq foundation (DSRR_P34404), NIH (1RO1HL139685-01), Torsten Söderberg Foundation, Cerebral Palsy Alliance Australia, Stroke-Riksförbundet, Åhlén Foundation and Wilhelm and Martina Lundgren Foundation.

Authors' contributions
LPS, HH, JE and CM made substantial contributions to conception and design. LPS, AM, PS and CJM made substantial contributions to acquisition and analysis of data. LPS, AM, HH, JE and CM made substantial contributions to interpretation of data. All authors read and approved the final manuscript.

Competing interests
The authors declare that they have no competing interests.

Author details
¹Institute of Neuroscience and Physiology, Department of Physiology, Sahlgrenska Academy, University of Gothenburg, Box 432, SE-405 30 Gothenburg, Sweden. ²Institute of Clinical Sciences, Department of Obstetrics and Gynaecology, Sahlgrenska Academy, University of Gothenburg, Gothenburg, Sweden.

References
1. Hagberg H, Mallard C, Ferriero DM, Vannucci SJ, Levison SW, Vexler ZS, Gressens P. The role of inflammation in perinatal brain injury. Nat Rev Neurol. 2015;11:192–208.
2. Degos V, Favrais G, Kaindl AM, Peineau S, Guerrot AM, Verney C, Gressens P. Inflammation processes in perinatal brain damage. J Neural Transm. 2010; 117:1009–17.
3. Bilbo SD, Schwarz JM. The immune system and developmental programming of brain and behavior. Front Neuroendocrinol. 2012;33: 267–86.
4. Hagberg H, Gressens P, Mallard C. Inflammation during fetal and neonatal

life: implications for neurologic and neuropsychiatric disease in children and adults. Ann Neurol. 2012;71:444–57.

5. Ginhoux F, Greter M, Leboeuf M, Nandi S, See P, Gokhan S, Mehler MF, Conway SJ, Ng LG, Stanley ER, et al. Fate mapping analysis reveals that adult microglia derive from primitive macrophages. Science. 2010;330:841–5.

6. Galea I, Bechmann I, Perry VH. What is immune privilege (not)? Trends Immunol. 2007;28:12–8.

7. Ransohoff RM, Kivisakk P, Kidd G. Three or more routes for leukocyte migration into the central nervous system. Nat Rev Immunol. 2003;3:569–81.

8. Hedtjarn M, Mallard C, Hagberg H. Inflammatory gene profiling in the developing mouse brain after hypoxia-ischemia. J Cereb Blood Flow Metab. 2004;24:1333–51.

9. Shi C, Pamer EG. Monocyte recruitment during infection and inflammation. Nat Rev Immunol. 2011;11:762–74.

10. McRae A, Gilland E, Bona E, Hagberg H. Microglia activation after neonatal hypoxic-ischemia. Brain Res Dev Brain Res. 1995;84:245–52.

11. Bona E, Andersson AL, Blomgren K, Gilland E, Puka-Sundvall M, Gustafson K, Hagberg H. Chemokine and inflammatory cell response to hypoxia-ischemia in immature rats. Pediatr Res. 1999;45:500–9.

12. Hudome S, Palmer C, Roberts RL, Mauger D, Housman C, Towfighi J. The role of neutrophils in the production of hypoxic-ischemic brain injury in the neonatal rat. Pediatr Res. 1997;41:607–16.

13. Nijboer CH, Kavelaars A, Vroon A, Groenendaal F, van Bel F, Heijnen CJ. Low endogenous G-protein-coupled receptor kinase 2 sensitizes the immature brain to hypoxia-ischemia-induced gray and white matter damage. J Neurosci. 2008;28:3324–32.

14. Jin Y, Silverman AJ, Vannucci SJ. Mast cells are early responders after hypoxia-ischemia in immature rat brain. Stroke. 2009;40:3107–12.

15. Perry VH, Hume DA, Gordon S. Immunohistochemical localization of macrophages and microglia in the adult and developing mouse brain. Neuroscience. 1985;15:313–26.

16. Sedgwick JD, Schwender S, Imrich H, Dorries R, Butcher GW, ter Meulen V. Isolation and direct characterization of resident microglial cells from the normal and inflamed central nervous system. Proc Natl Acad Sci U S A. 1991;88:7438–42.

17. Yamasaki R, Lu H, Butovsky O, Ohno N, Rietsch AM, Cialic R, Wu PM, Doykan CE, Lin J, Cotleur AC, et al. Differential roles of microglia and monocytes in the inflamed central nervous system. J Exp Med. 2014; 211:1533–49.

18. Geissmann F, Jung S, Littman DR. Blood monocytes consist of two principal subsets with distinct migratory properties. Immunity. 2003;19:71–82.

19. Mildner A, Mack M, Schmidt H, Bruck W, Djukic M, Zabel MD, Hille A, Priller J, Prinz M. CCR2+Ly-6Chi monocytes are crucial for the effector phase of autoimmunity in the central nervous system. Brain. 2009;132: 2487–500.

20. Auffray C, Fogg D, Garfa M, Elain G, Join-Lambert O, Kayal S, Sarnacki S, Cumano A, Lauvau G, Geissmann F. Monitoring of blood vessels and tissues by a population of monocytes with patrolling behavior. Science. 2007;317: 666–70.

21. Gliem M, Mausberg AK, Lee JI, Simiantonakis I, van Rooijen N, Hartung HP, Jander S. Macrophages prevent hemorrhagic infarct transformation in murine stroke models. Ann Neurol. 2012;71:743–52.

22. Yang J, Zhang L, Yu C, Yang XF, Wang H. Monocyte and macrophage differentiation: circulation inflammatory monocyte as biomarker for inflammatory diseases. Biomark Res. 2014;2(1).

23. Faust N, Varas F, Kelly LM, Heck S, Graf T. Insertion of enhanced green fluorescent protein into the lysozyme gene creates mice with green fluorescent granulocytes and macrophages. Blood. 2000;96:719–26.

24. Thawer SG, Mawhinney L, Chadwick K, de Chickera SN, Weaver LC, Brown A, Dekaban GA. Temporal changes in monocyte and macrophage subsets and microglial macrophages following spinal cord injury in the Lys-Egfp-ki mouse model. J Neuroimmunol. 2013;261:7–20.

25. Geissmann F, Manz MG, Jung S, Sieweke MH, Merad M, Ley K. Development of monocytes, macrophages, and dendritic cells. Science. 2010;327:656–61.

26. Hestdal K, Ruscetti FW, Ihle JN, Jacobsen SE, Dubois CM, Kopp WC, Longo DL, Keller JR. Characterization and regulation of RB6-8C5 antigen expression on murine bone marrow cells. J Immunol. 1991;147:22–8.

27. Daley JM, Thomay AA, Connolly MD, Reichner JS, Albina JE. Use of Ly6G-specific monoclonal antibody to deplete neutrophils in mice. J Leukoc Biol. 2008;83:64–70.

28. Mawhinney LA, Thawer SG, Lu WY, Rooijen N, Weaver LC, Brown A, Dekaban GA. Differential detection and distribution of microglial and hematogenous macrophage populations in the injured spinal cord of lys-EGFP-ki transgenic mice. J Neuropathol Exp Neurol. 2012;71:180–97.

29. Dommergues MA, Plaisant F, Verney C, Gressens P. Early microglial activation following neonatal excitotoxic brain damage in mice: a potential target for neuroprotection. Neuroscience. 2003;121:619–28.

30. Tahraoui SL, Marret S, Bodenant C, Leroux P, Dommergues MA, Evrard P, Gressens P. Central role of microglia in neonatal excitotoxic lesions of the murine periventricular white matter. Brain Pathol. 2001;11:56–71.

31. Derugin N, Wendland M, Muramatsu K, Roberts TP, Gregory G, Ferriero DM, Vexler ZS. Evolution of brain injury after transient middle cerebral artery occlusion in neonatal rats. Stroke. 2000;31:1752–61.

32. Denker SP, Ji S, Dingman A, Lee SY, Derugin N, Wendland MF, Vexler ZS. Macrophages are comprised of resident brain microglia not infiltrating peripheral monocytes acutely after neonatal stroke. J Neurochem. 2007;100: 893–904.

33. Towfighi J, Zec N, Yager J, Housman C, Vannucci RC. Temporal evolution of neuropathologic changes in an immature rat model of cerebral hypoxia: a light microscopic study. Acta Neuropathol. 1995;90:375–86.

34. Hellstrom Erkenstam N, Smith PL, Fleiss B, Nair S, Svedin P, Wang W, Bostrom M, Gressens P, Hagberg H, Brown KL, et al. Temporal characterization of microglia/macrophage phenotypes in a mouse model of neonatal hypoxic-ischemic brain injury. Front Cell Neurosci. 2016;10:286.

35. Palmer C, Roberts RL, Young PI. Timing of neutrophil depletion influences long-term neuroprotection in neonatal rat hypoxic-ischemic brain injury. Pediatr Res. 2004;55:549–56.

36. Winerdal M, Winerdal ME, Kinn J, Urmaliya V, Winqvist O, Aden U. Long lasting local and systemic inflammation after cerebral hypoxic ischemia in newborn mice. PLoS One. 2012;7:e36422.

37. Weston RM, Jones NM, Jarrott B, Callaway JK. Inflammatory cell infiltration after endothelin-1-induced cerebral ischemia: histochemical and myeloperoxidase correlation with temporal changes in brain injury. J Cereb Blood Flow Metab. 2007;27:100–14.

38. Yang D, Sun YY, Bhaumik SK, Li Y, Baumann JM, Lin X, Zhang Y, Lin SH, Dunn RS, Liu CY, et al. Blocking lymphocyte trafficking with FTY720 prevents inflammation-sensitized hypoxic-ischemic brain injury in newborns. J Neurosci. 2014;34:16467–81.

39. Geddes R, Vannucci RC, Vannucci SJ. Delayed cerebral atrophy following moderate hypoxia-ischemia in the immature rat. Dev Neurosci. 2001;23: 180–5.

40. Ek CJ, D'Angelo B, Baburamani AA, Lehner C, Leverin AL, Smith PL, Nilsson H, Svedin P, Hagberg H, Mallard C. Brain barrier properties and cerebral blood flow in neonatal mice exposed to cerebral hypoxia-ischemia. J Cereb Blood Flow Metab. 2015;35:818–27.

41. Mottahedin A, Smith PL, Hagberg H, Ek CJ, Mallard C. TLR2-mediated leukocyte trafficking to the developing brain. J Leukoc Biol. 2017;101: 297–305.

42. Liu L, Belkadi A, Darnall L, Hu T, Drescher C, Cotleur AC, Padovani-Claudio D, He T, Choi K, Lane TE, et al. CXCR2-positive neutrophils are essential for cuprizone-induced demyelination: relevance to multiple sclerosis. Nat Neurosci. 2010;13:319–26.

43. Ajami B, Bennett JL, Krieger C, McNagny KM, Rossi FM. Infiltrating monocytes trigger EAE progression, but do not contribute to the resident microglia pool. Nat Neurosci. 2011;14:1142–9.

44. Liesz A, Zhou W, Mracsko E, Karcher S, Bauer H, Schwarting S, Sun L, Bruder D, Stegemann S, Cerwenka A, et al. Inhibition of lymphocyte trafficking shields the brain against deleterious neuroinflammation after stroke. Brain. 2011;134:704–20.

45. Lee S, Chu HX, Kim HA, Real NC, Sharif S, Fleming SB, Mercer AA, Wise LM, Drummond GR, Sobey CG. Effect of a broad-specificity chemokine-binding protein on brain leukocyte infiltration and infarct development. Stroke. 2015;46:537–44.

46. Zattoni M, Mura ML, Deprez F, Schwendener RA, Engelhardt B, Frei K, Fritzschy JM. Brain infiltration of leukocytes contributes to the pathophysiology of temporal lobe epilepsy. J Neurosci. 2011;31:4037–50.

47. Mottahedin A, Svedin P, Nair S, Mohn CJ, Wang X, Hagberg H, Ek J, Mallard C. Systemic activation of Toll-like receptor 2 suppresses mitochondrial respiration and exacerbates hypoxic-ischemic injury in the developing brain. J Cereb Blood Flow Metab. 2017:271678X17691292.

48. Shechter R, London A, Schwartz M. Orchestrated leukocyte recruitment to immune-privileged sites: absolute barriers versus educational gates. Nat Rev Immunol. 2013;13:206–18.

49. Jin R, Yang G, Li G. Inflammatory mechanisms in ischemic stroke: role of inflammatory cells. J Leukoc Biol. 2010;87:779–89.

50. Perez-de-Puig I, Miro-Mur F, Ferrer-Ferrer M, Gelpi E, Pedragosa J, Justicia C, Urra X, Chamorro A, Planas AM. Neutrophil recruitment to the brain in mouse and human ischemic stroke. Acta Neuropathol. 2015;129:239–57.

51. Matsuo Y, Onodera H, Shiga Y, Nakamura M, Ninomiya M, Kihara T, Kogure K. Correlation between myeloperoxidase-quantified neutrophil accumulation and ischemic brain injury in the rat. Effects of neutrophil depletion. Stroke. 1994;25:1469–75.

52. Harris AK, Ergul A, Kozak A, Machado LS, Johnson MH, Fagan SC. Effect of neutrophil depletion on gelatinase expression, edema formation and hemorrhagic transformation after focal ischemic stroke. BMC Neurosci. 2005;6:49.

53. Klein SL, Flanagan KL. Sex differences in immune responses. Nat Rev Immunol. 2016;16:626–38.

54. Posillico C, Speirs I, Tronson N. Sex differences in the hippocampal cytokine response following systemic lipopolysaccharide. Brain Behavior and Immunity. 2017;66:e40.

55. Russi AE, Ebel ME, Yang Y, Brown MA. Male-specific IL-33 expression regulates sex-dimorphic EAE susceptibility. Proc Natl Acad Sci U S A. 2018; 115:E1520–9.

56. Schwarz JM, Sholar PW, Bilbo SD. Sex differences in microglial colonization of the developing rat brain. J Neurochem. 2012;120:948–63.

57. Thion MS, Low D, Silvin A, Chen J, Grisel P, Schulte-Schrepping J, Blecher R, Ulas T, Squarzoni P, Hoeffel G, et al. Microbiome influences prenatal and adult microglia in a sex-specific manner. Cell. 2018;172:500–16 e516.

58. Pace S, Rossi A, Krauth V, Dehm F, Troisi F, Bilancia R, Weinigel C, Rummler S, Werz O, Sautebin L. Sex differences in prostaglandin biosynthesis in neutrophils during acute inflammation. Sci Rep. 2017;7:3759.

59. Bain BJ, England JM. Normal haematological values: sex difference in neutrophil count. Br Med J. 1975;1:306–9.

60. Spitzer JA, Zhang P. Gender differences in neutrophil function and cytokine-induced neutrophil chemoattractant generation in endotoxic rats. Inflammation. 1996;20:485–98.

61. Jiang W, Gilkeson G. Sex differences in monocytes and TLR4 associated immune responses; implications for systemic lupus erythematosus (SLE). J Immunother Appl. 2014;1(1).

62. Hill CA, Fitch RH. Sex differences in mechanisms and outcome of neonatal hypoxia-ischemia in rodent models: implications for sex-specific neuroprotection in clinical neonatal practice. Neurol Res Int. 2012;2012:867531.

63. Mirza MA, Ritzel R, Xu Y, McCullough LD, Liu F. Sexually dimorphic outcomes and inflammatory responses in hypoxic-ischemic encephalopathy. J Neuroinflammation. 2015;12:32.

64. Nijboer CH, Groenendaal F, Kavelaars A, Hagberg HH, van Bel F, Heijnen CJ. Gender-specific neuroprotection by 2-iminobiotin after hypoxia-ischemia in the neonatal rat via a nitric oxide independent pathway. J Cereb Blood Flow Metab. 2007;27:282–92.

65. Nie X, Lowe DW, Rollins LG, Bentzley J, Fraser JL, Martin R, Singh I, Jenkins D. Sex-specific effects of N-acetylcysteine in neonatal rats treated with hypothermia after severe hypoxia-ischemia. Neurosci Res. 2016;108:24–33.

66. Rodriguez-Fanjul J, Duran Fernandez-Feijoo C, Lopez-Abad M, Lopez Ramos MG, Balada Caballe R, Alcantara-Horillo S, Camprubi Camprubi M. Neuroprotection with hypothermia and allopurinol in an animal model of hypoxic-ischemic injury: is it a gender question? PLoS One. 2017;12:e0184643.

67. Fleiss B, Nilsson MK, Blomgren K, Mallard C. Neuroprotection by the histone deacetylase inhibitor trichostatin A in a model of lipopolysaccharide-sensitised neonatal hypoxic-ischaemic brain injury. J Neuroinflammation. 2012;9:70.

8

Microglial response to increasing amyloid load saturates with aging: a longitudinal dual tracer in vivo µPET-study

Tanja Blume[1,2†], Carola Focke[1†], Finn Peters[2†], Maximilian Deussing[1], Nathalie L. Albert[1], Simon Lindner[1], Franz-Josef Gildehaus[1], Barbara von Ungern-Sternberg[1], Laurence Ozmen[3], Karlheinz Baumann[3], Peter Bartenstein[1], Axel Rominger[1,4,6], Jochen Herms[2,5,6†] and Matthias Brendel[1,6*†]

Abstract

Background: Causal associations between microglia activation and β-amyloid (Aβ) accumulation during the progression of Alzheimer's disease (AD) remain a matter of controversy. Therefore, we used longitudinal dual tracer in vivo small animal positron emission tomography (µPET) imaging to resolve the progression of the association between Aβ deposition and microglial responses during aging of an Aβ mouse model.

Methods: APP-SL70 mice ($N = 17$; baseline age 3.2–8.5 months) and age-matched C57Bl/6 controls (wildtype (wt)) were investigated longitudinally for 6 months using Aβ (18F-florbetaben) and 18 kDa translocator protein (TSPO) µPET (18F-GE180). Changes in cortical binding were transformed to Z-scores relative to wt mice, and microglial activation relative to amyloidosis was defined as the Z-score difference (TSPO—Aβ). Using 3D immunohistochemistry for activated microglia (Iba-1) and histology for fibrillary Aβ (methoxy-X04), we measure microglial brain fraction relative to plaque size and the distance from plaque margins.

Results: Aβ-PET binding increased exponentially as a function of age in APP-SL70 mice, whereas TSPO binding had an inverse U-shape growth function. Longitudinal Z-score differences declined with aging, suggesting that microglial response declined relative to increasing amyloidosis in aging APP-SL70 mice. Microglial brain volume fraction was inversely related to adjacent plaque size, while the proximity to Aβ plaques increased with age.

Conclusions: Microglial activity decreases relative to ongoing amyloidosis with aging in APP-SL70 mice. The plaque-associated microglial brain fraction saturated and correlated negatively with increasing plaque size with aging.

Keywords: TSPO µPET, Amyloid µPET, Alzheimer's disease, Neuroinflammation, Microglia, Aging

Background

The progressive accumulation of senile plaques composed of β-amyloid (Aβ) is a main pathological hallmark of Alzheimer's disease (AD), the most common dementing disorder in the elderly. The Aβ accumulation promotes synaptic loss and neuronal degeneration apparently by activating microglia, the resident macrophages of the brain [1–4]. In the healthy brain, microglia cells are long-lived cells using highly motile processes to survey parenchymal territory for the presence of pathogens and cell debris. In addition, microglia secrete factors that support neuronal survival and synaptogenesis [5]. In the early stages of AD, microglia migrate towards amyloid deposits and express certain cell-surface receptors to promote the clearance and phagocytosis of Aβ [6–8]. Furthermore, deficits in microglia activation favor accelerated amyloid deposition [9]. However, it has been hypothesized that microglial reactions are overwhelmed by the massive Aβ deposition in later AD stages [10, 11]. This suggestion is supported by the finding that plaque-associated microglia ultimately show decreased expression of Aβ-binding receptors, which leads to a significant reduction in Aβ degradation

* Correspondence: matthias.brendel@med.uni-muenchen.de
†Tanja Blume, Carola Focke, Finn Peters, Jochen Herms and Matthias Brendel contributed equally to this work.
[1]Department of Nuclear Medicine, University Hospital, LMU Munich, Marchioninistraße 15, 81377 Munich, Germany
[6]Munich Cluster for Systems Neurology (SyNergy), Munich, Germany
Full list of author information is available at the end of the article

by microglia in the aging brain [11]. Moreover, plaque-associated microglial cells show a threefold higher mortality rate compared to non-plaque-associated microglia in vivo [12].

The use of small animal positron emission tomography (μPET) with Aβ tracers enables longitudinal investigations of cerebral amyloidosis in rodents in vivo [13, 14]. Confirmation of the hypothesis of a ceiling effect in microglial reactions has been hampered by the technical difficulty in following the fate of aging microglial cells in living mice. The past decade has seen the introduction of Aβ-μPET in rodents [15, 16], using the same radioligands employed in the clinical routine for the differential diagnosis of AD [17, 18]. A series of PET radiotracers targeting the microglial marker 18-kDa translocator protein (TSPO), formerly known as the peripheral benzodiazepine receptor (PBR) [19–23], has been developed in recent years.

The basal availability of TSPO binding sites is low in the healthy living brain (21), such that local upregulation presents a sensitive marker for the detection of microglial activation in afflicted brain regions [24–26]. This is supported by findings of elevated TSPO expression in the hippocampus and the frontal, temporal, and parietal cortices of postmortem AD brain [25, 27, 28]. Our group has recently established cross-sectional dual tracer μPET imaging of Aβ and TSPO in transgenic AD mouse models [29]. Given this background, we aimed in the present longitudinal Aβ/TSPO double tracer μPET study to explore the longitudinal association between amyloidosis and microglial response during aging of an amyloid mouse model in vivo. By using mice with a range of baseline age, we were able to perform correlation analysis with the longitudinal biomarker progression over 7 months. Final immunohistochemistry supported the interpretation of μPET results by mapping of individual plaques and microglial cells.

Methods
Animals and study design
All experiments were carried out in compliance with the National Guidelines for Animal Protection, Germany, and with the approval of the regional animal care committee (Regierung Oberbayern) and were overseen by a veterinarian. Animals were housed in a temperature- and humidity-controlled environment with a 12 h light–dark cycle, with free access to food (Sniff, Soest, Germany) and water.

All experiments were performed in APP-SL70 mice, a mouse-line produced by Roche (Basel, Switzerland), ($N = 17$, baseline age: 3.2 to 8.5 months of age: 3.2 to 5.0 months ($N = 4$); 5.1 to 6.8 months ($N = 6$); and 6.9 to 8.5 months ($N = 7$)). First fibrillar Aβ deposits in this mouse-line appear as early as 2.5 months of age, similar to the mouse line used by Blanchard [30].

Congophilic plaques are observed starting from 5 to 6 months of age. Protein levels of Aβ40 and Aβ42 start to increase from 3 months of age and range around 1 ng/mg brain at 6 months, 25 ng/mg brain at 9 months, and 90 ng/mg brain at 12 months of age. μPET examinations (Aβ and TSPO) were performed in a longitudinal design at baseline (0 months), follow-up (+ 2.2 months/11 weeks) and terminal age (+ 6.3 months/29 weeks). Serial μPET scans of both tracers deriving from a total of 30 age-matched C57Bl6 mice (wt) served as control data. All mice were killed after terminal scanning, followed by rapid brain removal and performance of immunohistochemistry analyses. The study design is illustrated in Fig. 1.

Radiochemistry
Radiosynthesis of [18F]-GE180 was performed as previously described [23], with slight modifications [29]. This procedure yielded product with radiochemical purity exceeding 98%, and molar activity of 1400 ± 500 gigabecquerel (GBq)/μmol at end of synthesis. Radiosynthesis of [18F]-florbetaben was performed as described earlier [16, 31].

μPET data acquisition, reconstruction and preprocessing
All μPET procedures followed an established standardized protocol for radiochemistry, acquisition, and post-processing [29, 32]. Mice were anesthetized with isoflurane (1.5%, delivered at 3.5 l/min) and placed in the aperture of the Siemens Inveon DPET (Siemens, Knoxville, USA), as described previously [33]. In brief, we made TSPO-μPET emission recordings during 60–90 min (p.i.) per image of [18F]-GE180 (11.2 ± 1.5 megabecquerel (MBq)) beta-amyloid-μPET emission recordings during 30–60 min p.i. of [18F]-florbetaben (10.8 ± 1.5 MBq). All images were spatially normalized using automatic algorithms and tracer specific templates [32].

μPET data analyses
All μPET analyses were performed with PMOD (V3.5, PMOD technologies, Basel, Switzerland). Normalization of emission images to standardized uptake value ratio (SUVR) images was performed using a previously validated white matter reference region [29, 32]. A target volume of interest (VOI) was placed in the bilateral frontal cortex (46 mm^3) and $SUVR_{CTX/WM}$ values were extracted for each individual APP-SL70 and wt mouse at the serial imaging time points for both tracers. Differences of TSPO- and Aβ-μPET SUVR between terminal and baseline time points were calculated as percentage change ($\Delta\%$). Z-scores of the TSPO- and Aβ-μPET tracer uptake in individual APP-SL70 mice were calculated by normalization to age-matched wt mice. To this end, the mean uptake in age-matched wt

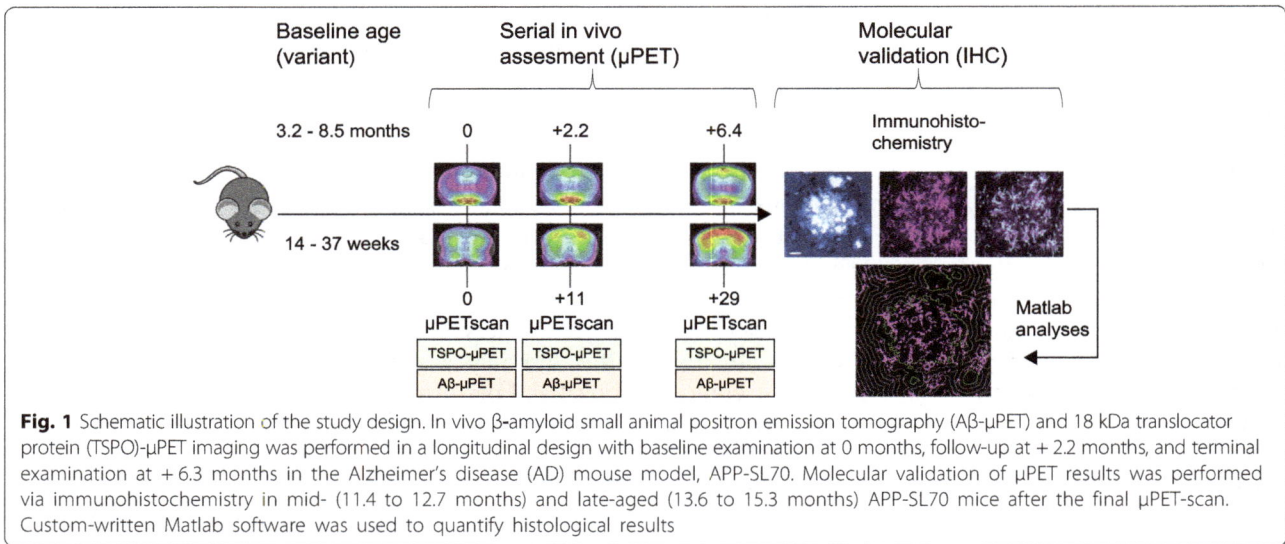

Fig. 1 Schematic illustration of the study design. In vivo β-amyloid small animal positron emission tomography (Aβ-μPET) and 18 kDa translocator protein (TSPO)-μPET imaging was performed in a longitudinal design with baseline examination at 0 months, follow-up at + 2.2 months, and terminal examination at + 6.3 months in the Alzheimer's disease (AD) mouse model, APP-SL70. Molecular validation of μPET results was performed via immunohistochemistry in mid- (11.4 to 12.7 months) and late-aged (13.6 to 15.3 months) APP-SL70 mice after the final μPET-scan. Custom-written Matlab software was used to quantify histological results

mice was subtracted from the individual value in APP-SL70 mice (APP-SL70$_{INDIVIDUAL}$ - wt$_{MEAN}$) and the resulting difference divided by the corresponding standard deviation for wt mice to generate an individual Z-score value.

$$Z\text{-score} = \frac{APPSL70(INDIVIDUAL) - wt(MEAN)}{wt(SD)}$$

To establish a readout of microglial activity relative to fibrillary amyloidosis we calculated Z-score differences between TSPO- and Aβ-μPET. Z-scores deriving from the same imaging time point of individual mice (gap 0.35 ± 1.62 weeks).

$$Z\text{-score difference} = Z\text{-score}\,(TSPO\text{-}\mu PET) - Z\text{-score}\,(A\beta\text{-}\mu PET)$$

Immunohistochemistry: acquisition and image analysis
Brains intended for immunohistochemistry were fixed by immersion in 4% paraformaldehyde at 4 °C for 15 h. Two representative 50-μm-thick slices per animal were then cut in the axial plane using a vibratome (VT 1000 S, Leica, Wetzlar, Germany). Free-floating sections were permeabilized with 2% Triton X-100 overnight and blocked with I-Block™ Protein-Based Blocking Reagent (Thermo Fischer Scientific, Waltham, USA). We obtained immunofluorescence labelling of microglia using an Iba-1 primary antibody (Wako, Richmond, USA) with a dilution of 1:200 in I-Block™ and the A-21244 secondary antibody (Invitrogen, Carlsbad, USA) with a dilution of 1:500 in I-Block™. For histological staining against fibrillar Aβ, we used methoxy-X04 (TOCRIS, Bristol, United Kingdom) with a dilution of 0.01 mg/ml. The unbound dye

was removed in three washing steps with PBS, and the slices were then mounted on microscope slides with fluorescent mounting medium (Dako, Santa Clara, USA). Images were acquired with a LSM 780 confocal microscope (Zeiss, Oberkochen, Germany) equipped with a 40x/1.4 oil immersion objective. The excitation wavelength for Iba-1 detection was 633 nm and emission was detected from 638 to 755 nm. For methoxy-X04, the excitation wavelength was 405 nm and emission was detected from 403 to 585 nm for each brain slice. We acquired three-dimensional 16-bit data stacks of $2048 \times 2048 \times 120$ pixels from five different positions in the frontal cortex at a lateral resolution of 0.17 μm/pixel and an axial resolution of 0.4 μm/pixel. To quantify Iba-1 positive brain volume fraction, hereinafter referred as microglia brain fraction, as well as plaque density and size, we utilized custom-written Matlab software (MathWorks, Natick, USA). The detailed method was described previously [34].

Local background subtraction was used to diminish intensity variations between different stacks. Subsequently, microglia cells were identified by applying the 90th percentile as minimal-intensity threshold. Noise was excluded by applying a connected component analysis excluding patches of contiguous voxels smaller than 1 μm^3. Analyses were performed by an operator who was blind to the μPET results.

Statistics
The associations between μPET readouts (Δ%, Z-score, Z-score difference) and age were characterized by applying linear, logarithmic, and quadratic regression analyses as implemented in SPSS (SPSS Version 24, IBM SPSS Software, IBM, Armonk, New York). In cases with several statistically significant fits ($p < 0.05$),

the best curve fitting model was determined by applying the Akaike Information Criterion (AIC) [35]. If the AIC proved indifferent between two models, we chose the one with the higher R^2 value. Statistics of histological analyses were calculated in Prism 7.01 (GraphPad Software, San Diego, CA, USA). Statistical comparison of the microglia fraction between different plaque radii was performed for the highest microglia occupancy in the vicinity to the plaque border [6]. Data was tested for normal distribution using the D'Agostino and Pearson omnibus test. Intergroup comparisons were performed using the two-tailed unpaired Student's t test. For correlation of plaque size and microglia brain fraction, the variables were compared across groups using one-way analysis of variance (ANOVA). All specifications of n state the number of biological replicates. All results are presented as mean ± standard error of mean (SEM).

Results

Microglial response saturates relatively to ongoing amyloidosis during aging

First, we analyzed serial changes of TSPO and fibrillar amyloidosis by dual tracer µPET to characterize the AD mouse model through molecular imaging. Both TSPO-µPET (+ 2.8 ± 2.4% per month) and Aβ-PET signals (+ 2.9 ± 2.5% per month direct comparison of TSPO-PET and Aβ-PET increase rates: $p = 0.897$) increased strongly during aging of individual APP-SL70 mice. At late time points, the two markers were distinctly elevated when compared to wt mice (Fig. 2a–c) and there was a strong direct association between SUVR values of both PET tracers (quadratic fit, $R = 0.90$, $p < 0.001$). However, the percentage change of PET SUVR between baseline and + 6.3 months as a function of starting age in APP-SL70 mice showed an inverted U-shape for TSPO binding (quadratic fit, $R = 0.69$, $p = 0.014$, Fig. 2d) but a linear positive association for amyloidosis (linear fit, $R = 0.50$, $p = 0.048$, Fig. 2e). Thus, increases of microglial activity in aged APP-SL70 mice tended to reach a plateau whereas amyloidosis continued to progress even at late follow-up. Given the differences by tracer in µPET alterations as functions of age, we aimed to compare directly the longitudinal time courses of TSPO activity and amyloidosis. To this end, we calculated standardized Z-scores for individual mice and for both tracers based on findings in age-matched wt controls. By this approach, we found the expected strong increases with age for TSPO activity (quadratic fit, $R = 0.68$, $p < 0.001$; Fig. 3a) and fibrillar amyloidosis (quadratic fit, $R = 0.86$, $p < 0.001$, Fig. 3b). Next, Z-score differences (TSPO—Aβ) for all serial imaging time points were introduced as a measure of microglial activity relative to fibrillar amyloidosis.

Importantly, we observed a decreasing Z-score difference as a function of age in APP-SL70 mice (quadratic fit, $R = 0.66$, $p < 0.001$, Fig. 3c), which clearly revealed that the microglial response to ongoing amyloid deposition is relatively attenuated at the later ages ((Z-score difference < 0) ≥ 12.2 months of age) of the mouse model. Notably, this effect was not only observed at the group level but was also distinguishable in single animals (Fig. 3d).

Plaque-associated microglial brain fraction decreases with increasing plaque size during aging

To confirm and extend observed in vivo results, methoxy-X04 staining of fibrillar Aβ as well as Iba-1 staining of microglia were performed in mid- (11.4 to 12.7 months) and late-aged (13.6 to 15.3 months) APP-SL70 mice after the final µPET-scans. In line with previous studies, our immunohistochemical analysis showed that the observed increase in the Aβ-µPET signal is indicative of plaque growth rather than increased plaque density (Fig. 4a, b). In late-aged APP-SL70, mice the mean plaque radius was significantly elevated by approximately 3 µm compared to that in mid-aged mice ($t_{(14)} = 5.86$, $p < 0.0001$, two-tailed Students t test, Fig. 4b), whereas plaque density in both age groups remained unchanged at approximately 3600/µm³ ($t_{(14)} = 0.33$, $p = 0.746$, two-tailed Students t test, Fig. 4c). Furthermore, plaque size distribution analysis showed a shift towards larger radii in late-aged compared to mid-aged transgenic mice (Fig. 4a).

Microglia proliferation in plaque-free areas and their migration towards Aβ plaques has already been shown to occur in AD model mice [12], which results in an increased number of microglial cells surrounding amyloid deposits [36]. However, our standardized µPET analysis revealed a decrease of the TSPO signal in direct relation to the increasing amyloid signal with aging (Fig. 3c). To assess the molecular relationship between plaque growth and microglial brain fraction, we applied custom-written MATLAB cluster analysis for automated morphological detection by applying the 90th percentile as the minimal intensity threshold for identifying microglial cells. We analyzed a total of 1312 plaques ranging in radius from 3 µm to 30 µm and identified their associated microglial cells via immunofluorescence. Representative plaques of several sizes are illustrated in Fig. 5. Interestingly, when we calculated the mean volume occupied by Iba1-positive microglia in consecutive 1-µm-thick layers around the plaque border up to 20 µm distance, we observed a maximum of microglial brain fraction near small plaques (radii between 3 and 4 µm), while the microglia brain fraction decreased with increasing plaque radius ($F_{(5,16)} = 11.87$, $p < 0.0001$, one-way ANOVA, (Fig. 4d, e, Fig. 5). We conclude that the observed age-related

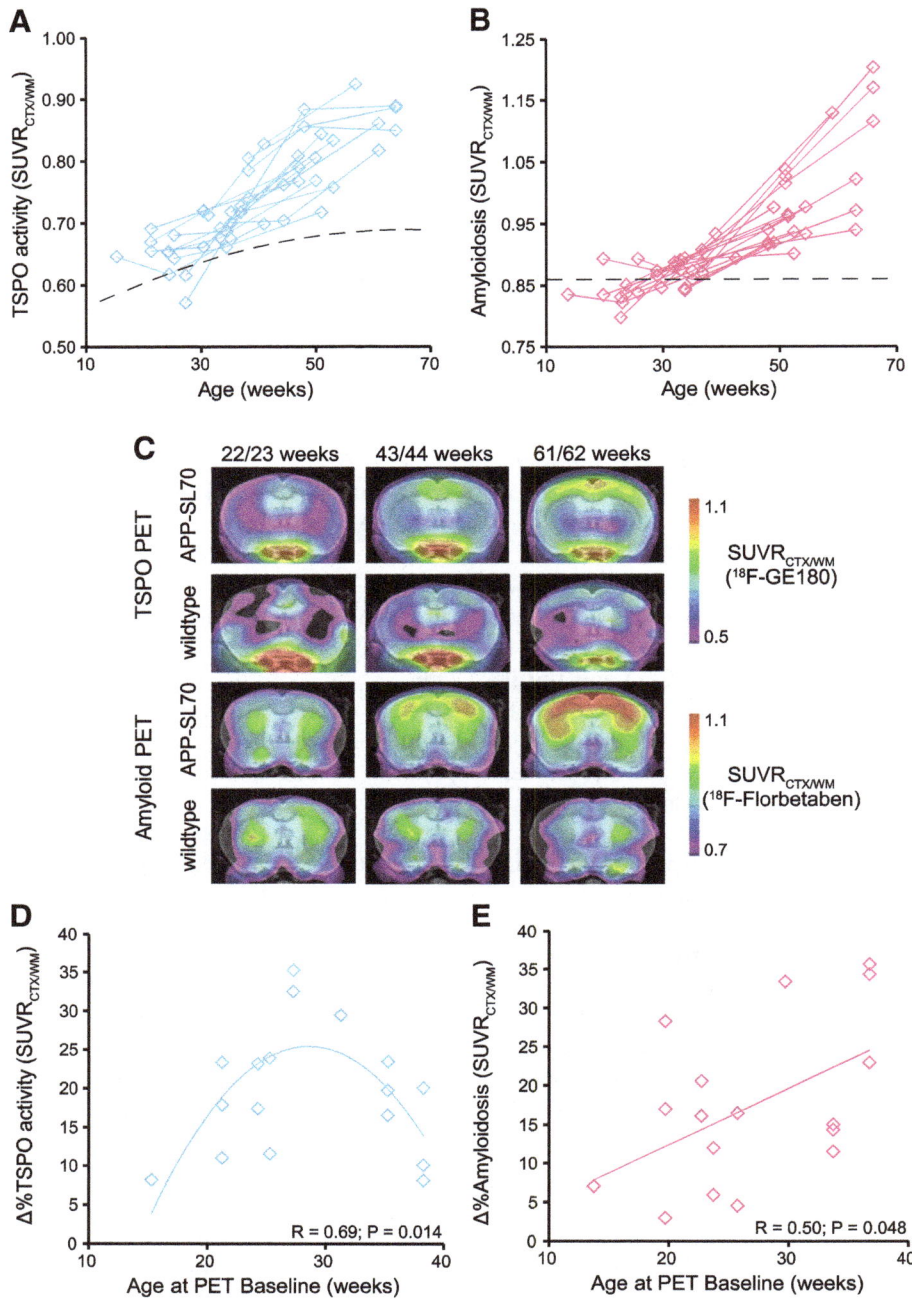

Fig. 2 Microglial response increased but saturated relative to ongoing amyloidosis during aging. Plots show cortical Standardized Uptake Value Ratio (SUVR) of [^{18}F]-GE180 (TSPO-activity) (**a**) and [^{18}F]-florbetaben (amyloidosis) (**b**) in APP-SL70 mice at different ages (B) APP-SL70 indicate increasing cortical amyloidosis and 18 kDa translocator protein (TSPO) binding during aging (**c**). Percentage change for both PET tracers between baseline and + 6.3 months as a function of baseline age in APP-SL70 mice and wt reveal an inverted U-shape for TSPO activity (quadratic fit, $R = 0.69$, $p = 0.014$ (**d**) but a linear positive association for amyloidosis in APP-SL70 (linear fit, $R = 0.50$, $p = 0.048$ (**e**). $N = 17$

decrease of the TSPO-μPET signal relative to the Aβ-μPET signal was likely driven by a decrease in the microglial brain fraction around large plaques, which came to predominate in late-aged APP-SL70 mice (Fig. 4b).

Microglial brain fraction in the plaque-free cortical brain parenchyma of APP-SL70 mice was less compared to wt mice

It is well acknowledged that microglial cells are essential for proper brain function and that microglia can

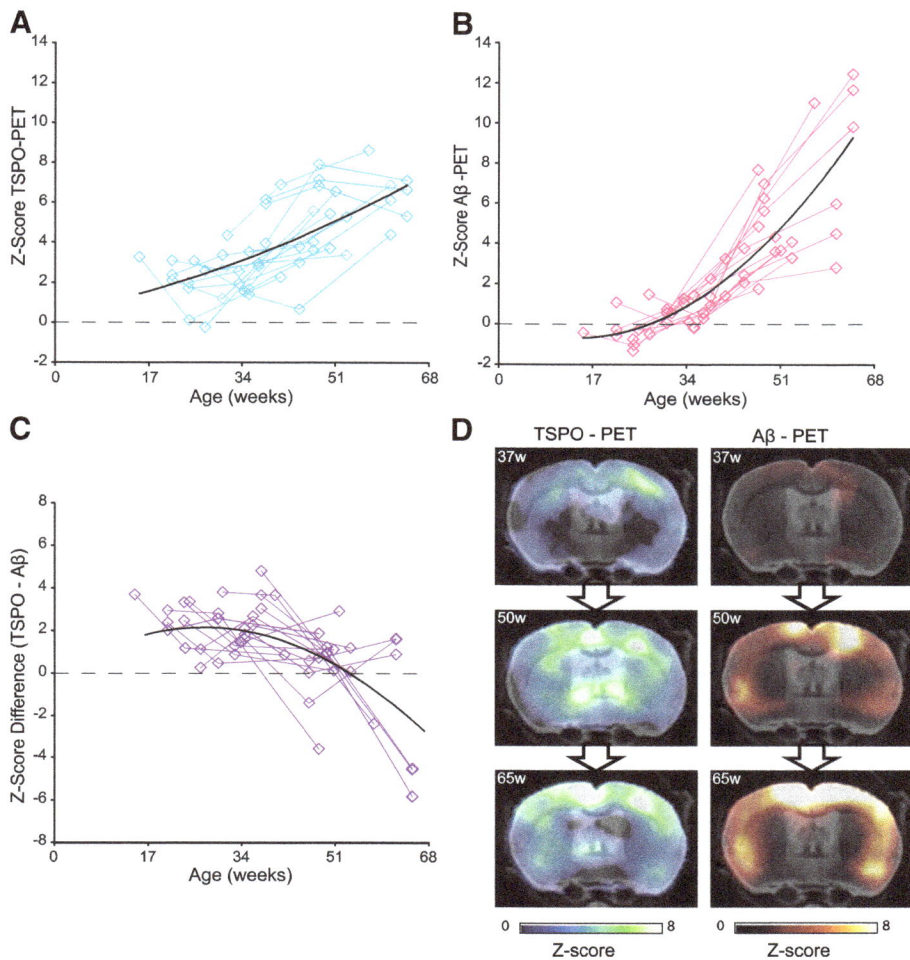

Fig. 3 Standardized µPET analysis (Z-scores) TSPO activity and amyloidosis. Standardized TSPO activity (**a**; quadratic fit, $R = 0.68$, $p < 0.001$) and standardized fibrillar amyloidosis (**b**; quadratic fit, $R = 0.86$, $p < 0.001$) indicate an increase with aging. The direct comparison of both standardized tracer signals reveals a decrease in the Z-score differences (TSPO—Aβ) with aging (**c**; quadratic fit, $R = 0.66$, $p < 0.001$). **d** Exemplary findings of a single APP-SL70 mouse show that microglia response is overwhelmed by ongoing amyloid deposition. $N = 16$

rapidly proliferate in response to a wide range of central nervous system insults [37, 38]. In this context, a recent study of microglial turnover and proliferation in AD showed comparable rates of proliferation and loss for plaque-associated microglial cells indicating a steady-state, while non-plaque-associated microglial cells showed a threefold higher proliferation rate. In contrast, wt mice show only moderate rates of microglial cell proliferation and loss [12]. In the present study, we observed an increase in microglial brain fraction in APP-SL70 mice only in proximity to the plaque border, starting at a maximal distance of 20 µm (Fig. 6a). Surprisingly, we detected a significantly lower microglial brain fraction distant to plaques in the APP-SL70 mice compared to the microglial brain fraction in wt mice ($t_{(25)} = 2.18$, $p < 0.05$, two-tailed Students t test, Fig. 6b). It is well-known that microglial

cells are activated by Aβ deposits and actively migrate towards the plaque within 1 to 2 days after the initial formation of an amyloid deposit [6, 39]. Regarding the threefold higher proliferation rate of non-plaque-associated microglial cells, the net microglial loss distal to plaques in APP-SL70 compared to wt mice, while surprising, is conspicuous in our double-labelling studies (Fig. 6c).

Discussion

We present the first longitudinal in vivo dual tracer µPET study aiming to directly compare the time courses of microglial activation and fibrillar amyloidosis with age in a transgenic amyloid mouse model. Our results clearly indicate that both biomarkers increase with age, but that microglial activation is disproportionately elevated at an early age and seems to

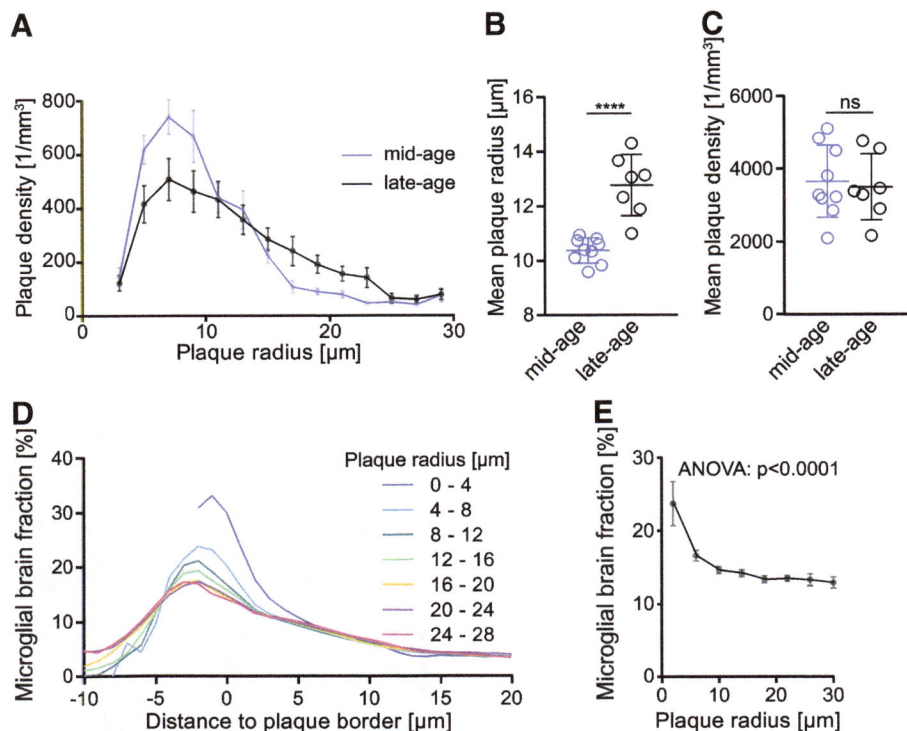

Fig. 4 Molecular elucidation of in vivo µPET findings by terminal immunohistochemistry. **a** Frequency distribution of plaque radii in mid-aged (11.4 to 12.7 months) and late-aged (13.6 to 15.3 months) APP-SL70 mice. The mean plaque radius (**b**) is significantly higher in the late-aged cohort when compared to mid-aged APP-SL70 mice ($p < 0.0001$, two-tailed Student's t test), whereas the plaque density (**c**) did not indicate changes during aging > 12 months in APP-SL70 mice ($p = 0.746$, two-tailed Student's t test). **d** Correlation of microglial brain fraction with distance to plaque border and plaque size. Each profile represents the change of microglial brain fraction with distance to the border of plaques with defined radius. **e** Microglial brain fraction in the vicinity to the plaque border (radius 1 µm) decreased significantly with increasing plaque radius (one-way ANOVA, $F(5,16) = 11.87$, $p < 0.0001$). Data presented as mean ± SEM; $n = 7$–9 mice

saturate relative to amyloidosis, which continues to progress. Detailed immunohistochemical analyses revealed a significant decrease of microglial brain fraction around amyloid plaques with increasing plaque radius to be the cellular correlate of our in vivo µPET findings. Moreover, we found that the microglia brain fraction in the plaque-free brain parenchyma of APP-SL70 mice was lower than in wt mice. This depletion of microglial cells distal to plaques is likely related to the massive microglial migration towards zones of fibrillar Aβ deposition [6, 39].

With this serial in vivo study, we aimed to investigate longitudinal relationships between microglial activation and amyloidosis during the life course of the APP-SL70 AD mouse model. We performed dual-tracer small animal µPET examinations with the novel tracer [18F]-GE180 for TSPO and [18F]-florbetaben for fibrillar amyloidosis, in conjunction with immunohistochemical analyses after the final imaging studies. To enable a reliable comparison of the relationship between the two µPET readouts, we took pains to develop a standard procedure for quantification, entailing

a biphasic calculation method: First, we calculated standardized tracer specific Z-scores of individual mice at different time points by considering mean and standard deviation values of age-matched wt mice. We next calculated differences between TSPO- and Aβ-µPET Z-scores as a measure of microglial activation relative to fibrillar amyloidosis. We deemed this calculation of a difference score to be more reliable than a ratio method, as values close to zero would potentially have distorted the results at the onset of fibrillar amyloidosis in young mice. The two radioligands have different sensitivities for their specific targets, resulting in distinct detection thresholds unequal magnitudes of signal alterations during the progression of the AD model. To address these issues, we used the standardized Z-score calculation as our main endpoint. In fact, our analysis showed positive Z-score differences at early ages of APP-SL70 mice, which suggest that microglial activation precedes fibrillar amyloidosis at the onset of amyloid pathology. However, even with standardized Z-scores, there remains some possibility that this effect may be related to a higher sensitivity of

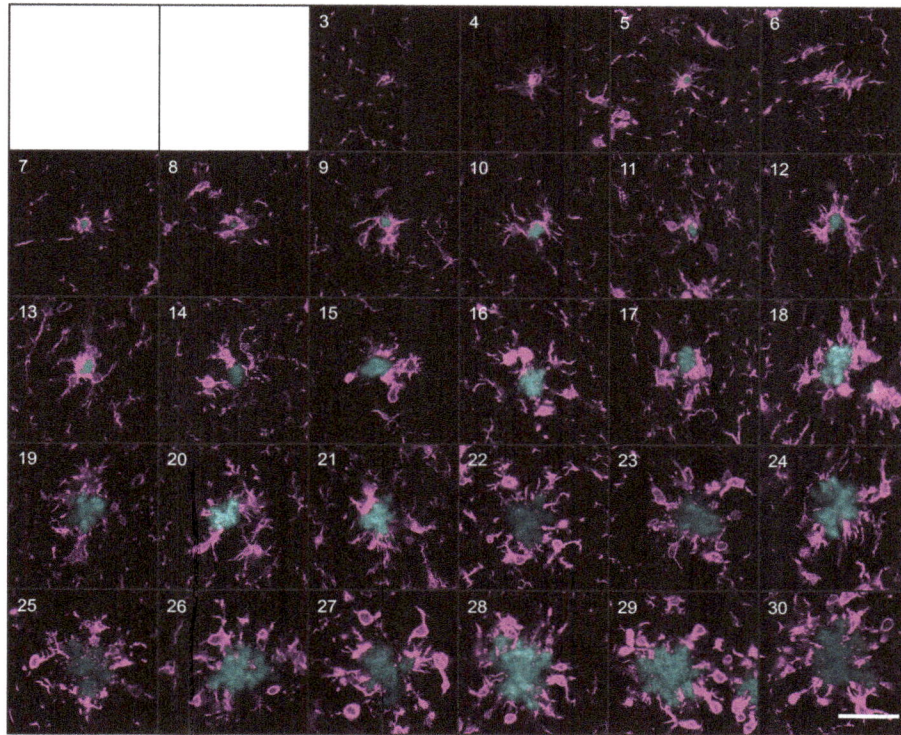

Fig. 5 Microglial brain fraction was maximal at small plaques. β-amyloid plaques of radius increasing from 3 to 30 μm are illustrated according to their size (white numeral in upper left corner). Each pane shows Methoxy-X04 stained plaque (cyan) together with the Iba-1 immunosignal (magenta). Scale bar 40 μm

the TSPO ligand to its target compared to the applied Aβ tracer. In contrast, due to its baseline dependency, the longitudinal decrease of the Z-score difference towards late ages is a rather compelling readout unlikely to be biased by possible tracer sensitivity differences. Furthermore, ceiling effects are unlikely as far higher magnitudes of TSPO activation and amyloidosis can be detected with these tracers in other circumstances [31, 40]. Thus, our serial dual tracer μPET imaging proves that microglial activation saturates during an ongoing fibrillar amyloid deposition in this mouse model (Figs. 2 and 3). Our PET findings are absolutely in line with a recently observed plateau during TSPO PET imaging in aged APP23 mice by the same radioligand [41]. The results are also in line with findings for other biomarkers of microglial function, i.e., the peak in sTrem2 levels in cerebrospinal fluid of patients with mild cognitive impairment [42], followed by a drop in patients who have converted to dementia [43]. Even more importantly, computed longitudinal courses of sTrem2 in individuals with dominantly inherited AD decrease after symptom onset whereas amyloid deposition continues to progress [44], thus concurring with the presently observed relations between TSPO expression and fibrillar amyloidosis in aging APP-SL70 mice.

Although an important strength of μPET lies in its fitness for longitudinal monitoring and target quantification, molecular imaging has limitations in spatial resolution and in its applicability for resolving mechanistic processes. For this reason, we supplemented μPET with a detailed immunohistochemical study of activated microglia and histological staining of fibrillar Aβ, which together supported automatized volumetric computations. Our data clearly indicate that microglia fraction adjacent to plaques declines with increasing plaque size (Fig. 4d). Given that plaque size but not density increases with advanced age (Fig. 4b, c), it seems obvious that the microglial activity must decrease relative to fibrillar amyloidosis over time. We validated these findings by comparing mid- and late aged APP-SL70 groups, concluding that the decreasing microglial brain fraction with increasing plaque size is consistent with our μPET results in vivo. Since a recent study showed that brain location of microglia is a relevant factor for its morphological classification [45], our specific analysis of frontal cortical microglia cells in wt and APP-SL70 mice seems appropriate as it matched to the regional PET analysis.

So far, it remains unclear when and why microglial activity decreases adjacent to plaques. It is known that

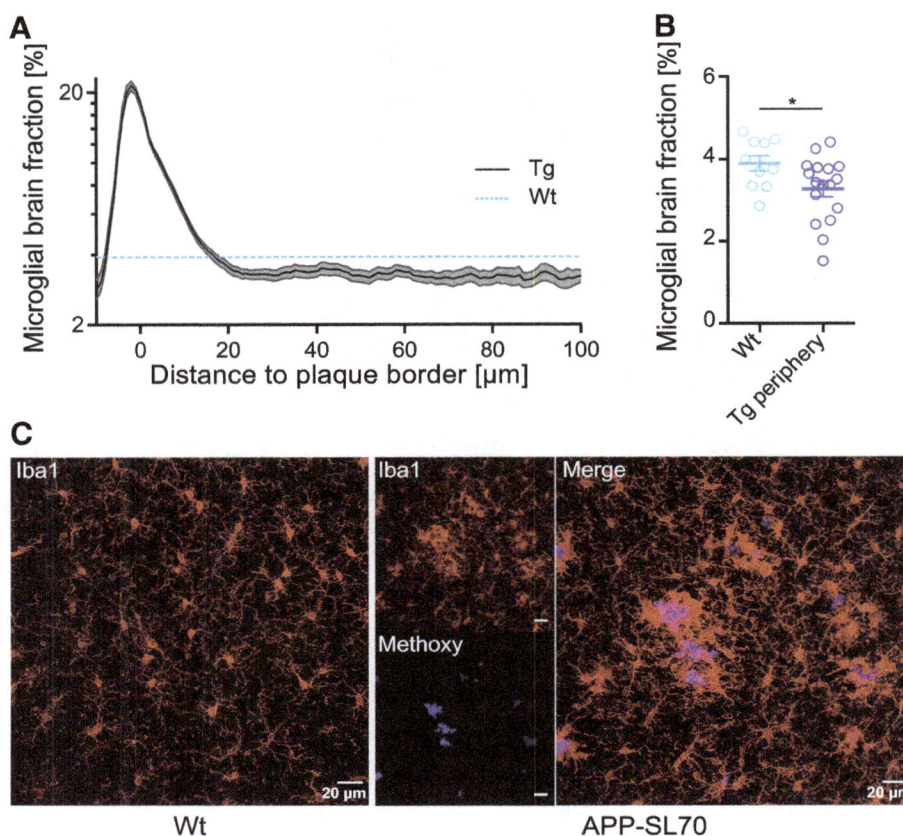

Fig. 6 Microglial brain fraction decreased in the plaque-free cortical brain parenchyma of APP-SL70 mice. **a** Microglial brain fraction as a function of the distance to the plaque border in APP-SL70 mice (black line) when compared to the mean microglial brain fraction in wildtype (wt) mice (dotted blue line). **b** Direct comparison of microglial brain fraction of APP-SL70 mice (> 30 μm from plaque borders) and wt mice (mean). Microglial brain fraction is significantly reduced compared to wt mice ($p < 0.05$, two-tailed Student's t test). **c** Iba-1 immunofluorescence staining in a wt mouse aged 16 months in comparison to a double staining of Iba-1 and methoxy-X04 stained plaque in APP-SL70 mouse aged 15 months. Data are presented as mean ± SEM; $n = 10$–17

microglia migrate within 1–2 days towards newly formed amyloid deposits, where they promote the clearance and phagocytosis of Aβ by expressing certain cell-surface receptors [6–8]. However, during disease progression, plaque-associated microglial cells show a decrease in fiber mobility [46], lower expression of Aβ-binding receptors [11], and moreover also show a threefold higher mortality rate compared to non-plaque associated microglial cells [12]. Nonetheless, the same in vivo study reported a threefold higher proliferation rate of microglia distal to plaques in AD compared to wt mice, suggesting that new microglial cells migrate from the periphery to the plaque border [12]. However, we observed even lower microglial brain fraction distal to plaques of aged APP-SL70 mice compared to wt animals (Fig. 6). We conclude that the rate of microglia cell migration towards Aβ depositions in APP-SL70 mice eventually exceeds the rate of proliferation of microglia cells staying in the peripheral zone. With aging, this potentially leads to an exhaustion of microglial cells for migration towards Aβ depositions and, together with the increased rate of microglial cell loss around plaques [12], this may explain the observed decrease in microglia brain fraction with increasing plaque radius.

As a limitation of this study, we note that the amyloid tracer does not distinguish soluble and oligomeric Aβ. Thus, we cannot disentangle if there is a stronger association between microglia and soluble or oligomeric proportions of Aβ, which could show different growth rates with aging. Furthermore, given the nature of our longitudinal PET design, we were not able to acquire immunohistochemistry from mice at younger ages but instead focused on the late stage of the disease. Proliferation rates, mortality, and spatial distribution of microglia during their whole life cycle should therefore receive attention in future cross-sectional designs.

Conclusion

Taken together, findings of this preclinical study in transgenic mice reveal the individual trajectories of microglial activation in relation to Aβ deposition, thus providing important information about the staging of AD-like pathology, which could guide human clinical research. The translation of findings in animal models to human disease is challenging, but the strong bidirectional translational science potential of μPET findings to clinical PET holds great promise to dramatically advance our understanding of AD.

Abbreviations

AD: Alzheimer's disease; AIC: Akaike Information Criterion; ANOVA: Analysis of variance; Aβ: β-amyloid; GBq: Gigabecquerel; MBq: Megabecquerel; p.i: Post injection; PBR: Peripheral benzodiazepine receptor; SEM: Standard error of mean; SUVR: Standardized uptake value ratio; TSPO: 18 kDa translocator protein; VOI: Volume of interest; wt: Wildtype; Δ%: Percentage change; μPET: Small animal positron emission tomography

Acknowledgements

We thank K. Bormann-Giglmaier and N. Lachner for their excellent technical support and animal care. Manuscript editing was provided by Inglewood Biomedical Editing. G.E. made GE-180 cassettes available through an early access model.

Funding

The study was financially supported by the SyNergy Cluster (J.H., P.B., C.H., and A.R.) and by the Deutsche Forschungsgemeinschaft (DFG) by a dedicated PET imaging grant to M.B. and A.R. (BR4580/1-1 & RO5194/1-1).

Authors' contributions

TB and CF performed the majority of PET and immunohistochemistry experiments. FP invented the Matlab driven 3D analysis of plaque and microglia. MB, TB, CF, MD, and FP analyzed and quantified the data. NLA and PB performed the interpretation of the PET data. SL and FJG performed and improved radiochemistry. KB and LO contributed to the generation of the mouse model and helped to interpret the findings in the context of the model. MB, TB, and FP interpreted the data. AR, JH, and MB contributed to the conception and design of the study. TB and MB wrote the manuscript. BU-S supervised the study as a veterinarian. All authors participated in the generation of the original data, added important intellectual content to the manuscript, and provided critical assessment of the current manuscript. All authors read and approved the final manuscript.

Competing interests

The authors Laurence Ozmen and Karlheinz Baumann are employed by company Roche, Basel, Switzerland. All other authors declare no financial or competing interests.

Author details

[1]Department of Nuclear Medicine, University Hospital, LMU Munich, Marchioninistraße 15, 81377 Munich, Germany. [2]German Center for Neurodegenerative Diseases (DZNE) Munich, Feodor-Lynen-Str. 17, 81377 Munich, Germany. [3]Roche, Pharma Research and Early Development, NORD DTA / Neuroscience Discovery, Roche Innovation Center Basel, F. Hoffmann-La Roche Ltd., Grenzacherstrasse 124, CH-4070 Basel, Switzerland. [4]Department of Nuclear Medicine, Inselspital, University Hospital Bern, Freiburgstrasse 4, 3010 Bern, Switzerland. [5]Center of Neuropathology and Prion Research, Feodor-Lynen-Straße 23, 81377 Munich, Germany. [6]Munich Cluster for Systems Neurology (SyNergy), Munich, Germany.

References

1. Perry VH, Gordon S. Macrophages and microglia in the nervous system. Trends Neurosci. 1988;11:273–7.
2. Dickson DW, Farlo J, Davies P, Crystal H, Fuld P, Yen SH. Alzheimer's disease. A double-labeling immunohistochemical study of senile plaques. Am J Pathol. 1988;132:86–101.
3. Selkoe DJ. The origins of Alzheimer disease: a is for amyloid. JAMA. 2000; 283:1615–7.
4. Mott RT, Hulette CM. Neuropathology of Alzheimer's disease. Neuroimaging Clin N Am. 2005;15:755–65, ix. https://doi.org/10.1016/j.nic.2005.09.003.
5. Nimmerjahn A, Kirchhoff F, Helmchen F. Resting microglial cells are highly dynamic surveillants of brain parenchyma in vivo. Science. 2005;308:1314–8. https://doi.org/10.1126/science.1110647.
6. Bolmont T, Haiss F, Eicke D, Radde R, Mathis CA, Klunk WE, et al. Dynamics of the microglial/amyloid interaction indicate a role in plaque maintenance. J Neurosci. 2008;28:4283–92. https://doi.org/10.1523/JNEUROSCI.4814-07.2008.
7. Yan SD, Chen X, Fu J, Chen M, Zhu H, Roher A, et al. RAGE and amyloid-beta peptide neurotoxicity in Alzheimer's disease. Nature. 1996;382:685–91. https://doi.org/10.1038/382685a0.
8. El Khoury J, Hickman SE, Thomas CA, Loike JD, Silverstein SC. Microglia, scavenger receptors, and the pathogenesis of Alzheimer's disease. Neurobiol Aging. 1998;19:S81–4.
9. El Khoury J, Toft M, Hickman SE, Means TK, Terada K, Geula C, Luster AD. Ccr2 deficiency impairs microglial accumulation and accelerates progression of Alzheimer-like disease. Nat Med. 2007;13:432–8. https://doi.org/10.1038/nm1555.
10. Lee CYD, Landreth GE. The role of microglia in amyloid clearance from the AD brain. J Neural Transm (Vienna). 2010;117:949–60. https://doi.org/10.1007/s00702-010-0433-4.
11. Hickman SE, Allison EK, El Khoury J. Microglial dysfunction and defective beta-amyloid clearance pathways in aging Alzheimer's disease mice. J Neurosci. 2008;28:8354–60. https://doi.org/10.1523/JNEUROSCI.0616-08.2008.
12. Füger P, Hefendehl JK, Veeraraghavalu K, Wendeln A-C, Schlosser C, Obermüller U, et al. Microglia turnover with aging and in an Alzheimer's model via long-term in vivo single-cell imaging. Nat Neurosci. 2017;20:1371–6. https://doi.org/10.1038/nn.4631.
13. Matthews PM, Rabiner EA, Passchier J, Gunn RN. Positron emission tomography molecular imaging for drug development. Br J Clin Pharmacol. 2012;73:175–86. https://doi.org/10.1111/j.1365-2125.2011.04085.x.
14. Zimmer ER, Parent MJ, Cuello AC, Gauthier S, Rosa-Neto P. MicroPET imaging and transgenic models: a blueprint for Alzheimer's disease clinical research. Trends Neurosci. 2014;37:629–41. https://doi.org/10.1016/j.tins.2014.07.002.
15. Rominger A, Brendel M, Burgold S, Keppler K, Baumann K, Xiong G, et al. Longitudinal assessment of cerebral β-amyloid deposition in mice overexpressing Swedish mutant β-amyloid precursor protein using 18F-florbetaben PET. J Nucl Med. 2013;54:1127–34. https://doi.org/10.2967/jnumed.112.114660.
16. Brendel M, Jaworska A, Herms J, Trambauer J, Rötzer C, Gildehaus F-J, et al. Amyloid-PET predicts inhibition of de novo plaque formation upon chronic γ-secretase modulator treatment. Mol Psychiatry. 2015;20:1179–87. https://doi.org/10.1038/mp.2015.74.
17. Barthel H, Gertz H-J, Dresel S, Peters O, Bartenstein P, Buerger K, et al. Cerebral amyloid-β PET with florbetaben (18F) in patients with Alzheimer's disease and healthy controls: a multicentre phase 2 diagnostic study. The Lancet Neurology. 2011;10:424–35. https://doi.org/10.1016/S1474-4422(11)70077-1.
18. Mirzaei N, Tang SP, Ashworth S, Coello C, Plisson C, Passchier J, et al. In vivo imaging of microglial activation by positron emission tomography with (11)CPBR28 in the 5XFAD model of Alzheimer's disease. Glia. 2016;64:993–1006. https://doi.org/10.1002/glia.22978.
19. Cumming P, Burgher B, Patkar O, Breakspear M, Vasdev N, Thomas P, et al. Sifting through the surfeit of neuroinflammation tracers. J Cereb Blood Flow Metab. 2018;38:204–24. https://doi.org/10.1177/0271678X17748786.

20. Dickens AM, Vainio S, Marjamäki P, Johansson J, Lehtiniemi P, Rokka J, et al. Detection of microglial activation in an acute model of neuroinflammation using PET and radiotracers 11C-(R)-PK11195 and 18F-GE-180. J Nucl Med. 2014;55:466–72. https://doi.org/10.2967/jnumed.113.125625.

21. James ML, Belichenko NP, Nguyen T-VV, Andrews LE, Ding Z, Liu H, et al. PET imaging of translocator protein (18 kDa) in a mouse model of Alzheimer's disease using N-(2,5-dimethoxybenzyl)-2-18F-fluoro-N-(2-phenoxyphenyl)acetamide. J Nucl Med. 2015;56:311–6. https://doi.org/10.2967/jnumed.114.141648.

22. Liu B, Le KX, Park M-A, Wang S, Belanger AP, Dubey S, et al. In vivo detection of age- and disease-related increases in neuroinflammation by 18F-GE180 TSPO MicroPET imaging in wild-type and Alzheimer's transgenic mice. J Neurosci. 2015;35:15716–30. https://doi.org/10.1523/JNEUROSCI.0996-15.2015.

23. Wickström T, Clarke A, Gausemel I, Horn E, Jørgensen K, Khan I, et al. The development of an automated and GMP compliant FASTlab™ synthesis of (18) FGE-180; a radiotracer for imaging translocator protein (TSPO). J Labelled Comp Radiopharm. 2014;57:42–8. https://doi.org/10.1002/jlcr.3112.

24. Chen M-K, Guilarte TR. Translocator protein 18 kDa (TSPO): molecular sensor of brain injury and repair. Pharmacol Ther. 2008;118:1–17. https://doi.org/10.1016/j.pharmthera.2007.12.004.

25. Cosenza-Nashat M, Zhao M-L, Suh H-S, Morgan J, Natividad R, Morgello S, Lee SC. Expression of the translocator protein of 18 kDa by microglia, macrophages and astrocytes based on immunohistochemical localization in abnormal human brain. Neuropathol Appl Neurobiol. 2009;35:306–28. https://doi.org/10.1111/j.1365-2990.2008.01006.x.

26. Scarf AM, Ittner LM, Kassiou M. The translocator protein (18 kDa): central nervous system disease and drug design. J Med Chem. 2009;52:581–92. https://doi.org/10.1021/jm8011678.

27. Venneti S, Wagner AK, Wang G, Slagel SL, Chen X, Lopresti BJ, et al. The high affinity peripheral benzodiazepine receptor ligand DAA1106 binds specifically to microglia in a rat model of traumatic brain injury: implications for PET imaging. Exp Neurol. 2007;207:118–27. https://doi.org/10.1016/j.expneurol.2007.06.003.

28. Venneti S, Wiley CA, Kofler J. Imaging microglial activation during neuroinflammation and Alzheimer's disease. J NeuroImmune Pharmacol. 2009;4:227–43. https://doi.org/10.1007/s11481-008-9142-2.

29. Brendel M, Probst F, Jaworska A, Overhoff F, Korzhova V, Albert NL, et al. Glial activation and glucose metabolism in a transgenic amyloid mouse model: a triple-tracer PET study. J Nucl Med. 2016;57:954–60. https://doi.org/10.2967/jnumed.115.167858.

30. Blanchard V, Moussaoui S, Czech C, Touchet N, Bonici B, Planche M, et al. Time sequence of maturation of dystrophic neurites associated with Aβ deposits in APP/PS1 transgenic mice. Exp Neurol. 2003;184:247–63. https://doi.org/10.1016/S0014-4886(03)00252-8.

31. Brendel M, Jaworska A, Grießinger E, Rötzer C, Burgold S, Gildehaus F-J, et al. Cross-sectional comparison of small animal 18F-florbetaben amyloid-PET between transgenic AD mouse models. PLoS One. 2015;10:e0116678. https://doi.org/10.1371/journal.pone.0116678.

32. Overhoff F, Brendel M, Jaworska A, Korzhova V, Delker A, Probst F, et al. Automated spatial brain normalization and hindbrain white matter reference tissue give improved (18)F-Florbetaben PET quantitation in Alzheimer's model mice. Front Neurosci. 2016;10:45. https://doi.org/10.3389/fnins.2016.00045.

33. Rominger A, Mille E, Zhang S, Böning G, Förster S, Nowak S, et al. Validation of the octamouse for simultaneous 18F-fallypride small-animal PET recordings from 8 mice. J Nucl Med. 2010;51:1576–83. https://doi.org/10.2967/jnumed.110.078451.

34. Peters F, Salihoglu H, Rodrigues E, Herzog E, Blume T, Filser S, et al. BACE1 inhibition more effectively suppresses initiation than progression of β-amyloid pathology. Acta Neuropathol. 2018;135:695–710. https://doi.org/10.1007/s00401-017-1804-9.

35. Akaike H. A new look at the statistical model identification. IEEE Trans Automat Contr. 1974;19:716–23. https://doi.org/10.1109/TAC.1974.1100705.

36. Radde R, Bolmont T, Kaeser SA, Coomaraswamy J, Lindau D, Stoltze L, et al. Abeta42-driven cerebral amyloidosis in transgenic mice reveals early and robust pathology. EMBO Rep. 2006;7:940–6. https://doi.org/10.1038/sj.embor.7400784.

37. Gómez-Nicola D, Fransen NL, Suzzi S, Perry VH. Regulation of microglial proliferation during chronic neurodegeneration. J Neurosci. 2013;33:2481–93. https://doi.org/10.1523/JNEUROSCI.4440-12.2013.

38. Graeber MB, López-Redondo F, Ikoma E, Ishikawa M, Imai Y, Nakajima K, et al. The microglia/macrophage response in the neonatal rat facial nucleus following axotomy. Brain Res. 1998;813:241–53.

39. Meyer-Luehmann M, Coomaraswamy J, Bolmont T, Kaeser S, Schaefer C, Kilger E, et al. Exogenous induction of cerebral beta-amyloidogenesis is governed by agent and host. Science. 2006;313:1781–4. https://doi.org/10.1126/science.1131864.

40. Zwergal A, Günther L, Brendel M, Beck R, Lindner S, Xiong G, et al. In vivo imaging of glial activation after unilateral labyrinthectomy in the rat: a 18FGE180-PET study. Front Neurol. 2017;8:665. https://doi.org/10.3389/fneur.2017.00665.

41. López-Picón FR, Snellman A, Eskola O, Helin S, Solin O, Haaparanta-Solin M, Rinne JO. Neuroinflammation appears early on PET imaging and then plateaus in a mouse model of Alzheimer disease. J Nucl Med. 2018;59:509–15. https://doi.org/10.2967/jnumed.117.197608.

42. Ulrich JD, Ulland TK, Colonna M, Holtzman DM. Elucidating the role of TREM2 in Alzheimer's disease. Neuron. 2017;94:237–48. https://doi.org/10.1016/j.neuron.2017.02.042.

43. Suárez-Calvet M, Kleinberger G, Araque Caballero MÁ, Brendel M, Rominger A, Alcolea D, et al. sTREM2 cerebrospinal fluid levels are a potential biomarker for microglia activity in early-stage Alzheimer's disease and associate with neuronal injury markers. EMBO Mol Med. 2016;8:466–76. https://doi.org/10.15252/emmm.201506123.

44. Suárez-Calvet M, Araque Caballero MÁ, Kleinberger G, Bateman RJ, Fagan AM, Morris JC, et al. Early changes in CSF sTREM2 in dominantly inherited Alzheimer's disease occur after amyloid deposition and neuronal injury. Sci Transl Med. 2016;8:369ra178. https://doi.org/10.1126/scitranslmed.aag1767.

45. Fernández-Arjona MDM, Grondona JM, Granados-Durán P, Fernández-Llebrez P, López-Ávalos MD. Microglia morphological categorization in a rat model of neuroinflammation by hierarchical cluster and principal components analysis. Front Cell Neurosci. 2017;11:235. https://doi.org/10.3389/fncel.2017.00235.

46. Krabbe G, Halle A, Matyash V, Rinnenthal JL, Eom GD, Bernhardt U, et al. Functional impairment of microglia coincides with beta-amyloid deposition in mice with Alzheimer-like pathology. PLoS One. 2013;8:e60921. https://doi.org/10.1371/journal.pone.0060921.

9

Anti-neuroinflammatory effects of GPR55 antagonists in LPS-activated primary microglial cells

Soraya Wilke Saliba[1], Hannah Jauch[1], Brahim Gargouri[1], Albrecht Keil[1], Thomas Hurrle[2,3], Nicole Volz[2], Florian Mohr[2,4], Mario van der Stelt[4], Stefan Bräse[2,3] and Bernd L. Fiebich[1,5*] (iD)

Abstract

Background: Neuroinflammation plays a vital role in Alzheimer's disease and other neurodegenerative conditions. Microglia are the resident mononuclear immune cells of the central nervous system, and they play essential roles in the maintenance of homeostasis and responses to neuroinflammation. The orphan G-protein-coupled receptor 55 (GPR55) has been reported to modulate inflammation and is expressed in immune cells such as monocytes and microglia. However, its effects on neuroinflammation, mainly on the production of members of the arachidonic acid pathway in activated microglia, have not been elucidated in detail.

Methods: In this present study, a series of coumarin derivatives, that exhibit GPR55 antagonism properties, were designed. The effects of these compounds on members of the arachidonic acid cascade were studied in lipopolysaccharide (LPS)-treated primary rat microglia using Western blot, qPCR, and ELISA.

Results: We demonstrate here that the various compounds with GPR55 antagonistic activities significantly inhibited the release of PGE_2 in primary microglia. The inhibition of LPS-induced PGE_2 release by the most potent candidate KIT 17 was partially dependent on reduced protein synthesis of mPGES-1 and COX-2. KIT 17 did not affect any key enzyme involved on the endocannabinoid system. We furthermore show that microglia expressed GPR55 and that a synthetic antagonist of the GPR receptor (ML193) demonstrated the same effect of the KIT 17 on the inhibition of PGE_2.

Conclusions: Our results suggest that KIT 17 is acting as an inverse agonist on GPR55 independent of the endocannabinoid system. Targeting GPR55 might be a new therapeutic option to treat neurodegenerative diseases with a neuroinflammatory background such as Alzheimer's disease, Parkinson, and multiple sclerosis (MS).

Keywords: GPR55, Prostaglandin E_2, Cyclooxygenase, Microglia, Neuroinflammation

Introduction

For many years, neuroinflammation has been known as a common phenomenon in the pathology of many brain diseases. Microglia, the principal cells involved in the innate immune response in the central nervous system (CNS), play essential roles in the maintenance of homeostasis and responses to inflammatory stimulus [1–3]. The over-activated

microglia has been associated with neurodegenerative diseases such as Alzheimer's disease (AD), Parkinson disease (PD), and traumatic brain injury or aging [4, 5].

The GPR55 is an orphan G-protein-coupled receptor, first described by Sawzdargo et al. in 1999 [6], and it is not only highly expressed in CNS, but also in peripheral tissue [7]. It can be activated by cannabinoids (CB) and non-CB, leading to the hypothesis that it might be a putative "type-3" cannabinoid receptor [8]. However, in contrast to the cannabinoid receptors CB1 and CB2, GPR55 only couples to $G\alpha_{12,13}$ proteins which leads to the activation of the ras homolog gene family member A (RhoA) and Rho-associated protein kinase (ROCK). The

* Correspondence: bernd.fiebich@uniklinik-freiburg.de
[1]Neuroimmunology and Neurochemistry Research Group, Department of Psychiatry and Psychotherapy, Medical Center - University of Freiburg, Faculty of Medicine, University of Freiburg, Freiburg, Germany
[5]Department of Psychiatry and Psychotherapy, Laboratory of Translational Psychiatry, University Hospital Freiburg, Hauptstr. 5, 79104 Freiburg, Germany
Full list of author information is available at the end of the article

phospholipase C pathway is triggered by these proteins, which increase the intercellular Ca^{2+} and extracellular signal-regulated kinase (ERK) phosphorylation [9].

GPR55 is expressed in immune cells, such as monocytes, natural killer (NK) cells [10], and microglia [11], and its involvement in inflammation has been reported [10, 12, 13]. Activation of GPR55 by the agonist O-1602 increased pro-inflammatory cytokines and cell cytotoxicity in monocytes and NK cells stimulated with LPS [10]. Corroborating with this, an antagonist of GPR55, CID16020046, and GPR55$^{-/-}$ knockout mice decreased the pro-inflammatory cytokines in colitis mice models comparable to human inflammatory bowel disease (IBD) [12]. In hyperalgesia associated with inflammatory and neuropathic pain, it was observed to increase anti-inflammatory cytokines, IL-4 and IL-10, and also pro-inflammatory IFN-γ in GPR55$^{-/-}$ knockout mice [13]. On the other hand, the GPR55 agonist O-1602 decreased IL-6 and TNF-α in a model of experimental acute pancreatitis [14].

The roles of GPR55 in the pathophysiology of the CNS are still not clear. In an excitotoxicity in vitro model of rat organotypic hippocampal slice cultures (OHSC), the activation of GPR55 receptor by L-α-Lysophosphatidylinositol (LPI) mediated neuroprotection through microglia [15]. In a mouse model of PD, the expression of GPR55 was downregulated in the striatum and the treatment with an agonist of GPR55, abnormal-cannabidiol, improved the motor behavior by neuroprotection of dopaminergic neuron cell bodies [16]. A molecular, anatomical, electrophysiological, and behavioral study of GPR55$^{-/-}$ knockout mice demonstrated a normal development of brain structure and did not affect the endocannabinoid system nor muscle strength and motor learning. However, these mice presented deficits in motor coordination and thermal sensitivity [17].

These studies suggest that GPR55 signaling can be involved in neurodegeneration and modulate certain cytokines and thus inflammation. However, its effects on neuroinflammation, especially on the production of members of the arachidonic acid pathway in activated microglia, have not been elucidated in detail. We therefore studied the effects of novel synthesized GPR55 antagonists in LPS-activated microglia by examining prostaglandin E$_2$ (PGE$_2$) production, COX/mPGES-1 mRNA, and protein levels. Furthermore, we evaluated the effect of KIT17 on key enzymes involved in the endocannabinoid system such as diacylglycerol lipase-α(DAGLα), monoacylglycerol lipase (MAGL), α,β-hydrolase domain-containing 6 and 12 (ABHD6 and ABHD12), and fatty acid amide hydrolase (FAAH).

Methods
Ethics statement
Animals were obtained from the Center for Experimental Models and Transgenic Services-Freiburg (CEMT-FR). All the experiments were approved and conducted according to the guidelines of the ethics committee of the University of Freiburg Medical School under protocol no. X-13/06A, and the study was carefully planned to minimize the number of animals used and their suffering. For the activity-based protein profiling (ABPP), the experiments were performed at Leiden University according to guidelines approved by the ethical committee of Leiden University (DEC#13191).

Chemicals
Synthetic GPR55 antagonists (Fig. 1) were synthesized at the Institute for Organic Chemistry Karlsruhe - KIT (Karlsruhe, Germany) [18] and dissolved in DMSO. The number of the corresponding compounds in the Rempel et al. 2013 paper are: KIT3 is 14, KIT17 is 37, and KIT21 is 41. ML193 and O-1602 were obtained from Tocris Biosciences. LPS from *Salmonella typhimurium* (Sigma Aldrich, Deissenhofen, Germany) was resuspended in sterile phosphate-buffered saline (PBS, 5 mg/mL) as stock and subsequently used at a final concentration (10 ng/mL) in the cultures.

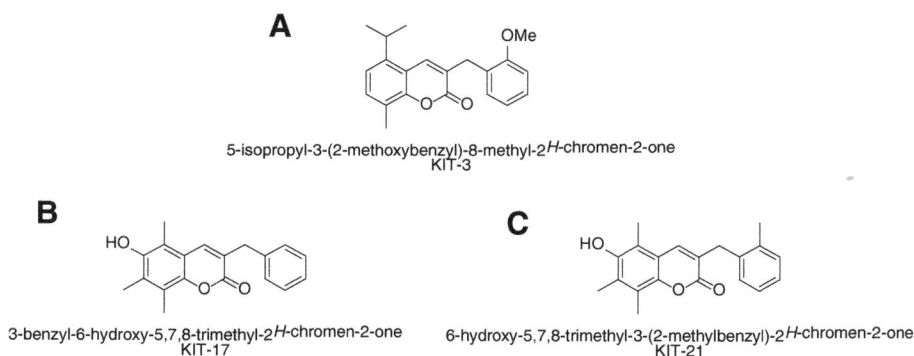

A

5-isopropyl-3-(2-methoxybenzyl)-8-methyl-2*H*-chromen-2-one
KIT-3

B

3-benzyl-6-hydroxy-5,7,8-trimethyl-2*H*-chromen-2-one
KIT-17

C

6-hydroxy-5,7,8-trimethyl-3-(2-methylbenzyl)-2*H*-chromen-2-one
KIT-21

Fig. 1 Molecular structure of the synthesized compounds **a** KIT 3: 8-isopropyl-3-(2-methoxybenzyl)-5-methyl-2*H*-chromen-2-one, MW = 336,1725 g/mol. **b** KIT 17: 3-benzyl-6-hydroxy-7,8-dimethyl-2*H*-chromen-2-one, MW = 294,1256 g/mol. **c** KIT 21: 6-hydroxy-7,8-dimethyl-3-(2-methylbenzyl)-2*H*-chromen-2-one, MW = 308,1412 g/mol

Primary microglia cultures

As described in our previous studies [19–24], primary mixed glial cell cultures were prepared from cerebral cortices of 1-day neonatal Sprague-Dawley rats. Under sterile conditions, the brains were carefully taken, and the cerebral cortices were isolated and the meninges removed. Then, the cortices were gently dissociated and filtered through a 70-μm nylon cell strainer (BD biosciences, Heidelberg, Germany). After centrifugation at 1000 rpm for 10 min, cells were collected and resuspended in Dulbecco's modified Eagle's medium (DMEM) containing 10% fetal calf serum (Biochrom AG, Berlin, Germany) and antibiotics (40 U/mL penicillin and 40 μg/mL streptomycin, both from PAA Laboratories, Linz, Austria). Cells were cultured on 10-cm cell culture dishes (Falcon, Heidelberg, Germany) with density of 5×10^5 cells/mL in 10% CO_2 at 37 °C (Heracell 240i, Thermo Scientific). After 12 days in vitro, floating microglia were harvested and re-seeded into 7 cm^2 culture flask to give pure microglial cultures. On the next day, medium was changed to remove non-adherent cells, and after 1 h, the cells were stimulated for respective experiments.

Determination of PGE_2 release from LPS-activated microglia

Cultured primary rat microglia were incubated with synthesized compounds (KITs) (0.1–25 μM) or commercial antagonist ML193 (10 μM) or agonist O-1602 (0.1–10 μM) for 30 min. Afterwards, the cells were treated with or without LPS (10 ng/mL) for the next 24 h. Supernatants were harvested and levels of PGE_2 were measured using a commercially available enzyme immunoassay (EIA) kit (Assay Designs Inc., Ann Arbor, MI, USA; distributed by Biotrend, Cologne, Germany). The results were normalized to LPS and presented as percentage of change in PGE_2 levels of at least three independent experiments.

Cell viability assay

Viability of primary rat microglia after treatment with the synthesized compounds was measured by the CellTiter-Glo® Luminescent Cell Viability Assay (Promega), which is used to determine the number of metabolically active and viable cells in cell culture based on quantitation of the ATP present in the cells. Briefly, cells were cultured in 96 well plates at the density of 25×10^3 cells/well for 24 h. Then, the medium was changed and after at least 1 h, the cells were incubated with KIT 3, KIT 17, and KIT 21 for 24 h. The compounds were dissolved in DMSO, and DMSO was used in the negative control wells at final concentration of 0.15% and as a positive control in a higher concentration (10%) during experiments. The concentration of ATP was measured after 24 h of incubation by adding 100 μL of reconstituted substrate and incubating for 10 min. Luminescence was measured using a Modulus™ II Microplate Multimode Reader (Turner BioSystems, USA).

RNA isolation and quantitative PCR

Quantitative real-time PCR (qPCR) was performed to determine the presence of *GPR55* in microglia and transcriptional regulation of *COX-1*, *COX-2*, and *mPGES-1* by synthesized compound (KIT17) in activated microglia. Cultured primary rat microglia were left untreated or incubated with LPS (10 ng/mL) in the presence or absence of KIT 17 (0.1–10 μM) which was added 30 min before LPS (10 ng/mL) treatment for 4 h. Total RNA was then extracted using the guanidine isothiocyanate method [25]. The cDNA synthesis were reverse transcribed from 1 μg of total RNA using Moloney Murine Leukemia Virus (M-MLV) reverse transcriptase (Promega, Mannheim, Germany), RNase Inhibitor rRNasin® (Promega), dNTP master mix (Invitek, Berlin, Germany), and random hexamer primers (Promega). The real-time PCR amplification was carried out by the CFX96 real-time PCR detection system (Bio-Rad Laboratories, Inc.) using iQ™ SYBR™ Green supermix (Bio-Rad Laboratories GmbH, Munich, Germany). Reaction conditions were 3 min at 95 °C, followed by 40 cycles of 15 s at 95 °C, 30 s at 50 °C, and 45 s at 72 °C, and every cycle was followed by plate reading. After that, 1 min at 95 °C, 1 min at 55 °C, followed by melt curve conditions of 65 °C, 95 °C with increment of 0.5 °C for 5 s, followed by final plate reading. Glyceraldehyde 3-phosphate dehydrogenase (GAPDH) served as an internal control for sample normalization, and the comparative cycle threshold Ct method was used for data quantification [26]. The primer sequences were as follows:

GPR55: Fwd 5′-ACGTGGAGTGCGAGAGTCTT-3′;
Rev 5′-TGCCCATAGGAAGGAGGAA-5′;
COX-1: Fwd 5'-GCTCTTCAAGGATGGGAAACT-3′;
Rev 5'-TTCTACGGAAGGTGGGTACAA-3′;
COX-2: Fwd 5′-GGCTTACAAGACGCCACATCAC CT-3′;
Rev 5′-TGGTTTAGGCGGCCGGGGAT-3′;
mPGES-1: Fwd 5′-TGCAGCACGCTGCTGGTCAT-3′;
Rev 5′-GTCGTTGCGGTGGGCTCTGAG-3′;
GAPDH: Fwd 5′-ATGCTGGTGCTGAGTATGTC-3′;
Rev 5′-AGTTGTCATATTTCTCGTGGGTT-3′.

Immunoblotting

Rat primary microglia were treated with KIT 17 (0.1–10 μM) and control for 30 min; then, the LPS (10 ng/mL) was added for 24 h. After the experiment, the cells were washed with cold PBS and lysed in the lysis buffer (42 mM Tris−HCl, 1.3% sodium dodecyl sulfate, 6.5% glycerin, 100-μM sodium orthovanadate, and 2%

phosphatase and protease inhibitors). Protein concentration of the samples was measured using the bicinchoninic acid (BCA) protein assay kit (Thermo Fisher Scientific, Bonn, Germany) according to the manufacturer's instructions. For Western blotting, 10–20 µg of total protein from each sample was subjected to sodium dodecyl sulfate-polyacrylamide gel electrophoresis (SDS-PAGE) under reducing conditions. Afterward, proteins were transferred onto polyvinylidene fluoride (PVDF) membranes (Merck Millipore, Darmstadt, Germany) by semi-dry blotting. After blocking with Roti-Block (Roth, Karlsruhe, Germany), membranes were incubated overnight with primary antibodies. Primary antibodies were goat anti-COX-2 (1:500; Santa Cruz Biotechnology, Heidelberg, Germany), rabbit anti-mPGES-1 (1:6000; Agrisera, Vännas, Sweden), and rabbit anti-actin (1:5000; Sigma Aldrich). The proteins were detected with horseradish peroxidase-coupled rabbit anti-goat IgG (Santa Cruz, 1:100,000 dilution) or goat anti-rabbit IgG (Amersham, 1:25,000 dilution) using enhanced chemiluminescence (ECL) reagents (GE Healthcare, Freiburg, Germany). Densitometric analysis was performed using ImageJ software (NIH, USA), and β-actin control was used to confirm equal sample loading and normalization of the data.

Cyclooxygenase activity assay in primary microglia culture

Under unstimulated conditions, primary microglial cells only express the COX-1 isoform [27]. To measure COX-1 activity, primary rat microglial cells were plated in 24-well cell culture plates. After 24 h, medium was removed and replaced with serum-free medium. KIT 17 (0.1–10 µM) or the selective reversible COX-1 inhibitor SC560 (1 and 10 µM) was added and left for 15 min. Then, 15 µM of arachidonic acid were supplemented for another 15 min. Supernatants were then collected and used for the determination of PGE_2.

To measure COX-2 activity, primary rat microglial cells were plated in 24-well cell culture plates and pre-incubated with LPS (10 ng/mL) for 24 h. Then, medium was removed and replaced with serum-free medium. KIT 17 (0.1–10 µM) or diclofenac sodium (preferential COX-2 inhibitor, 10 µM) was added and left for 15 min. Then, 15 µM of arachidonic acid was supplemented for another 15 min. Supernatants were then collected and used for determination of PGE_2.

Activity-based protein profiling (ABPP) in mouse brain proteome

The mouse brain proteome preparation and gel-based ABPP was performed as previously described [28, 29]. Mouse tissues were homogenized in lysis buffer A (20 mM HEPES pH 7.2, 2 mM DTT, 1 mM MgCl$_2$, 25 U/mL Benzonase) and incubated for 5 min on ice. To remove containing debris, the suspension was low speed centrifuged ($\times$ 2500g, 3 min, 4 °C). The resulting supernatant was subjected to ultracentrifugation ($\times$ 100.000g, 45 min. 4 °C, Beckman Coulter, Type Ti70 rotor) to separate the membrane fraction as a pellet and the cytosolic fraction in the supernatant. The pellet was resuspended in storage buffer (20 mM HEPES pH 7.2, 2 mM DTT). The total protein concentration was determined with Quick Start Bradford assay (Bio-Rad). Membranes and supernatant were stored in small aliquots at $-$ 80 °C until use. For the gel-based ABPP, mouse brain membrane proteome (2 mg/mL) were pre-incubated with 0.5 µL vehicle (DMSO) or 0.5 µL KIT 17 (in DMSO) for 30 min at room temperature. Followed by treatment with the activity-based probes tetramethylrodamine 5-carboxamdio fluorophosphonate (TAMRA-FP, 100 nM final concentration) and MB064 (250 nM final concentration) for 15 min at room temperature. The reactions were quenched by addition of 10 µL 3 $\times$ SDS-PAGE sample buffer, and the samples were directly loaded and resolved on SDS-PAGE gel (10% acrylamide). The gels were scanned with a Bio-Rad Chemidoc (Bio-Rad Laboratories B.V.) using settings for Cy3 and TAMRA (excitation wavelength 532 nm, emission wavelength 580 nm) and analyzed with ImageLab (5.2.1, Bio-Rad Laboratories B.V.).

Statistical analysis

Statistical analyses were performed using Prism 5 software (GraphPad software Inc., San Diego, CA, USA). Values of all experiments were represented as mean ± SEM of at least three independent experiments. Raw values were converted to percentage and compared using one-way ANOVA with post hoc Student-Newman-Keuls test (multiple comparisons). The level of significance was consider as $*p < 0.05$, $**p < 0.01$, and $***p < 0.001$.

Results

Expression of GPR55 in primary rat microglia

To prove that microglial cells express *GPR55*, we studied the mRNA levels of *GPR55* in primary rat microglia with or without LPS stimulation. We observed the *GPR55* mRNA is expressed in microglial cells and the stimulation with 10 ng/mL LPS did not affect the expression of this receptor (Additional file 1).

Effects of antagonists of the GPR55 receptor on PGE$_2$ release in LPS-stimulated primary microglial cells

We further investigated the effects of 21 chemical-related GPR55 receptor antagonists (KIT 1-KIT 21) on LPS-induced PGE$_2$ synthesis in microglia cells. We selected some of the active KIT compounds, KIT 3, KIT 17, and KIT 21 (Fig. 1), from the first screening (Additional file 2) due to activity of 90–100% PGE$_2$ inhibition and the availability of the compound for further studies.

When treated with LPS, primary microglial cells produced robust amounts of PGE_2 (2596.13 pg/mL, considered as 100%) compared to the untreated control (326.59 pg/mL) and this increase was inhibited by the three synthesized compounds (KIT 3, KIT 17, and KIT 21) in a concentration-dependent manner (Fig. 2).

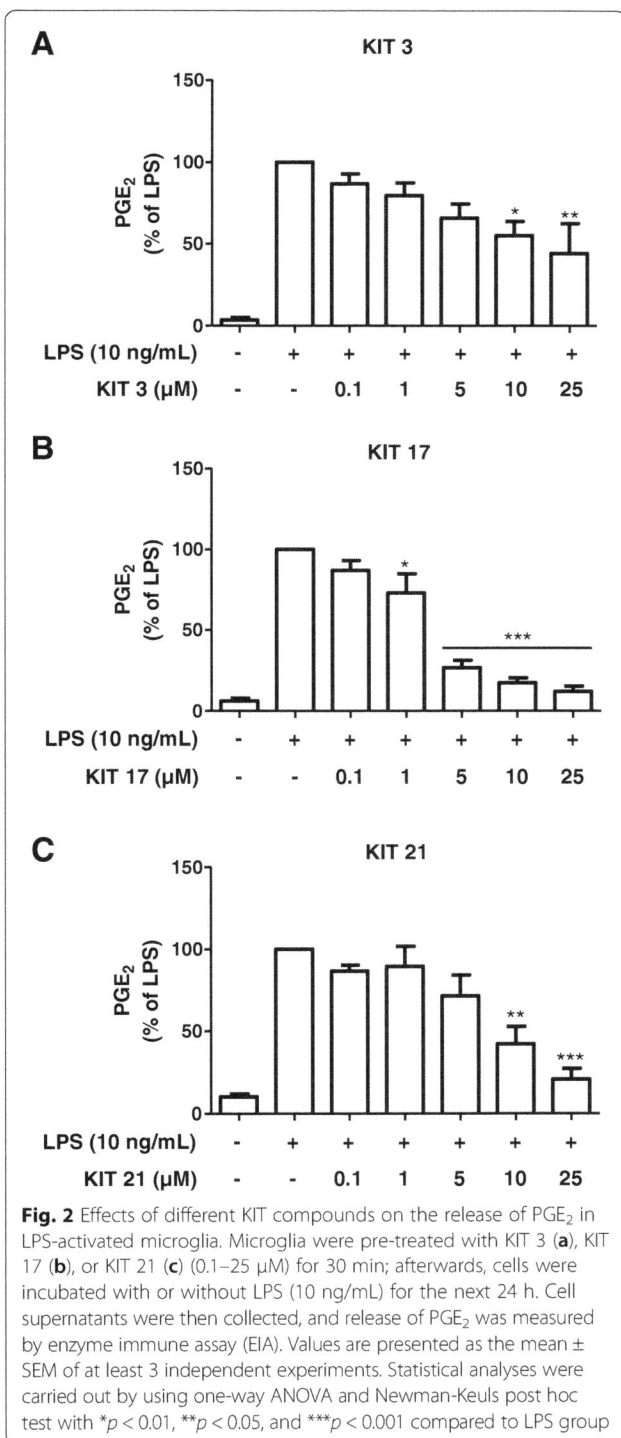

Fig. 2 Effects of different KIT compounds on the release of PGE_2 in LPS-activated microglia. Microglia were pre-treated with KIT 3 (a), KIT 17 (b), or KIT 21 (c) (0.1–25 μM) for 30 min; afterwards, cells were incubated with or without LPS (10 ng/mL) for the next 24 h. Cell supernatants were then collected, and release of PGE_2 was measured by enzyme immune assay (EIA). Values are presented as the mean ± SEM of at least 3 independent experiments. Statistical analyses were carried out by using one-way ANOVA and Newman-Keuls post hoc test with $*p < 0.01$, $**p < 0.05$, and $***p < 0.001$ compared to LPS group

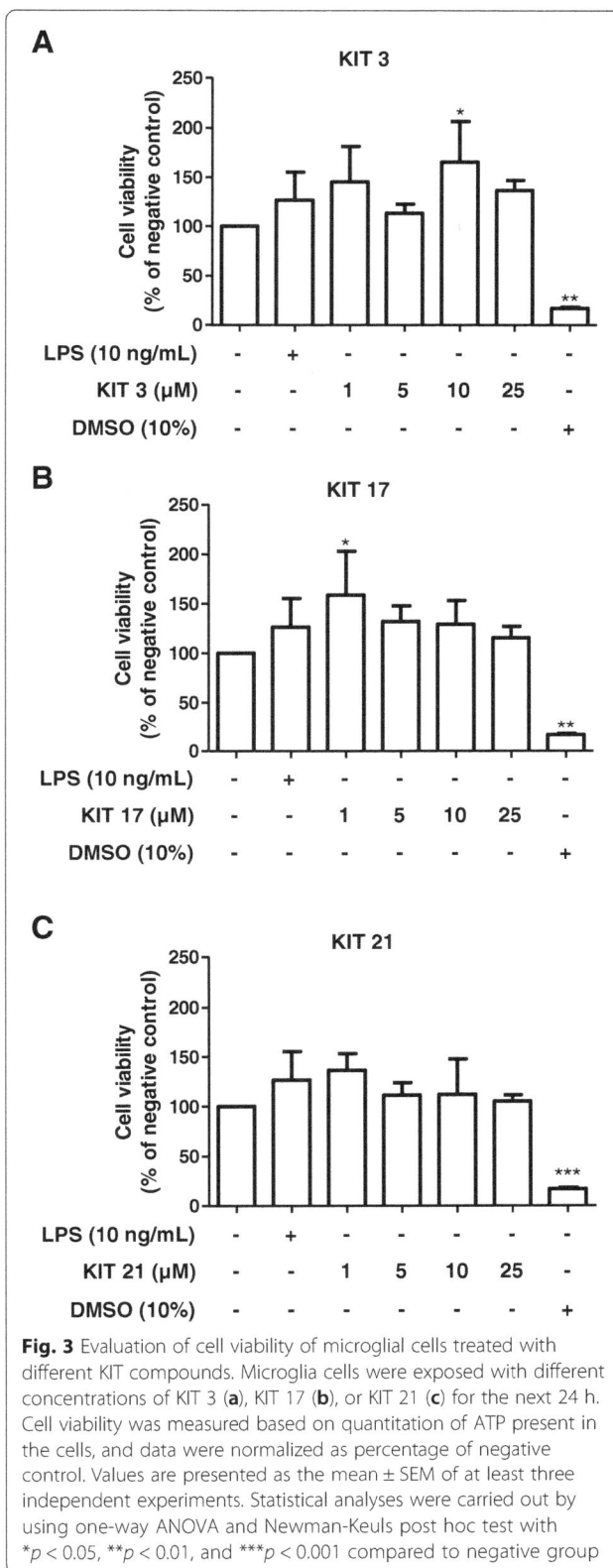

Fig. 3 Evaluation of cell viability of microglial cells treated with different KIT compounds. Microglia cells were exposed with different concentrations of KIT 3 (a), KIT 17 (b), or KIT 21 (c) for the next 24 h. Cell viability was measured based on quantitation of ATP present in the cells, and data were normalized as percentage of negative control. Values are presented as the mean ± SEM of at least three independent experiments. Statistical analyses were carried out by using one-way ANOVA and Newman-Keuls post hoc test with $*p < 0.05$, $**p < 0.01$, and $***p < 0.001$ compared to negative group

All three compounds tested, statistically, prevented the increase on levels of PGE_2 at the concentrations of 10 and 25 μM. Furthermore, the KIT 17 (Fig. 2b) also statistically prevented at the concentration of 1 and 5 μM.

Effects of GPR55 receptor antagonists on cell viability

We performed a cell viability assay to exclude the possibility that the inhibitory effects of the synthesized compounds observed were due to a reduction of cell viability. The effects of KIT 3, KIT 17, and KIT 21 on cell viability were studied using an ATP assay in primary microglial cells. The incubation with LPS or the compounds did not change cell viability compared to vehicle (DMSO) (Fig. 3). A significant increase in ATP was observed with the concentration of 10 μM KIT 3 (Fig. 3a) and 1 μM KIT 17 (Fig. 3b). DMSO in the high concentration of 10% was used as positive control, and it strongly affected cell viability of microglial cells (Fig. 3, right column).

Since KIT 17 showed a desirable inhibitory profile on PGE_2 release and had no negative impact on cell viability, even increased ATP levels, we used KIT 17 for the mechanistic follow-up experiments.

KIT 17 as well as the known GPR55 antagonist ML potently inhibited LPS-induced PGE_2 release whereas the GPR55 agonist O-1602 did not affect the PGE_2 levels in microglial cells

We further investigate the effects of a commercial antagonist (ML193) and an agonist of GPR55 (O-1602) on PGE_2 release in LPS-stimulated primary microglial cells. ML193 (10 μM) potently and statistically prevented LPS-induced increase of PGE_2 levels by 90%, and a comparable inhibition was observed using KIT 17 (85% inhibition) (Fig. 4a). A potent agonist of GPR55, O-1602 (0.1–10 μM), did not affect the LPS-induced PGE_2 release as well as did not interfere with the effects of ML193 and KIT 17. O-1602 also did not alter basal PGE_2 levels (Fig. 4b).

Activity-based protein profiling on mouse brain proteome for selectivity and off-target activity of KIT 17

Our previous study demonstrated the effects of KITs compounds on GPR55, CB1, CB2, and GPR18 receptors [18], in which KIT 17 showed inhibitory effects on GPR55 and CB2 receptors. To investigate its

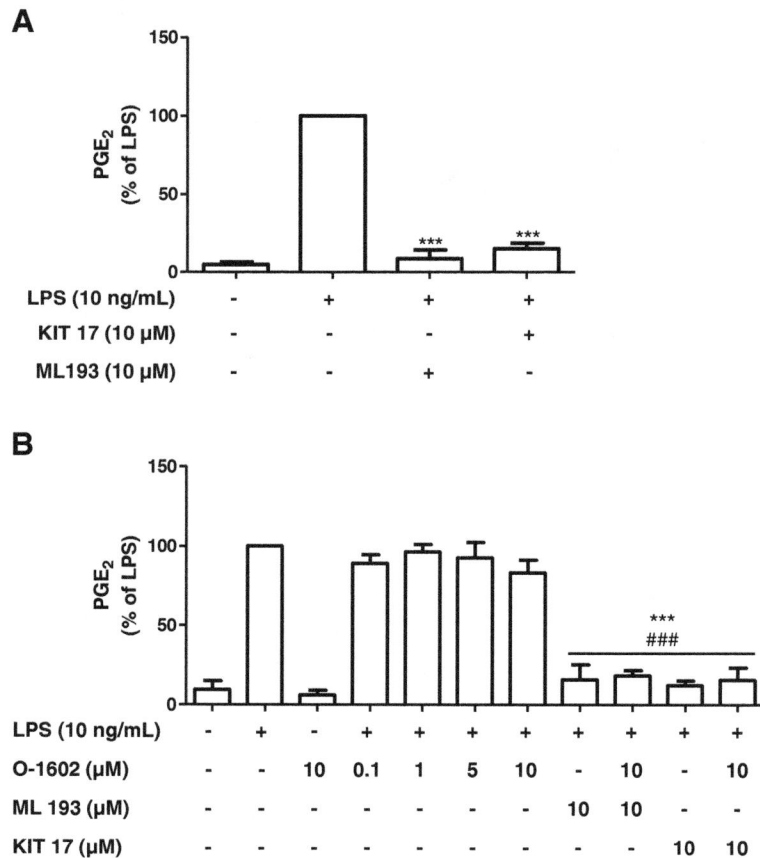

Fig. 4 Effects of the commercial GPR55 antagonist ML193 (**a**) and agonist O-1602 alone and in combination with ML 193 and KIT17 (**b**) on PGE2 release in LPS-stimulated primary microglial cells compared to KIT 17 alone

involvement on other members the endocannabinoid system, we further evaluated the selectivity of KIT 17 on key enzymes involved in the endocannabinoid system [diacylglycerol lipase-αDAGLα, monoacylglycerol lipase (MAGL), α,β-hydrolase domain-containing 6 and 12 (ABHD6 and ABHD12), and fatty acid amide hydrolase (FAAH)]. To this end, we used the approach of gel-based activity-based protein profiling (ABPP) on a mouse membrane brain proteome. As shown in Fig. 5, we did not find any off-target interactions of KIT 17 in the concentrations of 0.1–10 μM. This indicates that KIT 17 showed a highly selective profile against GPR55 and CB2, as no significant reduction of any other endocannabinoid enzyme in the mouse brain proteome was observed in this experimental setting.

Effects of KIT 17 on COX-2 and mPGES-1 mRNA and protein synthesis in LPS-stimulated primary microglial cells

Prostaglandins are synthesized through enzymes COX-2 and mPGES-1 under an inflammatory stimulus [30]. As shown in Fig. 6, LPS induced the expression and the protein synthesis of COX-2 and mPGES-1. We observed that LPS-induced mPGES-1 synthesis was significantly inhibited by KIT 17 in a concentration-dependent manner starting at the concentration of 5 μM and revealing maximal effects using 10 μM, which decreased mPGES-1 levels about approx. 70%, if compared to LPS control (Fig. 6c). However, no effects were observed on mRNA expression of *mPGES-1* at the 4-h time point (Fig. 6a).

Furthermore, we investigated whether KIT 17 affected COX-2 mRNA expression and protein synthesis. The pre-treatment with KIT 17 in microglial cells showed a significant concentration-dependent decrease of LPS-induced COX-2 mRNA expression (Fig. 6b) and protein synthesis (Fig. 6d) starting at 1 μM and maximal effects using 10 μM, which decreased approximately 60% and 30% of COX-2 mRNA and 70% and 40% of protein levels, respectively, if compared to the LPS control.

We also evaluated the effect of KIT 17 on *COX-1* mRNA expression (Additional file 3) showing a down-regulation of *COX-1* mRNA expression by LPS stimulation and no modulatory effect of KIT17.

Effects of KIT 17 on enzyme activity of COX-1 and COX-2

Thus, we extended our study to investigate if these robust inhibitory effects of KIT 17 on PGE$_2$ release were

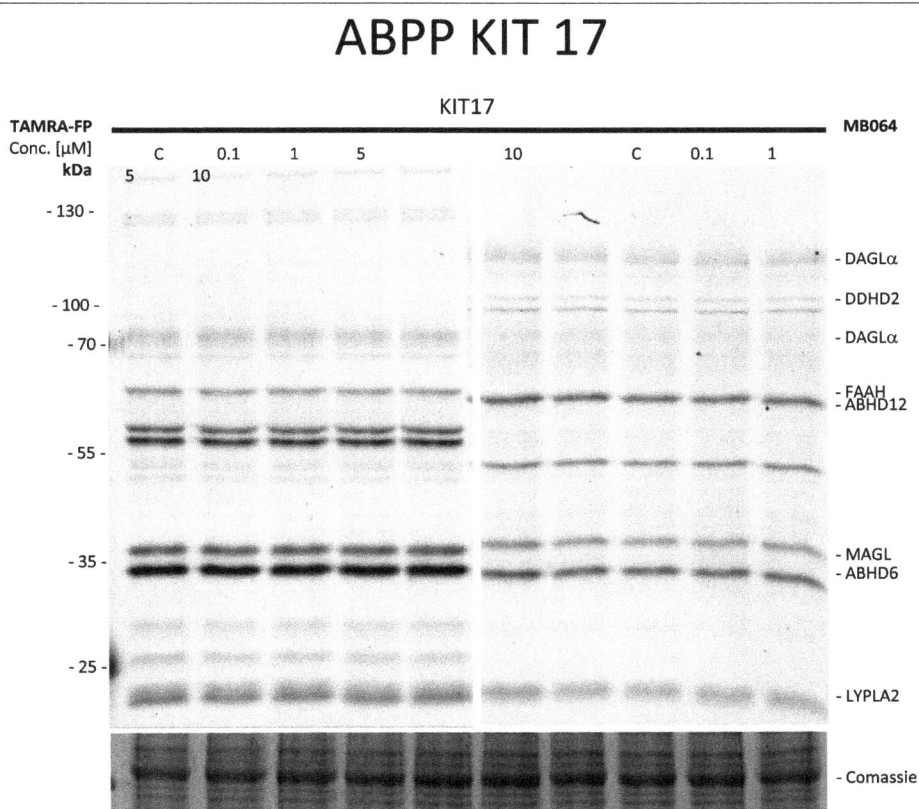

Fig. 5 Effects of KIT 17 on key enzymes involved in the endocannabinoid system. Dose-response gel-based ABPP on mouse membrane brain proteome with activity-based probes TAMRA-FP (left) and MB064 (right) (N = 3). ABHD6 and ABHD12 α,β-hydrolase domain-containing 6 and 12; DAGLα diacylglycerol lipase-α; FAAH fatty acid amide hydrolase, and MAGL monoacylglycerol lipase

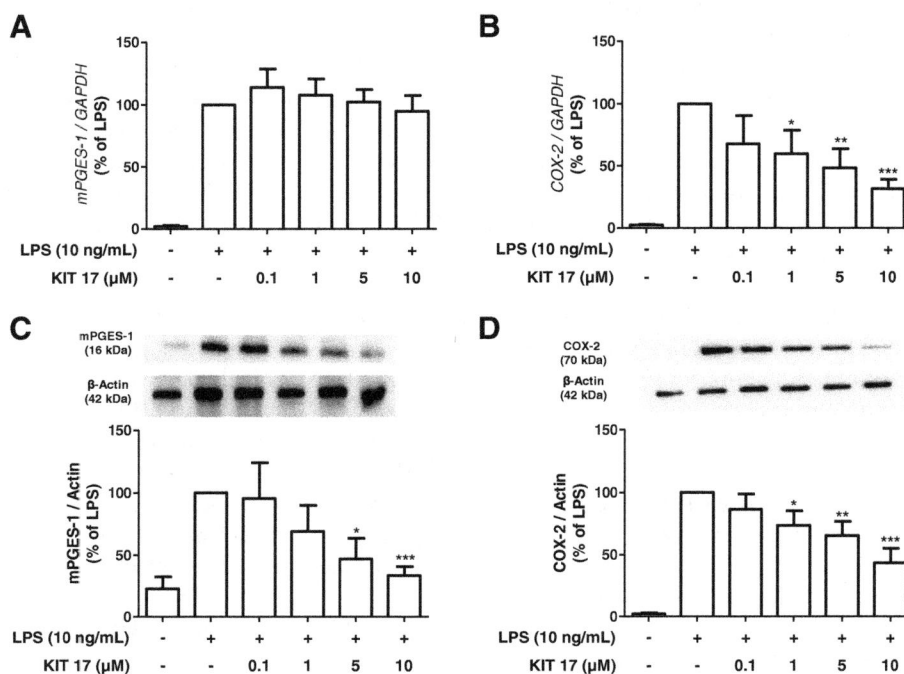

Fig. 6 Effects of KIT 17 on mRNA expression and protein synthesis of mPGES-1 (**a, c**) and COX-2 (**b, d**) in LPS-stimulated primary microglial cells. **a, b** Cells were pre-treated with different concentrations of KIT 17 for 30 min before stimulating with LPS. After 4 h, *mPGES-1* (**a**) and *COX-2* (**b**) were measured by qPCR. Western blot analysis of protein levels of mPGES-1 (**c**) or COX-2 (**d**) in cells pre-treated with different concentrations of KIT 17 for 30 min following LPS stimulation for 24 h. Protein levels were normalized to β-actin loading control ($n = 3–4$). $*p < 0.05$, $**p < 0.01$, and $***p < 0.001$ with respect to LPS (one-way ANOVA followed by the Newman-Keuls post hoc test)

additionally due to a direct suppression of COX enzymatic activity. As shown in Fig. 7a, COX-1 activity was even increased by KIT 17 in the concentrations of 0.1–10 μM, whereas in COX-2 activity was not affected (Fig. 7b). The control inhibitors for COX-1 (SC560) and COX-2 (diclofenac) showed the expected inhibitory effects (last 2 columns on the right).

Discussion

Neuroinflammatory processes are considered a double-edged sword, having both protective and detrimental effects in the brain [31–33]. Microglia, the resident innate immune cells of the brain, are a key component of neuroinflammatory response. There is a growing interest in developing drugs to target microglia and control neuroinflammatory processes [34, 35]. We have developed a new series of GPR55 receptor antagonist compounds derived from the coumarin structure which, in general, exhibit a promising profile as GPR55 receptor ligands with antagonistic activity [18].

In the current study, we demonstrated the anti-neuroinflammatory effect of these synthesized compounds in LPS-activated primary microglial cells by inhibiting PGE$_2$ release and downregulating mPGES-1 and COX-2 protein levels. We furthermore show that microglia expressed *GPR55* and that a synthetic antagonist of the

GPR55 receptor (ML193) revealed comparable effects as KIT 17 on the inhibition of LPS-induced PGE$_2$. Furthermore, we demonstrated that KIT 17 did not affect any enzyme involved in the endocannabinoid system in the mouse brain proteome.

Monocytes and macrophages express an extensive repertoire of G-protein-coupled receptors (GPCRs) that regulate inflammation and immunity [11, 36]. Among these receptors, the role of GPR55 in the perspective of neurological diseases and in microglia activation is controversial. GPR55 is expressed in many mammalian tissues including several brain regions [6, 37]. Pietr et al. (2009) showed that *GPR55* mRNA is significantly expressed in both, primary mouse microglia and the BV-2 mouse microglial cell line, and the stimulation with LPS downregulated *GPR55* expression [11]. However, in a study using primary rat microglial cells culture, the GPR55 transcript was detected in non-stimulated and LPS-stimulated cells, demonstrating no alterations of its levels [38]. Collaborating with this finding, we were able to confirm the expression of GPR55 in primary rat microglia and that the stimulation with LPS did not affect the expression of the receptor. Further studies, probably using microglia cell lines, have to be performed to demonstrate the functional GPR55 receptors on microglial cells.

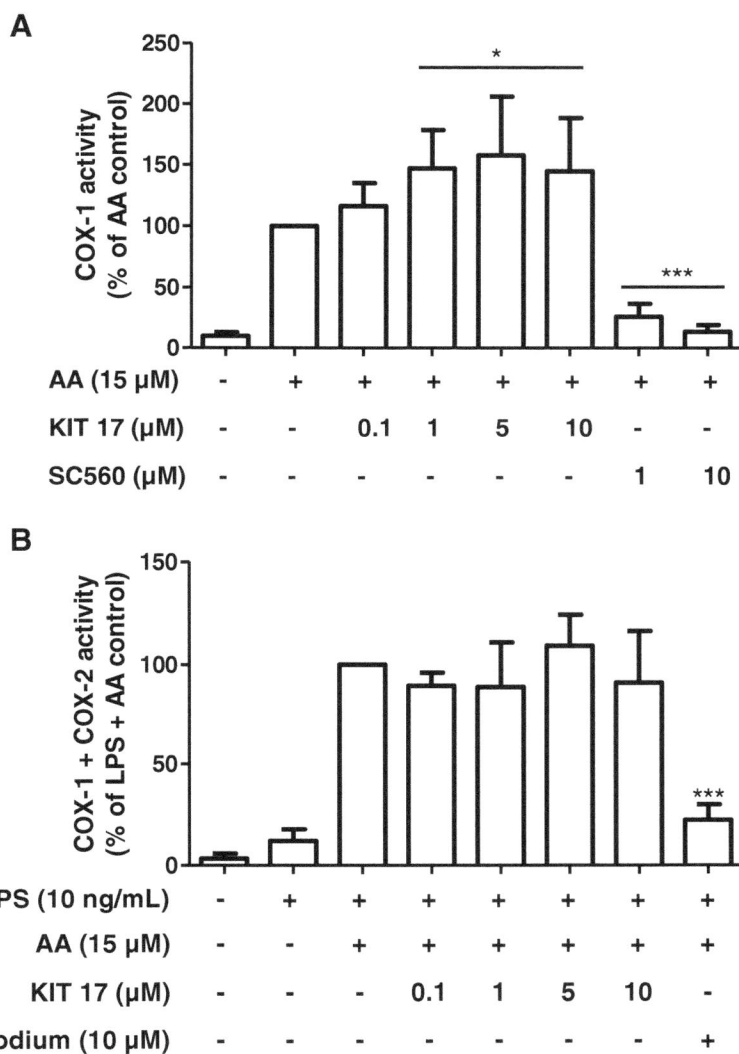

Fig. 7 Effects of KIT 17 on COX-1 (A) and COX-2 (b) enzyme activity in primary microglia cells. **a** For COX-1 activity assay, cells were treated with different concentrations of KIT 17 for 15 min before addition of 15 μM of arachidonic acid. PGE$_2$ in the supernatants was measured after additional 15 min. **b** Cells were stimulated for 24 h with LPS (10 ng/mL) and then treated with different concentrations of KIT 17 for 15 min. Then, 15 μM of arachidonic acid was added and PGE$_2$ in the supernatants was measured by enzyme immune assay (EIA). Data are expressed as mean ± S.E.M. of at least 3 independent experiments. *$p < 0.05$, **$p < 0.01$, and ***$p < 0.001$ with respect to control (one-way ANOVA followed by the Newman-Keuls post hoc test)

We next studied the potential role of GPR55 in microglia-mediated neuroinflammation by studying the effects of the KIT compounds on prostaglandin synthesis. Microglial cells are the resident macrophages of the CNS and the most important source of PGE$_2$ in neuroinflammation. As shown before, the stimulation of primary microglia with LPS strongly increases PGE$_2$ and COX-2 expression [39–41].

The main finding of our study is that the various synthesized KIT compounds decreased PGE$_2$ release in LPS-treated microglia and upstream members of the arachidonic acid pathway (COX-2/mPGES-1) without affecting the viability of microglia. Moreover, the similar

inhibition of PGE$_2$ was observed using the commercially available GPR55 antagonist ML193. Interestingly, the agonist O-1602 did not affect the inhibitory effect of ML193 as well as KIT 17 and also showed no effect on basal PGE$_2$ levels when applied without LPS.

KIT 17 and the other KIT compounds tested were synthesized by Rempel and collaborators (2013) as a series of coumarin derivatives (KITs) targeting GPR55 (formerly also known as CB3 receptor).

However, the compounds, including KIT 17, also bind to other receptors such as CB1, CB2, and GPR18 receptors, suggesting that the observed activities of KIT 17 are possible mediated also by other receptors [18]. The inhibitory values for KIT 17 on GPR55 is 9.32 ± 1.05 [IC50 ($\mu M \pm SEM$)] but it also binds to CB2 [Ki $\pm$ SEM (μM) 3.42 ± 0.90], whereas only weak binding was observed for CB1 and GPR18 [Ki $\pm$ SEM (μM)/IC50 ≥ 10] [18]. These data suggest that we can exclude CB1 and GPR18 as potential other receptors involved in the anti-inflammatory effects observed in microglial cells, but we cannot exclude an additional or exclusive involvement of CB2. The fact that KIT 17 as a GPR55 or CB2 antagonist is inhibiting TLR4-mediated inflammation, suggests an inverse agonistic activity of KIT 17 on GPR55 or CB2. To confirm this hypothesis and to prove a possible involvement of CB2, we used AM630, a compound with CB2 inverse agonistic activity with a Ki of 32 nM [42], also showing antagonistic activities on CB2. As shown in Additional file 4, AM630 also inhibited LPS-induced PGE_2 release in a comparable inhibitory profile on LPS-induced PGE_2 as KIT 17 with a slight more activity using 1 μM. However, the Ki of AM630 (32 nM) is 100 fold lower towards CB2 then the one of

KIT 17 (3.42 μM on CB2), implicating a more potent effect of AM630 on PGE_2 release induced by LPS then KIT 17, if we assume a CB2-mediated effect. Since the inhibitory activity of AM630 on LPS-induced PGE_2 release is only marginally higher than the effect of KIT 17, we conclude that CB2 is most likely not mediating the effects of KIT 17 and that AM630 might even also act via GPR55 on the observed effects. More studies have to be performed to support this conclusion, since there are to our knowledge no data available on the effects of AM630 on GPR55.

Since the GPR55 is described to be linked to the endocannabinoid system and due to the fact that the KIT compounds are also binding to CB1 and CB2, we were further interested in other interactions between KIT 17 and other members of the endocannabinoid system. Using the activity-based protein profiling on mouse brain proteome for selectivity and off-target activity approach, we did not find any interactions between KIT 17 and the endocannabinoid enzymes DAGLα, MAGL,

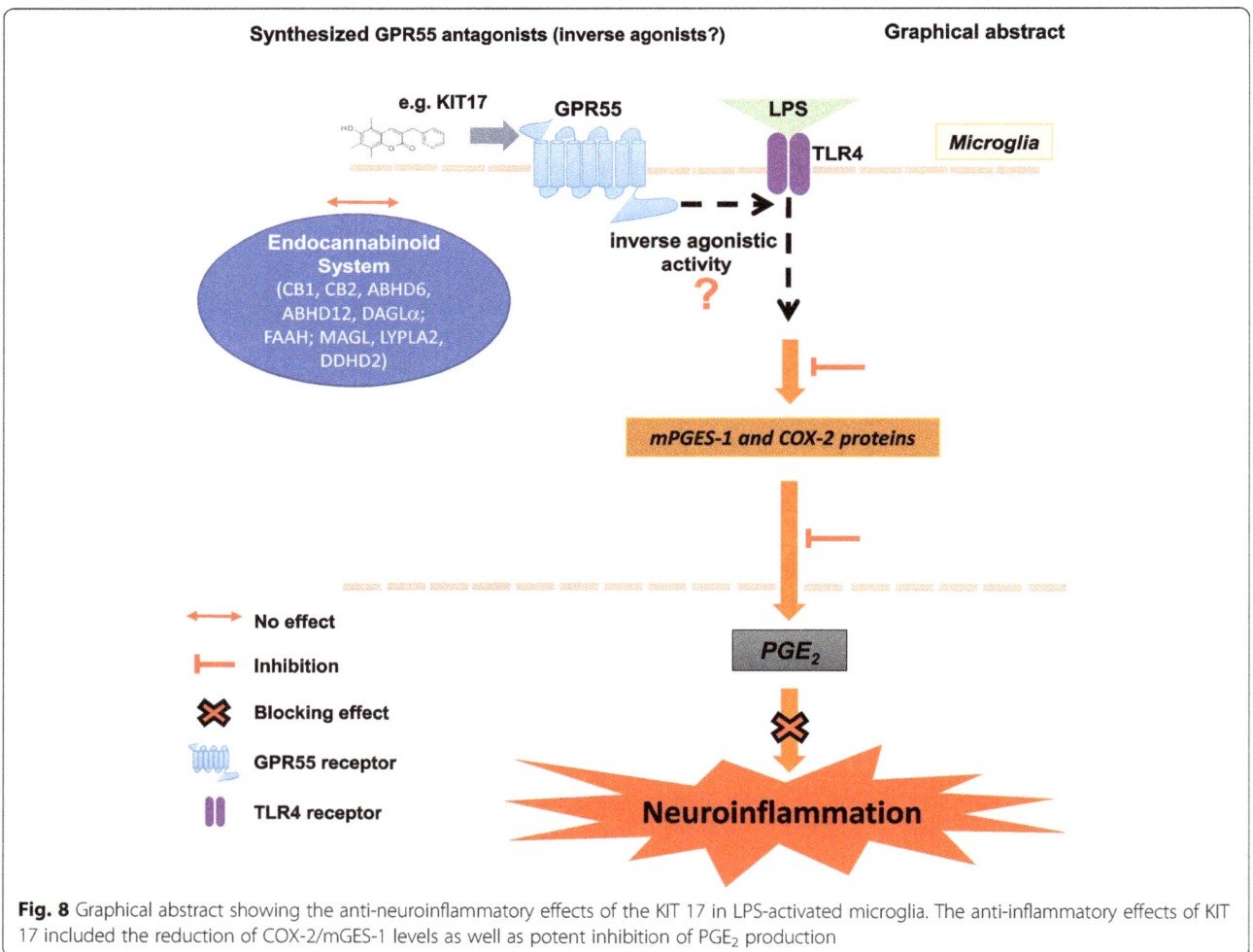

Fig. 8 Graphical abstract showing the anti-neuroinflammatory effects of the KIT 17 in LPS-activated microglia. The anti-inflammatory effects of KIT 17 included the reduction of COX-2/mGES-1 levels as well as potent inhibition of PGE_2 production

ABHD6, ABHD12, and FAAH. An interaction or effects of GPR55 activation on these enzymes have not been described to our knowledge in the literature yet.

Thus, our data strongly suggest that PGE_2 inhibitory effects in are most likely mediated by GPR55, although other mechanism independent of GPR55 and CBs in the observed effects cannot be excluded. The involvement of GPR55 in the activation of the arachidonic acid cascade during microglia activation and neuroinflammation has not been reported yet. The potential role in peripheral inflammation has been studied with GPR55 antagonists or knockout mice. The GPR55 inhibitor CID16020046 reduced TNF-α, IL-1β, IL-6, and COX-2 levels in a mouse model of intestinal inflammation [12]. In a mouse model of colorectal cancer, the levels of COX-2 and $PGF_{2\alpha}$ were decreased in GPR55$^{-/-}$ [43]. In hyperalgesia associated with inflammatory and neuropathic pain, an increase of anti-inflammatory cytokines, IL-4, and IL-10 has been observed in GPR55$^{-/-}$ knockout mice [13]. These data also suggest that GPR55 might be the mediator of the anti-neuroinflammatory effects of KIT17 as observed in this study.

In accordance with the diverse and complex pharmacology of GPR55, no data yet existed regarding the efficacy of GPR55 antagonists on COX-1/2 activity. Thus, we elucidated whether the robust inhibitory effects of KIT 17 on LPS-induced PGE_2 release is due to a direct inhibition of COX enzymatic activity, the mechanism of action of most NSAIDs. We demonstrate here, that COX-1 activity was increased by KIT 17 in the doses of 1–25 μM, whereas in COX-2 activity was not affected. The control inhibitors for COX-1 (SC560) and COX-2 (diclofenac) showed the expected inhibitory effects. This suggests that the PGE_2 inhibiting effects of KIT 17 and most likely by the other KIT compounds is not due a direct inhibition of COX activity. The COX-1 inducing effects might even have positive benefits, since COX-1 is protecting the gut mucosa and its inhibition by some NSAIDs cause gastro-intestinal side effects [44, 45].

Conclusions

As illustrated in the graphical abstract (Fig. 8), we provide the evidence that KIT 17 and the other KIT coumarin derivates and GPR55 antagonists effectively block microglia activation in terms of attenuation of both PGE_2 production and mPGES-1/COX-2 levels. Our data provide evidence that the anti-neuroinflammatory effects are mainly mediated by GPR55, most likely via an inverse agonist activity. However, further experiments are necessary to better comprehend the mechanistic effects of KIT compounds and the involvement of GPR55 receptors. Our study suggests that GPR55 antagonists might be a new therapeutic option for the treatment of neuroinflammation-, neurodegeneration-, and neuroinflammation-related diseases.

Additional files

Additional file 1: Expression of *GPR55* mRNA in primary rat microglia with or without LPS stimulation. Microglia were incubated with or without LPS (10 ng/mL) and after 4 h, *GPR55* mRNA expression was measured by qPCR. (PDF 7 kb)

Additional file 2: First screening of chemical-related synthesized compounds (KIT 1 - KIT 21) on LPS-induced PGE_2 synthesis in microglia cells. (PDF 16 kb)

Additional file 3: Effects of KIT 17 on mRNA expression of *COX-1* in LPS-stimulated primary microglial cells. Cells were pre-treated with different concentrations of KIT 17 for 30 min before stimulating with LPS. After 4 h, *COX-1* was measured by qPCR ($n = 5$). *$p < 0.01$ with respect to LPS (one-way ANOVA followed by the Newman-Keuls post hoc test). (PDF 9 kb)

Additional file 4: Effects of the AM630 on PGE_2 release in LPS-stimulated primary microglial cells. Microglia were pre-treated with AM630 (0.1–10 μM) for 30 min, afterwards cells were incubated with or without LPS (10 ng/mL) for the next 24 h. At the end of incubation, cell supernatants were collected and release of PGE_2 was measured by enzyme immune assay (EIA). Values are presented as the mean ± SEM of at least 3 independent experiments. Statistical analyses were carried out by using one-way ANOVA and Newman-Keuls post hoc test with ***$p < 0.001$ compared to LPS group. (PDF 9 kb)

Abbreviations
2-AG: 2-Arachidonoylglycerol; ABHD6 and ABHD12: α,β-Hydrolase domain-containing 6 and 12; ABPP: Activity-based protein profiling; AD: Alzheimer's disease; ATP: Adenosine triphosphate; BCA: Bicinchoninic acid; CB: Cannabinoids; CNS: Central nervous system; COX: Cyclooxygenase; DAG: Diacylglycerol; DAGLα: Diacylglycerol lipase-α; DMEM: Dulbecco's modified Eagle's medium; DMSO: Dimethyl sulfoxide; EIA: Enzyme immunoassay; ERK: Extracellular signal-regulated kinase; FAAH: Fatty acid amide hydrolase; GPR: G-protein-coupled receptor; IBD: Inflammatory bowel disease; IFN-γ: Interferon gamma; IL: Interleukin; LPI: L-α-Lysophosphatidylinositol; LPS: Lipopolysaccharide; MAGL: Monoacylglycerol lipase; mPGES: Microsomal prostaglandin E synthase; MS: Multiple sclerosis; NK: Natural killer; OHSC: Organotypic hippocampal slice cultures; PBS: Phosphate-buffered saline; PD: Parkinson disease; PG: Prostaglandin; PVDF: Polyvinylidene fluoride; RhoA: Ras homolog gene family member A; ROCK: Rho-associated protein kinase; SDS-PAGE: Sodium dodecyl sulfate-polyacrylamide gel electrophoresis; TAMRA-FP: Tetramethylrodamine 5-carboxamdio fluorophosphonate; TLR: Toll-like receptor; TNBS: Trinitrobenzene sulfonic acid; TNF: Tumor necrosis factor

Acknowledgements
We thank Ulrike Götzinger-Berger and Brigitte Günter for their excellent technical assistance. Soraya Wilke Saliba acknowledges CNPq/CSF (Brasília/Brazil) and DAAD (Germany) for the financial support. Brahim Gargouri and Bernd L. Fiebich acknowledge BMBF for supporting their research (TUNGER 036). Thomas Hurrle and Stefan Bräse want to acknowledge the Helmholtz program BIFTM (Karlsruhe/Teltow) for their support. Florian Mohr acknowledges the MWK Baden-Wuerttemberg and the KHYS for financial support, A.P.A. Janssen for providing the mouse brain proteome, and Ming Jiang for teaching the ABPP method. Moreover, we thank Franziska Gläser for the preliminary work. We thank the University of Freiburg Library for their support via the funding program "Open Access Publishing."

Funding
Soraya Wilke Saliba received a fellowship from CNPq/CSF (Brasília/Brazil) and DAAD (Germany). Brahim Gargouri received fellowships from BMBF/MESRS (TUNGER-36) and Alzheimer Forschungsinitiative (AFI). The project was in part supported by the AIF project GmbH (BMWi) (AGEsense) and BMBF (TUNGER-36). Thomas Hurrle and Stefan Bräse were supported by the Helmholtz program BIFTM (Karlsruhe/Teltow). Florian Mohr was financial supported by MWK Baden-Wuerttemberg and the KHYS. The article processing charge was funded by the University of Freiburg Library in the funding program "Open Access Publishing."

Authors' contributions

TH, NV, and SB designed and synthesized the GPR55 antagonists. HJ, AK, and BLF participated in research design. The experiments were performed by HJ, AK, and FM. Data were analyzed by SWS, HJ, TH, NV, AK, and FM. SWS, BG, TH, NV, SB, FM, MVDS, and BLF wrote or contributed to the writing of the manuscript. In addition, SWS, HJ, BG, AK, TH, NV, SB, FM, MVDS, and BLF reviewed the data and discussed the manuscript. All authors have read and approved the final version of the manuscript.

Competing interests

The authors declare that they have no competing interests.

Author details

[1]Neuroimmunology and Neurochemistry Research Group, Department of Psychiatry and Psychotherapy, Medical Center - University of Freiburg, Faculty of Medicine, University of Freiburg, Freiburg, Germany. [2]Institute of Organic Chemistry, Karlsruhe Institute of Technology (KIT), Karlsruhe, Germany. [3]Institute of Toxicology and Genetics, Karlsruhe Institute of Technology (KIT), Hermann-von-Helmholtz-Platz 1, 76344 Eggenstein-Leopoldshafen, Germany. [4]Department of Molecular Physiology, Leiden Institute of Chemistry, Leiden University, Leiden, the Netherlands. [5]Department of Psychiatry and Psychotherapy, Laboratory of Translational Psychiatry, University Hospital Freiburg, Hauptstr. 5, 79104 Freiburg, Germany.

References

1. Boche D, Perry VH, Nicoll JAR. Review: activation patterns of microglia and their identification in the human brain. Neuropathol Appl Neurobiol. 2013; 39:3–18.
2. Ransohoff RM, Perry VH. Microglial physiology: unique stimuli, specialized responses. Annu Rev Immunol. 2009;27:119–45.
3. Perry VH, Nicoll JAR, Holmes C. Microglia in neurodegenerative disease. Nat Rev Neurol. 2010;6:193–201.
4. Streit WJ, Conde JR, Fendrick SE, Flanary BE, Mariani CL. Role of microglia in the central nervous system's immune response. Neurol Res. 2005;27:685–91.
5. Town T, Nikolic V, Tan J. The microglial "activation" continuum: from innate to adaptive responses. J Neuroinflammation. 2005;2:24.
6. Sawzdargo M, Nguyen T, Lee DK, Lynch KR, Cheng R, Heng HH, et al. Identification and cloning of three novel human G protein-coupled receptor genes GPR52, ΨGPR53 and GPR55: GPR55 is extensively expressed in human brain. Mol Brain Res. 1999;64:193–8.
7. Yang H, Zhou J, Lehmann C. GPR55 – a putative "type 3" cannabinoid receptor in inflammation. J Basic Clin Physiol Pharmacol. 2016;27(3):297–302.
8. Ryberg E, Larsson N, Sjögren S, Hjorth S, Hermansson N-O, Leonova J, et al. The orphan receptor GPR55 is a novel cannabinoid receptor. Br J Pharmacol. 2007;152:1092–101.
9. Zhou J, Burkovskiy I, Yang H, Sardinha J, Lehmann C. CB2 and GPR55 receptors as therapeutic targets for systemic immune dysregulation. Front Pharmacol. 2016;7:264.
10. Chiurchiù V, Lanuti M, De Bardi M, Battistini L, Maccarrone M. The differential characterization of GPR55 receptor in human peripheral blood reveals a distinctive expression in monocytes and NK cells and a proinflammatory role in these innate cells. Int Immunol. 2015;27:153–60.
11. Pietr M, Kozela E, Levy R, Rimmerman N, Lin YH, Stella N, et al. Differential changes in GPR55 during microglial cell activation. FEBS Lett. 2009;583:2071–6.
12. Stančić A, Jandl K, Hasenöhrl C, Reichmann F, Marsche G, Schuligoi R, et al. The GPR55 antagonist CID16020046 protects against intestinal inflammation. Neurogastroenterol Motil. 2015;27:1432–45.
13. Staton PC, Hatcher JP, Walker DJ, Morrison AD, Shapland EM, Hughes JP, et al. The putative cannabinoid receptor GPR55 plays a role in mechanical hyperalgesia associated with inflammatory and neuropathic pain. Pain. 2008;139:225–36.
14. Li K, Feng J, Li Y, Yuece B, Lin X, Yu L, et al. Anti-inflammatory role of cannabidiol and O-1602 in cerulein-induced acute pancreatitis in mice. Pancreas. 2013;42:123–9.
15. Kallendrusch S, Kremzow S, Nowicki M, Grabiec U, Winkelmann R, Benz A, et al. The G protein-coupled receptor 55 ligand L-α-lysophosphatidylinositol exerts microglia-dependent neuroprotection after excitotoxic lesion: microglia-dependent GPR55-driven neuroprotection. Glia. 2013;61:1822–31.
16. Celorrio M, Rojo-Bustamante E, Fernández-Suárez D, Sáez E, Estella-Hermoso de Mendoza A, Müller CE, et al. GPR55: a therapeutic target for Parkinson's disease? Neuropharmacology. 2017;125:319–32.
17. Wu C-S, Chen H, Sun H, Zhu J, Jew CP, Wager-Miller J, et al. GPR55, a G-protein coupled receptor for lysophosphatidylinositol, plays a role in motor coordination. Tang Y-P, editor. PLoS One 2013;8:e60314.
18. Rempel V, Volz N, Gläser F, Nieger M, Bräse S, Müller CE. Antagonists for the orphan G-protein-coupled receptor GPR55 based on a coumarin scaffold. J Med Chem. 2013;56:4798–810.
19. Saliba SW, Marcotegui AR, Fortwängler E, Ditrich J, Perazzo JC, Muñoz E, et al. AM404, paracetamol metabolite, prevents prostaglandin synthesis in activated microglia by inhibiting COX activity. J Neuroinflammation. 2017;14:246.
20. Seregi A, Keller M, Jackisch R, Hertting G. Comparison of the prostanoid synthesizing capacity in homogenates from primary neuronal and astroglial cell cultures. Biochem Pharmacol. 1984;33:3315–8.
21. Bhatia HS, Baron J, Hagl S, Eckert GP, Fiebich BL. Rice bran derivatives alleviate microglia activation: possible involvement of MAPK pathway. J Neuroinflammation. 2016;13:148.
22. Bhatia HS, Roelofs N, Muñoz E, Fiebich BL. Alleviation of microglial activation induced by p38 MAPK/MK2/PGE2 Axis by capsaicin: potential involvement of other than TRPV1 mechanism/s. Sci Rep. 2017;7(1):116.
23. Kumar A, Bhatia HS, de Oliveira ACP, Fiebich BL. microRNA-26a modulates inflammatory response induced by toll-like receptor 4 stimulation in microglia. J Neurochem. 2015;135:1189–202.
24. Olajide OA, Bhatia HS, de Oliveira ACP, Wright CW, Fiebich BL. Inhibition of neuroinflammation in LPS-activated microglia by cryptolepine. Evid-Based Complement Altern Med. 2013;2013:459723.
25. Chomczynski P, Sacchi N. Single-step method of RNA isolation by acid guanidinium thiocyanate-phenol-chloroform extraction. Anal Biochem. 1987; 162:156–9.
26. Livak KJ, Schmittgen TD. Analysis of relative gene expression data using real-time quantitative PCR and the 2(−Delta Delta C(T)) method. Methods San Diego Calif. 2001;25:402–8.
27. Akundi RS, Candelario-Jalil E, Hess S, Hüll M, Lieb K, Gebicke-Haerter PJ, et al. Signal transduction pathways regulating cyclooxygenase-2 in lipopolysaccharide-activated primary rat microglia. Glia. 2005;51:199–208.
28. Baggelaar MP, Janssen FJ, van Esbroeck ACM, den Dulk H, Allarà M, Hoogendoorn S, et al. Development of an activity-based probe and in silico design reveal highly selective inhibitors for diacylglycerol lipase-α in brain. Angew Chem Int Ed Engl. 2013;52:12081–5.
29. Baggelaar MP, Chameau PJP, Kantae V, Hummel J, Hsu K-L, Janssen F, et al. Highly selective, reversible inhibitor identified by comparative chemoproteomics modulates diacylglycerol lipase activity in neurons. J Am Chem Soc. 2015;137:8851–7.
30. Kudo I, Murakami M. Prostaglandin E synthase, a terminal enzyme for prostaglandin E2 biosynthesis. J Biochem Mol Biol. 2005;38:633–8.
31. Colton CA. Heterogeneity of microglial activation in the innate immune response in the brain. J NeuroImmune Pharmacol. 2009;4:399–418.
32. Skokowa J, Cario G, Uenalan M, Schambach A, Germeshausen M, Battmer K, et al. LEF-1 is crucial for neutrophil granulocytopoiesis and its expression is severely reduced in congenital neutropenia. Nat Med. 2006;12:1191–7.
33. Akiyama H, Barger S, Barnum S, Bradt B, Bauer J, Cole GM. Inflammation and Alzheimer's disease. Neurobiol Aging. 2000;21:383–421.
34. Hunot S, Hirsch EC. Neuroinflammatory processes in Parkinson's disease. Ann Neurol. 2003;53(3):S49–58 discussion S58–60.
35. Koistinaho M, Koistinaho J. Interactions between Alzheimer's disease and cerebral ischemia--focus on inflammation. Brain Res Brain Res Rev. 2005;48: 240–50.
36. Lattin JE, Schroder K, Su AI, Walker JR, Zhang J, Wiltshire T, et al. Expression analysis of G protein-coupled receptors in mouse macrophages. Immunome Res. 2008;4:5.

37. Baker D, Pryce G, Davies WL, Hiley CR. In silico patent searching reveals a new cannabinoid receptor. Trends Pharmacol Sci. 2006;27:1–4.
38. Malek N, Popiolek-Barczyk K, Mika J, Przewlocka B, Starowicz K. Anandamide, acting via CB2 receptors, alleviates LPS-induced neuroinflammation in rat primary microglial cultures. Neural Plast. 2015;2015:130639.
39. Bauer MK, Lieb K, Schulze-Osthoff K, Berger M, Gebicke-Haerter PJ, Bauer J, et al. Expression and regulation of cyclooxygenase-2 in rat microglia. Eur J Biochem. 1997;243:726–31.
40. Minghetti L, Levi G. Induction of prostanoid biosynthesis by bacterial lipopolysaccharide and isoproterenol in rat microglial cultures. J Neurochem. 1995;65:2690–8.
41. Slepko N, Minghetti L, Polazzi E, Nicolini A, Levi G. Reorientation of prostanoid production accompanies "activation" of adult microglial cells in culture. J Neurosci Res. 1997;49:292–300.
42. Ross RA, Brockie HC, Stevenson LA, Murphy VL, Templeton F, Makriyannis A, Pertwee RG. Agonist-inverse agonist characterization at CB1 and CB2 cannabinoid receptors of L759633, L759656, and AM630. Br J Pharmacol. 1999 Feb;126(3):665–72.
43. Hasenoehrl C, Feuersinger D, Sturm EM, Bärnthaler T, Heitzer E, Graf R, et al. G protein-coupled receptor GPR55 promotes colorectal cancer and has opposing effects to cannabinoid receptor 1: GPR55 drives colorectal cancer. Int J Cancer. 2018;142:121–32.
44. Hirata T, Ukawa H, Kitamura M, Takeuchi K. Effects of selective cyclooxygenase-2 inhibitors on alkaline secretory and mucosal ulcerogenic responses in rat duodenum. Life Sci. 1997;61:1603–11.
45. Amagase K, Izumi N, Takahira Y, Wada T, Takeuchi K. Importance of cyclooxygenase-1/prostacyclin in modulating gastric mucosal integrity under stress conditions. J Gastroenterol Hepatol. 2014;29(4):3–10.

10

The small molecule CA140 inhibits the neuroinflammatory response in wild-type mice and a mouse model of AD

Ju-Young Lee[1], Jin Han Nam[1], Youngpyo Nam[1], Hye Yeon Nam[1], Gwangho Yoon[1], Eunhwa Ko[2], Sang-Bum Kim[2], Mahealani R Bautista[3], Christina C Capule[3], Takaoki Koyanagi[3], Geoffray Leriche[3], Hwan Geun Choi[2], Jerry Yang[3], Jeongyeon Kim[1]* and Hyang-Sook Hoe[1]* (iD)

Abstract

Background: Neuroinflammation is associated with neurodegenerative diseases, including Alzheimer's disease (AD). Thus, modulating the neuroinflammatory response represents a potential therapeutic strategy for treating neurodegenerative diseases. Several recent studies have shown that dopamine (DA) and its receptors are expressed in immune cells and are involved in the neuroinflammatory response. Thus, we recently developed and synthesized a non-self-polymerizing analog of DA (CA140) and examined the effect of CA140 on neuroinflammation.

Methods: To determine the effects of CA140 on the neuroinflammatory response, BV2 microglial cells were pretreated with lipopolysaccharide (LPS, 1 μg/mL), followed by treatment with CA140 (10 μM) and analysis by reverse transcription-polymerase chain reaction (RT-PCR). To examine whether CA140 alters the neuroinflammatory response in vivo, wild-type mice were injected with both LPS (10 mg/kg, intraperitoneally (i.p.)) and CA140 (30 mg/kg, i.p.), and immunohistochemistry was performed. In addition, familial AD (5xFAD) mice were injected with CA140 or vehicle daily for 2 weeks and examined for microglial and astrocyte activation.

Results: Pre- or post-treatment with CA140 differentially regulated proinflammatory responses in LPS-stimulated microglia and astrocytes. Interestingly, CA140 regulated D1R levels to alter LPS-induced proinflammatory responses. CA140 significantly downregulated LPS-induced phosphorylation of ERK and STAT3 in BV2 microglia cells. In addition, CA140-injected wild-type mice exhibited significantly decreased LPS-induced microglial and astrocyte activation. Moreover, CA140-injected 5xFAD mice exhibited significantly reduced microglial and astrocyte activation.

Conclusions: CA140 may be beneficial for preventing and treating neuroinflammatory-related diseases, including AD.

Keywords: Alzheimer's disease, Neuroinflammation, D1R, ERK, STAT3, LPS, CA140

Background

Increasing evidence indicates a critical role of the immune system in neurodegenerative diseases such as Alzheimer's disease (AD) [1]. Abnormal glial activation in patients with neurodegenerative diseases may be a hallmark diagnostic feature of these diseases, particularly AD [2]. Neuroinflammation or inflammation of the central nervous system (CNS) is mainly mediated by the activation of microglia [1]. In addition to releasing various neurotrophic factors that support neuronal cell survival and neurotoxic factors, activated microglia release proinflammatory cytokines such as interleukin-1β (IL-1β) and tumor necrosis factor-α (TNF-α) [3, 4]. The neuroinflammation induced by the release of these proinflammatory cytokines may eventually lead to neuronal cell death and synaptic dysfunction. Therefore, the elucidation of the regulation of glial activation and inactivation may provide a potential therapeutic strategy for treating neurodegenerative diseases.

Lipopolysaccharide (LPS) is a well-established stimulator that induces the activation of microglial cells and is widely used both in vivo and in vitro to induce neuroinflammation in animal models [5, 6]. The interaction

* Correspondence: jykim@kbri.re.kr; sookhoe72@kbri.re.kr
[1]Department of Neural Development and Disease, Korea Brain Research Institute (KBRI), 61 Cheomdan-ro, Dong-gu, Daegu 41068, South Korea
Full list of author information is available at the end of the article

between LPS and Toll-like receptor 4 (TLR4) activates inflammation-associated transcription factors [7] and the mitogen-activated protein kinase (MAPK) family [8, 9], which comprises at least three components: extracellular signal-regulated kinases (ERKs), c-Jun N-terminal kinase (JNK), and p38 MAPK. In addition, the association between LPS and TLR4 stimulates the release of both immune-related cytotoxic factors, including iNOS and COX-2, and proinflammatory cytokines (TNF-α, IL-1β, and IL-6) [10]. A chronic inflammatory response may be accompanied by amyloid beta (Aβ) production, and microglia have been identified near the Aβ plaques of AD patients [11, 12]. Aβ accumulation triggers AD pathogenesis through two mechanisms: neuronal apoptosis and glia-mediated inflammation leading to cell death [13]. Extracellular Aβ deposits in senile plaques trigger changes in glial reactivity and stimulate neuroinflammation. Thus, Aβ accumulation may lead to neuronal loss through the overproduction of reactive proinflammatory cytokines [14, 15]. CA140 is a chemically stable small-molecule analog of dopamine (DA) and is synthesized by acylation of the amine in DA with N-methylisatoic anhydride, which reduces the propensity of DA to undergo self-polymerization [16]. DA is a neurotransmitter that regulates a wide range of functions, including initiation of movement and learning and memory [17]. DA binds to several DA receptors, which are present on nearly all immune cells [18]. Activation of these receptors via DA or DA agonists modulates the activation, proliferation, and cytokine production of immune cells [19]. We therefore speculated that CA140 may also exhibit biological activity against the neuroinflammatory response.

In the present study, we examined whether CA140 regulates the neuroinflammatory response in vitro and in vivo. We discovered that CA140 reduced proinflammatory responses in LPS-stimulated BV2 microglial cells, primary microglial cells, and primary astrocytes. In addition, CA140 inhibited LPS-induced neuroinflammatory responses by inhibiting the dopamine D1 receptor (D1R)/ERK/STAT3 signaling pathways. Moreover, CA140 significantly decreased the activation of microglia and astrocytes in wild-type mice as well as a mouse model of AD. Taken together, our results indicate that CA140 is a potential therapeutic agent for treating and/or preventing neuroinflammation-related diseases, including AD.

Methods
Cell lines and culture conditions
BV2 microglial cells (a generous gift of Dr. Kyung-Ho Suk) or HEK cells (a generous gift of Dr. Hyung-Jun Kim) were maintained in high-glucose DMEM (Invitrogen, Carlsbad, CA, USA) with 5 or 10% fetal bovine serum (FBS, Invitrogen, Carlsbad, CA, USA) in a 5% CO_2 incubator.

Mouse primary microglial and astrocyte cultures
Mouse primary microglial and astrocyte cultures were prepared from mixed glial cultures as previously described [20]. Briefly, whole brains of post-natal 1-day-old C57BL/6 mice were chopped and mechanically disrupted using a 70-μm nylon mesh. The cells were seeded in 75 T culture flasks and grown in low-glucose DMEM supplemented with 10% FBS, 100 unit/mL penicillin, and 100 μg/mL streptomycin. The culture medium was changed after 7 days and every 3 days thereafter. After 14 days, mixed primary glial cells were obtained for use in subsequent experiments. To obtain mouse primary astrocytes, mixed glial cells were cultured with shaking at 250 rpm overnight. The next day, the culture medium was discarded, and the cells were washed three times with PBS. The cells were dissociated using trypsin-EDTA and collected by centrifugation at 1200 rpm for 10 min. Primary astrocytes were maintained in low-glucose DMEM supplemented with 10% FBS and penicillin-streptomycin. To obtain mouse primary microglial cells, mixed primary glial cells were incubated with trypsin solution (0.25% trypsin, 1 mM EDTA in Hank's balanced salt solution) diluted 1:4 in serum-free DMEM media [21]. After the mouse primary astrocyte layer was fully detached, low-glucose DMEM containing 10% FBS was added, the supernatant was aspirated, and the remaining primary microglial cells were used for experiments.

Rat primary microglial and astrocyte cultures
Rat primary mixed glial cells were cultured from the cerebral cortices of 1-day-old Sprague Dawley rats. Briefly, the cortices were triturated into single cells in high-glucose DMEM containing 10% FBS/penicillin-streptomycin solution (5000 units/mL penicillin, 5 mg/mL streptomycin, Corning, Mediatech Inc., Manassas, VA, USA) and plated into 75 T culture flasks (0.5 hemisphere/flask) for 2 weeks. To harvest rat primary microglial cells, the plate was shaken continuously at 120 rpm for 2 h to facilitate microglial detachment from the plate. The fluid medium was subsequently collected and centrifuged at 1500 rpm for 15 min, and the cell pellets were resuspended to plate 1×10^5 cells per well. The remaining cells in the flask were harvested using 0.1% trypsin to obtain rat primary astrocytes. These rat primary astrocytes and primary microglial cells were cultured in 12-well plates (35 mm) pre-coated with poly-D-lysine (Sigma).

Wild-type mice
All experiments were performed in accordance with the approved animal protocols and guidelines established by the Korea Brain Research Institute (IACUC-2016-0013). C57BL6/N mice were purchased from Orient-Bio

Company. Male C57BL6/N mice (8 weeks, 25–30 g) were housed in a pathogen-free facility with 12 h of light and dark per day at an ambient temperature of 22 °C. To determine if pretreatment with CA140 alters LPS-induced neuroinflammation, wild-type mice were intraperitoneally (i.p.) administered CA140 (30 mg/kg) or vehicle (10% DMSO) daily for 3 days and subsequently injected with LPS (Sigma, *Escherichia coli*, 10 mg/kg, i.p.) or PBS. After 3 h, immunostaining was performed with anti-IbaI or anti-GFAP antibodies. To examine whether post-treatment with CA140 regulates LPS-induced neuroinflammatory responses, wild-type mice were injected with LPS (10 mg/kg/day, i.p.) or PBS, followed 30 min later by injection with CA140 (30 mg/kg, i.p., twice with an interval of 1 h, followed 30 min later by a third injection) or vehicle (10% DMSO, i.p.). Immunohistochemistry was then performed with anti-Iba-1 and anti-GFAP antibodies.

Familial AD (5xFAD) mice

F1 generation 5xFAD mice (stock number 008730, B6SJL-Tg APPSwFlLon, PSEN1*M146 L*L286V6799Vas/ Mmjax) were purchased from The Jackson Laboratory. 5xFAD mice overexpress two mutant human proteins: APP (695) with KM670/671NL (Swedish), I716V (Florida), and V717I (London) FAD mutations and PS1 with M146 L and L286 V FAD mutations. To examine the effects of CA140 on the neuroinflammatory response in a mouse model of AD, 5xFAD mice were injected with CA140 (30 mg/kg, i.p.) or vehicle (10% DMSO, i.p.) daily for 2 weeks, and immunohistochemistry was conducted with anti-Iba-1 or anti-GFAP antibodies. The animal groups were randomized for all experiments. Data were analyzed in a semi-automated manner using ImageJ software and confirmed by an independent researcher who did not participate in the current experiments. Only male mice were used for this study because the pathology of 5xFAD female mice is more severe than that of male mice, leading to huge variations in in vivo experiments.

Synthesis of CA140

N-Methylisatoic anhydride (19.6 mg, 110 μmol) was added to 28.1 mg of 3,4-dimethoxyphenethylamine (155 μmol, 1.3 equiv) and 25 μL of triethylamine (339 μmol, 3 equiv) in dichloromethane (DCM). The reaction mixture was stirred for 2 h at room temperature and overnight at 20 °C. The mixture was warmed to room temperature, and a vacuum was subsequently applied to remove volatile organics. The amide product was purified by column chromatography (7% ethyl acetate in DCM; Rf = 0.27) to provide 31.5 mg of N-(3,4-dimethoxyphenethyl)-2-(methylamino)benzamide as a white solid (91% isolated yield). ^{1}H-NMR (400 MHz, CDCl$_3$) δ ppm = 7.30 (t, 1H, J = 7.7 Hz, Ar-H), 7.20 (d, 1H, J = 7.7 Hz, Ar-H), 6.82 (d, 1H, J = 8.1 Hz, Ar-H), 6.74 (m 2H, Ar-H), 6.55 (t, 1H, J = 7.5 Hz, Ar-H), 3.86 (s, 3H, OCH$_3$), 3.83 (s, 3H, OCH$_3$), 3.63 (t, 1H, J = 6.7 Hz, -HCH-), 3.61 (t, 1H, J = 6.7 Hz, -HCH-), 2.84 (s, 3H, CH$_3$), 2.84 (t, 2H, J = 6.8 Hz, CH$_2$). ^{13}C-NMR (100 MHz, CDCl$_3$) δ ppm = 169.6, 150.0, 148.9, 147.6, 132.7, 131.4, 127.0, 120.6, 115.4, 114.8, 111.9, 111.4, 111.3, 55.8, 55.7, 40.9, 35.1, 29.8.

N-(3,4-Dimethoxyphenethyl)-2-(methylamino)benzamide (9.2 mg, 29.3 μmol) was dissolved in 0.5 mL of anhydrous DCM, and 120 μL of 1 M BBr$_3$ in DCM (120 μmol, 4 equiv) was added. The reaction was stirred overnight under an inert atmosphere. Excess methanol was added to the mixture, and volatile organics were removed in vacuo. The addition and removal of methanol was repeated at least three times to remove boric acid as methyl borate. The target compound, N-(3,4-dihydroxyphenethyl)-2-(methylamino)benzamide (CA140), was obtained in quantitative yield. ^{1}H-NMR (400 MHz, CD$_3$OD) δ ppm = 7.91 (d, 1H, J = 8.0 Hz, Ar-H), 7.89 (t, 1H, J = 7.6 Hz, Ar-H), 7.74 (m, 2H, J = 7.6 Hz, Ar-H), 6.67 (d 2H, J = 9.6 Hz Ar-H), 6.56 (d, 1H, J = 8.0 Hz, Ar-H), 3.60 (t, 2H, J = 7.1 Hz, CH$_2$), 3.01 (s, 3H, NCH$_3$), 2.79 (t, 1H, J = 7.0 Hz, CH$_2$). LC-MS ESI positive mode m/z [M + H]$^+$ = 287.11 (calculated = 287.13).

Brain-to-plasma ratio in ICR (Institute for Cancer Research) mice

ICR mice (n = 3) were dosed with CA140 dissolved in DMSO/Tween-80/saline (10:5:85%) via a single intravenous administration (10 mg/kg). Blood was collected by cardiac puncture at 5 min and then centrifuged to isolate plasma. The brain was collected at 5 min and homogenized in PBS after washing with fresh PBS. The concentrations of CA140 in the plasma and brain were determined by LC-MS/MS. The LC-MS/MS system comprised a Nexera XR HPLC system (Shimadzu Co., Kyoto, Japan) coupled to a TSQ Vantage triple quadrupole mass spectrometer equipped with Xcalibur version 1.1.1 (Thermo Fisher Scientific Inc., Waltham, MA, USA).

Stability studies of CA140 and dopamine in vitro

To examine the stability of CA140 in vitro, samples were generated from stock solutions (30 mM in DMSO) of either dopamine (DA, as a control for CA140) or CA140 by dilution in 1 mL of preheated PBS buffer to yield final concentrations of 500 μM. The solutions were incubated at 37 °C in a thermoblock, and the concentration of CA140 or DA was followed over time in triplicate. Aliquots (50 μL) were taken at 0, 1, 2, 4, 6, 8, and 22 h and added to 200 μL of acetonitrile. The samples were mixed by vortexing for 30 s and then centrifuged at 4 °C for 15 min at 14,000 rpm. The clear supernatants were diluted in PBS (2-fold) and analyzed by HPLC at 254 and 280 nm for CA140 and DA, respectively.

Antibodies and inhibitors

The following primary antibodies were used throughout this study: rat anti-mouse CD11b (1:400, Abcam), rabbit anti-F-actin (1:1000, Abcam), rabbit anti-COX-2 (1:1000, Abcam), rabbit anti-IL-1β (1:200, Abcam), rabbit anti-GFAP (1:5000, Neuromics), rabbit anti-Iba-1 (1:1000, Wako), goat anti-Iba-1 (1:500, Wako), rabbit anti-AKT (1:1000, Santa Cruz), rabbit anti-p-AKT (Ser473, Thr308) (1:1000, Cell Signaling), rabbit anti-ERK (1:1000, Santa Cruz), rabbit anti-p-ERK (Thr42/44) (1:1000, Cell Signaling), rabbit anti-STAT3 (1:1000, Cell Signaling), rabbit anti-p-STAT3 (Ser727, Abcam), mouse anti-PCNA (1:1000, Santa Cruz), rabbit anti-D2R (1:1000, Abcam), and rabbit anti-D1R (1:1000, Millipore) antibodies. We used the following small molecules: D1R antagonists (LE300, 10 μM, Sigma-Aldrich; SCH23390, 30 μM, Tocris), D1R agonist (A77636 hydrochloride, 10 nM, Tocris), D2R antagonist (eticlopride hydrochloride, 100 nM, Sigma-Aldrich), a STAT3 inhibitor (S3I-201, 50 μM, Sigma-Aldrich), and an ERK inhibitor (PD98059, 10 μM, Millipore).

MTT assay

BV2 microglial cell viability was assessed using the 3-(4,5-dimethylthiazol-2-yl)-2,5-diphenyltetrazolium bromide (MTT) assay. BV2 microglial cells were seeded in 96-well plates and treated with various concentrations of CA140 (1–50 μM) or vehicle (1% DMSO) for 24 h in the absence of FBS. The cells were subsequently treated with 0.5 mg/mL MTT and incubated for 3 h at 37 °C in a 5% CO_2 incubator. The absorbance was read at 580 nm.

Reverse transcription-polymerase chain reaction (RT-PCR)

Total RNA was extracted from cells using TRIzol (Invitrogen) following the manufacturer's instructions. Total RNA was reverse transcribed into cDNA using a Superscript cDNA Premix Kit II with oligoDT (GeNetBio, Korea), and RT-PCR was performed using Prime Taq Premix (GeNetBio, Korea). RT-PCR products were separated by electrophoresis on 1.5% agarose gels with Eco Dye (1:5000, Korea) and photographed. Images were analyzed using ImageJ (NIH) and Fusion (Korea).

Immunocytochemistry

BV2 microglial cells were fixed in ice-cold methanol for 8 min, washed three times with 1 × PBS, and incubated with CD11b and COX-2 or CD11b and IL-1β antibodies in GDB buffer (0.1% gelatin, 0.3% Triton X-100, 16 mM sodium phosphate pH 7.4, and 450 mM NaCl) overnight at 4 °C. The next day, the cells were washed three times with 1 × PBS and incubated with the following secondary

antibodies for 1 h at room temperature: Alexa Fluor 488 and Alexa Fluor 555 (1:200, Molecular Probes, USA). Images were obtained on a single plane using a confocal microscope (Nikon, Japan) and analyzed using ImageJ software.

Immunohistochemistry and immunofluorescence

Animals were perfused and fixed with 4% paraformaldehyde (PFA) solution, and brain tissues were flash-frozen and dissected using a cryostat (35-mm-thick sections). Each brain section was processed for immunofluorescence or immunohistochemical staining. For immunofluorescence staining, sections were rinsed in PBS and incubated with rabbit anti-Iba-1 (1:1000, Wako, Japan) for microglia or rabbit anti-GFAP (1:5000, Neuromics) for astrocytes. Antibodies were diluted in 0.5% bovine serum albumin (BSA) and incubated at 4 °C overnight. The following day, tissues were rinsed with 0.5% BSA and incubated with Alexa Fluor 555-conjugated anti-rabbit IgG (1:200, Molecular Probes) for 1 h at room temperature. The tissues were subsequently mounted on a gelatin-coated cover glass and covered with DAPI-containing mounting solution (Vector Laboratories). Images of the stained tissues were captured using confocal microscopy (TI-RCP, Nikon).

For immunohistochemistry, sections were permeabilized for 1 h in PBS with 0.2% Triton X-100 and 1% BSA at room temperature. The sections were then incubated with primary antibodies at 4 °C overnight. The next day, the tissues were washed three times with 0.5% BSA and incubated with biotin-conjugated anti-rabbit antibody (1:400, Vector Laboratories) for 1 h at room temperature. After rinsing with 0.5% BSA, the sections were incubated for 1 h at room temperature in avidin-biotin complex solution (Vector Laboratories, Burlingame, CA), followed by rinsing three times in 0.1 M phosphate buffer (PB). The signal was detected by incubating the sections in 0.5 mg/mL 3,3′-diaminobenzidine (DAB, Sigma-Aldrich) in 0.1 M PB containing 0.003% H_2O_2. The sections were rinsed in 0.1 M PB and mounted on gelatin-coated slides, and images were obtained under a bright-field microscope (Leica).

Enzyme-linked immunosorbent assay (ELISA)

To measure the effects of pre- or post-treatment with CA140 on IL-1β, an enzyme-linked immunosorbent assay (ELISA) was performed. Briefly, BV2 microglial cells were treated with LPS (100 ng/mL) or PBS for 30 min, followed by treatment with CA140 (10 μM) or vehicle (1% DMSO). IL-1β ELISA was then performed using the conditioned medium. Mouse IL-1β ELISA kits (ELISA development reagents; R&D Systems, Minneapolis, MN) were used according to the manufacturer's recommendations. Recombinant mouse IL-1β protein

(R&D Systems) was used as a standard. The absorbance of the samples was measured at 450 nm using a microplate reader (BMG Labtech, Offenburg, Germany).

Griess assay
To examine the effects of CA140 on nitrite (NO) production, the Griess assay was performed. BV2 microglial cells were incubated with CA140 (10 μM) or vehicle (1% DMSO) for 30 min, followed by treatment with LPS (100 ng/mL) or PBS for 23.5 h. The conditioned medium was mixed with Griess reagent (0.1% N-(1-naphthyl)ethylenediamine dihydrochloride and 1% sulfanilamide in 2% phosphoric acid) in 96-well plates and incubated at room temperature for 5 min. The absorbance was measured at 540 nm using a microplate reader, and the level of nitrite was analyzed against a standard curve of sodium nitrite.

Western blotting
Cells were lysed using RIPA buffer containing protease and phosphatase inhibitor tablets (Roche, USA). Western blot analysis was performed as previously described [22]. Images were analyzed using Fusion software or ImageJ.

Cytosolic and nuclear fractionation
BV2 microglial cells were lysed in cytosolic fractionation buffer (10 mM HEPES pH 8.0, 1.5 mM $MgCl_2$, 10 mM KCl, 0.5 mM DTT, 300 mM sucrose, 0.1% NP-40, and 0.5 mM PMSF). After 5 min, the cell lysates were centrifuged at 10,000 rpm at 4 °C for 1 min, and the supernatant was stored as the cytosolic fraction. The pellet was lysed in nuclear fractionation buffer (10 mM HEPES pH 8.0, 20% glycerol, 100 mM KCl, 100 mM NaCl, 0.2 mM EDTA, 0.5 mM DTT, and 0.5 mM PMSF) on ice for 15 min, followed by centrifugation at 10,000 rpm at 4 °C for 15 min. The cytosolic and nuclear fractions were analyzed by western blot as previously described [23].

Statistical analyses
All data were analyzed using a two-tailed T test or ANOVA with GraphPad Prism 4 software. Post hoc analyses were performed using Tukey's multiple comparison test with significance set at $p < 0.05$. Data are presented as the mean ± S.E.M. (*$p < 0.05$, **$p < 0.01$, ***$p < 0.001$).

Results
CA140 has no cytotoxicity in BV2 microglial cells up to 25 μM
We recently synthesized CA140 formally by benzoylation of dopamine (DA) with N-Methylisatoic anhydride (Fig. 1a) and examined whether the newly developed CA140 crosses the blood-brain barrier. In a

pharmacokinetic study, we determined that the relevant brain-to-plasma ratio was 1.91 ± 0.22 (brain concentration, 2310–4457 ng/mL), which indicates a high brain distribution of CA140 (data not shown). In addition, we measured the stability of CA140 in vitro and found that the rates of disappearance of CA140 and DA (as a control for CA140) were comparable within the first 8 h. However, after 22 h, more than 40% of CA140 remained in solution, whereas DA was no longer detectable (Fig. 1b).

To examine the effects of CA140 on the LPS-induced neuroinflammatory response, we initially assessed the cytotoxicity of CA140 in BV2 microglial cells. BV2 microglial cells were treated with vehicle (1% DMSO) or CA140 (1, 5, 10, 25, or 50 μM) for 24 h, and MTT assays were performed. CA140 did not affect cell viability up to a concentration of 25 μM; however, CA140 exhibited some toxicity at 50 μM in BV2 microglial cells (Fig. 1c).

We then assessed whether CA140 can alter cell morphology in LPS-stimulated BV2 microglial cells. BV2 microglial cells were pretreated with LPS (1 μg/mL) or PBS for 30 min and treated with vehicle (1% DMSO) or CA140 (10 μM) for 5.5 h. After 6 h, BV2 microglial cells were fixed and immunostained with anti-CD11b and anti-F-actin antibodies. LPS treatment produced aberrant cell morphology of BV2 microglial cells, such as thin fibroblast-like processes from the cell body (Fig. 1d, middle panel). However, treatment with LPS followed by CA140 appeared to rescue this abnormal cell morphology (Fig. 1d, lower panel).

CA140 reduces proinflammatory cytokine levels in LPS-stimulated BV2 microglial cells
To determine whether post-treatment with CA140 reduces proinflammatory responses in LPS-stimulated BV2 microglial cells, cells were pretreated with LPS (1 μg/mL) or PBS for 30 min, followed by treatment with CA140 (5 or 10 μM) or vehicle (1% DMSO) for 5.5 h. Proinflammatory cytokine levels were then measured by RT-PCR. Interestingly, we observed that 5 μM CA140 only significantly decreased LPS-induced IL-1β mRNA levels (Additional file 1: Figure S1a–g). To determine if post-treatment with a higher concentration of CA140 could alter LPS-stimulated increase in proinflammatory cytokine levels, BV2 microglial cells were subjected to the same procedure but with 10 μM CA140, and proinflammatory cytokine levels were measured by RT-PCR. Post-treatment with 10 μM CA140 significantly reduced LPS-induced IL-1β and COX-2 mRNA levels in BV2 microglial cells (Fig. 2a–g). As a complementary study, BV2 microglial cells were treated with LPS (1 μg/mL) or PBS for 30 min, followed by treatment with vehicle (1% DMSO) or CA140 (10 μM) for 5.5 h and analysis by immunocytochemistry. Consistent with our findings above,

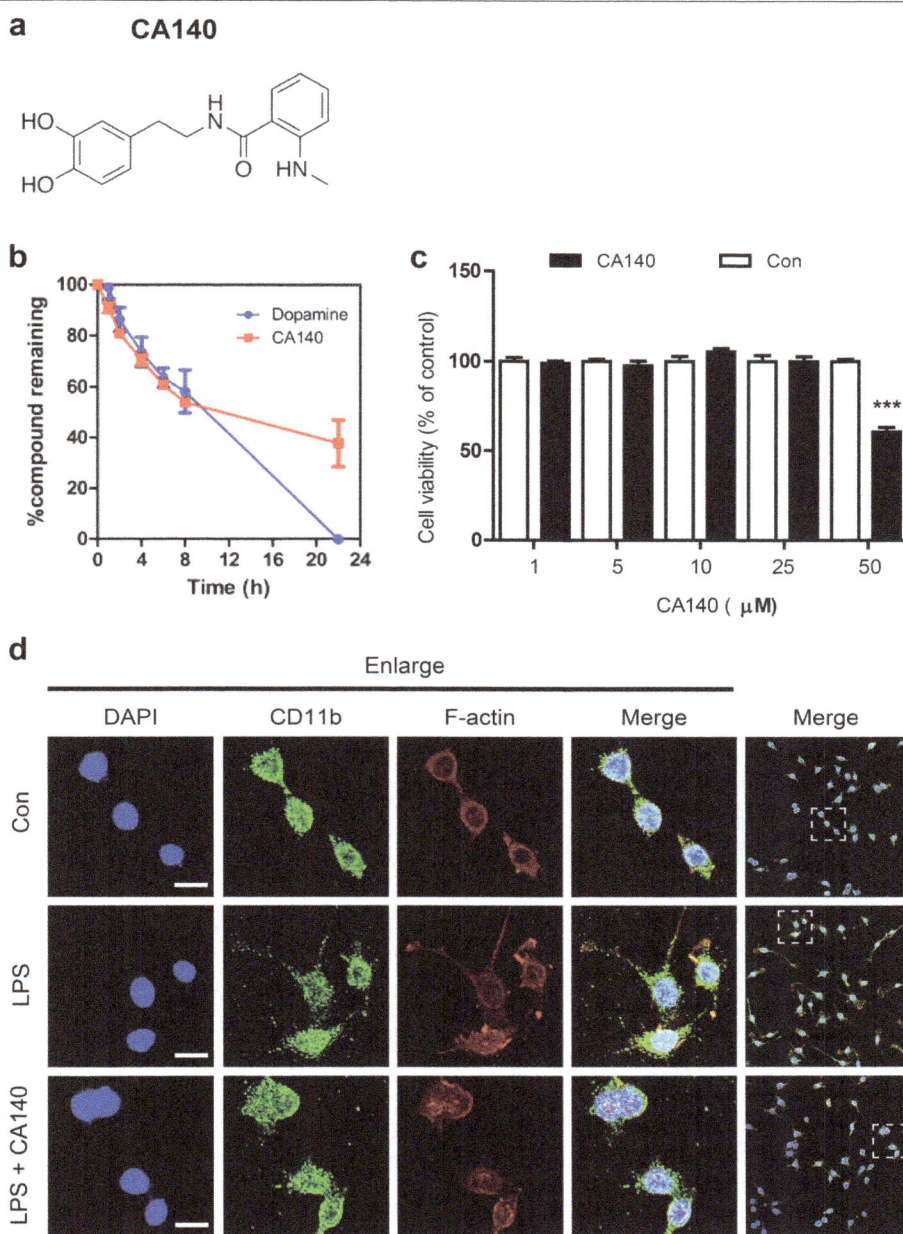

Fig. 1 Concentrations of CA140 up to 25 μM were not toxic in BV2 microglial cells. **a** Structure of CA140. **b** Stability studies of CA140 and dopamine (DA) in vitro. **c** BV2 microglial cells were treated with vehicle (1% DMSO) or CA140 at various concentrations (1, 5, 10, 25, or 50 μM) for 24 h, and cell viability was measured ($n = 8$ for each dose). **d** BV2 microglial cells were pretreated with LPS (1 μg/mL) or PBS for 30 min, followed by treatment with vehicle (1% DMSO) or CA140 (10 μM) for 6 h and immunostaining with anti-CD11b and anti-F-actin antibodies. ***$p < 0.001$

post-treatment with CA140 also significantly reduced the levels of COX-2 and IL-1β in LPS-stimulated BV2 microglial cells (Fig. 2h–k). To further confirm these findings, we conducted an IL-1β ELISA assay. For this experiment, BV2 microglial cells were pretreated with LPS (100 ng/mL) or PBS for 30 min, followed by treatment with CA140 (10 μM) or vehicle (1% DMSO) for 23.5 h. The IL-1β ELISA assay was then performed. Consistent with the findings above,

post-treatment with CA140 significantly decreased LPS-induced IL-1β levels compared with LPS treatment alone (Fig. 2l).

We then examined whether post-treatment with CA140 can further regulate LPS-induced proinflammatory cytokine levels in a longer treatment. BV2 microglial cells were pretreated with LPS (1 μg/mL) or PBS for 30 min, followed by treatment with CA140 (10 μM) or vehicle (1% DMSO) for 11.5 or 23.5 h.

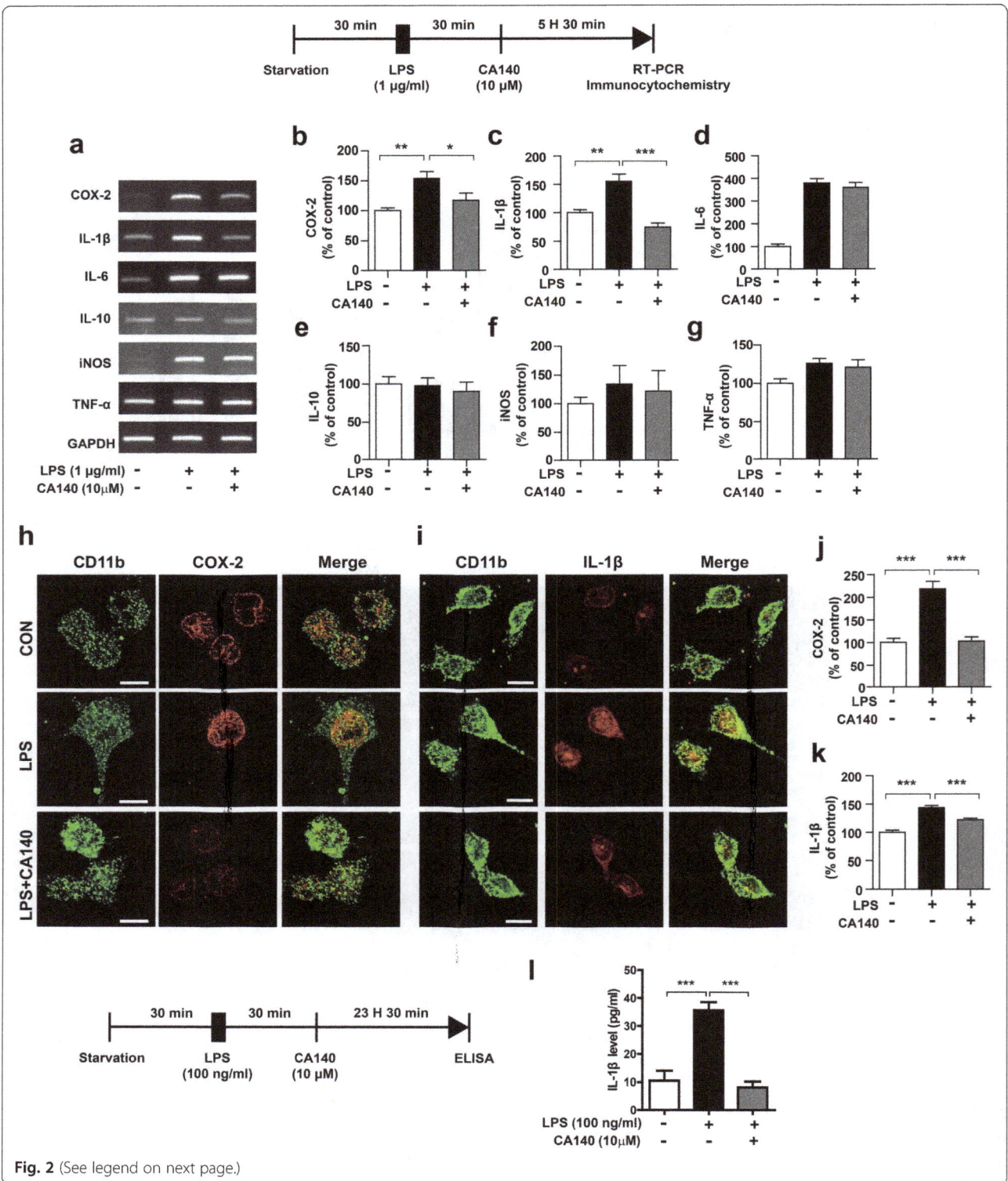

Fig. 2 (See legend on next page.)

(See figure on previous page.)
Fig. 2 Pretreatment with LPS followed by CA140 treatment decreased LPS-induced proinflammatory cytokine levels. **a–g** BV2 microglial cells were pretreated with LPS (1 μg/mL) or PBS for 30 min, followed by treatment with vehicle (1% DMSO) or CA140 (10 μM) for 5.5 h. Total RNA was then isolated, and proinflammatory cytokine levels were measured by RT-PCR (COX-2: con, $n = 17$; LPS, $n = 17$; LPS + CA140, $n = 17$; IL-1β: con, $n = 8$; LPS, $n = 8$; LPS + CA140, $n = 8$; IL-6, IL-10, iNOS, and TNF-alpha: con, $n = 4$; LPS, $n = 4$; LPS + CA140, $n = 4$). **h, j** BV2 microglial cells were pretreated with LPS (1 μg/mL) or PBS for 30 min, followed by treatment with vehicle (1% DMSO) or CA140 (10 μM) for 5.5 h and immunostaining with anti-CD11b and anti-COX-2 antibodies (con, $n = 74$; LPS, $n = 78$; LPS + CA140, $n = 84$). **i, k** BV2 microglial cells were pretreated with LPS (1 μg/mL) or PBS for 30 min, followed by treatment with vehicle (1% DMSO) or CA140 (10 μM) for 5.5 h and immunostaining with anti-CD11b and anti-IL-1β antibodies (con, $n = 314$; LPS, $n = 268$; LPS + CA140, $n = 234$). **l** BV2 microglial cells were pretreated with LPS (100 ng/mL) or PBS for 30 min, followed by treatment with vehicle (1% DMSO) or CA140 (10 μM) for 23.5 h and measurement of IL-1β levels using IL-1β ELISA (con, $n = 8$; LPS, $n = 8$; LPS + CA140, $n = 8$). *$p < 0.05$, **$p < 0.001$, ***$p < 0.0001$

Proinflammatory cytokine levels were then measured by RT-PCR. Interestingly, post-treatment with CA140 significantly suppressed LPS-induced proinflammatory cytokine levels in a time-dependent manner (Additional file 1: Figure S2a–l).

We subsequently examined whether pretreatment with CA140 prevents LPS-induced neuroinflammatory responses. BV2 microglial cells were incubated with CA140 (5 μM) or vehicle (1% DMSO) for 30 min, followed by LPS (1 μg/mL) or PBS for 5.5 h. Proinflammatory cytokine levels were evaluated by RT-PCR. Pretreatment with 5 μM CA140 followed by LPS treatment did not decrease proinflammatory cytokine levels (Additional file 1: Figure S3a–g). However, pretreatment with 10 μM CA140 significantly reduced the mRNA levels of COX-2, IL-1β, and iNOS (Additional file 1: Figure S3h–n). In addition, pretreatment with CA140 at 10 μM significantly decreased LPS-induced IL-1β and NO levels as assessed by IL-1β ELISA or the Griess assay (Additional file 1: Figure S3o–p).

We then investigated whether pretreatment with CA140 further regulates LPS-induced proinflammatory cytokine levels in a longer treatment. BV2 microglial cells were incubated with CA140 (10 μM) or vehicle (1% DMSO) for 30 min, followed by LPS (1 μg/mL) or PBS for 11.5 or 23.5 h. Longer pretreatment with CA140 further reduced LPS-induced mRNA levels of the proinflammatory cytokines COX-2, IL-1β, and iNOS compared with pretreatment for 6 h (Additional file 1: Figure S4a–h). These results suggest that CA140 both reduces and prevents proinflammatory responses in LPS-induced BV2 microglial cells. Based on these findings, we selected 10 μM CA140 as our optimal working concentration for further experiments.

CA140 reduces LPS-induced proinflammatory cytokine levels in primary microglial cells and primary astrocytes

Although BV2 microglial cells have been extensively used as an alternative model system for investigating microglial function in neuroinflammation [24], we aimed to examine whether pre- or post-treatment with CA140 modulates proinflammatory responses in different cell types, such as primary microglial cells or primary astrocytes. For these experiments, rat primary microglial or primary astrocyte cultures in high-glucose DMEM were used. Rat primary microglial cells were treated with LPS (1 μg/mL) or PBS for 30 min, followed by vehicle (1% DMSO) or CA140 (10 μM) for 5.5 h. Proinflammatory cytokine levels were measured by RT-PCR. Post-treatment with CA140 significantly decreased the mRNA levels of COX-2 and IL-1β in LPS-stimulated rat primary microglial cells (Additional file 1: Figure S5a–f) but failed to lower proinflammatory cytokine levels in LPS-induced rat primary astrocytes (Additional file 1: Figure S5g–l).

We subsequently examined whether pretreatment with CA140 differentially regulates LPS-induced proinflammatory responses in rat primary microglial cells and primary astrocytes. Rat primary microglial cells or primary astrocytes were pretreated with CA140 (10 μM) or vehicle (1% DMSO) for 30 min, followed by treatment with LPS (1 μg/mL) or PBS for 5.5 h. Proinflammatory cytokine levels were then measured by RT-PCR. Interestingly, pretreatment with CA140 reduced LPS-induced COX-2, IL-1β, iNOS, and TNF-α mRNA levels in rat primary microglial cells (Additional file 1: Figure S6a–f). In addition, pretreatment with CA140 significantly decreased the mRNA levels of IL-6 and iNOS in rat primary astrocytes (Additional file 1: Figure S6g–l).

Several recent studies have demonstrated that primary glial cells can be activated by high glucose levels [25–28]. Thus, we cultured primary glial cells under low-glucose DMEM conditions to test whether pre-or post-treatment with CA140 can differentially affect LPS-induced neuroinflammatory responses under low-glucose conditions. Mouse primary microglial cells were treated with LPS (1 μg/mL) or PBS for 30 min, followed by vehicle (1% DMSO) or CA140 (10 μM) for 5.5 h, and proinflammatory cytokine levels were measured by RT-PCR. Post-treatment with CA140 significantly reduced IL-6, iNOS, and TNF-alpha mRNA levels in LPS-stimulated mouse primary microglial cells (Fig. 3a–f). Interestingly, post-treatment with CA140 significantly suppressed LPS-stimulated iNOS mRNA levels in primary astrocytes but not the levels of other proinflammatory cytokines

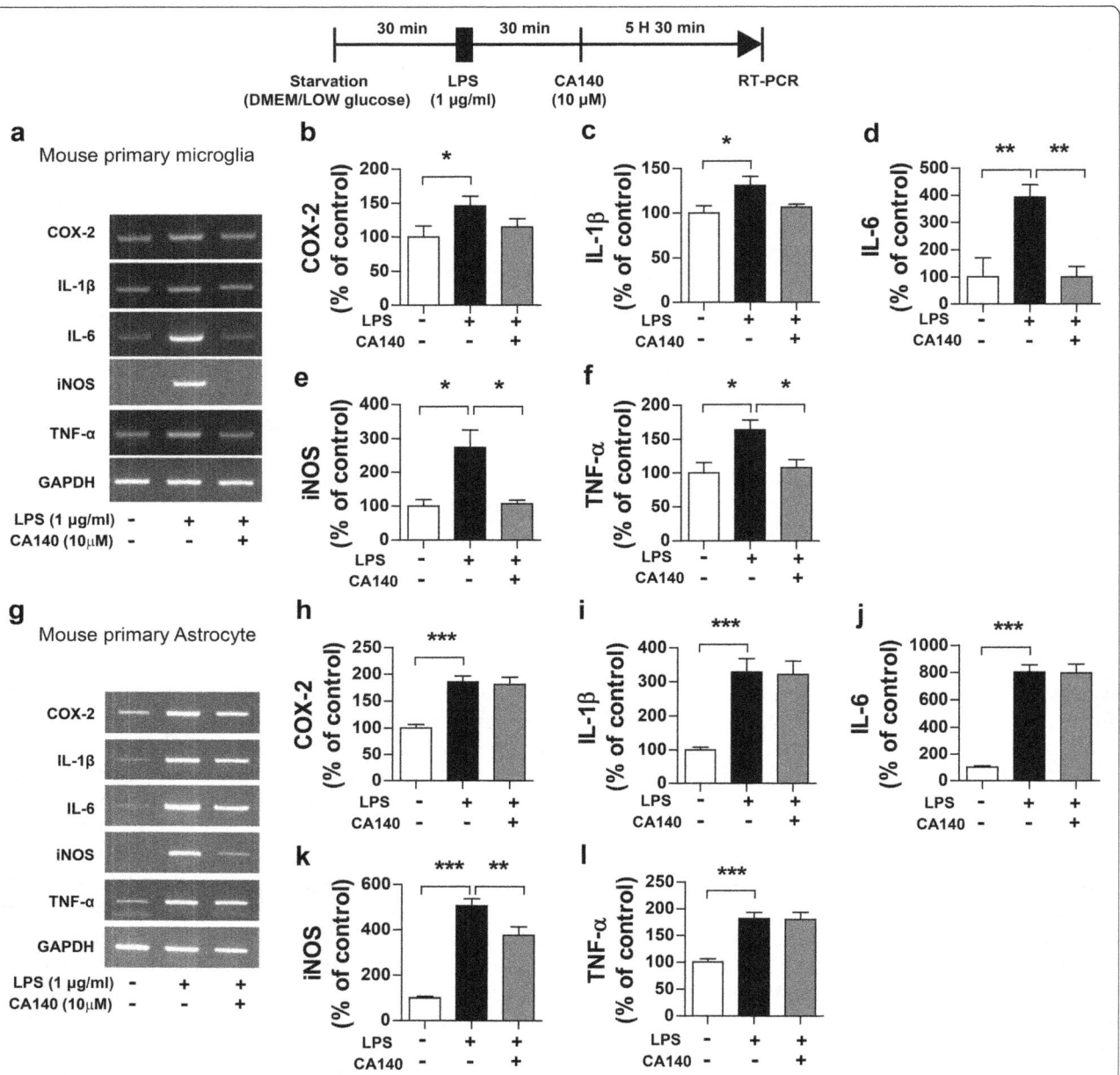

Fig. 3 Pretreatment with LPS followed by CA140 treatment decreased LPS-induced proinflammatory cytokine levels in mouse primary microglial cells. **a–f** Mouse primary microglial cells were pretreated with LPS (1 µg/mL) or PBS for 30 min, followed by treatment with vehicle (1% DMSO) or CA140 (10 µM) for 5.5 h. Total RNA was then isolated, and proinflammatory cytokine levels were measured by RT-PCR (con, $n = 4$; LPS, $n = 4$; LPS + CA140, $n = 4$). **g–l** Mouse primary astrocytes were pretreated with LPS (1 µg/mL) or PBS for 30 min, followed by treatment with vehicle (1% DMSO) or CA140 (10 µM) for 5.5 h. Total RNA was then isolated, and proinflammatory cytokine levels were measured by RT-PCR (COX-2: con, $n = 20$; LPS, $n = 20$; LPS + CA140, $n = 20$; IL-1β: con, $n = 20$; LPS, $n = 20$; LPS + CA140, $n = 20$; IL-6, iNOS, and TNF-alpha: con, $n = 16$; LPS, $n = 16$; LPS + CA140, $n = 16$). *$p < 0.05$, **$p < 0.001$, ***$p < 0.0001$

(Fig. 3g–l). In addition, pretreatment with CA140 significantly decreased LPS-induced proinflammatory cytokine levels in mouse primary microglial cells and primary astrocytes (Additional file 1: Figure S7a–l). These results indicate that the timing of CA140 treatment and culture conditions (high vs low glucose) can differentially affect the LPS-induced proinflammatory response depending on cell type. The alleviatory effect of CA140 was specific to microglial cells.

CA140 regulates the dopamine D1 receptor to alter proinflammatory cytokine levels

Because CA140 is structurally related to DA, we hypothesized that CA140 may directly or indirectly interact with DA receptors (i.e., D1R, D2R) to alter the neuroinflammatory response. To test this idea, we initially investigated whether BV2 microglial cells present endogenous dopamine D1 receptor (D1R) or dopamine D2 receptor (D2R). For the initial experiment, BV2 microglial cells were pretreated with LPS (1 μg/mL) or PBS for 30 min, followed by treatment with CA140 (10 μM) or vehicle (1% DMSO) for 5.5 h, and the mRNA levels of D1R were measured by RT-PCR. Interestingly, LPS treatment significantly increased D1R mRNA levels, whereas treatment with LPS followed by CA140 significantly downregulated D1R mRNA levels (Additional file 1: Figure S8a–b). To further confirm these findings, we performed immunocytochemistry with anti-CD11b and anti-D1R antibodies and determined that post-treatment with CA140 reduced D1R levels compared with LPS treatment (Additional file 1: Figure S8c, d).

We subsequently examined whether post-treatment with CA140 can alter D2R levels. BV2 microglial cells were pretreated with LPS (1 μg/mL) or PBS for 30 min, followed by treatment with CA140 (10 μM) or vehicle (1% DMSO) for 5.5 h and immunocytochemistry with anti-CD11b and anti-D2R antibodies. Interestingly, LPS treatment significantly increased D2R levels in BV2 microglial cells (Additional file 1: Figure S8e, f). However, post-treatment with CA140 did not alter D2R levels compared with LPS treatment (Additional file 1: Figure S8e, f), which suggests that CA140 modulates only LPS-induced D1R expression levels in BV2 microglial cells.

To examine whether D1R or D2R affects the LPS-stimulated proinflammatory response, BV2 microglial cells were treated with LPS (1 μg/mL) or PBS for 30 min, followed by treatment with a D1R antagonist (LE300, 10 μM) or vehicle (1% DMSO) for 5.5 h. Proinflammatory cytokine levels were then measured by RT-PCR. LE300 treatment significantly reduced LPS-stimulated COX-2 and IL-1β mRNA levels (Fig. 4a–f), which suggests that inhibition of D1R regulates the proinflammatory response in LPS-induced BV2 microglial cells.

Next, to investigate whether CA140 further regulates the neuroinflammatory response in the presence of a D1R antagonist, BV2 microglial cells were pretreated with LPS (1 μg/mL) or PBS for 30 min, followed by treatment with LE300 (a D1R antagonist, 10 μM) or vehicle (1% DMSO) for 30 min and finally CA140 (10 μM) or vehicle (1% DMSO) for 5 h. Subsequent RT-PCR analysis revealed that treatment with LE300, CA140, and LPS further inhibited IL-1β mRNA levels compared with treatment with LE300 and LPS or CA140 and LPS (Fig. 4g–h).

To further confirm these findings, BV2 microglial cells were treated with LPS (1 μg/mL) or PBS for 30 min, followed by another D1R antagonist (SCH23390, 30 μM)

or vehicle (1% DMSO) for 5.5 h, and proinflammatory cytokine levels were measured by RT-PCR. SCH23390 treatment significantly decreased LPS-induced COX-2 and IL-1β mRNA levels (Fig. 4i–n). In addition, treatment with SCH23390, CA140, and LPS further inhibited LPS-stimulated COX-2 and IL-1β mRNA levels compared with treatment with LPS and SCH23390 (Fig. 4o–p).

Next, to examine whether D1R agonist treatment alters neuroinflammatory responses, BV2 microglial cells were treated with LPS (1 μg/mL) or PBS for 30 min, followed by a D1R agonist (A77636, 10 nM) or PBS for 5.5 h and measurement of proinflammatory cytokine levels by RT-PCR. A77636 treatment did not decrease any LPS-induced proinflammatory cytokine levels (Fig. 5a–f).

We then investigated whether CA140 modulates neuroinflammatory responses in the presence of a D1R agonist. BV2 microglial cells were pretreated with LPS (1 μg/mL) or PBS for 30 min, followed by treatment with A77636 (a D1R agonist, 10 nM) or PBS for 30 min and finally CA140 (10 μM) or vehicle (1% DMSO) for 5 h; we subsequently performed RT-PCR. Consistent with our findings above, post-treatment with CA140 dramatically reduced LPS-induced IL-1β mRNA levels (Fig. 5g–h). Most importantly, treatment with LPS, A77636, and CA140 significantly reduced LPS-induced IL-1β mRNA levels compared with treatment with A77636 and LPS (Fig. 5g–h).

We subsequently examined whether D2R inhibition affects the proinflammatory response in LPS-induced BV2 microglial cells and found that treatment with D2R antagonist did not suppress LPS-induced proinflammatory cytokine levels (Additional file 1: Figure S9a–f). In addition, treatment with LPS, EH, and CA140 did not decrease LPS-induced IL-1β mRNA levels compared with treatment with EH and LPS or CA140 and LPS (Additional file 1: Figure S9g–h). Taken together, these results suggest that CA140 may modulate D1R to alter proinflammatory responses.

CA140 alters LPS-induced ERK signaling in BV2 microglial cells

Several studies have shown that ERK and AKT signaling plays an important role in regulating proinflammatory cytokines in microglial cells [29]. Thus, we investigated whether pre- or post-treatment with CA140 regulates ERK and AKT signaling to alter the LPS-induced neuroinflammatory response. BV2 microglial cells were pretreated with LPS (1 μg/mL) or PBS for 45 min, followed by treatment with CA140 (10 μM) or vehicle (1% DMSO) for 45 min and western blotting with anti-p-ERK/ERK or anti-p-AKT/AKT antibodies. Post-treatment with CA140 did not significantly alter p-AKT levels (Fig. 6a–c), whereas post-treatment with

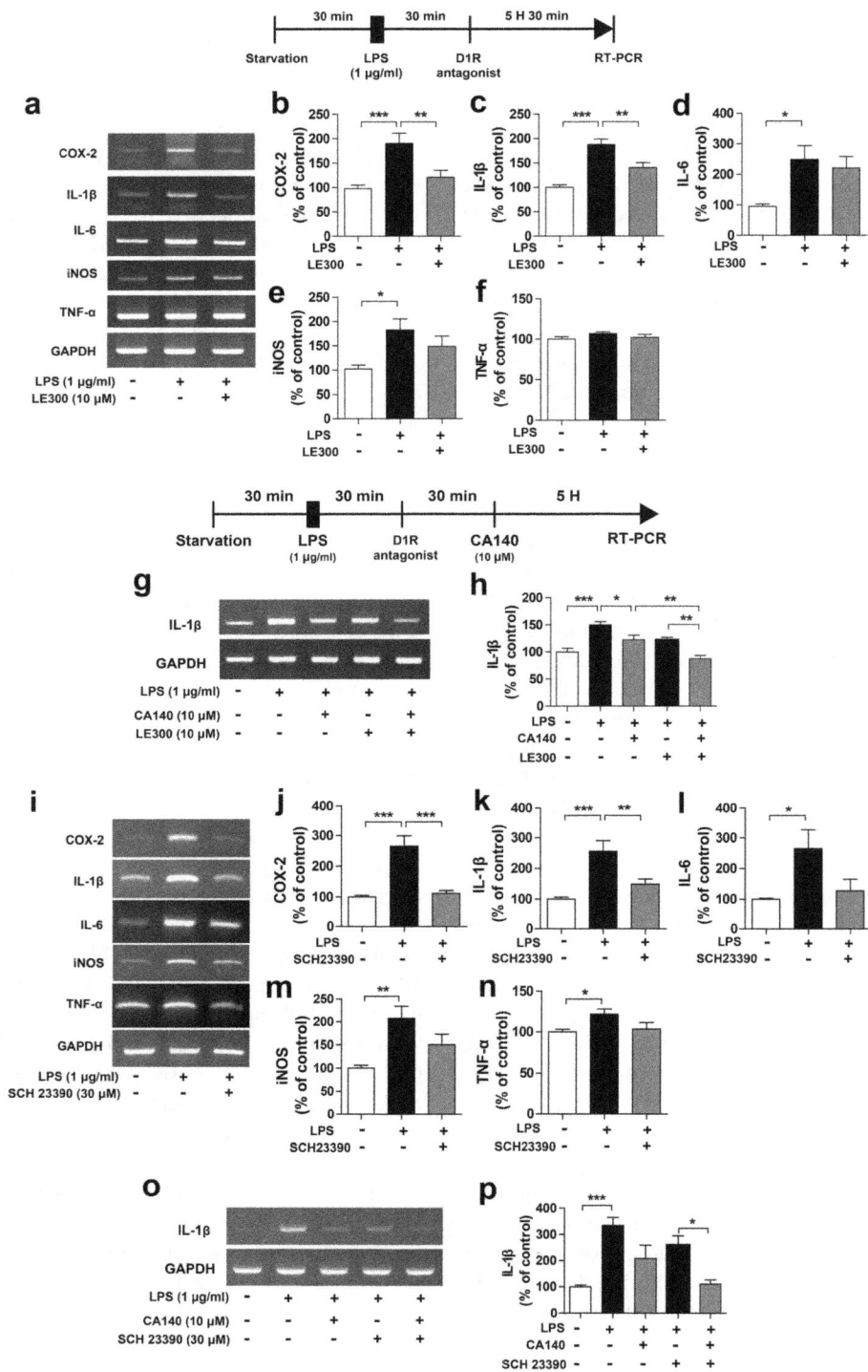

Fig. 4 (See legend on next page.)

(See figure on previous page.)
Fig. 4 CA140 downregulated LPS-induced neuroinflammatory responses with D1R inhibition. **a** Representative images of proinflammatory cytokine mRNA levels in BV2 microglial cells. **b–f** BV2 microglial cells were pretreated with LPS (1 μg/mL) or PBS for 30 min, followed by treatment with vehicle (1% DMSO) or LE300 (a D1R antagonist, 10 μM) for 5.5 h 30 min. Total RNA was then isolated, and proinflammatory cytokine levels were measured by RT-PCR (IL-1β: con, $n = 20$; LPS, $n = 20$; LPS + CA140, $n = 20$; COX-2, IL-6, iNOS, and TNF-alpha: con, $n = 10$; LPS, $n = 10$; LPS + CA140, $n = 10$). **g–h** BV2 microglial cells were pretreated with LPS (1 μg/mL) or PBS for 30 min, followed by treatment with vehicle (1% DMSO) or LE300 (10 μM) for 30 min and finally CA140 (10 μM) or vehicle (1% DMSO) for 5 h. Total RNA was then isolated, and IL-1β mRNA levels were measured by RT-PCR (con, $n = 16$; LPS, $n = 16$; LPS + CA140, $n = 16$). **i–n** BV2 microglial cells were pretreated with LPS (1 μg/mL) or PBS for 30 min, followed by treatment with vehicle (1% DMSO) or SCH23390 (a D1R antagonist, 30 μM) for 5.5 h. Total RNA was then isolated, and proinflammatory cytokine levels were measured by RT-PCR (con, $n = 12$; LPS, $n = 12$; LPS + CA140, $n = 12$). **o–p** BV2 microglial cells were pretreated with LPS (1 μg/ml) or PBS for 30 min, followed by treatment with SCH23390 (30 μM) or vehicle (1% DMSO) for 30 min and finally CA140 (10 μM) or vehicle (1% DMSO) for 5 h. Total RNA was then isolated, and IL-1β mRNA levels were measured by RT-PCR (con, $n = 14$; LPS, $n = 14$; LPS + CA140, $n = 14$). $*p < 0.05$, $**p < 0.001$, $***p < 0.0001$

CA140 significantly decreased p-ERK levels in LPS-stimulated BV2 microglial cells (Fig. 6d–f).

We subsequently assessed whether post-treatment with CA140 regulates the LPS-stimulated proinflammatory response through ERK signaling. BV2 microglial cells were pretreated with LPS (1 μg/mL) or PBS for 30 min, followed by treatment with PD98059 (an ERK inhibitor, 10 μM) or vehicle (1% DMSO) for 30 min and finally vehicle (1% DMSO) or CA140 (10 μM) for 5 h. The mRNA levels of COX-2 and IL-1β were measured by RT-PCR. Consistent with our previously described findings, post-treatment with CA140 significantly decreased the mRNA levels of COX-2 and IL-1β (Fig. 6g–i). In addition, compared with LPS and PD98059 treatment, treatment with LPS, PD98059, and CA140 further decreased COX-2 and IL-1β mRNA levels (Fig. 6g–i).

We then examined whether pretreatment with CA140 alters ERK and AKT signaling. BV2 cells were pretreated with vehicle (1% DMSO) or CA140 (10 μM) for 45 min, followed by LPS (1 μg/mL) or PBS treatment for 45 min and western blotting with anti-p-ERK/ERK or anti-p-AKT/AKT antibodies. Interestingly, pretreatment with CA140 significantly suppressed the phosphorylation of ERK and AKT in LPS-treated BV2 microglial cells (Additional file 1: Figure S10a–f). These data suggest that pre- or post-treatment with CA140 differentially affects ERK and AKT signaling.

CA140 suppresses LPS-induced cytosolic and nuclear p-STAT3 in BV2 microglial cells

STAT3 plays an important role in the regulation of proinflammatory cytokine levels induced by LPS [30]. Thus, we examined whether CA140 regulates STAT3 expression in the nucleus and cytosol. BV2 microglial cells were pretreated with LPS (1 μg/mL) or PBS for 30 min, followed by treatment with vehicle (1% DMSO) or CA140 (10 μM) for 5.5 h and subcellular fractionation. LPS treatment significantly increased p-STAT3 (Ser727) levels in the cytosol and nucleus (Fig. 7a–d). In addition, post-treatment with CA140 significantly reduced LPS-induced cytosolic and nuclear p-STAT3 (Ser727) levels (Fig. 7a–d). As a

complementary study, we conducted immunocytochemistry with anti-CD11b and anti-p-STAT3 (Ser727) antibodies and determined that post-treatment with CA140 significantly decreased LPS-induced p-STAT3 (Ser727) levels in the nucleus (Fig. 7e–f).

In addition, we investigated whether pretreatment with CA140 alters LPS-stimulated p-STAT3 levels in the cytosol and nucleus. For this experiment, BV2 microglial cells were pretreated with vehicle (1% DMSO) or CA140 (10 μM) for 30 min, followed by treatment with LPS (1 μg/mL) or PBS for 5.5 h and subcellular fractionation. Pretreatment with CA140 also significantly decreased LPS-induced cytosolic and nuclear p-STAT3 (Ser727) levels (Additional file 1: Figure S11a–d).

We then examined whether CA140 further regulates the LPS-induced proinflammatory response in the presence of a STAT3 inhibitor. BV2 microglial cells were pretreated with LPS (1 μg/mL) or PBS for 30 min, followed by treatment with S31-201 (a STAT3 inhibitor, 50 μM) or vehicle (1% DMSO) for 30 min and finally vehicle (1% DMSO) or CA140 (10 μM) for 5 h. The mRNA levels of COX-2 and IL-1β were then measured by RT-PCR. Compared with treatment with LPS and S3I-201 or with LPS and CA140, treatment with LPS, S3I-201, and CA140 further decreased IL-1β and COX-2 mRNA levels (Fig. 7g–i). These data suggest that CA140 modulates STAT3 signaling to regulate the LPS-stimulated neuroinflammatory response.

CA140 significantly reduces the activation of microglia and astrocytes in LPS-injected wild-type mice

Numerous studies have shown that activated microglia and astrocytes are involved in neuroinflammatory responses [31]. To examine whether post-treatment with CA140 alters microglial and astrocyte activation in vivo, wild-type mice were injected with LPS (10 mg/kg/day, i.p.) or PBS, followed 30 min later by injection with CA140 (30 mg/kg, i.p., twice with an interval of 1 h, followed 30 min later by a third injection) or vehicle (10% DMSO), and immunohistochemistry was performed with anti-Iba-1 and anti-GFAP antibodies. As expected, LPS-injected wild-type mice exhibited

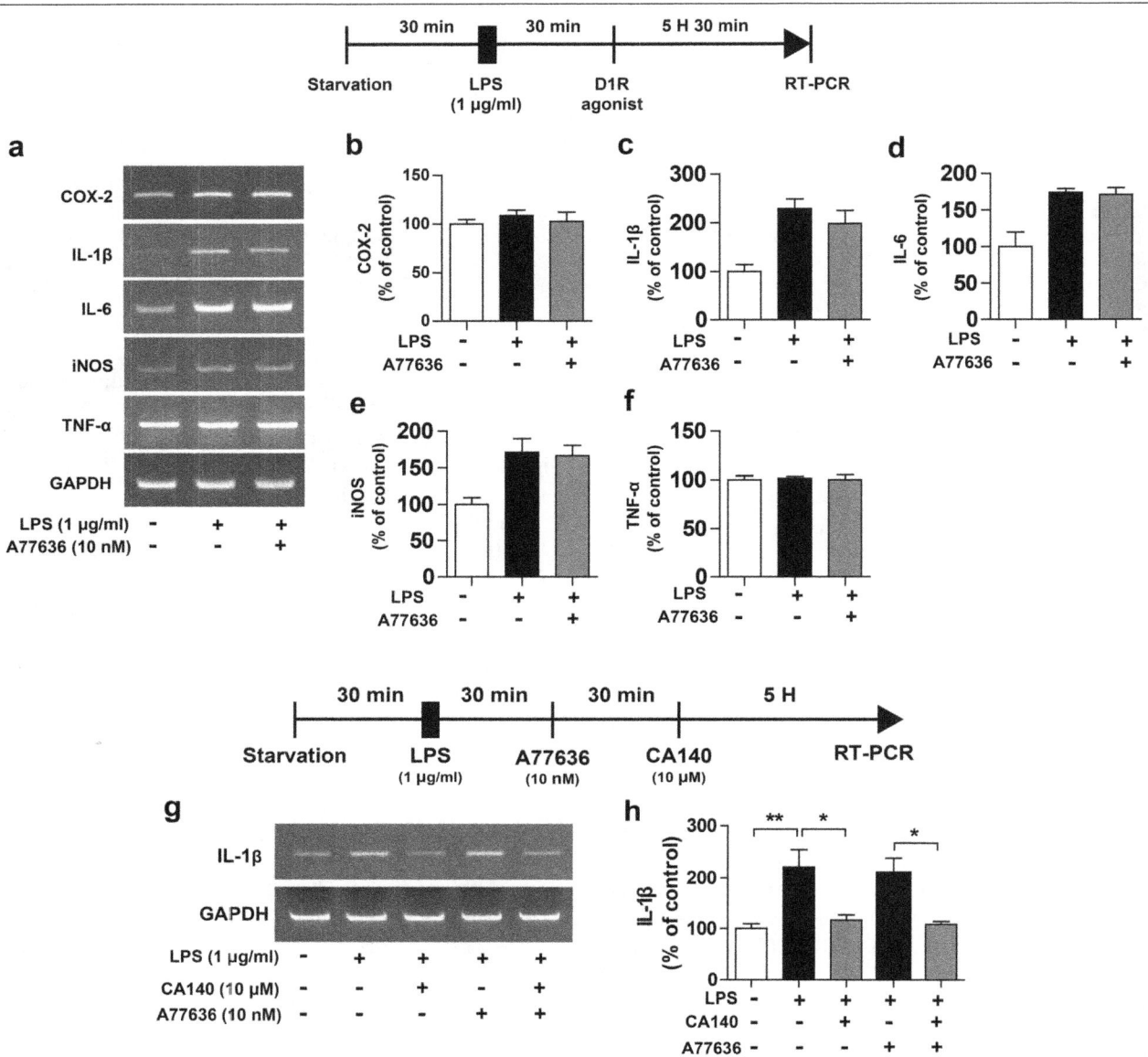

Fig. 5 Post-treatment with CA140 significantly reduced LPS-induced IL-1β mRNA levels in the presence of a D1R agonist. **a** Representative images of proinflammatory cytokine mRNA levels in BV2 microglial cells. **b–f** BV2 microglial cells were pretreated with LPS (1 μg/mL) or PBS for 30 min, followed by treatment with vehicle (1% DMSO) or A77636 (a D1R agonist, 10 nM) for 5.5 h. Total RNA was then isolated, and proinflammatory cytokine levels were measured by RT-PCR (COX-2, IL-1β, IL-6, iNOS, and TNF-alpha: con, $n = 4$; LPS, $n = 4$; LPS + CA140, $n = 4$).
g–h BV2 microglial cells were pretreated with LPS (1 μg/mL) or PBS for 30 min, followed by treatment with vehicle (1% DMSO) or A77636 (10 nM) for 30 min and finally CA140 (10 μM) or vehicle (1% DMSO) for 5 h. Total RNA was then isolated, and IL-1β mRNA levels were measured by RT-PCR (con, $n = 6$; LPS, $n = 6$; LPS + CA140, $n = 5$). *$p < 0.05$, **$p < 0.001$

significantly increased Iba-1 (Fig. 8a–c) and GFAP (Fig. 8d–f) immunoreactivity in the hippocampus and cortex. In addition, post-treatment with CA140 significantly reduced microglial (Fig. 8a–c) and astrocyte (Fig. 8d–f) immunoreactivity compared with LPS-injected wild-type mice.

We subsequently examined whether post-treatment with CA140 alters LPS-stimulated proinflammatory cytokine levels in wild-type mice. For this experiment, wild-type mice were injected with LPS (10 mg/kg/day, i.p.) or PBS, followed 30 min later by injection with CA140 (30 mg/kg, i.p., twice with an interval of 1 h, followed 30 min later by a third injection) or vehicle (10% DMSO, i.p). Immunohistochemistry was performed with anti-IL-1β and anti-COX-2 antibodies. Post-treatment with CA140 significantly downregulated LPS-stimulated IL-1β (Fig. 9a–e) and COX-2 (Fig. 9f–h) immunoreactivity in the cortex and hippocampus.

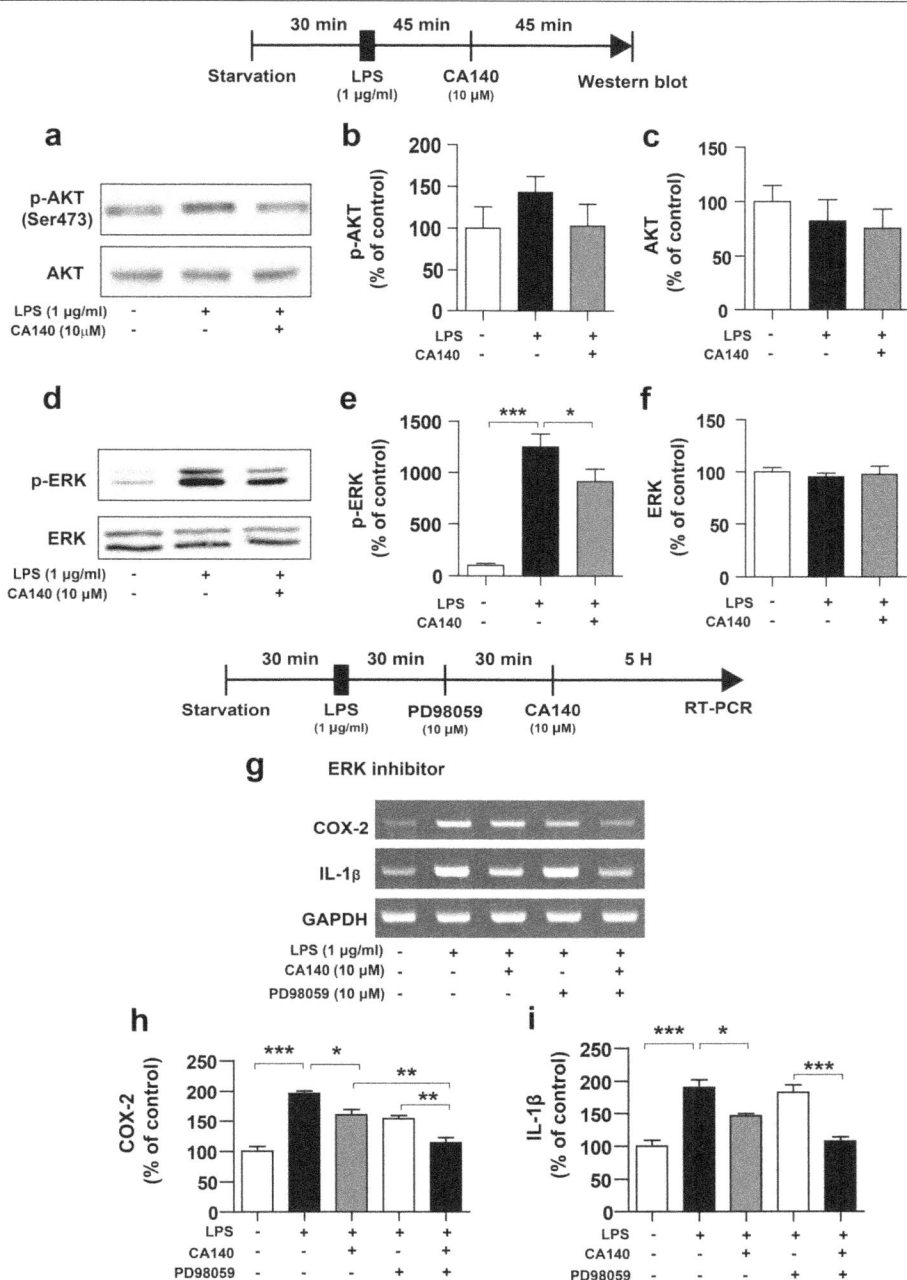

Fig. 6 Pretreatment with LPS followed by CA140 treatment decreased ERK signaling in LPS-stimulated BV2 cells. **a–c** BV2 microglial cells were pretreated with LPS (1 µg/mL) or PBS for 45 min, followed by treatment with vehicle (1% DMSO) or CA140 (10 µM) for 45 min and western blotting with anti-p-AKT and anti-AKT antibodies (p-AKT and AKT; con, $n = 5$; LPS, $n = 5$; LPS + CA140, $n = 5$). **d–f** BV2 cells were pretreated with LPS (1 µg/ml) or PBS for 45 min, followed by treatment with vehicle (1% DMSO) or CA140 (10 µM) for 45 min and western blotting with anti-p-ERK and anti-ERK antibodies (p-ERK and ERK; con, $n = 6$; LPS, $n = 6$; LPS + CA140, $n = 6$). **g–i** BV2 microglial cells were pretreated with LPS (1 µg/mL) or PBS for 30 min, followed by treatment with an ERK inhibitor (PD98059, 10 µM) or vehicle (1% DMSO) for 30 min and finally CA140 (10 µM) or vehicle (1% DMSO) for 5 h. Total RNA was then isolated, and IL-1β or COX-2 mRNA levels were measured by RT-PCR (COX-2 and IL-1β: con, $n = 4$; LPS, $n = 4$; LPS + CA140, $n = 4$). *$p < 0.05$, **$p < 0.001$, ***$p < 0.0001$

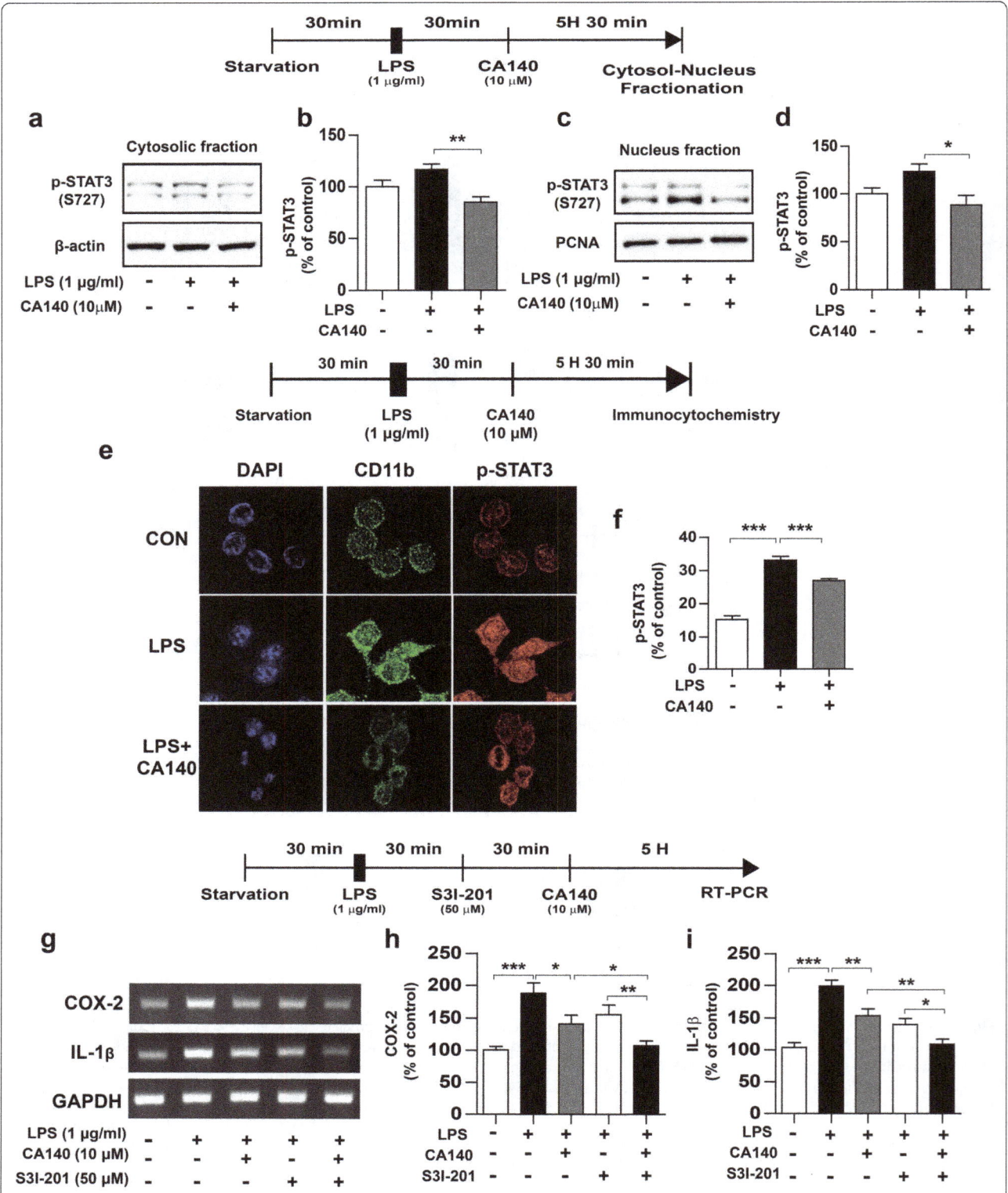

Fig. 7 (See legend on next page.)

(See figure on previous page.)
Fig. 7 Pretreatment with LPS followed by CA140 treatment decreased phosphorylation of STAT3 in the nucleus and cytosol. **a** BV2 microglial cells were pretreated with LPS (1 μg/mL) or PBS for 45 min, followed by treatment with vehicle (1% DMSO) or CA140 (10 μM) for 5.5 h and subcellular fractionation (nuclear and cytosolic fractions). Western blotting was performed on the cytosolic fraction using antibodies against p-STAT3 (Ser727) and β-actin. **b** Quantification of data from **a** (con, $n = 12$; LPS, $n = 12$; LPS + CA140, $n = 12$). **c, d** Western blotting was performed on the nuclear fraction using anti-p-STAT3 (Ser727) and anti-PCNA antibodies (con, $n = 12$; LPS, $n = 12$; LPS + CA140, $n = 12$). **e, f** BV2 microglial cells were pretreated with LPS (1 μg/ml) or PBS for 30 min, followed by treatment with vehicle (1% DMSO) or CA140 (10 μM) for 5.5 h and immunostaining with anti-p-STAT3 (Ser727) and anti-CD11b antibodies (con, $n = 202$; LPS, $n = 169$; LPS + CA140, $n = 397$). **g–i** BV2 microglial cells were pretreated with LPS (1 μg/mL) or PBS for 30 min, followed by treatment with a STAT3 inhibitor (S3I-301, 10 μM) or vehicle (1% DMSO) for 30 min and finally CA140 (10 μM) or vehicle (1% DMSO) for 5 h. Total RNA was then isolated, and IL-1β or COX-2 mRNA levels were measured by RT-PCR (COX-2 and IL-1β: con, $n = 17$; LPS, $n = 17$; LPS + CA140, $n = 17$). $*p < 0.05$, $**p < 0.01$, $***p < 0.0001$

To further examine whether pretreatment with CA140 attenuates microglial and astrocyte activation, wild-type mice were injected with CA140 (30 mg/kg, i.p.) or vehicle (10% DMSO, i.p.) daily for 3 days, followed by injection with LPS (10 mg/kg/day, i.p.) or PBS. Three hours later, immunohistochemistry was conducted with anti-Iba-1 and anti-GFAP antibodies. We observed that pretreatment with CA140 also significantly decreased microglial and astrocyte immunoreactivity (Additional file 1: Figure S12a–f). These results suggest that CA140 may be beneficial for the prevention and treatment of neuroinflammatory-related disease.

CA140 significantly decreases the activation of microglia and astrocytes in a mouse model of AD

Neuroinflammation and microglial activation are closely associated with neurodegenerative diseases, including AD [32–34]. Thus, we aimed to examine whether CA140 regulates microglial and astrocyte activation in a mouse model of AD. 5xFAD mice (3 months old) were injected with CA140 (30 mg/kg, i.p.) or vehicle (10% DMSO, i.p.) daily for 2 weeks. After 2 weeks, immunohistochemistry was performed with anti-Iba-1 (a microglial cell marker, Fig. 10a–e) and anti-GFAP (an astrocyte marker, Fig. 10f–j) antibodies. CA140-injected 5xFAD mice had significantly reduced Iba-1 immunoreactivity in the hippocampus CA1 (Fig. 10a, b) and cortex (Fig. 10d, e) but not the dentate gyrus (Fig. 10a, c). Furthermore, CA140-injected 5xFAD mice had significantly suppressed GFAP immunoreactivity in the hippocampus DG (Fig. 10f, h) and cortex (Fig. 10i, j) but not the hippocampus CA1 (Fig. 10f, g). These data suggest that CA140 modulates microglial and astrocyte activation in a mouse model of AD.

Discussion

Increasing evidence is highlighting the critical role of the immune system in neurodegenerative diseases such as AD. Unchecked glial activation and neuroinflammation may represent hallmark diagnostic features of neurodegenerative diseases. However, research to explicate the mechanisms underlying neuroinflammation has been limited.

Several recent studies have demonstrated that microglia and astrocytes release proinflammatory cytokines, leading to neuronal cell death and synaptic dysfunction in neurodegenerative diseases, including AD [35, 36]. The release of these cytokines may be induced by LPS in vivo and in vitro via Toll-like receptors [37, 38]. McGeer et al. determined that neuroinflammation stimulated by a single intraperitoneal injection of LPS lasted 10 months in the mouse brain and eventually led to neurodegeneration. Therefore, the identification of agents that reduce proinflammatory cytokine levels may represent a promising strategy for developing drugs to treat neurodegenerative diseases.

In this study, we synthesized a novel analog of dopamine, CA140 that can penetrate the blood-brain barrier. We determined that 10 μM CA140 was effective for lowering LPS-induced proinflammatory cytokine levels in BV2 microglial cells regardless of the timing of treatment (Fig. 2, Additional file 1: Figure S1). However, post-treatment with 5 μM CA140 only reduced the mRNA levels of LPS-induced IL-1β and not those of other proinflammatory cytokines. Our findings imply that an appropriate concentration of CA140 may be efficiently employed to both reduce and prevent neuroinflammatory responses in LPS-stimulated BV2 microglial cells. In addition, we observed that pretreatment with CA140 significantly reduced LPS-induced proinflammatory cytokine levels in rat primary microglia and primary astrocytes under high-glucose conditions (Additional file 1: Figure S6). However, post-treatment with CA140 only affected the LPS-stimulated proinflammatory response in rat primary microglial cells and not primary astrocytes under high-glucose conditions (Additional file 1: Figure S6). Why do pre- and post-treatment with CA140 have different effects on LPS-induced proinflammatory responses? Several recent studies have reported that high glucose levels induce primary glial cell activation [25–28]. Thus, we conducted additional experiments to assess the anti-inflammatory effects of CA140 on primary glial cells under low-glucose conditions. Pre- or post-treatment with CA140 significantly reduced LPS-stimulated proinflammatory cytokine levels in mouse primary microglial cells

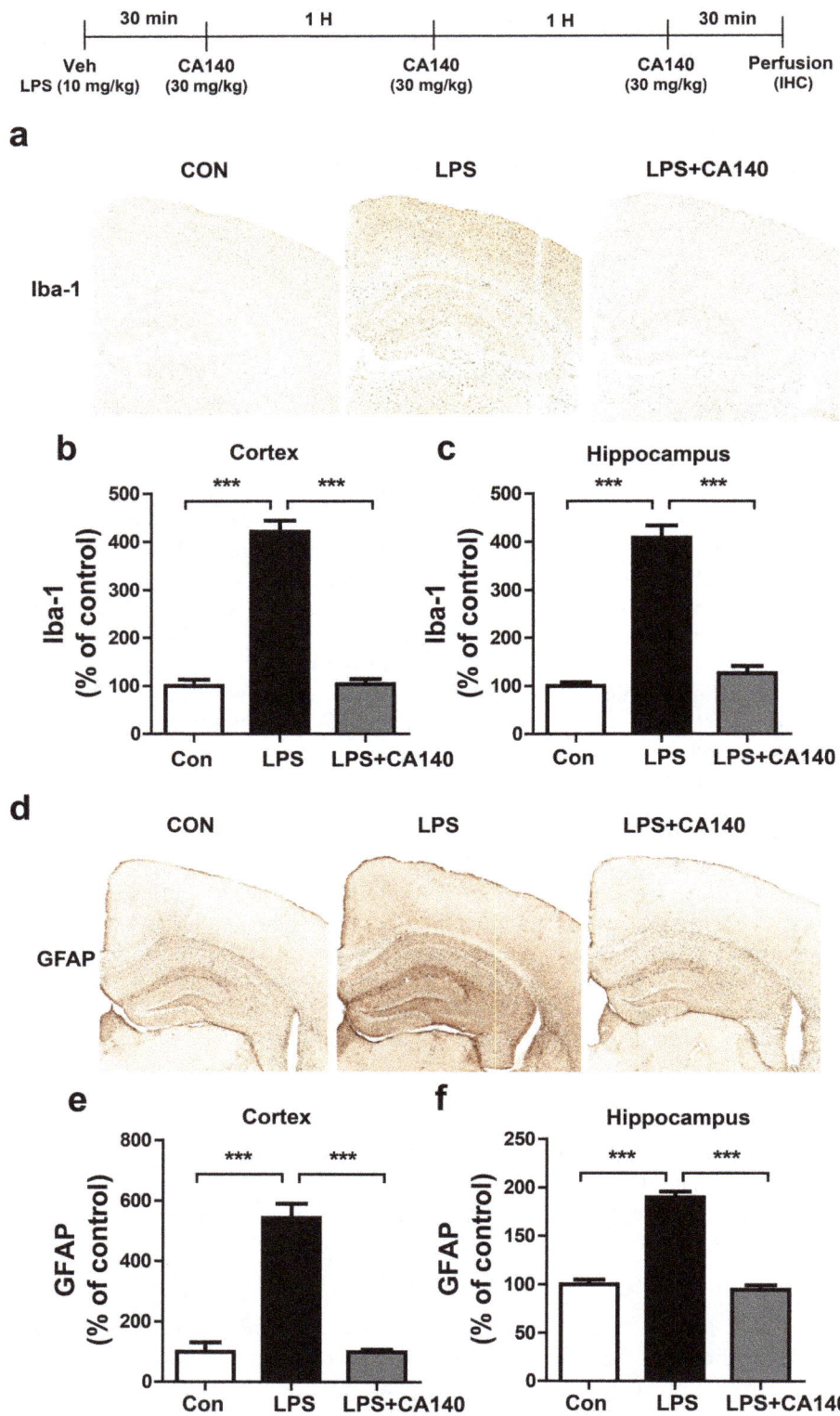

Fig. 8 (See legend on next page.)

(See figure on previous page.)
Fig. 8 Pretreatment with LPS followed by CA140 treatment significantly decreased microglial and astrocyte activation in wild-type mice. **a** Wild-type mice were injected with LPS (10 mg/kg, i.p.), followed 30 min later by injection twice with CA140 (30 mg/kg, i.p.) at an interval of 1 h and a third injection (30 mg/kg, i.p.) at an interval of 30 min. The mice were perfused, fixed, and immunostained with anti-Iba-1 antibody. **b**, **c** Quantification of data from **a** (con, n = 5 mice; LPS, n = 5 mice; LPS + CA140, n = 5 mice). **d** Wild-type mice were injected with LPS (10 mg/kg, i.p.), followed 30 min later by injection twice with CA140 (30 mg/kg, i.p.) at an interval of 1 h and a third injection (30 mg/kg, i.p.) at an interval of 30 min. The mice were perfused, fixed, and immunostained with anti-GFAP antibody. **e**, **f** Quantification of data from **d** (con, n = 5 mice; LPS, n = 5 mice; LPS + CA140, n = 5 mice). ***$p < 0.0001$

under low-glucose conditions (Fig. 3a–f, Additional file 1: Figure S7). In addition, pretreatment with CA140 significantly reduced LPS-induced proinflammatory cytokine levels in mouse primary astrocytes (Additional file 1: Figure S7). Interestingly, post-treatment with CA140 only reduced LPS-induced iNOS mRNA levels in mouse primary astrocytes under low-glucose conditions (Fig. 3). These data suggest that pre- or post-treatment with CA140 may have different effects depending on cell type and culture conditions (e.g., low vs high glucose).

The physiological functions of the catecholaminergic neurotransmitter DA, which range from voluntary movement and reward to hormonal regulation and hypertension, are mediated by G-protein-coupled DA receptors (D1, D2, D3, D4, and D5) [39, 40]. DA receptors have also been identified as important factors for controlling immunity in the CNS [41]. Importantly, D1R and D2R are expressed in rodent and human microglia from brains damaged by stroke or neurodegeneration [41–43]. Here, we observed that D1R and D2R were expressed in BV2 microglial cells and upregulated by LPS treatment (Additional file 1: Figure S8). Previous studies and our results may imply that the upregulation of DA receptors in microglia contributes to neuroinflammation in pathological conditions. Spiperone, a D1/D2R antagonist, inhibits DA-induced chemotaxis in cultured human microglia [44]. Pretreatment with SCH23390, an antagonist of D1R, suppresses NO production by microglia in LPS-injected mice [45]. Consistent with these findings, pretreatment with LE300 or SCH23390, antagonists of D1R, significantly suppressed COX-2 and IL-1β mRNA levels in LPS-stimulated BV2 microglial cells (Fig. 4). A68930, an agonist of D1R, inhibits the production of proinflammatory cytokines in mice [46], and pretreatment with SKF83959, an atypical D1R agonist, reduces proinflammatory cytokine levels in LPS-stimulated BV2 microglia [47]. However, in the present study, pretreatment with A77636, a selective agonist of D1R, did not reduce LPS-induced proinflammatory cytokine levels (Fig. 5). More importantly, treatment with A77636, LPS, and CA140 significantly suppressed LPS-stimulated IL-1β mRNA levels compared with treatment with A77636 and LPS, suggesting that CA140 regulates D1R to alter the LPS-induced neuroinflammatory response (Fig. 5).

With respect to the effects of D2R on neuroinflammation, the D2R agonist pramipexole increases nitrites in cultured primary microglia [42]. In addition, sulpiride, an antagonist of D2R, reduces LPS-induced TNF-α and NO production [45]. In astrocytes, D2R contributes to the suppression of neuroinflammation; however, microglial D2R is not involved in neuroinflammation according to studies of D2R-deficient mice or an ischemic mouse model [48, 49]. In our study, the D2R antagonist eticlopride hydrochloride (EH) did not alter LPS-stimulated proinflammatory cytokine levels in BV2 microglial cells (Additional file 1: Figure S9). This discrepancy may be a result of differences in the details of the experimental procedures, such as treatment duration (i.e., 6 h compared with 24 h), the effective dose of antagonist or agonist, and/or pre- or post-treatment with a DA receptor antagonist. Based on the existing literature and our current findings, we suggest that CA140 may directly or indirectly interact with D1R and thereby regulate neuroinflammatory responses. However, we do not exclude other possibilities; for example, CA140 may regulate other neuroinflammation-related receptors (e.g., TLR4, other DA receptors) to modulate neuroinflammatory responses. Additional studies are required to fully dissect the molecular mechanisms involved in the CA140/DA receptors-induced neuroinflammatory response in vivo.

Activation of TLR receptors via LPS turns on downstream signaling cascades, such as MAP kinases, including ERK and AKT signaling in microglia and astrocytes [10, 50, 51]. Therefore, inhibiting the MAP kinase signaling pathway has been suggested as a potential target for therapeutic drugs for anti-inflammation. Moreover, MAP kinase has been suggested as a downstream effector of both D1R and D2R stimulation [52, 53]. Treatment with the D1R agonist SKF 38393 and the D2R agonist quinpirole activates ERK signaling in primary cultured striatal neurons [54], and in cultured neuroblastoma cells, treatment with the D1R agonist SKF 38393 results in oxidative stress and cytotoxicity via ERK activation [55]. Interestingly, our results indicated that pre- or post-treatment with CA140 significantly suppressed LPS-stimulated ERK signaling in BV2 microglial cells (Fig. 6, Additional file 1: Figure S10). In addition, we found that CA140 further reduced proinflammatory

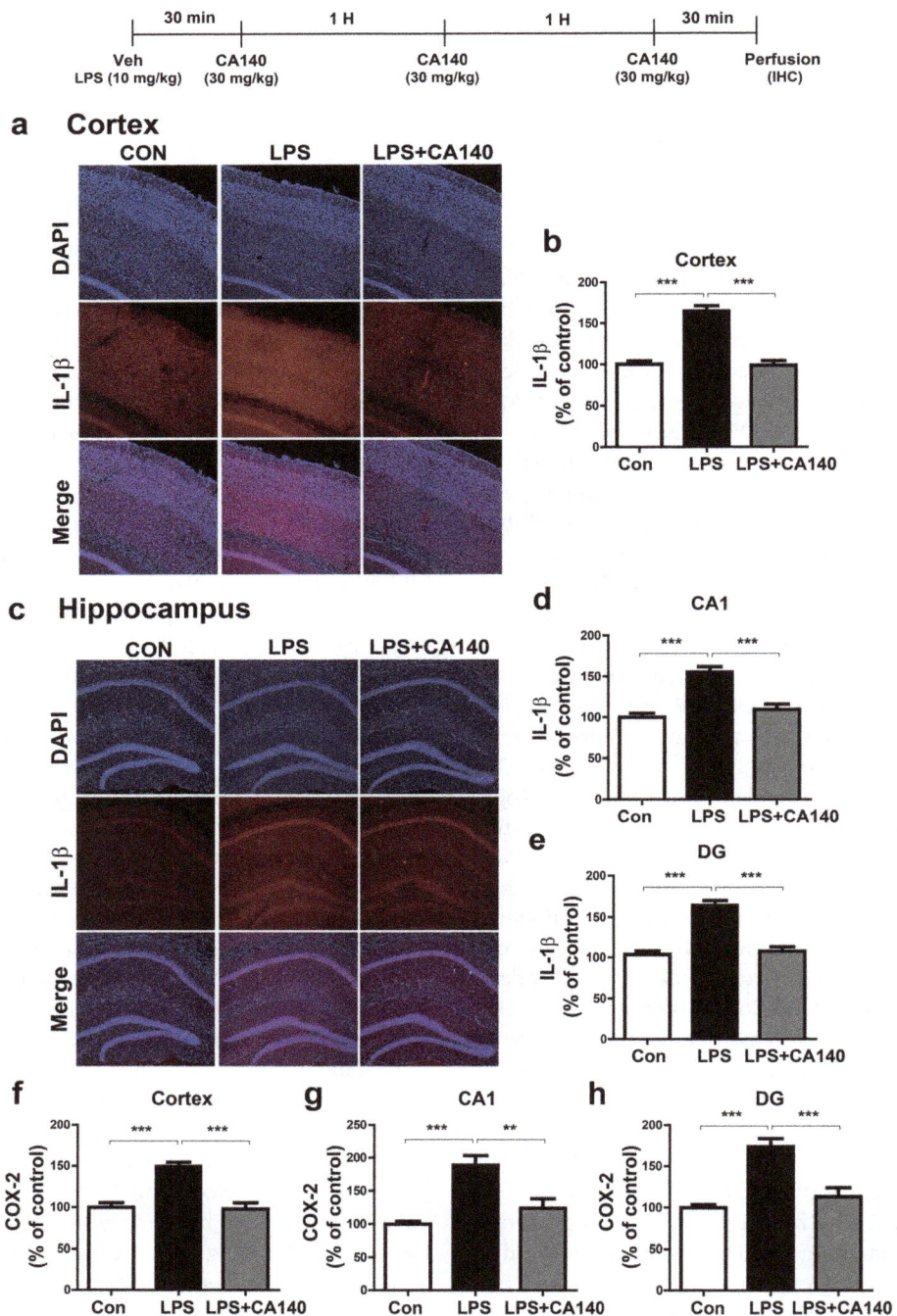

Fig. 9 Pretreatment with LPS followed by CA140 treatment significantly reduced IL-1β and COX-2 levels in wild-type mice. **a**, **c** Wild-type mice were injected with LPS (10 mg/kg, i.p.), followed 30 min later by injection twice with CA140 (30 mg/kg, i.p.) at an interval of 1 h and a third injection (30 mg/kg, i.p.) at an interval of 30 min. The mice were perfused, fixed, and immunostained with anti-IL-1β antibody in the cortex (**a**) and hippocampus (**c**). **b**, **d**, **e** Quantification of data from **a** (cortex: con, $n = 5$ mice; LPS, $n = 5$ mice; LPS + CA140, $n = 5$ mice) and **c** (hippocampus CA1 and DG: con, $n = 5$ mice; LPS, $n = 5$ mice; LPS + CA140, $n = 5$ mice). **f–h** Wild-type mice were injected with LPS (10 mg/kg, i.p.), followed 30 min later by injection twice with CA140 (30 mg/kg, i.p.) at an interval of 1 h and a third injection (30 mg/kg, i.p.) at an interval of 30 min. The mice were perfused, fixed, and immunostained with anti-IL-1β antibody in the cortex (con, $n = 5$ mice; LPS, $n = 5$ mice; LPS + CA140, $n = 5$ mice), hippocampus CA1 (**g**, con, $n = 5$ mice; LPS, $n = 5$ mice; LPS + CA140, $n = 5$ mice), and dentate gyrus (**h**, con, $n = 5$ mice; LPS, $n = 5$ mice; LPS + CA140, $n = 5$ mice). ***$p < 0.0001$

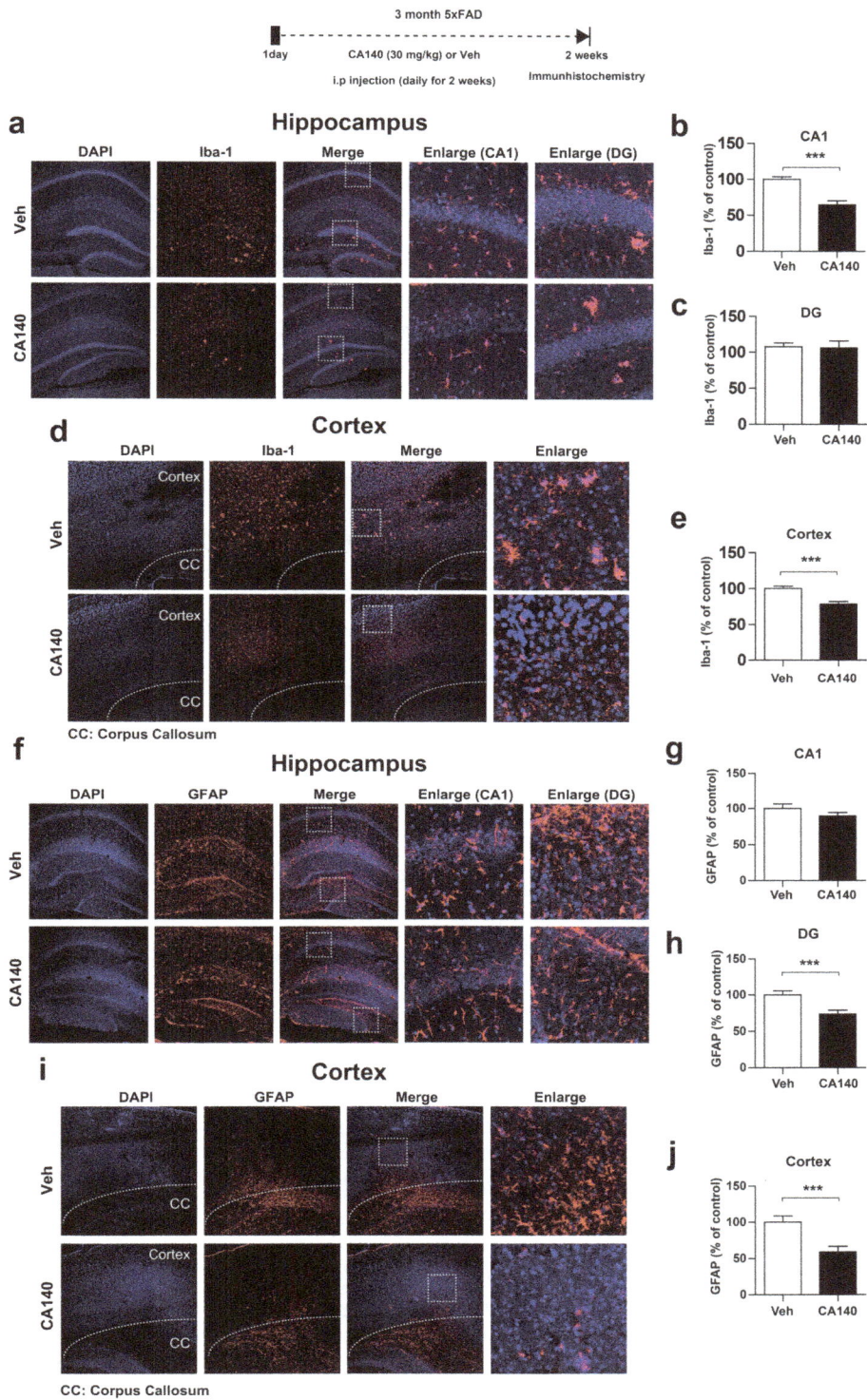

Fig. 10 (See legend on next page.)

cytokine levels when combined with an ERK inhibitor, which suggests that CA140 alters LPS-induced ERK phosphorylation to modify the neuroinflammatory response.

STAT3, a member of the STAT family, is a transcription factor that plays a critical role in regulating microglial activation and inflammatory responses [56, 57]. STAT3 levels in microglia are enhanced in brain injury and a neurodegenerative disease model [58, 59]. Thus, we examined whether CA140 alters the nuclear localization of STAT3 to regulate the neuroinflammatory response and found that pre- or post-treatment with CA140 reduced cytosolic and nuclear p-STAT3 levels in LPS-stimulated BV2 microglial cells (Fig. 7, Additional file 1: Figure S11). Taken together, our data suggest that CA140 may alter neuroinflammation by regulating the ERK/STAT3 signaling pathway.

Systemic injection of LPS in wild-type mice significantly induces astrocyte and microglial activation and proinflammatory cytokine expression [60–62]. Moreover, a single injection of LPS induces robust expression of IL-1β and TNF-α mRNA in various brain regions of wild-type mice [63]. Intracerebral LPS injection in rats induces inflammatory responses and β-secretase-1 (BACE1) in the cortex and hippocampus, with axonal and dendritic pathologies similar to those present in AD [64, 65]. Other studies have also demonstrated that LPS treatment exacerbates the accumulation of amyloid beta and tau pathology in a mouse model of AD [59, 66, 67]. Interestingly, a recent study has shown that both SCH23390, a D1R antagonist, and sulpiride, a D2R antagonist, suppress proinflammatory cytokine levels in LPS-injected mice [45]. DA released by electroacupuncture reduces proinflammatory cytokine levels through D1R in LPS-injected mice [68]. In addition, the regulation of catecholamines by pharmacological agents, such as methylphenidate, enhances neuroinflammatory responses and microgliosis in 5xFAD mice, a transgenic AD mouse model [32, 69]. In the present study, our novel drug CA140, which is structurally related to DA, also substantially reduced astrocyte and microglial activation as well as proinflammatory cytokine levels in LPS-injected wild-type mice and 5xFAD mice (Fig. 8–10, Additional file 1: Figure S12). Taken together, our results suggest that

CA140 may serve as a therapeutic agent for the prevention/treatment of neuroinflammation-related diseases, including AD.

Conclusions

In the present study, we have demonstrated that CA140 exhibits novel anti-inflammatory effects and provided initial evidence for its mechanism of action. We discovered that CA140 suppresses LPS-induced proinflammatory cytokine levels in BV2 microglial cells, primary microglia, and primary astrocytes. In addition, CA140 modulates D1R to regulate LPS-induced neuroinflammation in BV2 microglial cells. Moreover, CA140 affects ERK/STAT3 signaling to alter the LPS-induced neuroinflammatory response. In in vivo experiments, CA140 significantly reduced microglial and astrocyte activation in LPS-injected wild-type mice and 5xFAD mice. This study reveals that CA140 is a promising compound with anti-inflammatory effects and subsequent attenuation of neurotoxins such as LPS.

Additional file

Additional file 1: Figure S1. Post-treatment with CA140 at 5 μM only significantly reduced LPS-induced IL-1β mRNA levels. Figure S2. Post-treatment with CA140 significantly reduced LPS-induced proinflammatory cytokine levels in a longer treatment. Figure S3. Pretreatment with CA140 significantly decreased LPS-induced COX-2, IL-1β, and iNOS mRNA levels in BV2 microglial cells. Figure S4. Pretreatment with CA140 significantly decreased LPS-induced COX-2, IL-1β, and iNOS mRNA levels in a longer treatment. Figure S5. Post-treatment with CA140 significantly decreased LPS-mediated proinflammatory cytokine levels in rat primary microglial cells. Figure S6. Pretreatment with CA140 decreased LPS-induced proinflammatory cytokine levels in rat primary microglial cells and primary astrocytes. Figure S7. Pretreatment with CA140 decreased LPS-mediated proinflammatory cytokine levels in mouse primary microglial cells and primary astrocytes. Figure S8. Post-treatment with CA140 downregulated LPS-induced dopamine D1 receptor (D1R) levels in BV2 microglial cells. Figure S9. Inhibition of dopamine D2 receptor (D2R) did not reduce LPS-stimulated proinflammatory cytokine levels in BV2 microglial cells. Figure S10 Pretreatment with CA140 significantly decreased phosphorylation of ERK and AKT in LPS-stimulated BV2 microglial cells. Figure S11. Pretreatment with CA140 significantly decreased cytosolic and nuclear p-STAT3 levels in LPS-induced BV2 microglial cells. Figure S12. Pretreatment with CA140 significantly reduced microglia and astrocyte activation in wild-type mice. (DOCX 22915 kb)

Abbreviations

AD: Alzheimer's disease; BBB: Blood-brain barrier; CNS: Central nervous system; D1R: Dopamine D1 receptor; D2R: Dopamine D2 receptor; DA: Dopamine; ERK: Extracellular signal-regulated kinase; IL-1β: Interleukin-1β; JNK: c-Jun N-terminal kinase; LPS: Lipopolysaccharide; MAPK: Mitogen-activated protein kinase; TLR4: Toll-like receptor 4; TNF-α: Tumor necrosis factor-α

Acknowledgements
Confocal microscopy (Nikon, TI-RCP) and bright-field microscopy (Carl Zeiss) data were acquired at the Advanced Neural Imaging Center of the Korea Brain Research Institute (KBRI).

Funding
This work was supported by the KBRI basic research program through KBRI funded by the Ministry of Science, ICT and Future Planning (grant number 18-BR-02-04, H.S.H.), the National Research Foundation of Korea (grant number 2016R1A2B4011393, H.S.H.), and the National Research Council of Science and Technology (grant number CAP-12-1-KIST, W.G.C.). Research reported in this publication was also supported by the National Institute on Aging of the National Institutes of Health under Award Number R01AG053577 (M.R.B., C.C.C., T.K., and J.Y.).

Authors' contributions
JYL, HGC, JY, JK, and HSH conceived the study, participated in the design of the study, and wrote the manuscript. JYL, JHN, and HYN performed molecular/cellular experiments, in vivo experiments, and statistical analyses. EK, SBK, and HGC performed blood-brain barrier experiments. MRB, CCC, TK, GL, and JY synthesized and developed CA140. YPN and GY conducted the ELISA studies (cAMP, IL-1β, NO), time-dependent experiments, functional assays of CA140/DIR by treatment with DIR agonist or antagonist in vitro and in vivo, and data analysis and contributed to writing the revised manuscript. All authors read and approved the final manuscript.

Competing interests
The authors declare that they have no competing interests.

Author details
[1]Department of Neural Development and Disease, Korea Brain Research Institute (KBRI), 61 Cheomdan-ro, Dong-gu, Daegu 41068, South Korea. [2]New Drug Development Center, Daegu-Gyeongbuk Medical Innovation Foundation, 80 Cheombok-ro, Dong-gu, Daegu 41061, South Korea. [3]Department of Chemistry and Biochemistry, University of California, San Diego, La Jolla, CA 92093-0358, USA.

References
1. Balducci C, Forloni G. Novel targets in Alzheimer's disease: a special focus on microglia. Pharmacol Res. 2018.
2. Fan Z, Okello AA, Brooks DJ, Edison P. Longitudinal influence of microglial activation and amyloid on neuronal function in Alzheimer's disease. Brain. 2015;138:3685–98.
3. Kirkley KS, Popichak KA, Afzali MF, Legare ME, Tjalkens RB. Microglia amplify inflammatory activation of astrocytes in manganese neurotoxicity. J Neuroinflammation. 2017;14:99.
4. La Rosa F, Saresella M, Baglio F, Piancone F, Marventano I, Calabrese E, Nemni R, Ripamonti E, Cabinio M, Clerici M. Immune and imaging correlates of mild cognitive impairment conversion to Alzheimer's disease. Sci Rep. 2017;7:16760.
5. Badshah H, Ali T, Kim MO. Osmotin attenuates LPS-induced neuroinflammation and memory impairments via the TLR4/NFkappaB signaling pathway. Sci Rep. 2016;6:24493.
6. Li JJ, Wang B, Kodali MC, Chen C, Kim E, Patters BJ, Lan L, Kumar S, Wang X, Yue J, Liao FF. In vivo evidence for the contribution of peripheral circulating inflammatory exosomes to neuroinflammation. J Neuroinflammation. 2018;15:8.
7. Lester SN, Li K. Toll-like receptors in antiviral innate immunity. J Mol Biol. 2014;426:1246–64.
8. Cheng B, Lin Y, Kuang M, Fang S, Gu Q, Xu J, Wang L. Synthesis and anti-neuroinflammatory activity of lactone benzoyl hydrazine and 2-nitro-1-phenyl-1h-indole derivatives as p38alpha MAPK inhibitors. Chem Biol Drug Des. 2015;86:1121–30.
9. Xu P, Huang MW, Xiao CX, Long F, Wang Y, Liu SY, Jia WW, Wu WJ, Yang D, Hu JF, et al. Matairesinol suppresses neuroinflammation and migration associated with Src and ERK1/2-NF-kappaB pathway in activating BV2 microglia. Neurochem Res. 2017;42:2850–60.
10. Guo C, Yang L, Wan CX, Xia YZ, Zhang C, Chen MH, Wang ZD, Li ZR, Li XM, Geng YD, Kong LY. Anti-neuroinflammatory effect of Sophoraflavanone G from Sophora alopecuroides in LPS-activated BV2 microglia by MAPK, JAK/STAT and Nrf2/HO-1 signaling pathways. Phytomedicine. 2016;23:1629–37.
11. Choo XY, Alukaidey L, White AR, Grubman A. Neuroinflammation and copper in Alzheimer's disease. Int J Alzheimers Dis. 2013;2013:145345.
12. Schlachetzki JC, Hull M. Microglial activation in Alzheimer's disease. Curr Alzheimer Res. 2009;6:554–63.
13. Fang XX, Sun GL, Zhou Y, Qiu YH, Peng YP. TGF-beta1 protection against Abeta1-42-induced hippocampal neuronal inflammation and apoptosis by TbetaR-I. Neuroreport. 2018;29:141–6.
14. Valles SL, Dolz-Gaiton P, Gambini J, Borras C, Lloret A, Pallardo FV, Vina J. Estradiol or genistein prevent Alzheimer's disease-associated inflammation correlating with an increase PPAR gamma expression in cultured astrocytes. Brain Res. 2010;1312:138–44.
15. von Bernhardi R. Glial cell dysregulation: a new perspective on Alzheimer disease. Neurotox Res. 2007;12:215–32.
16. Liu Y, Ai K, Lu L. Polydopamine and its derivative materials: synthesis and promising applications in energy, environmental, and biomedical fields. Chem Rev. 2014;114:5057–115.
17. Grigoryan G, Hodges H, Mitchell S, Sinden JD, Gray JA. 6-OHDA lesions of the nucleus accumbens accentuate memory deficits in animals with lesions to the forebrain cholinergic projection system: effects of nicotine administration on learning and memory in the water maze. Neurobiol Learn Mem. 1996;65:135–53.
18. Femenia T, Qian Y, Arentsen T, Forssberg H, Diaz Heijtz R. Toll-like receptor-4 regulates anxiety-like behavior and DARPP-32 phosphorylation. Brain Behav Immun. 2017.
19. Basu B, Sarkar C, Chakroborty D, Ganguly S, Shome S, Dasgupta PS, Basu S. D1 and D2 dopamine receptor-mediated inhibition of activated normal T cell proliferation is lost in T leukemic cells, Jurkat. J Biol Chem. 2010;285:27026–32.
20. Lee S, Park JY, Lee WH, Kim H, Park HC, Mori K, Suk K. Lipocalin-2 is an autocrine mediator of reactive astrocytosis. J Neurosci. 2009;29:234–49.
21. Saura J, Tusell JM, Serratosa J. High-yield isolation of murine microglia by mild trypsinization. Glia. 2003;44:183–9.
22. Nam JH, Cho HJ, Kang H, Lee JY, Jung M, Chang YC, Kim K, Hoe HS. A mercaptoacetamide-based class II histone deacetylase inhibitor suppresses cell migration and invasion in monomorphic malignant human glioma cells by inhibiting FAK/STAT3 signaling. J Cell Biochem. 2017;118:4672–85.
23. Song JM, Sung YM, Nam JH, Yoon H, Chung A, Moffat E, Jung M, Pak DT, Kim J, Hoe HS. A mercaptoacetamide-based class II histone deacetylase inhibitor increases dendritic spine density via RasGRF1/ERK pathway. J Alzheimers Dis. 2016;51:591–604.
24. Henn A, Lund S, Hedtjarn M, Schrattenholz A, Porzgen P, Leist M. The suitability of BV2 cells as alternative model system for primary microglia cultures or for animal experiments examining brain inflammation. ALTEX. 2009;26:83–94.
25. Wang J, Li G, Wang Z, Zhang X, Yao L, Wang F, Liu S, Yin J, Ling EA, Wang L, Hao A. High glucose-induced expression of inflammatory cytokines and reactive oxygen species in cultured astrocytes. Neuroscience. 2012;202:58–68.
26. Nagai K, Fukushima T, Oike H, Kobori M. High glucose increases the expression of proinflammatory cytokines and secretion of TNFalpha and beta-hexosaminidase in human mast cells. Eur J Pharmacol. 2012;687:39–45.
27. Quincozes-Santos A, Bobermin LD, de Assis AM, Goncalves CA, Souza DO. Fluctuations in glucose levels induce glial toxicity with glutamatergic, oxidative and inflammatory implications. Biochim Biophys Acta. 1863;2017:1–14.
28. Lange SC, Bak LK, Waagepetersen HS, Schousboe A, Norenberg MD. Primary cultures of astrocytes: their value in understanding astrocytes in health and disease. Neurochem Res. 2012;37:2569–88.
29. Kim EK, Choi EJ. Compromised MAPK signaling in human diseases: an update. Arch Toxicol. 2015;89:867–82.
30. Fourrier C, Remus-Borel J, Greenhalgh AD, Guichardant M, Bernoud-Hubac N, Lagarde M, Joffre C, Laye S. Docosahexaenoic acid-containing choline

phospholipid modulates LPS-induced neuroinflammation in vivo and in microglia in vitro. J Neuroinflammation. 2017;14:170.

31. Bellaver B, Souza DG, Bobermin LD, Goncalves CA, Souza DO, Quincozes-Santos A. Guanosine inhibits LPS-induced pro-inflammatory response and oxidative stress in hippocampal astrocytes through the heme oxygenase-1 pathway. Purinergic Signal. 2015;11:571–80.

32. Ardestani PM, Evans AK, Yi B, Nguyen T, Coutellier L, Shamloo M. Modulation of neuroinflammation and pathology in the 5XFAD mouse model of Alzheimer's disease using a biased and selective beta-1 adrenergic receptor partial agonist. Neuropharmacology. 2017;116:371–86.

33. Benzing WC, Wujek JR, Ward EK, Shaffer D, Ashe KH, Younkin SG, Brunden KR. Evidence for glial-mediated inflammation in aged APP(SW) transgenic mice. Neurobiol Aging. 1999;20:581–9.

34. Frank-Cannon TC, Alto LT, McAlpine FE, Tansey MG. Does neuroinflammation fan the flame in neurodegenerative diseases? Mol Neurodegener. 2009;4:47.

35. Downen M, Amaral TD, Hua LL, Zhao ML, Lee SC. Neuronal death in cytokine-activated primary human brain cell culture: role of tumor necrosis factor-alpha. Glia. 1999;28:114–27.

36. Norden DM, Godbout JP. Review: microglia of the aged brain: primed to be activated and resistant to regulation. Neuropathol Appl Neurobiol. 2013;39:19–34.

37. Font-Nieves M, Sans-Fons MG, Gorina R, Bonfill-Teixidor E, Salas-Perdomo A, Marquez-Kisinousky L, Santalucia T, Planas AM. Induction of COX-2 enzyme and down-regulation of COX-1 expression by lipopolysaccharide (LPS) control prostaglandin E2 production in astrocytes. J Biol Chem. 2012;287:6454–68.

38. Parajuli B, Sonobe Y, Kawanokuchi J, Doi Y, Noda M, Takeuchi H, Mizuno T, Suzumura A. GM-CSF increases LPS-induced production of proinflammatory mediators via upregulation of TLR4 and CD14 in murine microglia. J Neuroinflammation. 2012;9:268.

39. Missale C, Nash SR, Robinson SW, Jaber M, Caron MG. Dopamine receptors: from structure to function. Physiol Rev. 1998;78:189–225.

40. Beaulieu JM, Gainetdinov RR. The physiology, signaling, and pharmacology of dopamine receptors. Pharmacol Rev. 2011;63:182–217.

41. Pocock JM, Kettenmann H. Neurotransmitter receptors on microglia. Trends Neurosci. 2007;30:527–35.

42. Huck JH, Freyer D, Bottcher C, Mladinov M, Muselmann-Genschow C, Thielke M, Gladow N, Bloomquist D, Mergenthaler P, Priller J. De novo expression of dopamine D2 receptors on microglia after stroke. J Cereb Blood Flow Metab. 2015;35:1804–11.

43. Farber K, Pannasch U, Kettenmann H. Dopamine and noradrenaline control distinct functions in rodent microglial cells. Mol Cell Neurosci. 2005;29:128–38.

44. Mastroeni D, Grover A, Leonard B, Joyce JN, Coleman PD, Kozik B, Bellinger DL, Rogers J. Microglial responses to dopamine in a cell culture model of Parkinson's disease. Neurobiol Aging. 2009;30:1805–17.

45. Hasko G, Szabo C, Merkel K, Bencsics A, Zingarelli B, Kvetan V, Vizi ES. Modulation of lipopolysaccharide-induced tumor necrosis factor-alpha and nitric oxide production by dopamine receptor agonists and antagonists in mice. Immunol Lett. 1996;49:143–7.

46. Wang T, Nowrangi D, Yu L, Lu T, Tang J, Han B, Ding Y, Fu F, Zhang JH. Activation of dopamine D1 receptor decreased NLRP3-mediated inflammation in intracerebral hemorrhage mice. J Neuroinflammation. 2018;15:2.

47. Wu Z, Li L, Zheng LT, Xu Z, Guo L, Zhen X. Allosteric modulation of sigma-1 receptors by SKF83959 inhibits microglia-mediated inflammation. J Neurochem. 2015;134:904–14.

48. Shao W, Zhang SZ, Tang M, Zhang XH, Zhou Z, Yin YQ, Zhou QB, Huang YY, Liu YJ, Wawrousek E, et al. Suppression of neuroinflammation by astrocytic dopamine D2 receptors via alphaB-crystallin. Nature. 2013;494:90–4.

49. Qiu J, Yan Z, Tao K, Li Y, Li Y, Li J, Dong Y, Feng D, Chen H. Sinomenine activates astrocytic dopamine D2 receptors and alleviates neuroinflammatory injury via the CRYAB/STAT3 pathway after ischemic stroke in mice. J Neuroinflammation. 2016;13:263.

50. Dang Y, Xu Y, Wu W, Li W, Sun Y, Yang J, Zhu Y, Zhang C. Tetrandrine suppresses lipopolysaccharide-induced microglial activation by inhibiting NF-kappaB and ERK signaling pathways in BV2 cells. PLoS One. 2014;9:e102522.

51. Kaminska B, Gozdz A, Zawadzka M, Ellert-Miklaszewska A, Lipko M. MAPK signal transduction underlying brain inflammation and gliosis as therapeutic target. Anat Rec (Hoboken). 2009;292:1902–13.

52. Yan Z, Feng J, Fienberg AA, Greengard P. D(2) dopamine receptors induce mitogen-activated protein kinase and cAMP response element-binding protein phosphorylation in neurons. Proc Natl Acad Sci U S A. 1999;96:11607–12.

53. Zanassi P, Paolillo M, Feliciello A, Avvedimento EV, Gallo V, Schinelli S. cAMP-dependent protein kinase induces cAMP-response element-binding protein phosphorylation via an intracellular calcium release/ERK-dependent pathway in striatal neurons. J Biol Chem. 2001;276:11487–95.

54. Brami-Cherrier K, Valjent E, Garcia M, Pages C, Hipskind RA, Caboche J. Dopamine induces a PI3-kinase-independent activation of Akt in striatal neurons: a new route to cAMP response element-binding protein phosphorylation. J Neurosci. 2002;22:8911–21.

55. Chen J, Rusnak M, Luedtke RR, Sidhu A. D1 dopamine receptor mediates dopamine-induced cytotoxicity via the ERK signal cascade. J Biol Chem. 2004;279:39317–30.

56. Huang C, Ma R, Sun S, Wei G, Fang Y, Liu R, Li G. JAK2-STAT3 signaling pathway mediates thrombin-induced proinflammatory actions of microglia in vitro. J Neuroimmunol. 2008;204:118–25.

57. Dinapoli VA, Benkovic SA, Li X, Kelly KA, Miller DB, Rosen CL, Huber JD, O'Callaghan JP. Age exaggerates proinflammatory cytokine signaling and truncates signal transducers and activators of transcription 3 signaling following ischemic stroke in the rat. Neuroscience. 2010;170:633–44.

58. Chen S, Dong Z, Cheng M, Zhao Y, Wang M, Sai N, Wang X, Liu H, Huang G, Zhang X. Homocysteine exaggerates microglia activation and neuroinflammation through microglia localized STAT3 overactivation following ischemic stroke. J Neuroinflammation. 2017;14:187.

59. Carret-Rebillat AS, Pace C, Gourmaud S, Ravasi L, Montagne-Stora S, Longueville S, Tible M, Sudol E, Chang RC, Paquet C, et al. Neuroinflammation and Abeta accumulation linked to systemic inflammation are decreased by genetic PKR down-regulation. Sci Rep. 2015;5:8489.

60. Qin L, Wu X, Block ML, Liu Y, Breese GR, Hong JS, Knapp DJ, Crews FT. Systemic LPS causes chronic neuroinflammation and progressive neurodegeneration. Glia. 2007;55:453–62.

61. Jeong HK, Jou I, Joe EH. Systemic LPS administration induces brain inflammation but not dopaminergic neuronal death in the substantia nigra. Exp Mol Med. 2010;42:823–32.

62. Catorce MN, Gevorkian G. LPS-induced murine neuroinflammation model: main features and suitability for pre-clinical assessment of nutraceuticals. Curr Neuropharmacol. 2016;14:155–64.

63. Skelly DT, Hennessy E, Dansereau MA, Cunningham C. A systematic analysis of the peripheral and CNS effects of systemic LPS, IL-1beta, [corrected] TNF-alpha and IL-6 challenges in C57BL/6 mice. PLoS One. 2013;8:e69123.

64. Deng X, Li M, Ai W, He L, Lu D, Patrylo PR, Cai H, Luo X, Li Z, Yan X. Lipolysaccharide-induced neuroinflammation is associated with Alzheimer-like amyloidogenic axonal pathology and dendritic degeneration in rats. Adv Alzheimer Dis. 2014;3:78–93.

65. Kitazawa M, Oddo S, Yamasaki TR, Green KN, LaFerla FM. Lipopolysaccharide-induced inflammation exacerbates tau pathology by a cyclin-dependent kinase 5-mediated pathway in a transgenic model of Alzheimer's disease. J Neurosci. 2005;25:8843–53.

66. Lee DC, Rizer J, Hunt JB, Selenica ML, Gordon MN, Morgan D. Review: experimental manipulations of microglia in mouse models of Alzheimer's pathology: activation reduces amyloid but hastens tau pathology. Neuropathol Appl Neurobiol. 2013;39:69–85.

67. LaFerla FM, Green KN. Animal models of Alzheimer disease. Cold Spring Harb Perspect Med. 2012;2.

68. Torres-Rosas R, Yehia G, Pena G, Mishra P, del Rocio T-BM, Moreno-Eutimio MA, Arriaga-Pizano LA, Isibasi A, Ulloa L. Dopamine mediates vagal modulation of the immune system by electroacupuncture. Nat Med. 2014;20:291–5.

69. Schneider F, Baldauf K, Wetzel W, Reymann KG. Effects of methylphenidate on the behavior of male 5xFAD mice. Pharmacol Biochem Behav. 2015;128:68–77.

11

Adult neurogenic deficits in HIV-1 Tg26 transgenic mice

Raj Putatunda[1,2], Yonggang Zhang[1,2], Fang Li[1,2], Xiao-Feng Yang[1,4], Mary F Barbe[3] and Wenhui Hu[1,2*] ⓘ

Abstract

Background: Even in the antiretroviral treatment (ART) era, HIV-1-infected patients suffer from milder forms of HIV-1-associated neurocognitive disorders (HAND). While the viral proteins Tat and gp120 have been shown to individually inhibit the proliferation and neural differentiation of neural stem cells (NSCs), no studies have characterized the effects of all the combined viral proteins on adult neurogenesis.

Methods: The HIV-1 Tg26 transgenic mouse model was used due to its clinical relevance to ART-controlled HIV-1-infected patients who lack active viral replication but suffer from continuous stress from the viral proteins. Quantitative RT-PCR analysis was performed to validate the expression of viral genes in the neurogenic zones. In vitro stemness and lineage differentiation assays were performed in cultured NSCs from HIV-1 Tg26 transgenic mice and their wild-type littermates. Hippocampal neurogenic lineage analysis was performed to determine potential changes in initial and late differentiation of NSCs in the subgranular zone (SGZ). Finally, fluorescent retroviral labeling of mature dentate granule neurons was performed to assess dendritic complexity and dendritic spine densities.

Results: Varying copy numbers of partial *gag* (p17), *tat* (unspliced and spliced variants), *env* (gp120), *vpu*, and *nef* transcripts were detected in the neurogenic zones of Tg26 mice. Significantly fewer primary neurospheres and a higher percentage of larger sized primary neurospheres were generated from Tg26 NSCs than from littermated wild-type mouse NSCs, implying that Tg26 mouse NSCs exhibit deficits in initial differentiation. In vitro differentiation assays revealed that Tg26 mouse NSCs have reduced neuronal differentiation and increased astrocytic differentiation. In the SGZs of Tg26 mice, significantly higher amounts of quiescent NSCs, as well as significantly lower levels of active NSCs, proliferating neural progenitor cells, and neuroblasts, were observed. Finally, newborn mature granule neurons in the dentate gyri of Tg26 mice had deficiencies in dendritic arborization, dendritic length, and dendritic spine density.

Conclusions: Both in vitro and in vivo studies demonstrate that HIV-1 Tg26 mice have early- and late-stage neurogenesis deficits, which could possibly contribute to the progression of HAND. Future therapies should be targeting this process to ameliorate, if not eliminate HAND-like symptoms in HIV-1-infected patients.

Keywords: HIV-1, HAND, Tg26 mouse, Neurogenesis, Neural stem cells, Stemness, Differentiation, Dendritic spine density

Background

Since the start of the antiretroviral treatment (ART) era, HIV-1-associated co-morbidities have manifested in the clinical population, most notably HIV-associated neurocognitive disorders (HAND), accelerated aging, cardiovascular diseases, and metabolic dysfunction [1]. HAND continues to affect over 50% of all HIV-1-infected patients, even while undergoing ART treatment [2, 3]. This disorder describes a specific spectrum of neurocognitive impairments such as asymptomatic neurocognitive impairment (ANI), mild neurocognitive disorder (MND), and HIV-associated dementia (HAD) [4]. Although the incidence of HAD has decreased due to ART, the incidence of MND continues to rise [5–8]. It is widely accepted that a key contributing factor of neuronal dysfunction in HIV-1 infection is attributed to the "Trojan Horse" mechanism of HIV-1 neuroinvasion via infected immune cells into the central nervous system (CNS) [9–11]. However, recent reports point to the

* Correspondence: whu@temple.edu
[1]Center for Metabolic Disease Research, Temple University Lewis Katz School of Medicine, 3500 N Broad Street, Philadelphia, PA 19140, USA
[2]Department of Pathology and Laboratory Medicine, Temple University Lewis Katz School of Medicine, 3500 N Broad Street, Philadelphia, PA 19140, USA
Full list of author information is available at the end of the article

possibility that chronic neuroinflammation from HIV-1 negatively impacts adult neurogenesis, thus contributing to the evolution of HAND [2, 12].

Neurogenesis describes the process in which neuronal and glial cells are generated from neural precursors that includes neural stem cells (NSCs) and neural progenitor cells (NPCs). This process takes place during prenatal development and throughout adult life [13, 14]. In the context of adult neurogenesis, there are two main neurogenic niches: the subgranular zone (SGZ) in the dentate gyrus of the hippocampus and the subventricular zone (SVZ) lining the lateral ventricles [15–17]. In both neurogenic niches, slowly proliferating NSCs differentiate into rapidly proliferating NPCs, which then differentiate into neuroblasts and glioblasts that form neurons and glial cells respectively. Subsequently, these newborn neurons integrate into neural circuits to modulate olfactory processing and memory acquisition/maintenance [16].

Neurogenesis is important to study in the context of HAND, because HIV-1 virions have been found in the hippocampal formation of pediatric AIDS patients [18], and impaired neurogenesis has been observed in both HIV-1-infected patients and SIV-infected macaques [19, 20], as well as glial fibrillary acidic protein (GFAP)-driven gp120 transgenic mice [21–25] and GFAP-Tat transgenic mice [26, 27]. More importantly, NSCs have been shown to be targets of active HIV-1 infection [25, 27–32]. Additionally, well-known antiretroviral drugs such as AZT, efavirenz, and a tenofovir/emtricitabine/raltegravir cocktail inhibit NSC proliferation and differentiation in vitro and in vivo at pharmacologically relevant doses [33–35].

While previous studies hallmark the roles of active viral infection or viral protein production in neurogenic dysfunction [22, 24, 25, 27, 31], the role of chronic/latent HIV-1 infection in the CNS remains poorly understood. Here, we utilized the HIV-1 Tg26 mouse model to evaluate adult neurogenesis. The Tg26 mouse line expresses seven of the nine HIV-1 viral proteins under the viral long terminal repeat (LTR) promoter [36–39]. Because the replication-deficient proviral HIV-1 DNA randomly integrates into the host genome and the viral transcripts are spontaneously driven by the LTRs, the Tg26 mice serve as an appropriate model for studying the long-term effects of viral proteins on the host. This model is clinically relevant to ART-controlled HIV-1-infected patients who lack active viral replication, but suffer from continuous stress from HIV-1 viral protein exposure. The aim of this study is to characterize the effects of the combined HIV-1 viral proteins on adult neurogenesis.

Methods

Transgenic mice

The Institutional Animal Care and Use Committee (IACUC) at Temple University (Philadelphia, PA)

approved all procedures detailed in this study that required the use of vertebrate animals prior to initiating any experimental objectives. Additionally, all methods were performed in full compliance with Temple University's IACUC policies and the National Institutes of Health (NIH) ethical guidelines. Inbred HIV-1 Tg26 transgenic mice (Jackson Lab, #022354) and their wild-type (WT) gender and age-matched littermates were utilized in this study. These mice harbor truncated HIV-1 NL4-3 genome with a 3.1-kb deletion in the *Gag* and *Pol* regions, rendering the latent provirus replication deficient [36]. The Tg26 mice were originally generated on the FV/B background and develop a well-characterized kidney disease. As a result, most mice are moribund between 2 and 6 months of age [36, 37]. Since Tg26 mice on the C57BL/6J background do not develop kidney disease and have longer life expectancies [40–42], we generated Tg26 mice on a complete C57BL/6J background by backcrossing FVB/N-Tg(HIV)26Aln/PkltJ mice [36] with C57BL/6J mice (Jackson Lab, #000664) for at least eight generations. Since Tg26 homozygous (+/+) mice are runted and rarely survive to weaning [36], the Tg26 mice were maintained as heterozygotes (+/–) throughout the study. Mice were utilized between 8 and 12 weeks old for all the proposed studies.

Quantitative reverse transcription PCR (RT-qPCR)

Total RNA was extracted from the brains of four Tg26 mice. Specifically, the SVZs, SGZs, olfactory bulbs, and kidneys were microdissected and stored in Trizol reagent (Thermo Fischer Scientific). The kidneys have been characterized to express proviral transcripts and served as an appropriate positive control for our studies [36, 37]. Littermated WT mice were used as negative controls. The RNA was then purified with the Direct-zol RNA Miniprep Kit according to the manufacturer's instructions (Zymo Research Cat. # R2052). Equal amounts (100 ng) of RNA from each sample was used for reverse transcription with the High Capacity cDNA Reverse Transcription Kit (Thermo Fischer Scientific Cat.# 4368814), and 2 ng of cDNA was applied for qPCR using specific primers (Table 1, Fig. 1a) targeting partial *gag* (*p17*), *tat* (spliced and unspliced variants), *env* (*gp120*), *vpu*, and *nef* based on previously published reports [43, 44]. Absolute quantification assays were performed using an HIV-1 pNL4-3 plasmid or reverse transcribed 2 or 4 kb HIV-1 cDNA fragments as the standards.

Immunohistochemistry (IHC) and immunocytochemistry (ICC)

The following antibodies were used in this study: chicken anti-GFAP (IHC and ICC 1:500, Aves Labs Cat# GFAP, RRID:AB_2313547), Goat Sox2 (IHC and ICC 1:250, Santa

Table 1 List of primers used for RT-qPCR and Tg26 mouse genotyping

Gene target	Direction	Sequence (5' to 3')
Partial Gag (p17)	T760—forward	GGATAGATGTAAAAGACACCA
	T946—reverse	ACCTGGCTGTTGTTTCCTGTGTC
Env (gp120)	T876—forward	CCGAAGGAATAGAAGAAGAAG
	T691—reverse	AGAGTAAGTCTCTCAAGCGG
Tat$_2$ (spliced variant)	T1002—forward	TGGAAGCATCCAGGAAGTCAGCC
	T1003—reverse	TTCTTCTTCTATTCCTTCGGGCC
Tat$_1$ (unspliced variant)	T1002—forward	TGGAAGCATCCAGGAAGTCAGCC
	T1007—reverse	GAGAAGCTTGATGAGTCTGACTG
Nef	F3.3—forward	CCGAAGGAATAGAAGAAGAAG
	R3.3—reverse	CTTGTAGCACCATCCAAAGG
Vpu	T1002—forward	TGGAAGCATCCAGGAAGTCAGCC
	R1.3—reverse	GTGGTGGTTGCTTCCTTCC
PCR for mouse genotyping	T361—Tg26 forward	GATCTGTGGATCTACCACACACA
	T363—Tg26 reverse	GCTGCTTATATGCAGCATCTGAG

Cruz Biotechnology Cat# sc-54517, RRID:AB_2195807), rabbit anti-Ki67 (IHC 1:500, Abcam Cat# ab92353, RRID:AB_2049848), rabbit anti-eGFP (IHC 1:1000, Molecular Probes Cat# A-6455, RRID:AB_221570), goat anti-doublecortin (DCX,1:500, Santa Cruz Biotechnology Cat# sc-8066, RRID:AB_2088494), and rabbit anti-β3-tubulin (Tuj1, ICC 1:1000, Sigma-Aldrich Cat# T2200, RRID:AB_262133).

The IHC and ICC procedures have been conducted in a similar manner as described previously [45]. For ICC, cells were fixed in 4% paraformaldyhyde in phosphate-buffered saline (PBS) for 20 min. After three consecutive PBS washes, the cells were permeabilized for 30 min with 0.5% Triton X-100 mixed with PBS. After permeabilization, the cells were blocked with 2% bovine serum albumin (BSA) dissolved in PBS with 0.1% Triton X-100 for 1 h. NSCs were then treated with primary antibodies diluted in blocking buffer overnight at 4 °C. NSCs were washed three times with PBS and then treated with the appropriate Alexa fluorescent secondary antibodies at room temperature for 1 h, followed by counterstaining with DAPI for 5 min and coverslipping with Fluoroshield (Sigma-Aldrich). Fluorescent confocal microscopy images were acquired and analyzed using the Leica SP8 confocal system.

For IHC, mice were euthanized with an overdose of avertin solution and transcardially perfused with 4% paraformaldehyde. The brains were dissected, postfixed overnight in the same fixative, and cryopreserved with buffered 30% sucrose. A series of coronal sections of brain at 40 μm thickness were cut cryostatically and stored at − 20 °C. Then, standard multiple-labeled fluorescent IHC was performed. Briefly, the floating brain sections (40 μm) were washed three times with 0.5% Triton X-100/tris-buffered saline (TBS) and blocked for 30 min in blocking buffer containing 2% BSA in TBS with 0.5% Triton X-100. Then, primary antibodies were added and the sections were incubated overnight at 4 °C. After three washes, the brain sections were treated with the corresponding Alexa fluorescent labeled secondary antibodies in blocking buffer for 1 h at room temperature. After washing and DAPI counterstaining (Sigma Aldrich Cat. #D9542), brain sections were mounted onto glass microscope slides and then coverslipped with Fluoroshield (Sigma Aldrich Cat. #F6182). Image acquisition and analysis was also performed with the Leica SP8 confocal system.

To assess in vivo hippocampal neurogenic dynamics, specific antibody combinations were used to label different cellular types. Generally, GFAP and Sox2 co-localization is used to histologically mark NSCs, while Sox2 immunoreactivity only marks NPCs [46]. Additional Ki67 immunoreactivity would help distinguish quiescent NSCs from the actively dividing NSCs [47]. DCX is a microtubule-associated protein that is prominently expressed in neuroblasts, and becomes lost once the neuroblast terminally differentiates into a neuron, which usually expresses NeuN and β3-tubulin. All these cell types during adult neurogenesis were quantified in an unbiased stereological manner as described previously [24, 27, 46].

In vitro NSC stemness and differentiation assay
The isolation and culture of NSCs from 8- to 12-week-old WT or Tg26 mice were performed as described previously [45, 48]. First, the mice were euthanized by cervical dislocation, and their brains were rapidly dissected and placed in dissection wash buffer (Hanks buffered salt solution containing 0.6% glucose, 10 mM HEPES, 2 mM L-glutamine, and 1% penicillin/streptomycin, all from Corning CellGro). Their SVZs were microdissected, placed in wash buffer, and

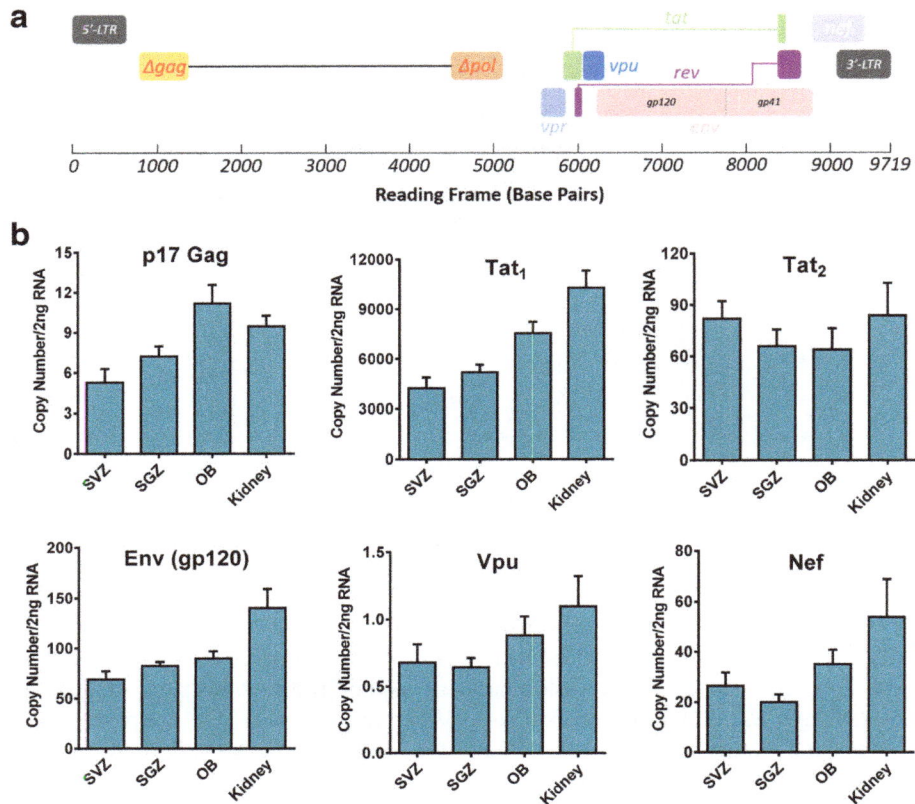

Fig. 1 HIV-1 Tg26 transgenic mice express viral mRNA in neurogenic regions. **a** Diagram of the truncated HIV-1 NL4-3 proviral genome in HIV-1 Tg26 mice, showing a deletion of 3.1 kb DNA spanning a majority of the Gag and Pol genes, and the predicted presence of seven viral gene transcripts. **b** RT-qPCR analysis of viral gene transcripts in neurogenic regions of HIV-1 Tg26 mice. Equal amount of RNA from the SVZs, SGZs, olfactory bulbs (OB), and kidneys of HIV-1 Tg26 mice was reverse transcribed, with 2 ng of the generated cDNA used for real-time PCR with primers covering *p17 gag*, *tat₁* (unspliced variant), *tat₂* (spliced variant), *env* (*gp120*), *vpu*, and *nef*. Samples were collected from four HIV-1 Tg26 mice (two males and two females), and reactions were run in triplicate. Values are expressed as mean ± SEM

digested with Type IV Collagenase (Worthington Biochemical, Cat. # CLS-4) and 0.05% Trypsin (Thermo Fisher Scientific Cat. # 25300054) diluted in wash buffer. After tissue digestion, the SVZ tissue was gently triturated with a P1000 pipette tip approximately 20 times until a homogenous cell suspension was achieved. The dissociated cells were then seeded in NSC culture media consisting of 0.2% heparin (Stem Cell Technologies Cat. # 07980) (diluted 10,000×), 20 ng/ml epidermal growth factor (EGF) (Stem Cell Technologies Cat.# 78016), 10 ng/ml basic fibroblast growth factor (bFGF) (Stem Cell Technologies Cat.# 78003), 2 mM L-glutamine (Corning), and 1% penicillin/streptomycin (Corning) in DMEM/F12 media (Corning). Primary neurospheres were grown in culture for 7 days, followed by microscopy and imaging to determine size and quantity of the neurospheres present.

The primary neurospheres were further digested with Accutase (Sigma) to obtain a single cell suspension for in vitro lineage differentiation studies as described previously [45, 48]. Briefly, 20,000 cells were seeded in 4 well Matrigel-coated 8-well chamber slides per genotype in

NSC proliferation media. The next day, neural differentiation was induced by removal of bFGF and EGF [45, 49] and maintained for 5 days before fixation in 4% paraformaldyhyde. ICC was performed with antibodies against DCX (neuroblasts), β3-tubulin (neurons), and GFAP (astrocytes). Confocal images were taken at five to eight fields per well, and the percentage of differentiated cells over DAPI-positive cells was quantified in a genotype-blinded manner.

Retrovirus production and stereotaxic injection into the hippocampus

Packaging of the eGFP-containing retrovirus was performed in GP2-293 cells (Clonetech Cat. # 631458) in accordance with previously established protocols [50, 51]. Briefly, 15 μg of the pUX-eGFP vector (a gift from Dr. Shaoyu Ge at State University of New York) was co-transfected via the calcium phosphate method with 15 μg of pVSVG per 100 mm dish when the GP2-293 cells were 70–80% confluent. At 48 and 72 h after transfection, the cell media, which contained infectious retroviral particles, was collected and pooled together for concentration via ultracentrifugation at 25,000 RPM for 2 h at 4 °C. The viral pellet was resuspended in PBS and agitated overnight on a shaker in 4 °C. Viral titering was performed on HEK293T cells, with titers ranging up to 1×10^8 colony-forming units (cfu)/ml.

Stereotaxic surgery was performed on 10-week-old mice. Before the injections, the mice were anesthetized with Avertin (Sigma Aldrich Cat. #T48402-25G) (180 µl/10 g body weight). Surgery was initiated when lack of tactile response was observed. The mice were mounted onto a stereotaxic frame, and the hair on the head was shaved to expose the scalp. After dissection of the scalp, four shallow holes were drilled into the skull using a dental drill (0.5 mm drill bit) at the following stereotaxic coordinates:

AP, – 2.0 mm from bregma; lateral, ± 1.5 mm
AP, – 3.0 mm from bregma; lateral, ± 2.5 mm

After the holes were drilled, 2 µl of concentrated retrovirus was injected at each of these stereotaxic coordinates with a 10-µl Hamilton microsyringe:

AP, – 2.0 mm from bregma; lateral, ± .5 mm; ventral, – 2.0 mm
AP, – 3.0 mm from bregma; lateral, ± 2.5 mm; ventral, – 3.0 mm

After the stereotaxic injections were completed, the wound was closed with sterile surgical sutures, and the mice were returned back to their cages until further analysis at 4 weeks after injection.

Confocal imaging and Sholl/dendritic spine analysis of retroviral eGFP-labeled dentate granule neurons

Imaging of eGFP-labeled dentate granule neurons for Sholl analysis and dendritic spine analysis was performed using a Leica SP8 confocal microscopy system. For Sholl analysis, images were taken at a × 63 objective with a Z-stack thickness of 1.0 µm. For dendritic spine analysis, images were acquired with a × 63 objective with a Z-stack thickness of 0.2 µm. For each granule neuron, three to four apical dendritic segments totaling approximately 200 µm were used for dendritic spine analysis as described previously [52]. Neurolucida360 software (MBF Bioscience, RRID:SCR_001775) was used for Sholl and dendritic spine analysis, using maximum projection Z-stack images of the granule neurons or dendritic spines [53].

Statistical analysis

All statistical analysis was performed using GraphPad Prism 6.0. An unpaired two-tailed Student's t test was performed between two groups of different treatments or genotypes. The p value thresholds for statistical significance were set at < 0.05, < 0.01, and < 0.001.

Results

HIV-1 Tg26 transgenic mice express viral mRNA in the neurogenic regions

Various transgenic animal models have been used for the study of HIV-1 [3]. While the HIV-1 transgenic rat has shown varying levels of proviral gene expression in the CNS [54], no studies to date have characterized the extent of proviral gene expression in the brains of HIV-1 Tg26 mice. To this end, absolute quantitative RT-PCR was performed using the primers targeting specific viral transcripts (Fig. 1a, Table 1) in the neurogenic regions. With this method, varying copy numbers of transcripts for partial *gag* (p17), *tat* (unspliced and spliced variants), *env* (gp120), *vpu*, and *nef* were detected in Tg26 mice (Fig. 1b), specifically in the SVZ and SGZ neurogenic regions. The unspliced *tat1* transcript showed the highest level of expression in all the neurogenic zones and the kidney. The e*nv* (*gp120*), the spliced *tat2*, and the *nef* transcripts showed the second highest levels of expression, though it is interesting to note that their expression levels were relatively similar. Finally, the *p17 gag* transcript and the *vpu* transcript showed the lowest levels of expression in the neurogenic zones and the kidney. However, C_t values for the *vif* or *vpr* transcripts were not detected in the tested tissues or the kidney samples, most likely due to their relatively low expression levels. The PCR efficiency for *vif* and *vpr* was validated using the cDNA, which was reverse transcribed from the RNA of HIV-1 latent J-Lat cells. Interestingly, the expression levels of all the viral gene transcripts in the kidney were less than twofold higher than the expression levels in the neurogenic zones in the Tg26 mice with a pure C57BL/6J background.

Neural stem cells (NSCs) from HIV-1 Tg26 transgenic mice exhibit in vitro NSC quiescence and neuronal lineage differentiation deficits

To explore whether Tg26 transgenic mice exhibit early and late differentiation deficits, primary neurospheres were cultured from both Tg26 mice and WT littermated mice in accordance with previously established protocols [45]. The stemness assay [45] revealed significantly fewer number of primary neurospheres in Tg26 mice than that of littermated WT mice (Fig. 2a, b) ($t_6 = 5.836$; $p = 0.0011$). When the primary neurospheres were stratified by size (Fig. 2b), Tg26 mouse NSCs formed significantly less smaller sized neurospheres (< 75 µm) ($t_5 = 4.049$; $p = 0.0098$), but significantly more large-sized neurospheres (> 150 µm) ($t_6 = 2.829$; $p = 0.0281$). Since larger sized neurospheres typically contain more NSCs and smaller sized

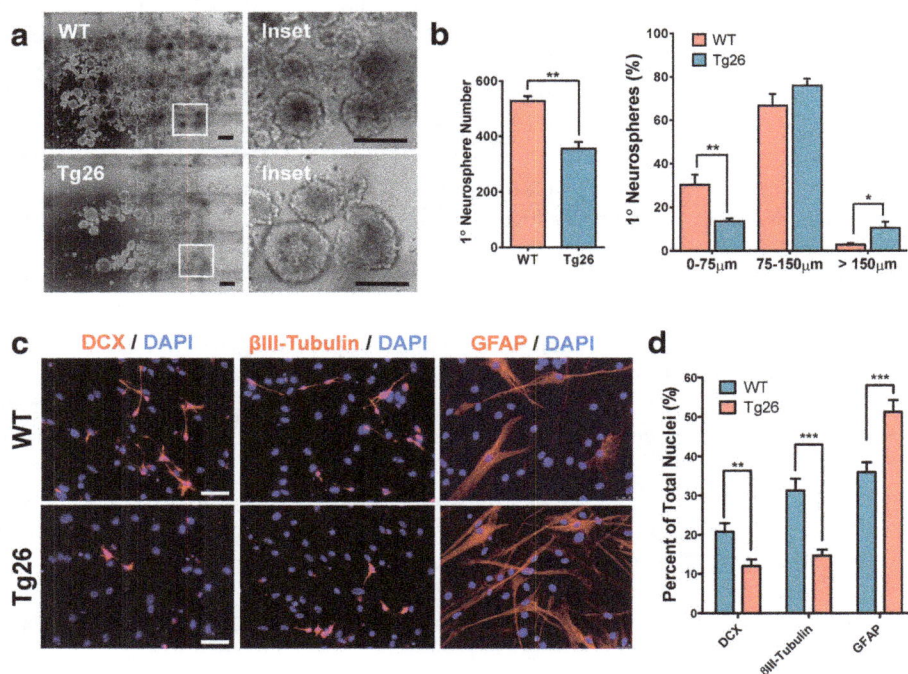

Fig. 2 In vitro stemness and neural lineage differentiation are impaired in HIV-1 Tg26 transgenic mice. **a, b** Fewer number of primary neurospheres but higher proportion of larger sized neurospheres in Tg26 mice. Representative tiled images of SVZ-derived primary neurospheres at 7 days in vitro are shown (**a**), and the number of the size stratified primary neurospheres was quantified using ImageJ software (**b**). Data is presented as the mean ± SEM from four mice per genotype. **c, d** Reduced neuronal lineage differentiation but increased astroglial lineage differentiation in Tg26 mouse NSCs/ NPCs. Dissociated NSCs/NPCs from primary neurospheres were differentiated for 5 days followed by immunocytochemistry with cell lineage-specific antibodies to assess for neuroblast (DCX) and neuronal (β3 tubulin) differentiation, and astrocytic (GFAP) formation (**c**). Tg26 mouse NSCs were unable to form as many neuroblasts or neurons as wild-type (WT) mouse NSCs, but instead formed more astrocytes (**d**). The quantitative differentiation data is presented as the Mean ± SEM from 4 mice (2 males and 2 females per genotype), with five to eight random fields per mouse for each cellular marker. Scale bar in **a**, 300 μm; inset, 150 μm. Scale bar in **c** 50 μm. $*p < 0.05$, $**p < 0.01$, $***p < 0.001$

neurospheres contain more NPCs [45, 48, 54, 55], these results suggest that Tg26 NSCs have significantly increased quiescence, implying that Tg26 mouse NSCs exhibit deficits in initial differentiation of NSCs to NPCs.

After the initial differentiation of NSCs to NPCs, the differentiation of NPCs to neuroblasts and finally the immature/mature neural cells continues throughout the middle/late stages of adult neurogenesis [16]. To explore whether the chronic stress induced by HIV-1 viral proteins affects neural lineage differentiation, multi-labeled ICC analysis of cultured differentiated NSCs was performed. As shown in Fig. 2c, d, Tg26 NSCs were unable to form as many neuroblasts ($t_{48} = 3.222$; $p = 0.0023$) and neurons ($t_{58} = 6.4989$; $p < 0.0001$) as WT NSCs. However, Tg26 NSCs had an increased incidence of astrocyte formation ($t_{58} = 3.889$; $p = 0.0003$). These results show that Tg26 NSCs exhibit hampered neuronal differentiation and aberrant astrocytic differentiation.

HIV-1 Tg26 mice exhibit hippocampal neurogenic deficits in vivo

To validate the in vitro findings that Tg26 NSCs exhibit stemness and neuronal differentiation impairments, multi-labeled fluorescent IHC with cell-specific markers and confocal imaging analysis (Fig. 3a, b) were performed in serial brain sections from WT and Tg26 mice. Stereological quantification (Fig. 3c) showed that the SGZs of Tg26 mice had significantly higher numbers of quiescent NSCs ($t_8 = 2.447$; $p = 0.0401$) and significantly lower levels of NSC proliferation ($t_9 = 3.523$; $p = 0.0065$). Additionally, Tg26 mouse SGZs showed fewer numbers of NPCs than WT mouse SGZs ($t_7 = 4.04$; $p = 0.0049$). Finally, Tg26 mouse SGZs had lower neuroblast formation (Fig. 3d, e), as depicted by significantly fewer numbers of DCX immunostained cells in the SGZ ($t_8 = 3.061$; $p = 0.0156$). Altogether, these studies suggest that Tg26 mice have significantly increased NSC quiescence and impaired initial differentiation of NSCs into NPCs as well as decreased neuronal lineage differentiation in vivo. This further

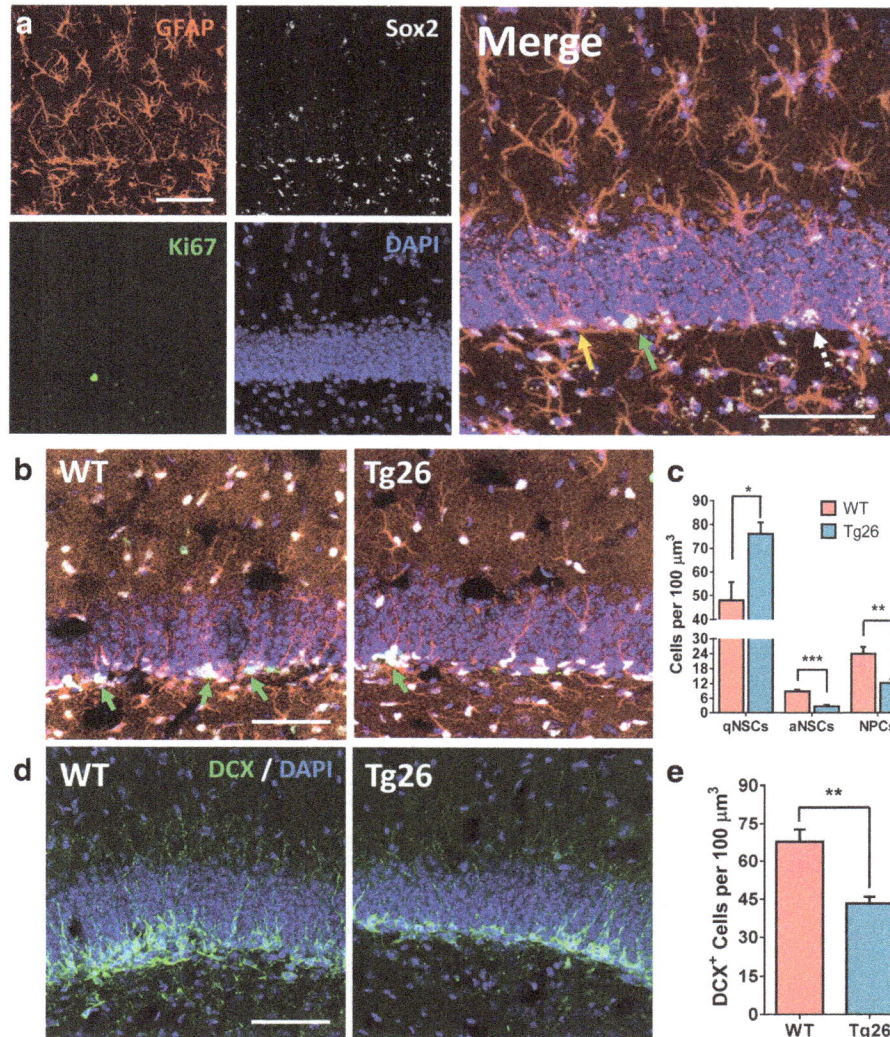

Fig. 3 Tg26 mice exhibit hippocampal neurogenesis deficits. **a** Representative confocal image showing quiescent NSCs (qNSCs, orange arrow, GFAP$^+$/Sox2$^+$/Ki67$^-$), active NSCs (aNSCs, green arrow, GFAP$^+$/Sox2$^+$/Ki67$^+$), and NPCs (dashed arrow, GFAP$^-$/Sox2$^+$) in the SGZ. **b** Comparative SGZ images from WT and littermated Tg26 mice showing less aNSCs (green arrows) in Tg26 mice. **c** Stereological quantification revealed significantly increased numbers of qNSCs, decreased numbers of aNSCs, and decreased numbers of NPCs in Tg26 mouse SGZs. **d** Representative confocal images showing DCX-positive neuroblasts in WT and Tg26 SGZs. **e** Stereological quantification revealing less neuroblast formation in Tg26 mice. Data in **c** and **e** represent the mean ± SEM from five to six mice per genotype (all females). Scale bars in **a**, **b**, and **d**, 50 μm. *$p < 0.05$ and **$p < 0.01$ indicate statistical changes compared with the corresponding WT SGZ

confirms the in vitro results from the primary neurosphere assays and the in vitro lineage differentiation assays.

Newborn dentate granule neurons in HIV-1 Tg26 mice exhibit dendritic arborization deficits, decreased dendritic length, and decreased dendritic spine density

Both the in vitro and in vivo studies, as described above, have shown that HIV-1 transgenic viral proteins significantly perturbed NSC initial differentiation and neuroblast/neuronal linage differentiation during adult neurogenesis. Next, experiments were performed to determine whether chronic stress from HIV-1 viral proteins in Tg26 mice had effects on late-stage neuronal maturation. Therefore, the maturation of newborn granule neurons in the dentate gyrus was analyzed using a well-established retroviral eGFP labeling technology [24, 50, 51]. Here, actively dividing cells (i.e., active NSCs, proliferating NPCs, and a few dividing neuroblasts) were instantly labeled with the eGFP reporter after stereotaxic injection of the retrovirus into the dentate gyrus. The fate of the labeled cells was mapped at different times after injection as described previously [24, 50, 51]. Studies have shown that maturation of newborn granule neurons from SGZ NSCs can be viewed by eGFP IHC and confocal image analysis approximately 4 weeks after retroviral injection in mice [50]. To identify any potential effects of chronic HIV-1 viral protein stress on dendritic arborization and spinogenesis during neuronal maturation [50], Sholl analysis on eGFP-labeled granule neurons in SGZ of WT and Tg26 mice at 4 weeks after retroviral injection into the dentate gyrus was performed using Neurolucida360 software (Fig. 4a). The eGFP-labeled newborn neurons in Tg26 mice exhibited significantly lower levels of dendritic arborization and complexity (Fig. 4b) at 20 μm (t_{56} = 2.557; p = 0.0133), 30 μm (t_{56} = 3.116; p = 0.0029), 40 μm (t_{64} = 2.753; p = 0.0077), 50 μm (t_{56} = 2.590; p = 0.0122), 60 μm (t_{56} = 2.115; p = 0.0389), 70 μm (t_{56} = 2.401; p = 0.0197), 160 μm (t_{31} = 2.492; p = 0.0182), and 170 μm (t_{27} = 2.411; p = 0.0230) away from the cell soma. This decrease in dendritic complexity also correlated with Tg26 granule neurons having a lower dendritic length (Fig. 4c) (t_{48} = 2.035; p = 0.0474). However, total dendritic surface area and dendritic volume remained unchanged (Fig. 4d, e). In addition to dendritic arborization deficits, several studies have

shown that HIV-1-infected patients exhibit synapto-dendritic damage, even while on ART [56, 57]. To examine whether Tg26 mouse dentate granule neurons have any changes in dendritic spine integrity, dendritic spine density analysis was conducted to assess any differences in total spine density, thin spine density, stubby spine density, and mushroom spine density (Fig. 5a). The eGFP-labeled granule neurons from HIV-1 Tg26 mice had significantly less apical dendritic spine densities (t_{43} = 5.681; p < 0.0001) compared to that from WT mice (Fig. 5b). Dendritic spines come in a variety of shapes and sizes, with the more common classifications being designated as thin spines, stubby spines, and mushroom-shaped spines [53]. Quantification of these specific spine types revealed that Tg26 granule neurons had a significantly lower thin spine density (Fig. 5c) (t_{40} = 2.047; p = 0.0473) and stubby spine density (Fig. 5d) (t_{41} = 2.884; p = 0.0062). However, quantification of mushroom spine density revealed that there were no differences between WT and Tg26 granule neurons (Fig. 5e). This data suggests that low-level chronic HIV-1 expression induces synaptodendritic damage in a manner similarly observed in HIV-1-infected patients [5].

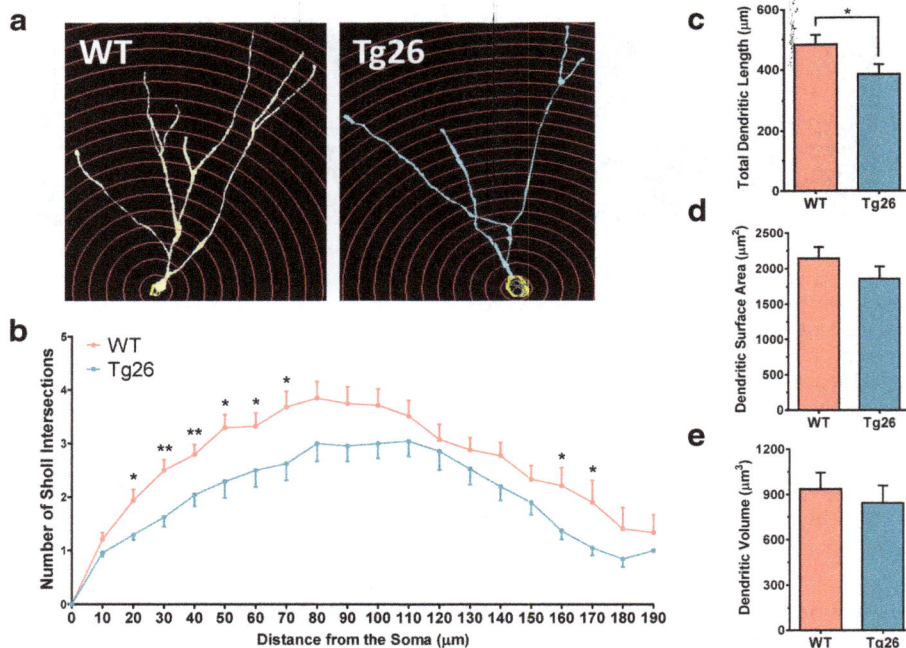

Fig. 4 Newborn dentate granule neurons in Tg26 mice have lower dendritic complexity and length. **a** Representative retroviral eGFP-labeled dentate granule neurons from WT and Tg26 mice with the Sholl analysis. Each Sholl circle increases in diameter by 10 μm from the cell soma. **b** Quantitative data of Sholl intersections. **c–e** Retroviral eGFP-labeled dentate granule neurons in WT and Tg26 mice were also assessed for total dendritic length (**c**), dendritic surface area (**d**), and dendritic volume (**e**). Data is presented as the mean ± SEM from four mice (three males and one female per genotype), with six to eight granule neurons being analyzed per mouse. *p < 0.05 and **p < 0.01 indicate statistical changes compared with corresponding WT granule neuron

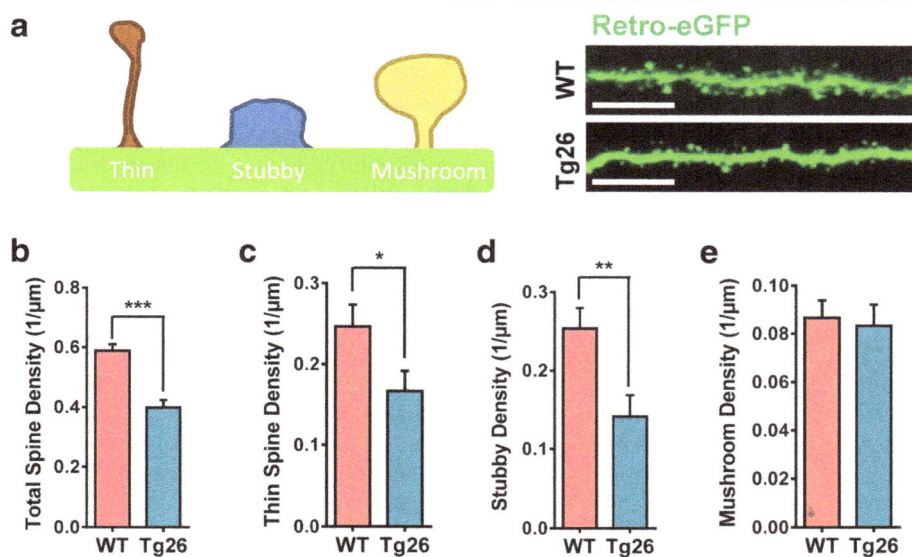

Fig. 5 Newborn dentate granule neurons in Tg26 mice harbor decreased apical dendritic spine density. **a** Diagram of dendritic spine types and representative images of retroviral eGFP-labeled apical dendritic arbors from WT and Tg26 granule neurons. **b–e** Quantitative analysis of total dendritic density as well as densities for specific spine types. Data is presented as the mean ± SEM from four mice (three males and one female per genotype), with at least 200 μm of apical dendritic arbors from six to eight granule neurons being analyzed per mouse. Scale bar in **a**, 6.25 μm. *$p < 0.05$, **$p < 0.01$, and ***$p < 0.001$ indicate statistical changes compared with the corresponding WT dendritic arbor

Discussion

In the ART era, HIV-1 infection continues to elicit mild to moderate forms of HAND, more notably ANI and MND [5, 6]. Many mechanisms have been characterized that explain some of the pathogenesis underlying ANI/MND, but recently, compromised adult neurogenic changes have been proposed as a newer mechanism for HIV-induced CNS injury [2, 3, 27, 31]. The salient findings of this study include (1) varying levels of HIV-1 proviral transcripts in the neurogenic zones of HIV-1 Tg26 mice, (2) deficits in initial NSC differentiation into NPCs in vitro and in vivo, (3) decreased neuronal lineage differentiation in vitro and in vivo, and (4) impairment of neuronal maturation and spinogenesis in newborn dentate granule neurons. These findings solidify the HIV-1 Tg26 mouse model as an appropriate approach to study the milder forms of HAND, which are clinically relevant to the HIV-1 latently infected population under ART today [6, 58].

Several pioneering studies have shown mosaic levels of HIV-1 proviral expression in peripheral organs such as the spleen, thymus, kidney, and muscle of Tg26 mice [36, 37, 59]. However, no previous studies have assessed viral gene expression levels in Tg26 mouse brains. To our knowledge, we are the first group to show the presence of the unspliced and spliced transcripts of HIV-1 viral genes not just in the brain, but specifically in different neurogenic niches. Our RT-PCR analysis revealed mosaic levels of p17 Gag, Tat (unspliced and spliced variants), Env (gp120), Vpu, and Nef transcripts in the

different neurogenic zones. These mosaic levels of proviral gene transcript expression are consistent with previous reports in HIV-1 transgenic rats using the same truncated pNL4-3 construct with all the transcripts driven by the HIV-1 5′-LTR promoter [54]. Interestingly, the unspliced Tat1 transcript showed a dramatically higher expression level than the spliced Tat2 transcript and other viral transcripts, implying that Tat1 might be the major contributor to CNS neurotoxicity [60–62]. Due to replication deficiency, the expression of these viral transcripts is relatively lower but constitutively persistent, implicating its clinical relevance to chronic HIV-1 infection in the ART era. The presence of HIV-1 viral transcripts in neurogenic zones also supports an earlier clinical finding by in situ hybridization in the SVZ and SGZ of a post-mortem patient with severe NeuroAIDS, showing that HIV-1 RNA transcripts localized to the neurogenic zones [18]. Further analysis using more sensitive technologies such as RNA/DNAscope [63, 64] and barcoded single-cell sequencing [65, 66] are warranted to distinguish the cellular distribution of HIV-1 viral transcripts in the neurogenic zones.

Most cases of HAND consist of subtle or milder forms of neurocognitive deficits. Since neurogenic defects have been shown to contribute to developing many subtle neurocognitive changes after CNS injury or neurodegenerative diseases [67, 68], it has been hypothesized that neurogenic impairment may contribute to the more subtle forms of HAND. This neurogenic impairment by HIV-1 single viral proteins has been demonstrated by several previous studies using in vitro cell cultures [25, 28, 31] and in vivo transgenic animal models [22, 24, 27, 56, 69]. For example, treating cultured NSCs/NPCs with Tat has been shown to inhibit NSC proliferation and differentiation through attenuation of the ERK pathway [70] and the p38-MAPK pathway [71] or through activation of the Notch pathway [27]. Additionally, treating NSCs/NPCs with gp120 suppresses NSC proliferation via activation of p38 MAPK pathway [25]. In this study, we performed a more comprehensive evaluation of impaired neurogenesis at both the in vitro and in vivo levels using a clinically relevant HIV-1 transgenic mouse model that harbors seven of nine HIV-1 viral genes. Our in vitro NSC stemness assays revealed a significantly diminished NSC pool in Tg26 mice compared to their WT littermates, as assessed by the reduced number of the primary neurospheres generated. Additionally, we found that chronic HIV-1 viral protein stress increased the formation of larger sized primary neurospheres, implying the impairment of initial differentiation of NSCs into NPCs. Primary neurospheres contain a mixed population of de novo NSCs and NPCs [45, 48], and larger sized neurospheres represent the existence of the tri-potential, self-renewing NSCs [55, 72]. These in vitro findings were validated in vivo, as Tg26 mouse SGZs had a higher level of quiescent NSCs, while having a diminished proliferating NSC population as well as a lower NPC pool. This increased NSC quiescence due to the hampered initial activation and differentiation into NPCs is consistent with previous reports on cultured NSCs treated with Tat and other viral proteins [70, 71, 73–75] and using in vivo animal models [20, 25, 73, 74, 76].

NSCs/NPCs terminally differentiate into neurons and glial cells. This lineage differentiation process is regulated by a series of environmental niche factors. Inflammatory mediators such as cytokines and chemokines have been widely shown to regulate this tri-potential lineage differentiation pattern in varying ways. The direct effects of chronic HIV-1 infection or viral proteins on NSC lineage differentiation have yet to be comprehensively understood. Our in vitro and in vivo neural lineage differentiation studies have shown that Tg26 NSCs have a decreased affinity towards neuronal lineage differentiation, but exhibit increased astroglial lineage differentiation. Similar effects have been observed in cultured NSCs/NPCs treated with Tat [70, 77] or direct HIV-1 infection [76], as well as in mice with HIV-1 encephalitis [78], doxycycline-inducible GFAP-Tat transgenic mice [27], and GFAP-gp120 mice [24, 25, 79]. However, a recent in vitro study has shown that active HIV-1 infection of human NSCs promotes both neuronal and astroglial lineage differentiation, when compared to uninfected human NSCs [31]. One possible explanation could be intrinsic mechanistic difference between

various HIV-1 strains: the CCR5-tropic HIV-1 BaL viral strain in previous study [31] vs the CXCR4-tropic NL4-3 strain in Tg26 mice. CCR5-tropic viruses represent the predominant viral population right after initial infection, but CXCR4 tropic viruses are associated with progressive CNS injury [80, 81]. In the clinical setting, CXCR4 tropic viruses may contribute more to the milder forms of HAND than CCR5 tropic viruses [3], which would make our in vivo HIV-1 Tg26 mouse model more clinically relevant. Another explanation may be the type of infection being performed: active infection vs. low-level chronic/latent infection. The supernatant from HIV-infected peripheral blood mononuclear cells may induce a more robust and confounding effect on NSC differentiation due to the combination of active virial particles, HIV-1 viral proteins, growth factors, and inflammatory mediators secreted by the infected cells [31].

Adult neurogenesis is a process that describes the generation of neural lineage cells from NSCs and NPCs. However, it is important to recognize the neuronal maturation and synaptic integration into this process. As of now, no studies have examined the effects of chronic HIV-1 infection and proviral protein stress on newborn neuronal formation and maturation. Retroviral eGFP labeling of newborn granule neurons in the dentate gyrus revealed that Tg26 mouse granule neurons have significantly decreased dendritic morphology, decreased total dendritic length, and decreased dendritic spine densities. These findings are notable, as these are the first to implicate the combined HIV-1 viral proteins in dendritic arborization deficits in newborn dentate granule neurons. Our observed decrease in dendritic spine density in dentate granule neurons is consistent with a previous study analyzing dendritic spine damage in layer II/III pyramidal prefrontal cortical neurons of both HIV-1 transgenic rats and gp120 infused rats [52], as well as aberrant dendritic development of newborn neurons in GFAP-gp120 transgenic mice [24]. Our Neurolucida360 studies further elaborated on the detrimental effects on various types of dendritic spines (thin, stubby, or mushroom spines) instead of only total dendritic spine density [52]. Additionally, our Sholl analysis identified dendritic morphological deficits of newborn hippocampal dentate granule neurons in Tg26 mice, while no differences in pyramidal cortical neuron dendritic length or branching were observed in HIV-1 transgenic rats [52]. This abnormal dendritic arborization in HIV-1 Tg26 mouse dentate granule neurons also supports a previous study using similar retroviral labeling technology of newborn dentate granule neurons in GFAP-gp120 mice [24]. However, further electrophysiological and circuit tracing experiments are needed to assess any functional differences in the newborn matured granule neurons between WT and Tg26 mice. Additionally, the molecular mechanisms behind the abnormal dendritic spine density in HIV-1 Tg26 mice remain to be determined.

Conclusions

Our in vitro and in vivo studies demonstrate that HIV-1 Tg26 transgenic mice manifest early-state and late-stage neurogenic deficits, when compared to their WT littermates. Additionally, these neurogenic deficits lead to deficient dentate granule neuron morphology as well as decreased dendritic spine densities. These neurogenic deficits may possibly play a role modulating learning and memory function in these mice, which is an interesting topic for further investigation.

Abbreviations

ANI: Asymptomatic neurocognitive impairment; ART: Antiretroviral treatment; bFGF: Basic fibroblast growth factor; CNS: Central nervous system; DCX: Doublecortin; EGF: Epidermal growth factor; eGFP: Enhanced green fluorescent protein; GFAP: Glial fibrillary acidic protein; HAD: HIV-associated dementia; HAND: HIV-associated neurocognitive disorders; HIV: Human immunodeficiency virus; ICC: Immunocytochemistry; IHC: Immunohistochemistry; LTR: Long terminal repeat; MND: Mild neurocognitive disorder; NPCs: Neural progenitor cells; NSCs: Neural stem cells; PBS: Phosphate-buffered saline; RT-PCR: Reverse transcription-polymerase chain reaction; SGZ: Subgranular zone; SVZ: Subventricular zone; TBS: Tris-buffered saline; TG: Transgenic; WT: Wild-type

Acknowledgements

We thank Dr. Shaoyu Ge at State University of New York at Stony Brook for the retroviral pUX-eGFP vector and critical comment.

Funding

This work was supported by the National Institutes of Health (R01DK075964 to W.H. and T32MH079785 to R.P).

Authors' contributions

RP, YZ, and WH designed the research. RP, YZ, and FL performed the cell culture, immunohistochemistry, confocal imaging, and quantitative analysis. RP and FL performed RT-qPCR analysis. RP, WH, and XFY analyzed the data and prepared figures. RP, MFB, and WH wrote and edited the manuscript. All authors read and approved the final manuscript.

Competing interests

The authors declare that they have no competing interests.

Author details

[1]Center for Metabolic Disease Research, Temple University Lewis Katz School of Medicine, 3500 N Broad Street, Philadelphia, PA 19140, USA. [2]Department of Pathology and Laboratory Medicine, Temple University Lewis Katz School of Medicine, 3500 N Broad Street, Philadelphia, PA 19140, USA. [3]Department of Anatomy and Cell Biology, Temple University Lewis Katz School of Medicine, 3500 N Broad Street, Philadelphia, PA 19140, USA. [4]Department of Pharmacology, Temple University Lewis Katz School of Medicine, 3500 N Broad Street, Philadelphia, PA 19140, USA.

References

1. Rodriguez-Penney AT, Iudicello JE, Riggs PK, Doyle K, Ellis RJ, Letendre SL, Grant I, Woods SP, Group HIVNRPH. Co-morbidities in persons infected with HIV: increased burden with older age and negative effects on health-related quality of life. AIDS Patient Care STDs. 2013;27:5–16.

2. Ferrell D, Giunta B. The impact of HIV-1 on neurogenesis: implications for HAND. Cell Mol Life Sci. 2014;71:4387–92.

3. Saylor D, Dickens AM, Sacktor N, Haughey N, Slusher B, Pletnikov M, Mankowski JL, Brown A, Volsky DJ, McArthur JC. HIV-associated neurocognitive disorder--pathogenesis and prospects for treatment. Nat Rev Neurol. 2016;12:234–48.

4. Antinori A, Arendt G, Becker JT, Brew BJ, Byrd DA, Cherner M, Clifford DB, Cinque P, Epstein LG, Goodkin K, et al. Updated research nosology for HIV-associated neurocognitive disorders. Neurology. 2007;69:1789–99.

5. Ellis RJ, Deutsch R, Heaton RK, Marcotte TD, McCutchan JA, Nelson JA, Abramson I, Thal LJ, Atkinson JH, Wallace MR, Grant I. Neurocognitive impairment is an independent risk factor for death in HIV infection. San Diego HIV Neurobehavioral Research Center Group. Arch Neurol. 1997; 54:416–24.

6. Heaton RK, Clifford DB, Franklin DR Jr, Woods SP, Ake C, Vaida F, Ellis RJ, Letendre SL, Marcotte TD, Atkinson JH, et al. HIV-associated neurocognitive disorders persist in the era of potent antiretroviral therapy: CHARTER study. Neurology. 2010;75:2087–96.

7. Kaul M, Garden GA, Lipton SA. Pathways to neuronal injury and apoptosis in HIV-associated dementia. Nature. 2001;410:988–94.

8. Kaul M, Zheng J, Okamoto S, Gendelman HE, Lipton SA. HIV-1 infection and AIDS: consequences for the central nervous system. Cell Death Differ. 2005; 12(Suppl 1):878–92.

9. Gonzalez-Scarano F, Martin-Garcia J. The neuropathogenesis of AIDS. Nat Rev Immunol. 2005;5:69–81.

10. Liu NQ, Lossinsky AS, Popik W, Li X, Gujuluva C, Kriederman B, Roberts J, Pushkarsky T, Bukrinsky M, Witte M, et al. Human immunodeficiency virus type 1 enters brain microvascular endothelia by macropinocytosis dependent on lipid rafts and the mitogen-activated protein kinase signaling pathway. J Virol. 2002;76:6689–700.

11. Williams KC, Hickey WF. Central nervous system damage, monocytes and macrophages, and neurological disorders in AIDS. Annu Rev Neurosci. 2002; 25:537–62.

12. Kaul M. HIV's double strike at the brain: neuronal toxicity and compromised neurogenesis. Front Biosci. 2008;13:2484–94.

13. Duan X, Kang E, Liu CY, Ming GL, Song H. Development of neural stem cell in the adult brain. Curr Opin Neurobiol. 2008;18:108–15.

14. Ming GL, Song H. Adult neurogenesis in the mammalian central nervous system. Annu Rev Neurosci. 2005;28:223–50.

15. Ihrie RA, Alvarez-Buylla A. Lake-front property: a unique germinal niche by the lateral ventricles of the adult brain. Neuron. 2011;70:674–86.

16. Ming GL, Song H. Adult neurogenesis in the mammalian brain: significant answers and significant questions. Neuron. 2011;70:687–702.

17. Riquelme PA, Drapeau E, Doetsch F. Brain micro-ecologies: neural stem cell niches in the adult mammalian brain. Philos Trans R Soc Lond Ser B Biol Sci. 2008;363:123–37.

18. Schwartz L, Civitello L, Dunn-Pirio A, Ryschkewitsch S, Berry E, Cavert W, Kinzel N, Lawrence DM, Hazra R, Major EO. Evidence of human immunodeficiency virus type 1 infection of nestin-positive neural progenitors in archival pediatric brain tissue. J Neuro-Oncol. 2007;13: 274–83.

19. Curtis K, Rollins M, Carryl H, Bradshaw K, Van Rompay KK, Abel K, Burke MW. Reduction of pyramidal and immature hippocampal neurons in pediatric simian immunodeficiency virus infection. Neuroreport. 2014;25:973–8.

20. Krathwohl MD, Kaiser JL. HIV-1 promotes quiescence in human neural progenitor cells. J Infect Dis. 2004;190:216–26.

21. Thaney VE, Sanchez AB, Fields JA, Minassian A, Young JW, Maung R, Kaul M. Transgenic mice expressing HIV-1 envelope protein gp120 in the brain as an animal model in neuroAIDS research. J Neuro-Oncol. 2018;24:156–67.

22. Avraham HK, Jiang S, Fu Y, Rockenstein E, Makriyannis A, Wood J, Wang L, Masliah E, Avraham S. Impaired neurogenesis by HIV-1-Gp120 is rescued by genetic deletion of fatty acid amide hydrolase enzyme. Br J Pharmacol. 2015;172:4603–14.

23. Lee MH, Amin ND, Venkatesan A, Wang T, Tyagi R, Pant HC, Nath A. Impaired neurogenesis and neurite outgrowth in an HIV-gp120 transgenic model is reversed by exercise via BDNF production and Cdk5 regulation. J Neuro-Oncol. 2013;19:418–31.

24. Lee MH, Wang T, Jang MH, Steiner J, Haughey N, Ming GL, Song H, Nath A, Venkatesan A. Rescue of adult hippocampal neurogenesis in a mouse model of HIV neurologic disease. Neurobiol Dis. 2011;41:678–87.

25. Okamoto S, Kang YJ, Brechtel CW, Siviglia E, Russo R, Clemente A, Harrop A, McKercher S, Kaul M, Lipton SA. HIV/gp120 decreases adult neural progenitor cell proliferation via checkpoint kinase-mediated cell-cycle withdrawal and G1 arrest. Cell Stem Cell. 2007;1:230–6.

26. Langford D, Oh Kim B, Zou W, Fan Y, Rahimain P, Liu Y, He JJ. Doxycycline-inducible and astrocyte-specific HIV-1 Tat transgenic mice (iTat) as an HIV/neuroAIDS model. J Neuro-Oncol. 2018;24:168–79.

27. Fan Y, Gao X, Chen J, Liu Y, He JJ. HIV Tat impairs neurogenesis through functioning as a notch ligand and activation of notch signaling pathway. J Neurosci. 2016;36:11362–73.

28. Lawrence DM, Durham LC, Schwartz L, Seth P, Maric D, Major EO. Human immunodeficiency virus type 1 infection of human brain-derived progenitor cells. J Virol. 2004;78:7319–28.

29. Schwartz L, Major EO. Neural progenitors and HIV-1-associated central nervous system disease in adults and children. Curr HIV Res. 2006;4: 319–27.

30. Tran PB, Ren D, Miller RJ. The HIV-1 coat protein gp120 regulates CXCR4-mediated signaling in neural progenitor cells. J Neuroimmunol. 2005;160: 68–76.

31. Balinang JM, Masvekar RR, Hauser KF, Knapp PE. Productive infection of human neural progenitor cells by R5 tropic HIV-1: opiate co-exposure heightens infectivity and functional vulnerability. AIDS. 2017;31:753–64.

32. Skowronska M, McDonald M, Velichkovska M, Leda AR, Park M, Toborek M. Methamphetamine increases HIV infectivity in neural progenitor cells. J Biol Chem. 2018;293:296–311.

33. Demir M, Laywell ED. Neurotoxic effects of AZT on developing and adult neurogenesis. Front Neurosci. 2015;9:93.

34. Jin J, Grimmig B, Izzo J, Brown LA, Hudson C, Smith AJ, Tan J, Bickford PC, Giunta B. HIV non-nucleoside reverse transcriptase inhibitor efavirenz reduces neural stem cell proliferation in vitro and in vivo. Cell Transplant. 2016;25:1967–77.

35. Xu P, Wang Y, Qin Z, Qiu L, Zhang M, Huang Y, Zheng JC. Combined medication of antiretroviral drugs tenofovir disoproxil fumarate, emtricitabine, and raltegravir reduces neural progenitor cell proliferation in vivo and in vitro. J Neuroimmune Pharmacol. 2017;12:682–92.

36. Dickie P, Felser J, Eckhaus M, Bryant J, Silver J, Marinos N, Notkins AL. HIV-associated nephropathy in transgenic mice expressing HIV-1 genes. Virology. 1991;185:109–19.

37. Kopp JB, Klotman ME, Adler SH, Bruggeman LA, Dickie P, Marinos NJ, Eckhaus M, Bryant JL, Notkins AL, Klotman PE. Progressive glomerulosclerosis and enhanced renal accumulation of basement membrane components in mice transgenic for human immunodeficiency virus type 1 genes. Proc Natl Acad Sci U S A. 1992;89:1577–81.

38. Carroll VA, Lafferty MK, Marchionni L, Bryant JL, Gallo RC, Garzino-Demo A. Expression of HIV-1 matrix protein p17 and association with B-cell lymphoma in HIV-1 transgenic mice. Proc Natl Acad Sci U S A. 2016;113: 13168–73.

39. Lu TC, He JC, Klotman P. Animal models of HIV-associated nephropathy. Curr Opin Nephrol Hypertens. 2006;15:233–7.

40. Gharavi AG, Ahmad T, Wong RD, Hooshyar R, Vaughn J, Oller S, Frankel RZ, Bruggeman LA, D'Agati VD, Klotman PE, Lifton RP. Mapping a locus for susceptibility to HIV-1-associated nephropathy to mouse chromosome 3. Proc Natl Acad Sci U S A. 2004;101:2488–93.

41. Mallipattu SK, Liu R, Zhong Y, Chen EY, D'Agati V, Kaufman L, Ma'ayan A, Klotman PE, Chuang PY, He JC. Expression of HIV transgene aggravates kidney injury in diabetic mice. Kidney Int. 2013;83:626–34.

42. Zhong J, Zuo Y, Ma J, Fogo AB, Jolicoeur P, Ichikawa I, Matsusaka T. Expression of HIV-1 genes in podocytes alone can lead to the full spectrum of HIV-1-associated nephropathy. Kidney Int. 2005;68:1048–60.

43. Ocwieja KE, Sherrill-Mix S, Mukherjee R, Custers-Allen R, David P, Brown M, Wang S, Link DR, Olson J, Travers K, et al. Dynamic regulation of HIV-1 mRNA populations analyzed by single-molecule enrichment and long-read sequencing. Nucleic Acids Res. 2012;40:10345–55.

44. Yin C, Zhang T, Qu X, Zhang Y, Putatunda R, Xiao X, Li F, Xiao W, Zhao H, Dai S, et al. In vivo excision of HIV-1 provirus by saCas9 and multiplex single-guide RNAs in animal models. Mol Ther. 2017;25: 1168 86.

45. Zhang Y, Liu J, Yao S, Li F, Xin L, Lai M, Bracchi-Ricard V, Xu H, Yen W, Meng W, et al. Nuclear factor kappa B signaling initiates early differentiation of neural stem cells. Stem Cells. 2012;30:510–24.

46. Beckervordersandforth R, Ebert B, Schaffner I, Moss J, Fiebig C, Shin J, Moore DL, Ghosh L, Trinchero MF, Stockburger C, et al. Role of mitochondrial metabolism in the control of early lineage progression and aging phenotypes in adult hippocampal neurogenesis. Neuron. 2017;93:560–73 e566.

47. von Bohlen Und Halbach O. Immunohistological markers for staging neurogenesis in adult hippocampus. Cell Tissue Res. 2007;329:409–20.

48. Azari H, Rahman M, Sharififar S, Reynolds BA. Isolation and expansion of the adult mouse neural stem cells using the neurosphere assay. J Vis Exp. 2010; 45:2393.

49. Ostenfeld T, Svendsen CN. Requirement for neurogenesis to proceed through the division of neuronal progenitors following differentiation of epidermal growth factor and fibroblast growth factor-2-responsive human neural stem cells. Stem Cells. 2004;22:798–811.

50. Ge S, Goh EL, Sailor KA, Kitabatake Y, Ming GL, Song H. GABA regulates synaptic integration of newly generated neurons in the adult brain. Nature. 2006;439:589–93.

51. van Praag H, Schinder AF, Christie BR, Toni N, Palmer TD, Gage FH. Functional neurogenesis in the adult hippocampus. Nature. 2002;415: 1030–4.

52. Festa L, Gutoskey CJ, Graziano A, Waterhouse BD, Meucci O. Induction of interleukin-1beta by human immunodeficiency virus-1 viral proteins leads to increased levels of neuronal ferritin heavy chain, synaptic injury, and deficits in flexible attention. J Neurosci. 2015;35:10550–61.

53. Dickstein DL, Dickstein DR, Janssen WG, Hof PR, Glaser JR, Rodriguez A, O'Connor N, Angstman P, Tappan SJ. Automatic dendritic spine quantification from confocal data with Neurolucida 360. Curr Protoc Neurosci. 2016;77:1.27.1–1.27.21.

54. Peng J, Vigorito M, Liu X, Zhou D, Wu X, Chang SL. The HIV-1 transgenic rat as a model for HIV-1 infected individuals on HAART. J Neuroimmunol. 2010; 218:94–101.

55. Siebzehnrubl FA, Vedam-Mai V, Azari H, Reynolds BA, Deleyrolle LP. Isolation and characterization of adult neural stem cells. Methods Mol Biol. 2011;750:61–77.

56. Fitting S, Knapp PE, Zou S, Marks WD, Bowers MS, Akbarali HI, Hauser KF. Interactive HIV-1 Tat and morphine-induced synaptodendritic injury is triggered through focal disruptions in Na(+) influx, mitochondrial instability, and Ca(2)(+) overload. J Neurosci. 2014;34:12850–64.

57. Masliah E, Heaton RK, Marcotte TD, Ellis RJ, Wiley CA, Mallory M, Achim CL, McCutchan JA, Nelson JA, Atkinson JH, Grant I. Dendritic injury is a pathological substrate for human immunodeficiency virus-related cognitive disorders. HNRC Group. The HIV Neurobehavioral Research Center. Ann Neurol. 1997;42:963–72.

58. Johnson TP, Patel K, Johnson KR, Maric D, Calabresi PA, Hasbun R, Nath A. Induction of IL-17 and nonclassical T-cell activation by HIV-Tat protein. Proc Natl Acad Sci U S A. 2013;110:13588–93.

59. Bruggeman LA, Thomson MM, Nelson PJ, Kopp JB, Rappaport J, Klotman PE, Klotman ME. Patterns of HIV-1 mRNA expression in transgenic mice are tissue-dependent. Virology. 1994;202:940–8.

60. Rahimian P, He JJ. HIV-1 Tat-shortened neurite outgrowth through regulation of microRNA-132 and its target gene expression. J Neuroinflammation. 2016;13:247.

61. Fields J, Dumaop W, Eleuteri S, Campos S, Serger E, Trejo M, Kosberg K, Adame A, Spencer B, Rockenstein E, et al. HIV-1 Tat alters neuronal autophagy by modulating autophagosome fusion to the lysosome: implications for HIV-associated neurocognitive disorders. J Neurosci. 2015;35:1921–38.

62. Zhou BY, Liu Y, Kim B, Xiao Y, He JJ. Astrocyte activation and dysfunction and neuron death by HIV-1 Tat expression in astrocytes. Mol Cell Neurosci. 2004;27:296–305.

63. Vasquez JJ, Hussien R, Aguilar-Rodriguez B, Junger H, Dobi D, Henrich TJ, Thanh C, Gibson E, Hogan LE, McCune J, et al. Elucidating the burden of HIV in tissues using multiplexed immunofluorescence and in situ hybridization: methods for the single-cell phenotypic characterization of cells harboring HIV in situ. J Histochem Cytochem. 2018;66:427–46.

64. Deleage C, Wietgrefe SW, Del Prete G, Morcock DR, Hao XP, Piatak M Jr, Bess J, Anderson JL, Perkey KE, Reilly C, et al. Defining HIV and SIV reservoirs in lymphoid tissues. Pathog Immun. 2016;1:68–106.

65. Zilionis R, Nainys J, Veres A, Savova V, Zemmour D, Klein AM, Mazutis L. Single-cell barcoding and sequencing using droplet microfluidics. Nat Protoc. 2017;12:44–73.

66. Cole C, Byrne A, Beaudin AE, Forsberg EC, Vollmers C. Tn5Prime, a Tn5 based 5' capture method for single cell RNA-seq. Nucleic Acids Res. 2018;46: 62.

67. Iascone DM, Padidam S, Pyfer MS, Zhang X, Zhao L, Chin J. Impairments in neurogenesis are not tightly linked to depressive behavior in a transgenic mouse model of Alzheimer's disease. PLoS One. 2013;8:e79651.

68. Mu Y, Gage FH. Adult hippocampal neurogenesis and its role in Alzheimer's disease. Mol Neurodegener. 2011;6:85.

69. Carey AN, Sypek EI, Singh HD, Kaufman MJ, McLaughlin JP. Expression of HIV-Tat protein is associated with learning and memory deficits in the mouse. Behav Brain Res. 2012;229:48–56.

70. Mishra M, Taneja M, Malik S, Khalique H, Seth P. Human immunodeficiency virus type 1 Tat modulates proliferation and differentiation of human neural precursor cells: implication in NeuroAIDS. J Neuro-Oncol. 2010;16:355–67.

71. Chao J, Yang L, Yao H, Buch S. Platelet-derived growth factor-BB restores HIV Tat -mediated impairment of neurogenesis: role of GSK-3beta/beta-catenin. J Neuroimmune Pharmacol. 2014;9:259–68.

72. Azari H, Louis SA, Sharififar S, Vedam-Mai V, Reynolds BA. Neural-colony forming cell assay: an assay to discriminate bona fide neural stem cells from neural progenitor cells. J Vis Exp. 2011;49:2639.

73. Fatima M, Kumari R, Schwamborn JC, Mahadevan A, Shankar SK, Raja R, Seth P. Tripartite containing motif 32 modulates proliferation of human neural precursor cells in HIV-1 neurodegeneration. Cell Death Differ. 2016;23:776–86.

74. Hahn YK, Podhaizer EM, Hauser KF, Knapp PE. HIV-1 alters neural and glial progenitor cell dynamics in the central nervous system: coordinated response to opiates during maturation. Glia. 2012;60:1871–87.

75. Yao H, Duan M, Yang L, Buch S. Platelet-derived growth factor-BB restores human immunodeficiency virus Tat-cocaine-mediated impairment of neurogenesis: role of TRPC1 channels. J Neurosci. 2012;32:9835–47.

76. Das S, Basu A. Viral infection and neural stem/progenitor cell's fate: implications in brain development and neurological disorders. Neurochem Int. 2011;59:357–66.

77. Yang L, Chen X, Hu G, Cai Y, Liao K, Buch S. Mechanisms of platelet-derived growth factor-BB in restoring HIV Tat-cocaine-mediated impairment of neuronal differentiation. Mol Neurobiol. 2016;53:6377–87.

78. Peng H, Sun L, Jia B, Lan X, Zhu B, Wu Y, Zheng J. HIV-1-infected and immune-activated macrophages induce astrocytic differentiation of human cortical neural progenitor cells via the STAT3 pathway. PLoS One. 2011;6:e19439.

79. Avraham HK, Jiang S, Fu Y, Rockenstein E, Makriyannis A, Zvonok A, Masliah E, Avraham S. The cannabinoid CB(2) receptor agonist AM1241 enhances neurogenesis in GFAP/Gp120 transgenic mice displaying deficits in neurogenesis. Br J Pharmacol. 2014;171:468–79.

80. Connor RI, Sheridan KE, Ceradini D, Choe S, Landau NR. Change in coreceptor use correlates with disease progression in HIV-1--infected individuals. J Exp Med. 1997;185:621–8.

81. Scarlatti G, Tresoldi E, Bjorndal A, Fredriksson R, Colognesi C, Deng HK, Malnati MS, Plebani A, Siccardi AG, Littman DR, et al. In vivo evolution of HIV-1 co-receptor usage and sensitivity to chemokine-mediated suppression. Nat Med. 1997;3:1259–65.

12

Reduced gut microbiome protects from alcohol-induced neuroinflammation and alters intestinal and brain inflammasome expression

Patrick P. Lowe, Benedek Gyongyosi, Abhishek Satishchandran, Arvin Iracheta-Vellve, Yeonhee Cho, Aditya Ambade and Gyongyi Szabo*ⓘ

Abstract

Background: The end-organ effects of alcohol span throughout the entire body, from the gastrointestinal tract to the central nervous system (CNS). In the intestine, alcohol use changes the microbiome composition and increases gut permeability allowing translocation of microbial components into the circulation. Gut-derived pathogen-associated signals initiate inflammatory responses in the liver and possibly elsewhere in the body. Because previous studies showed that the gut microbiome contributes to alcohol-induced liver disease, we hypothesized that antibiotic administration to reduce the gut microbiome would attenuate alcohol-induced inflammation in the brain and small intestine (SI).

Methods: Six- to 8-week-old C57BL/6J female mice were fed alcohol in a liquid diet or a calorie-matched control diet for 10 days with an acute alcohol binge or sugar on the final day (acute-on-chronic alcohol administration). Some mice were treated with oral antibiotics daily to diminish the gut microbiome. We compared serum levels of TNFα, IL-6, and IL-1β by ELISA; expression of cytokines *Tnfa*, *Mcp1*, *Hmgb1*, *Il-17*, *Il-23*, *Il-6*, and *Cox2*; and inflammasome components *Il-1β*, *Il-18*, *Casp1*, *Asc*, and *Nlrp3* in the CNS and SI by qRT-PCR. Microglial morphology was analyzed using immunohistochemical IBA1 staining in the cortex and hippocampus.

Results: Antibiotics dramatically reduced the gut microbiome load in both alcohol- and pair-fed mice. Alcohol-induced neuroinflammation and increase in SI cytokine expression were attenuated in mice with antibiotic treatment. Acute-on-chronic alcohol did not induce serum TNFα, IL-6, and IL-1β. Alcohol feeding significantly increased the expression of proinflammatory cytokines such as *Tnfa*, *Mcp1*, *Hmgb1*, *Il-17*, and *Il-23* in the brain and intestine. Reduction in the gut bacterial load, as a result of antibiotic treatment, attenuated the expression of all of these alcohol-induced proinflammatory cytokines in both the brain and SI. Alcohol feeding resulted in microglia activation and morphologic changes in the cortex and hippocampus characterized by a reactive phenotype. These alcohol-induced changes were abrogated following an antibiotic-induced reduction in the gut microbiome. Unexpectedly, antibiotic treatment increased the mRNA expression of some inflammasome components in both the brain and intestine.

Conclusions: Our data show for the first time that the acute-on-chronic alcohol administration in mice induces both neuroinflammation and intestinal inflammation and that reduction in the intestinal bacterial load can attenuate alcohol-associated CNS and gut inflammation. Gut microbiome-derived signals contribute to neuroinflammation in acute-on-chronic alcohol exposure.

Keywords: Neuroinflammation, Alcohol, Microglia, Cytokines, Microbiome, Inflammasome

* Correspondence: Gyongyi.Szabo@umassmed.edu
Department of Medicine, University of Massachusetts Medical School, 364 Plantation Street, Worcester, MA 01605, USA

Background

Prolonged alcohol consumption leads to translocation of gut bacterial components, such as endotoxin, from the intestinal lumen into the circulation [1–3]. Once absorbed, alcohol along with gut-derived endotoxin is delivered via the portal circulation to the liver where metabolism begins and an inflammatory cascade is initiated. However, endotoxin, unmetabolized alcohol, and alcohol metabolites also pass through the liver and reach the systemic circulation and other organs, including the peripheral immune system and the central nervous system (CNS). While previous studies have investigated the direct effects of alcohol on the brain [4–6], little is known about the role of gut-derived microbial products and their impact on the nervous system and neuroinflammation.

Microglia play a critical role in sensing and responding to alcohol consumption and are involved in multiple immune signaling pathways [7–10]. Microglia express Toll-like receptor 4 (TLR4), a pattern recognition receptor critical in alcohol-induced neuroinflammation [11–13] as well as the NLR family pyrin domain containing 3 (NLRP3) inflammasome [9]. Previous studies showed that TLR4 knockout mice are protected from increased cytokine expression in various regions of the brain and from increased activation of microglia [14–16]. TLR4 recognizes endogenous danger signals such as HMGB1 [17, 18] and is the major pattern recognition receptor of bacterial endotoxin (also known as lipopolysaccharide (LPS)) [19]. Although endotoxin is not generally believed to cross the blood-brain barrier [20], data from TLR4 knockout mice suggests that signaling through TLR4 is an important component influencing alcohol-induced neuroinflammation. Neuroinflammation is mediated by the inflammasome complex, a multiprotein complex that senses pathogens and danger signals leading to cleavage and release of proinflammatory IL-1β and IL-18 [9].

LPS signaling is also a critical component of liver pathology associated with alcohol consumption. Alcohol metabolism leads to cell stress, hepatocyte damage, and release of sterile danger signals in the liver [21, 22]. Endotoxins, derived from the intestinal microbiome into the portal circulation, are recognized by pattern recognition receptors such as TLR4 and initiate an inflammatory response secondary to the hepatocyte stress and damage caused by the release of reactive oxygen species and other cellular stresses induced by alcohol metabolism. Interestingly, we and others have shown that treating mice with antibiotics to reduce the bacterial load in the gastrointestinal tract (and thereby reducing endotoxin levels) attenuates liver inflammation and steatosis after alcohol use [23–25]. This reduction in gut bacterial load could ameliorate the alcohol-induced changes in the brain.

To further explore the critical role of the gut microbiome in the gut-brain axis, we used antibiotics to reduce the intestinal bacterial load in mice. Following acute-on-chronic alcohol consumption in mice (10 days of alcohol followed by an acute alcohol binge), we show that alcohol induces neuroinflammation in the CNS and also increases cytokine expression in the small intestine. Inflammation in both organs was attenuated with antibiotic-induced microbiome reduction. Interestingly, although cytokine expression was reduced, antibiotic treatment induced the mRNA expression of inflammasome components and cytokines processed by the inflammasome in the CNS and intestine. These results show for the first time that manipulation of the gut microbiome via reduction of the microbial load protects from alcohol-induced CNS and intestinal inflammation. Our study provides important insights into the interactions of the intestinal microbiome and brain in the gut-brain axis induced by alcohol.

Methods

Mouse alcohol feeding

All animal studies were approved by the Institutional Animal Care and Use Committee at the University of Massachusetts Medical School (UMMS). Wild-type C57BL/6J 6- to 8-week-old female mice were purchased from Jackson Laboratories and co-housed in the UMMS Animal Medicine Facility. Female mice were chosen because they are more susceptible to alcohol-induced liver injury than male mice [26–28]. Alcohol feeding followed the acute-on-chronic model previously described by Bertola et al. [29]. Briefly, all mice received the pair-fed Lieber-DeCarli (Bio-Serv) liquid diet for 5 days. Some mice then received 5% alcohol and maltose dextran in a liquid diet while pair-fed mice remained on the control liquid diet. Pair-fed mice were calorie-matched with the alcohol-fed mice. Nine hours prior to sacrifice, alcohol-fed mice received alcohol via oral gavage (5 g kg^{-1} body weight) and pair-fed mice received isocaloric maltose dextran.

Antibiotic treatment

Mice were either treated twice daily with an oral intragastric gavage of water or a broad spectrum antibiotic cocktail (Abx) containing ampicillin (100 mg/kg body weight (BW); Sigma), neomycin (100 mg/kg BW; Gibco), metronidazole (100 mg/kg BW; Sigma), and vancomycin (50 mg/kg BW; Sigma). Gavages began on the first day of liquid diet and continued daily until the completion of alcohol feeding. Significant reduction in bacterial load was confirmed by bacterial culture (described below) similar to previous reports [23].

Bacterial culture

Mouse feces were collected directly from the anus and suspended in thioglycolate media. Suspensions were plated on non-selective LB agar plates (EMD Millipore) and incubated for 24 h at 37 °C for assessment of bacterial load reduction.

qPCR analysis

RNA extraction from the small intestine and brain cortical tissue was performed using miRNeasy Extraction Kit (Qiagen) according to the manufacturer's instructions, including on-column DNase digestion (Zymo Research). Reverse transcription for cDNA was completed from 1 µg of RNA and subsequent 1:5 dilution in nuclease-free water. Real-time qPCR using SYBR Green (BioRad) was performed according to the manufacturer's instructions. RT-qPCR primers are listed in Table 1, and *18S* mRNA expression was used as a housekeeping gene for $2^{-\Delta\Delta Ct}$ method of RNA expression analysis. For 16S comparison between antibiotic-treated and non-treated animals, stool bacterial DNA was extracted using QIAamp DNA Stool Mini Kit (Qiagen) according to the manufacturer's protocol. After running a qPCR reaction using 16S primers similar to described above, a ΔCt was calculated using the average Ct value of each sample duplicate and subtracting the average ΔCt of untreated pair-fed mice. The bacterial 16S PCR product was run on a 1% agarose gel to visualize the relative reduction in bacterial load.

Serum cytokine measurement

Mice were cheek-bled prior to sacrifice, and serum was isolated. TNFα and IL-6 (Biolegend, San Diego, CA, USA) and IL-1β (R&D Systems, Minneapolis, MN, USA) were measured by ELISA.

Immunohistochemistry

Following sacrifice, brain tissue was dissected and fixed in 10% formalin overnight before paraffin embedding. Immunohistochemical staining was completed at the UMMS Morphology Core using anti-ionized calcium-binding adapter molecule (IBA1) antibody (Wako; 1:1000) and subsequently labeled with streptavidin-biotin immunoenzymatic antigen for detection with 3,3′-diaminobenzidine (DAB) (UltraVision Mouse Tissue Detection System Anti-Mouse HRP/DAB; Lab Vision). Images were acquired from the described CNS areas by light microscopy (cortex; CA1, CA3, and DG of the hippocampus) at × 40 magnification for process length and cell body size measurements of microglia using ImageJ. Cell process length for each microglial cell was measured by tracing all extensions off of the soma to their distal termination using ImageJ's freehand measuring tool. For each microglia, the length of all processes was summed to obtain the total cell process length. The soma area was measured by tracing the perimeter of the cell body and measuring the contained area using ImageJ's freehand tracer and the area measurement function. Microglia were analyzed from five to nine images taken randomly from each CNS region from each mouse. The investigator was blinded to the sample groups during staining, image acquisition, and ImageJ analysis. IBA1 positivity was measured using the *Color Deconvolution* plug-in in ImageJ.

Statistical analysis

Statistical analysis was carried out using GraphPad Prism Version 7.0 using Mann-Whitney test. $p < 0.05$ was considered statistically significant. Outlier exclusion was calculated using Grubbs' outlier test with alpha set to 0.05.

Table 1 Real-time PCR primers

Primer	Forward (5′–3′)	Reverse (5′–3′)
18S	GTAACCCGTTGAACCCCATT	CCATCCAATCGGTAGTAGCG
16S	TCCTACGGGAGGCAGCAGT	GGACTACCAGGGTATCTAATCCTGTT
Tnfa	GAAGTTCCCAAATGGCCTCC	GTGAGGGTCTGGGCCATAGA
Mcp-1	CAG GTC CCT GTC ATG CTT CT	TCTGGACCCATTCCTTCTTG
Il-1β	TCTTTGAAGTTGACGGACCC	TGAGTGATACTGCCTGCCTG
Il-17	CAGGGAGAGCTTCATCTGTGT	GCTGAGCTTTGAGGGATGAT
Il-23	AAGTTCTCTCCTCTTCCCTGTCGC	TCTTGTGGAGCAGCAGATGTGAG
Hmgb1	CGCGGAGGAAAATCAACTAA	TCATAACGAGCCTTGTCAGC
Il-6	ACAACCACGGCCTTCCCTACTT	CACGATTTCCCAGAGAACATGTG
Cox2	AACCGAGTCGTTCTGCCAAT	CTAGGGAGGGGACTGCTCAT
Nlrp3	AGCCTTCCAGGATCCTCTTC	CTTGGGCAGCAGTTTCTTTC
Asc	GAAGCTGCTGACAGTGCAAC	GCCACAGCTCCAGACTCTTC
Casp1	AGATGGCACATTTCCAGGAC	GATCCTCCAGCAGCAACTTC
Il-18	CAGGCCTGACATCTTCTGCAA	TCTGACATGGCAGCCATTGT

The above forward and reverse sequences of primers were used in real-time PCR

Abbreviations: *Tnfa* tumor necrosis factor-α, *Mcp-1* monocyte chemoattractant protein 1 (encoded by *CCL2*), *Il-1β* interleukin-1β, *Il-17* interleukin-17, *Il-23* interleukin-23, *Hmgb1* high-mobility group box 1, *Il-6* interleukin 6, *Cox2* cyclooxygenase 2, *Nlrp3* NLR family pyrin domain containing 3, *Asc* apoptosis-associated speck-like protein (encoded by *PYCARD*), *Casp1* caspase-1 (encoded by *CASP1*), *Il-18* interleukin-18

Results

Antibiotic treatment dramatically decontaminates gut bacterial load

While the modulating effects of chronic alcohol administration have been studied in the gut microbiome, alcoholic liver disease, and neuroinflammation, it is unclear how shorter alcohol use and/or alcohol binge affect inflammation signaling in the CNS and what role the gut microbiome plays in this process. In this study, mice received 5% alcohol (EtOH) in a liquid diet for 10 days (after a 5-day liquid diet acclimation period), followed by a one-time alcohol binge or a calorie-matched pair-fed (PF) diet [29]. Female mice were chosen because they have greater sensitivity to alcohol, and previous studies have focused on female animals [26–28]. To elucidate the importance of the gut microbiome in the translocation of pathogen-associated molecular patterns (PAMPs) from the intestine to extra-enteric organs, we used oral administration of a cocktail of antibiotics (ampicillin, neomycin, vancomycin, and metronidazole) to drastically reduce the bacterial load in the gut (Fig. 1a). Oral antibiotic treatment (Abx) caused a significant reduction in endotoxin in the circulation at the time of sacrifice both in pair-fed and alcohol-fed mice (Fig. 1b). The expression of 16S bacterial DNA, measured from mice stools collected immediately prior to sacrifice, was dramatically reduced by antibiotic treatment (Fig. 1c, d). Stool bacteria cultured on non-selective agar plates also revealed almost complete elimination of culturable colonies after 5 days of antibiotic treatment (Fig. 1e). Some recovery of bacteria in the stool was observed by the conclusion of the 15-day study, likely due to the development of antibiotic resistance (Fig.1e). However, bacterial colony-forming units (CFUs) were dramatically reduced in the stool obtained on the day of sacrifice in antibiotic-treated animals compared with untreated mice (Fig.1f). Together, these data indicate that antibiotic treatment successfully suppressed gut bacterial load and reduced circulating endotoxin in both pair- and alcohol-fed mice.

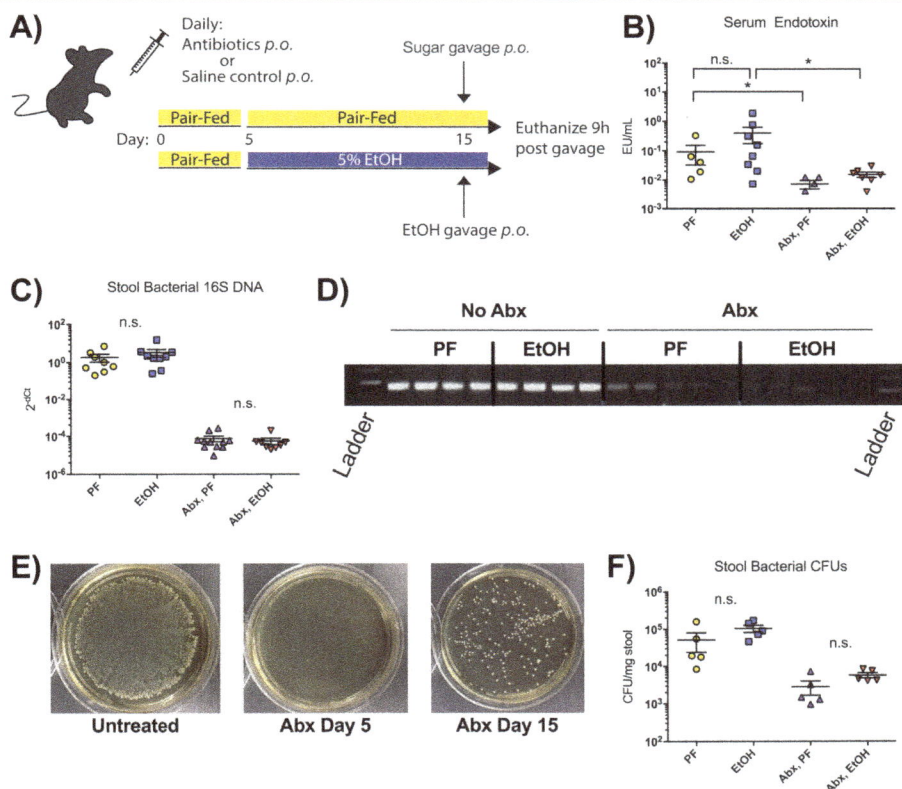

Fig. 1 Oral antibiotics significantly reduce the gut bacterial load. **a** Four groups of wild-type C57BL/6J female mice were treated with pair-fed diet (PF; $n = 5$), 5% alcohol diet (EtOH; $n = 10$), oral antibiotics (Abx) with PF ($n = 6$), or Abx with EtOH ($n = 9$). An acute sugar or alcohol binge was given 9 h before sacrifice. **b** Serum endotoxin was measured at sacrifice to determine translocation of gut bacterial products into systemic circulation. **c** DNA was isolated from the stool of PF and EtOH mice before sacrifice, and 16S DNA was measured by qPCR using universal 16S primers. **d** The PCR products from **c** were run on an agarose gel for a general comparison of the four groups. **e** Stools were resuspended in thioglycolate and plated on non-selective agar to measure gut bacterial load prior to antibiotic treatment (untreated), after 5 days of Abx treatment (Abx day 5), and at the end of the experiment (Abx day 15). **f** Colony-forming units (CFUs) were quantified from stool extracted at sacrifice on day 15. Data are mean ± SEM, $n = 5$–10 mice/group. *$p < 0.05$; n.s., not significant

Gut decontamination abrogates alcohol-induced proinflammatory cytokine expression in the brain cortex

Chronic alcohol induces circulating proinflammatory cytokines in both animal models and in human patients [30, 31]. To determine whether this systemic cytokine induction also occurs in the acute-on-chronic model in mice, we measured circulating TNFα and IL-6 in the serum (Fig. 2a). While alcohol did not induce statistically significant increases in either cytokine, antibiotic treatment significantly reduced circulating TNFα in both pair-fed and alcohol-fed mice (Fig. 2a).

Chronic alcohol use results in neuroinflammation both in humans and in mice [7, 12]. We found that 10 days of chronic alcohol feeding followed by a one-time binge in mice, a model of acute-on-chronic alcohol consumption not previously used to study neuroinflammation, induced significantly higher expression of proinflammatory cytokine genes including *Mcp-1*, *Hmgb1*, and *Il-17* and non-significant trends toward increased expression of *Tnfα* and *Il-23* in the brain cortex (Fig. 2b). *Tnfα*, *Mcp-1*, *Hmgb1*, *Il-17*, and *Il-23* are proinflammatory cytokines that can be released by multiple cell types, and each has previously been associated with alcohol-induced neuroinflammation [9, 14, 32, 33]. Alcohol did not induce expression of *Il-6* or *Cox2*. Interestingly, *Il-6* was induced in pair-fed antibiotic-treated mice compared to non-treated mice, and alcohol feeding reduced this induction (Fig. 2b).

Previous studies indicate that antibiotic treatment that reduces intestinal bacterial load also reduces alcohol-induced inflammation in the liver [23]. Here, we hypothesized that translocation of gut bacterial products to the CNS contributes to alcohol-induced neuroinflammation and that this process is regulated by the gut microbial load. Therefore, we sought to investigate whether gut decontamination could protect from neuroinflammation associated with alcohol consumption. We observed that the proinflammatory cytokine expression increase in the cortex in alcohol-fed mice compared to PF controls was markedly reduced in mice treated with Abx (Fig. 2b). Antibiotic treatment fully prevented alcohol-related induction of *Mcp1*, *Il-17*, and *Il-23* mRNA expression in the cortex. *Tnfα* was induced in antibiotic-treated, alcohol-fed mice compared to antibiotic-treated pair-fed mice, but its expression was still significantly lower compared to alcohol-fed mice without antibiotic treatment. Expression of *Tnfα*, *Mcp1*, *Il-17*, and *Il-23* was also reduced in the cortex of antibiotic-treated pair-fed mice compared to those without antibiotic treatment. These results indicate that acute-on-chronic alcohol feeding in mice increases proinflammatory cytokine induction that is prevented by the reduction in gut-derived PAMPs and the gut microbiome.

Cortical expression of inflammasome components increase with bacterial decontamination

Because we found that multiple proinflammatory cytokines were reduced in the cortex of antibiotic-treated mice (Fig. 2), we next measured inflammasome-related transcripts to elucidate if alcohol or antibiotics influenced inflammasome-mediated cytokine expression. The inflammasome is a multiprotein complex containing NOD-like receptors (NLRs, including NLRP3) that can sense pathogens and danger signals, the adaptor molecule, ASC, and the effector molecule, caspase-1. Inflammasome activation leads to cleavage of pro-IL-1β and pro-IL-18 to their respective bioactive forms, IL-1β and IL-18 [9]. We found that although alcohol did not induce IL-1β, antibiotic treatment increased circulating serum IL-1β in pair-fed mice ($p < 0.05$) and trended toward an increase in alcohol-fed mice ($p = 0.055$) (Fig. 3a). Interestingly, although chronic alcohol consumption models have led to increased expression of inflammasome components and *Il-1β* [9], we found no significant increase in alcohol-induced *Il-1β* mRNA expression in this acute-on-chronic alcohol model (Fig. 3b). However, cortical *Il-1β* mRNA expression in antibiotic-treated pair-fed mice was significantly increased and we observed an increasing trend in *Il-1β* in antibiotic-treated alcohol-fed compared to untreated mice. Interestingly, in antibiotic-treated mice, alcohol administration significantly increased *Il-1β* mRNA expression compared to pair-fed mice. Expression of *Il-18* was induced in alcohol-fed mice in the cortex, and similar to the increase in pair-fed *Il-1β*, we also found that *Il-18* and *Asc* were elevated in antibiotic-treated, PF mice compared to untreated PF mice (Fig. 3b). Acute-on-chronic alcohol administration reduced the expression of *Nlrp3* and *Asc* and increased the expression of *Il-18* in untreated alcohol-fed mice compared to untreated PF controls. *Asc* and *Il-18* mRNA expression were reduced in antibiotic-treated compared to untreated alcohol-fed mice (Fig. 3b). *Caspase-1* mRNA levels did not change significantly in any of the treatment groups (Fig. 3b). These observations suggest that regulation of the inflammasome and IL-1β depends on the gut microbiome and is minimally influenced in the acute-on-chronic alcohol model in mice.

Gut decontamination alters cortical and hippocampal microglia

To characterize the effects of the acute-on-chronic alcohol model in the CNS, we next examined the microglia activation. Microglia are the resident macrophages of the CNS capable of expressing proinflammatory cytokines in response to an insult, such as alcohol [34]. Activated microglia are characterized by altered cell morphology, taking on an amoeboid shape with enlarged cell bodies (soma) and shortened peripheral processes [35]. We used immunohistochemistry to identify IBA1-positive microglia (representative images shown in Fig. 4a, b). The soma size and

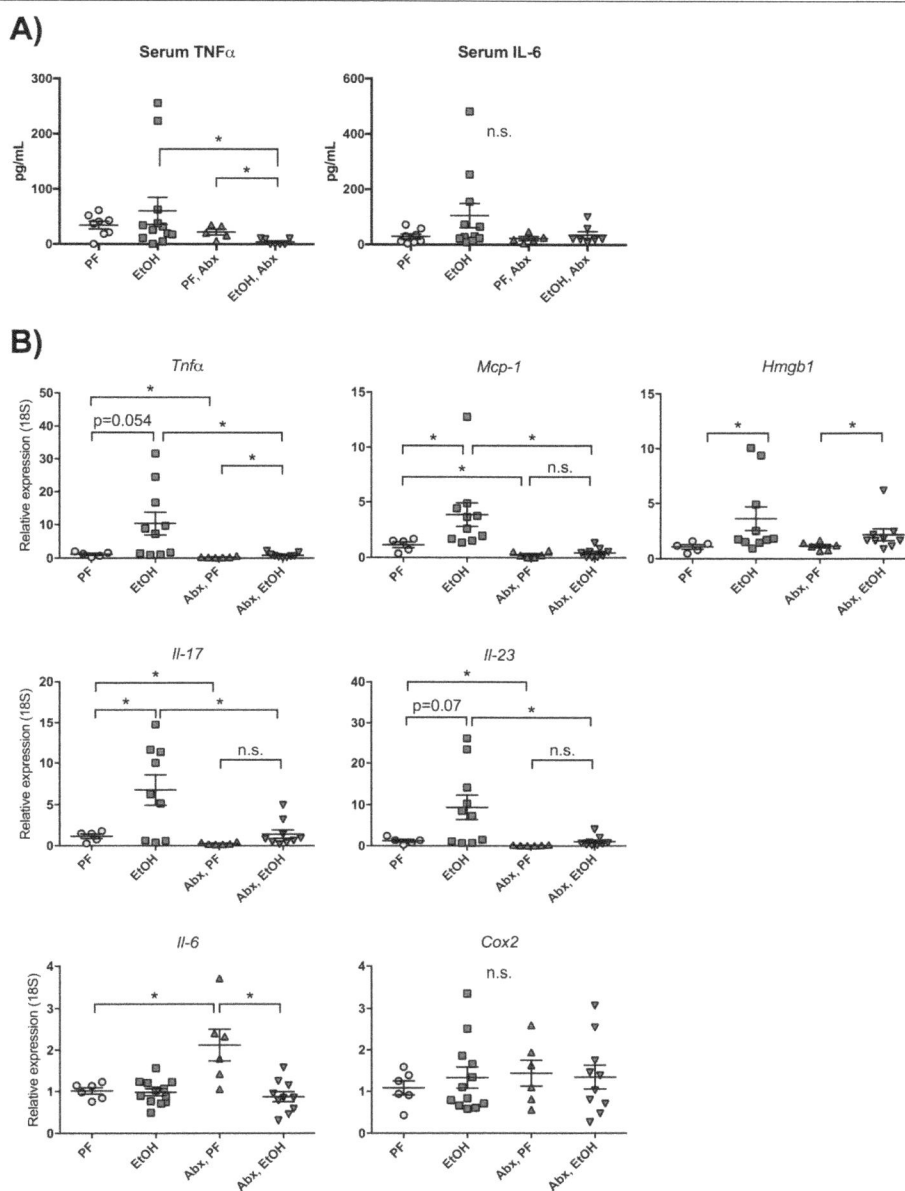

Fig. 2 Antibiotic treatment protects from alcohol-induced inflammatory cytokine expression in the cortex. **a** Serum TNFα and IL-6 were measured by ELISA. **b** Expression levels of proinflammatory cytokines *Tnfa*, *Mcp1*, *Hmgb1*, *Il-17*, *Il-23*, *Il-6*, and *Cox2* were measured from the cortex of pair-fed (PF) or alcohol-fed (EtOH) mice with or without daily antibiotic treatment (Abx). Data are mean ± SEM, *n* = 5–10 mice/group. *$p < 0.05$; n.s., not significant

length of cell extensions off the soma were measured in the cortical and hippocampal microglia in all treatment groups and normalized to PF mice. No significant differences in soma size were observed in the cortex (Fig. 4c). Investigation of the sub-regions of the hippocampus, such as the CA1, CA3, and dentate gyrus (DG) areas, revealed that alcohol increased the soma area only in the microglia of the CA3 region. There was no change in the soma area for CA3 microglia in EtOH-fed mice compared to PF controls that were both treated with antibiotics (Fig. 4d).

Importantly, we found that alcohol reduced the total process length compared to pair-fed mice in the cortex (Fig. 4e), consistent with the condensed cell morphology characteristic of microglial activation [35]. Antibiotic treatment eliminated this alcohol-induced reduction in process length in cortical microglia. Hippocampal microglia process length in alcohol-fed mice was significantly reduced compared to pair-fed controls in all regions investigated, and as in the cortex, antibiotic treatment eliminated this morphological change (Fig. 4f). The number of

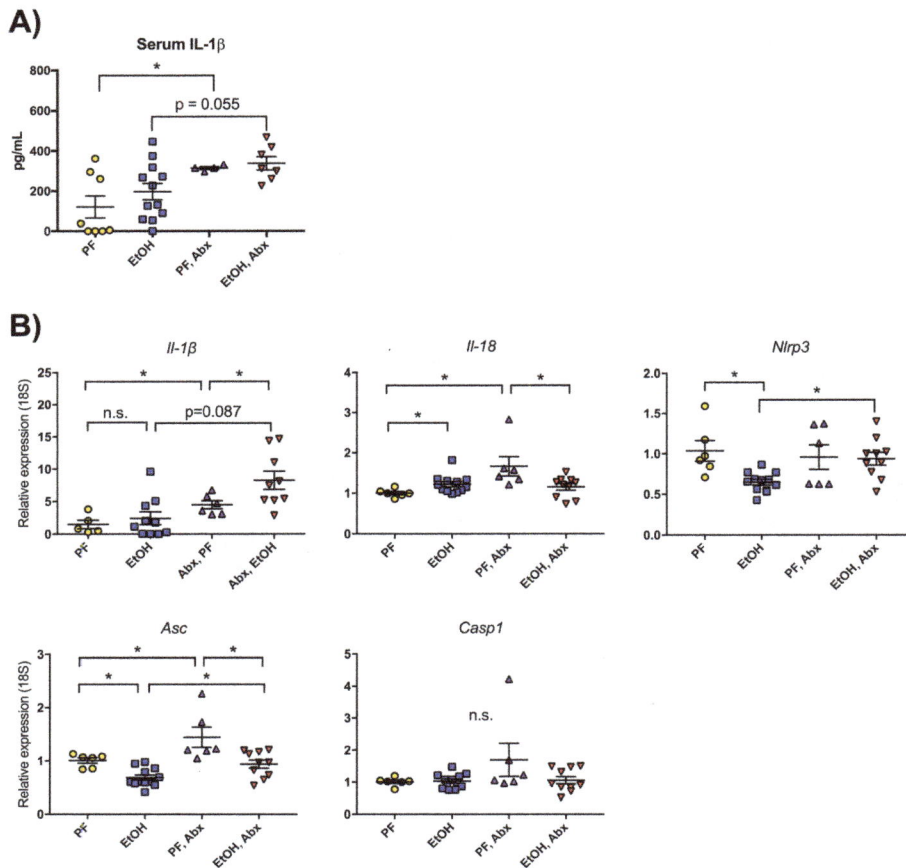

Fig. 3 The expression levels of inflammasome components and *Il-1β* are increased in the cortex after antibiotic decontamination. **a** Serum IL-1β was measured by ELISA. **b** Cortical expression of the inflammasome components *Nlrp3*, *Asc*, and *Casp1* as well as the cytokines *Il-1β* and *Il-18* were measured from the brains of pair-fed (PF) or alcohol-fed (EtOH) mice with or without daily antibiotic treatment (Abx). Data are mean ± SEM, *n* = 5–10 mice/group. *$p < 0.05$

microglia in the cortex was not changed in EtOH-fed compared to PF mice in either treatment group, although antibiotic treatment in PF mice modestly reduced the number of cortical microglia compared to untreated PF mice (Fig. 4g). There was no change in microglial numbers in the hippocampus (Fig. 4h).

Alcohol-induced cytokine expression in the small intestine is attenuated by antibiotic administration

The alcohol-induced changes we observed in the brain could be due to a loss of integrity of the gut barrier. Previous studies have shown that intestinal cytokine expression can reduce gut barrier integrity and may allow leakage of pathogen-associated molecules from the intestinal lumen into the systemic circulation [36]. Therefore, we measured the intestinal expression of various proinflammatory cytokines and found that they were increased after the acute-on-chronic alcohol administration compared to calorie-matched pair-fed mice (Fig. 5a). The expression of

Tnfα, *Mcp1*, and *Hmgb1* mRNA was significantly increased in the small intestine following alcohol consumption, and *Il-17* and *Il-23* expression also showed an increasing trend in EtOH mice. Treatment with the antibiotic cocktail reduced the bacterial load in the intestine (Fig. 1) and led to significantly attenuated alcohol-induced *Mcp1* and *Hmgb1* mRNA levels. Antibiotic treatment reduced the baseline expression of the inflammatory cytokines including *Tnfα*, *Il-17*, and *Il-23* in PF mice compared to untreated PF mice (Fig. 5a). Interestingly, even with antibiotic treatment, alcohol feeding still increased the expression of *Tnfα*, *Il-17*, and *Il-23* in the small intestine of antibiotic-treated alcohol-fed mice compared to antibiotic-treated pair-fed mice (Fig. 5a).

Recent research has highlighted an important connection between the intestinal microbiome and inflammasomes [37], particularly the NLRP3 inflammasome [38]. Therefore, we investigated whether antibiotic decontamination of the gut impacted the expression of inflammasome components in the small intestine. Alcohol induced

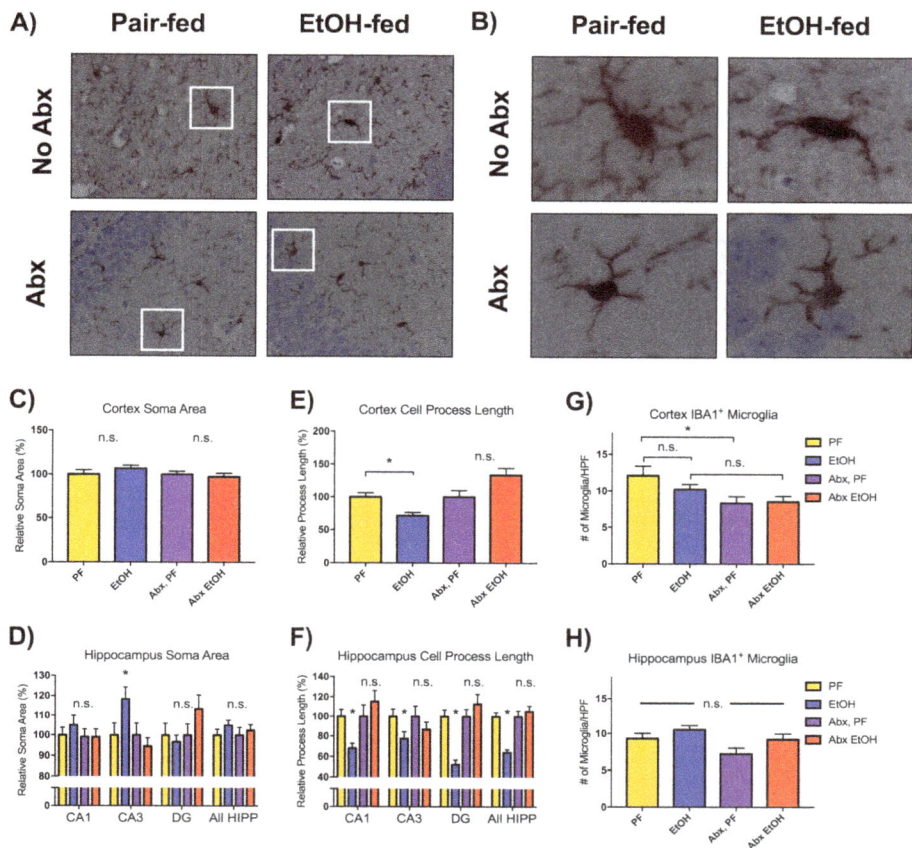

Fig. 4 Antibiotic treatment prevents alcohol-induced morphological changes in cortical and hippocampal microglia. **a** Microglia were immunohistochemically stained for IBA1 and visualized at ×40 magnification in the cortex of pair-fed (PF) or alcohol-fed (EtOH) mice. Representative microglia from the insets are shown in **b**. **c–d** For both the cortex and hippocampus, microglial soma area was measured by tracing the perimeter of the cell body and calculating the area. **e–f** Cell process length was measured in cortical and hippocampal microglia by summing the length of all extensions off of the soma to their distal termination and normalized to the respective PF controls. IBA1-positive staining microglia were quantified in the cortex (**g**) and hippocampus (**h**). Data are mean ± SEM, n = 3 mice/group and 5–9 images/region. *p < 0.05

expression of *Il-1β*, *Nlrp3*, and *Asc* compared to pair-fed controls (Fig. 5b). Antibiotic treatment abrogated the alcohol induction of *Il-1β*, *Nlrp3*, and *Asc*, and antibiotics also increased the baseline expression in pair-fed mice of *Il-1β*, *Il-18*, *Asc*, and *Casp1* (Fig. 5b).

Discussion

In this study, we show that acute-on-chronic alcohol administration results in the central nervous system and small intestinal inflammation and that reducing the gut microbial load with antibiotics protects against alcohol-induced neuroinflammation. The cocktail of oral antibiotics dramatically reduced the gut bacterial load and circulating endotoxin levels. Alcohol-induced neuroinflammation, including microglial morphologic changes and proinflammatory gene expression, was significantly attenuated in oral antibiotic-treated mice, providing novel evidence for the importance of gut bacterial load and PAMPs in the gut-brain axis in alcohol use. We also describe increased proinflammatory cytokine expression in the small intestine after alcohol consumption that can be reduced by treatment with intragastric antibiotics that drastically reduced the bacterial load in the intestine. Interestingly, reduction in the gut microbiome was associated with increased expression of inflammasome components in both the CNS and intestine.

Previously, we have shown that antibiotic treatment in the acute-on-chronic alcohol model protects the liver from alcohol-induced inflammation (including cytokine expression), immune cell infiltration, and steatosis [23]. In the present study, we found evidence of microglial activation by acute-on-chronic alcohol administration in mice. CNS proinflammatory cytokine expression was increased, and average cell process length was decreased in EtOH mice indicating microglia activation. Activated microglia take on an amoeboid-like morphology with reduced process length and, typically, an increased soma size [35].

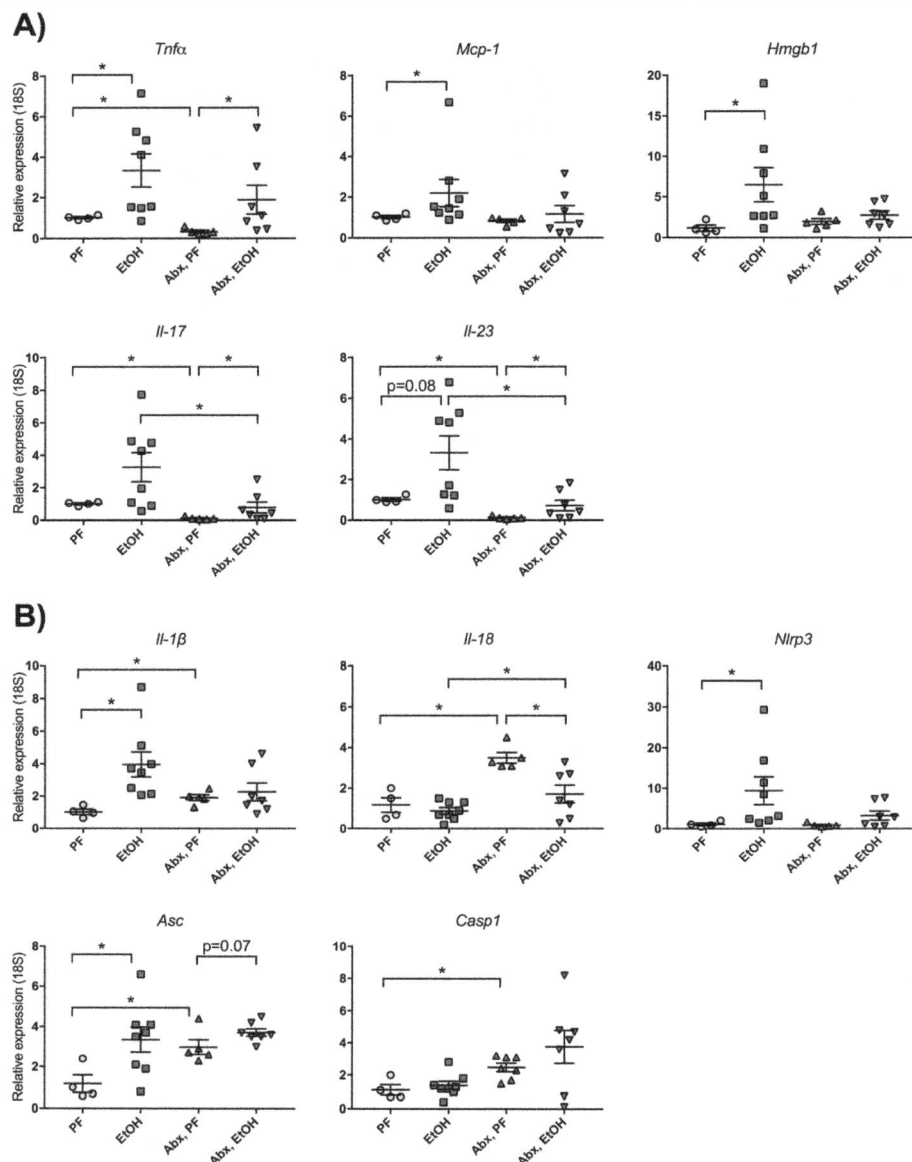

Fig. 5 Alcohol-induced small intestinal inflammation is reduced with gut bacterial load reduction. **a** Expression of proinflammatory cytokines *Tnfa*, *Mcp1*, *Hmgb1*, *Il-17*, and *Il-23* was measured from the small intestine of pair-fed (PF) or alcohol-fed (EtOH) mice with or without daily antibiotic treatment (Abx). **b** Expression of inflammasome components *Nlrp3*, *Asc*, and *Casp1* as well as the cytokines *Il-1β* and *Il-18* were measured by qPCR. Data are mean ± SEM, *n* = 5–10 mice/group. **p < 0.05*

Acute-on-chronic alcohol reduced cell process length in both the cortex and hippocampus and significantly increased the soma size in part of the hippocampus. Interestingly, although acute-on-chronic alcohol-induced proinflammatory cytokine expression in the CNS, alcohol feeding did not increase circulating levels of TNFα, IL-6, and IL-1β. This indicates that alcohol-induced neuroinflammation may occur independent of systemic inflammation, although further investigation of other peripheral signals will be necessary to rule out contributions from circulating factors.

Similar to observations in the liver [23], antibiotic gut decontamination protected the CNS from proinflammatory gene expression and changes in the resident macrophage population. Interestingly, germ-free mice do not show the same protection from alcohol-induced liver damage that we have previously described using antibiotic decontamination [39]. A possible explanation for these different observations is that some baseline bacterial load and/or presence of bacteria during development is critical for the alcohol-induced response of the immune system as well as for organ-specific immunity.

Indeed, previous research has highlighted a role for antibiotic treatment during development in affecting the function of adaptive immune cells [40]. Although multiple studies demonstrated alcohol-induced neuroinflammation after chronic, prolonged alcohol administration in mice and rats, here, we show that a 10-day alcohol feeding followed by an acute binge also results in alcohol-related neuroinflammation. Furthermore, this NIAAA model of alcohol administration results in common end-organ effects of inflammation on the brain, small intestine and liver.

Our data are consistent with previous studies examining the role of TLR4 signaling in alcohol-related organ pathology. While some have suggested that alcohol may interact directly with TLR4 or affect lipid membrane interactions required for proper TLR4 signal transduction [41, 42], TLR4 also recognizes endogenous (including HMGB1) [17, 18] and exogenous (i.e., bacterial components such as LPS) [19] danger signals. Studies show that TLR4 knockout and knockdown mice are protected from numerous inflammation-related sequelae of alcohol exposure in the liver [43] and in the brain [14–16]. Rather than focusing on TLR4 and its signaling pathway, we used antibiotics to reduce bacterial LPS, one of the prominent ligands of TLR4, and reveal a similar reduction in tissue inflammation from the gut to the brain. Our study adds critical evidence to the understanding of the gut-brain axis that relates multifocal pathology in the body after chronic alcohol exposure.

An important remaining question is whether gut bacteria or their products are primarily responsible for organ damage. A direct link between LPS and organ inflammation is possible; leakage of live or dead bacteria or bacterial-derived products into the systemic circulation has been documented in various alcohol administration settings [1, 2, 44, 45]. These bacterial signals could be directly responsible for inducing inflammation in the gut and in the brain, as well as the associated organ damage. Although LPS does not cross the blood-brain barrier at significant levels [20], it could be interacting with juxta-cerebrovascular cells to transmit an immune signal across the barrier. Evidence of blood-brain barrier disruption in alcohol models and human patients provides another explanation for a possible direct mechanism of LPS-induced neuroinflammation [46]. Alternatively, gut-derived signals, such as LPS, bacterial metabolites, or other undescribed intestinal signals, could lead to a systemic reaction. This reaction could include inflammatory cytokines or activated immune cells in the liver or in the circulation that then induce organ-specific inflammation in the CNS and elsewhere in the body. In the present study, we did not detect alcohol-induced increases in circulating TNFα, IL-6, or IL-1β which suggests that alcohol-induced neuroinflammation can be induced by alcohol in the absence of systemic cytokine increases. Developing models to investigate possible peripheral signaling to the CNS leading to neuroinflammation will be a critical area of further study to explain inter-organ communication after alcohol consumption.

Our data supports previous studies showing that alcohol can induce inflammatory signaling in the intestine. This inflammation may be a key factor in the breakdown of the intestinal barrier integrity and ensuing leakage of bacterial products into the circulation associated with alcohol. Using both in vitro and in vivo models, Al-Sadi et al. have shown that proinflammatory cytokines are capable of reducing tight junctions and gut barrier integrity, leading to breakdown and molecule translocation across the gastrointestinal tract [47–49]. Other mechanisms of alcohol-induced loss of intestinal barrier integrity have been explored and include bacterial dysbiosis [50, 51], luminal homeostasis [45, 52], enterocyte cellular stress, and dysregulation of structural proteins [53]. Furthermore, the relationship between proinflammatory gene expression and gut barrier dysfunction appears to be critical [36, 54], and our data further emphasize the role of alcohol and intestinal bacteria in regulating intestinal cytokine levels.

Conclusion

Our study shows for the first time that acute-on-chronic alcohol induces neuroinflammation and small intestinal proinflammatory cytokine expression. Reducing the gut bacterial load with oral antibiotics protects mice from proinflammatory cytokine expression in the CNS and small intestine and highlights critical connections between intestinal microbiome and the gut-brain axis following alcohol consumption.

Abbreviations

Abx: Broad spectrum antibiotic cocktail; *Asc*: Apoptosis-associated speck-like protein;; *Casp1*: Caspase-1; CFUs: Colony-forming units; CNS: Central nervous system; *Cox2*: Cyclooxygenase 2; *Hmgb1*: High-mobility group box 1; *Il-17*: Interleukin-17; *Il-18*: Interleukin-18; *Il-1β*: Interleukin-1β; *Il-23*: Interleukin-23; *Il-6*: Interleukin-6; *Mcp-1*: Monocyte chemoattractant protein 1; *Nlrp3*: NLR family pyrin domain containing 3; PAMPs: Pathogen-associated molecular patterns; SI: Small intestine; TLR4: Toll-like receptor 4; *Tnfa*: Tumor necrosis factor-α

Acknowledgements

The authors thank Dr. Liu of the University of Massachusetts Morphology Core, Karen Kodys, Donna Catalano, and Jeeval Mehta for their technical assistance as well as Candice Dufour and Melanie Trombly for their assistance in preparing the manuscript.

Funding

Research reported in this publication was supported by the National Institute on Alcohol Abuse and Alcoholism of the National Institutes of Health under award numbers F30AA024680 (to PL), F30AA022283 (to AS), F31AA025545 (to AIV), and 5R01AA017729-05 (to GS). The content is solely the responsibility of the authors and does not necessarily represent the official views of the National Institutes of Health.

Authors' contributions

PL, BG, and GS conceived and designed the experiments. PL, BG, AIV, AS, YC, and AA performed the experiments. PL, AS, AIV, and GS obtained funding for the project. PL and GS analyzed the data and wrote the paper. All authors read and approved the final manuscript.

Competing interests

The authors declare that they have no competing interests.

References

1. Bode C, Kugler V, Bode JC. Endotoxemia in patients with alcoholic and non-alcoholic cirrhosis and in subjects with no evidence of chronic liver disease following acute alcohol excess. J Hepatol. 1987;4:8–14.

2. Lippai D, Bala S, Catalano D, Kodys K, Szabo G. Micro-RNA-155 deficiency prevents alcohol-induced serum endotoxin increase and small bowel inflammation in mice. Alcohol Clin Exp Res. 2014;38:2217–24. https://doi.org/10.1111/acer.12483.

3. Parlesak A, Schafer C, Schutz T, Bode JC, Bode C. Increased intestinal permeability to macromolecules and endotoxemia in patients with chronic alcohol abuse in different stages of alcohol-induced liver disease. J Hepatol. 2000;32:742–7.

4. Zorumski CF, Mennerick S, Izumi Y. Acute and chronic effects of ethanol on learning-related synaptic plasticity. Alcohol. 2014;48:1–17. https://doi.org/10.1016/j.alcohol.2013.09.045.

5. Roberto M, Varodayan FP. Synaptic targets: chronic alcohol actions. Neuropharmacology. 2017;122:85–99. https://doi.org/10.1016/j.neuropharm.2017.01.013.

6. Harrison NL, et al. Effects of acute alcohol on excitability in the CNS. Neuropharmacology. 2017;122:36–45. https://doi.org/10.1016/j.neuropharm.2017.04.007.

7. He J, Crews FT. Increased MCP-1 and microglia in various regions of the human alcoholic brain. Exp Neurol. 2008;210:349–58. https://doi.org/10.1016/j.expneurol.2007.11.017.

8. Walter TJ, Crews FT. Microglial depletion alters the brain neuroimmune response to acute binge ethanol withdrawal. J Neuroinflammation. 2017;14:86. https://doi.org/10.1186/s12974-017-0856-z.

9. Lippai D, et al. Alcohol-induced IL-1beta in the brain is mediated by NLRP3/ASC inflammasome activation that amplifies neuroinflammation. J Leukoc Biol. 2013;94:171–82. https://doi.org/10.1189/jlb.1212659.

10. Qin L, Crews FT. NADPH oxidase and reactive oxygen species contribute to alcohol-induced microglial activation and neurodegeneration. J Neuroinflammation. 2012;9:5. https://doi.org/10.1186/1742-2094-9-5.

11. Szabo G, Lippai D. Converging actions of alcohol on liver and brain immune signaling. Int Rev Neurobiol. 2014;118:359–80. https://doi.org/10.1016/B978-0-12-801284-0.00011-7.

12. Crews FT, Lawrimore CJ, Walter TJ, Coleman LG Jr. The role of neuroimmune signaling in alcoholism. Neuropharmacology. 2017;122:56–73. https://doi.org/10.1016/j.neuropharm.2017.01.031.

13. Pascual M, Montesinos J, Guerri C. Role of the innate immune system in the neuropathological consequences induced by adolescent binge drinking. J Neurosci Res. 2018;96:765–80. https://doi.org/10.1002/jnr.24203.

14. Lippai D, Bala S, Csak T, Kurt-Jones EA, Szabo G. Chronic alcohol-induced microRNA-155 contributes to neuroinflammation in a TLR4-dependent manner in mice. PLoS One. 2013;8:e70945. https://doi.org/10.1371/journal.pone.0070945.

15. Alfonso-Loeches S, Urena-Peralta J, Morillo-Bargues MJ, Gomez-Pinedo U, Guerri C. Ethanol-induced TLR4/NLRP3 neuroinflammatory response in microglial cells promotes leukocyte infiltration across the BBB. Neurochem Res. 2016;41:193–209. https://doi.org/10.1007/s11064-015-1760-5.

16. Pascual M, Balino P, Aragon CM, Guerri C. Cytokines and chemokines as biomarkers of ethanol-induced neuroinflammation and anxiety-related behavior: role of TLR4 and TLR2. Neuropharmacology. 2015;89:352–9. https://doi.org/10.1016/j.neuropharm.2014.10.014.

17. Akira S, Takeda K. Toll-like receptor signalling. Nat Rev Immunol. 2004;4:499–511. https://doi.org/10.1038/nri1391.

18. Yang H, et al. A critical cysteine is required for HMGB1 binding to Toll-like receptor 4 and activation of macrophage cytokine release. Proc Natl Acad Sci U S A. 2010;107:11942–7. https://doi.org/10.1073/pnas.1003893107.

19. Park BS, Lee JO. Recognition of lipopolysaccharide pattern by TLR4 complexes. Exp Mol Med. 2013;45:e66. https://doi.org/10.1038/emm.2013.97.

20. Banks WA, Robinson SM. Minimal penetration of lipopolysaccharide across the murine blood-brain barrier. Brain Behav Immun. 2010;24:102–9. https://doi.org/10.1016/j.bbi.2009.09.001.

21. Iracheta-Vellve A, et al. Inhibition of sterile danger signals, uric acid and ATP, prevents inflammasome activation and protects from alcoholic steatohepatitis in mice. J Hepatol. 2015;63:1147–55. https://doi.org/10.1016/j.jhep.2015.06.013.

22. Petrasek J, et al. Metabolic danger signals, uric acid and ATP, mediate inflammatory cross-talk between hepatocytes and immune cells in alcoholic liver disease. J Leukoc Biol. 2015;98:249–56. https://doi.org/10.1189/jlb.3AB1214-590R.

23. Lowe PP, et al. Alcohol-related changes in the intestinal microbiome influence neutrophil infiltration, inflammation and steatosis in early alcoholic hepatitis in mice. PLoS One. 2017;12:e0174544. https://doi.org/10.1371/journal.pone.0174544.

24. Chen P, Starkel P, Turner JR, Ho SB, Schnabl B. Dysbiosis-induced intestinal inflammation activates tumor necrosis factor receptor I and mediates alcoholic liver disease in mice. Hepatology. 2015;61:883–94. https://doi.org/10.1002/hep.27489.

25. Adachi Y, Moore LE, Bradford BU, Gao W, Thurman RG. Antibiotics prevent liver injury in rats following long-term exposure to ethanol. Gastroenterology. 1995;108:218–24.

26. Iimuro Y, et al. Female rats exhibit greater susceptibility to early alcohol-induced liver injury than males. Am J Phys. 1997;272:G1186–94. https://doi.org/10.1152/ajpgi.1997.272.5.G1186.

27. Frezza M, et al. High blood alcohol levels in women. The role of decreased gastric alcohol dehydrogenase activity and first-pass metabolism. N Engl J Med. 1990;322:95–9. https://doi.org/10.1056/NEJM199001113220205.

28. Ikejima K, et al. Estrogen increases sensitivity of hepatic Kupffer cells to endotoxin. Am J Phys. 1998;274:G669–76.

29. Bertola A, Mathews S, Ki SH, Wang H, Gao B. Mouse model of chronic and binge ethanol feeding (the NIAAA model). Nat Protoc. 2013;8:627–37. https://doi.org/10.1038/nprot.2013.032.

30. Achur RN, Freeman WM, Vrana KE. Circulating cytokines as biomarkers of alcohol abuse and alcoholism. J Neuroimmune Pharmacol. 2010;5:83–91. https://doi.org/10.1007/s11481-009-9185-z.

31. Leclercq S, De Saeger C, Delzenne N, de Timary P, Starkel P. Role of inflammatory pathways, blood mononuclear cells, and gut-derived bacterial products in alcohol dependence. Biol Psychiatry. 2014;76:725–33. https://doi.org/10.1016/j.biopsych.2014.02.003.

32. Zou JY, Crews FT. Release of neuronal HMGB1 by ethanol through decreased HDAC activity activates brain neuroimmune signaling. PLoS One. 2014;9:e87915. https://doi.org/10.1371/journal.pone.0087915.

33. Pascual M, et al. TLR4 response mediates ethanol-induced neurodevelopment alterations in a model of fetal alcohol spectrum disorders. J Neuroinflammation. 2017;14:145. https://doi.org/10.1186/s12974-017-0918-2.

34. Fernandez-Lizarbe S, Pascual M, Guerri C. Critical role of TLR4 response in the activation of microglia induced by ethanol. J Immunol. 2009;183:4733–44. https://doi.org/10.4049/jimmunol.0803590.

35. Lehmann ML, Cooper HA, Maric D, Herkenham M. Social defeat induces depressive-like states and microglial activation without involvement of peripheral macrophages. J Neuroinflammation. 2016;13:224. https://doi.org/10.1186/s12974-016-0672-x.

36. Al-Sadi R, Boivin M, Ma T. Mechanism of cytokine modulation of epithelial tight junction barrier. Front Biosci (Landmark Ed). 2009;14:2765–78.

37. Zmora N, Levy M, Pevsner-Fischer M, Elinav E. Inflammasomes and intestinal inflammation. Mucosal Immunol. 2017;10:865–83. https://doi.org/10.1038/mi.2017.19.

38. Yao X, et al. Remodelling of the gut microbiota by hyperactive NLRP3 induces regulatory T cells to maintain homeostasis. Nat Commun. 2017;8:1896. https://doi.org/10.1038/s41467-017-01917-2.

39. Chen P, et al. Microbiota protects mice against acute alcohol-induced liver injury. Alcohol Clin Exp Res. 2015;39:2313–23. https://doi.org/10.1111/acer.12900.

40. Scheer S, et al. Early-life antibiotic treatment enhances the pathogenicity of CD4(+) T cells during intestinal inflammation. J Leukoc Biol. 2017;101:893–900. https://doi.org/10.1189/jlb.3MA0716-334RR.

41. Fernandez-Lizarbe S, Montesinos J, Guerri C. Ethanol induces TLR4/TLR2 association, triggering an inflammatory response in microglial cells. J Neurochem. 2013;126:261–73. https://doi.org/10.1111/jnc.12276.

42. Szabo G, Dolganiuc A, Dai Q, Pruett SB. TLR4, ethanol, and lipid rafts: a new mechanism of ethanol action with implications for other receptor-mediated effects. J Immunol. 2007;178:1243–9.

43. Uesugi T, Froh M, Arteel GE, Bradford BU, Thurman RG. Toll-like receptor 4 is involved in the mechanism of early alcohol-induced liver injury in mice. Hepatology. 2001;34:101–8. https://doi.org/10.1053/jhep.2001.25350.

44. Bala S, Marcos M, Gattu A, Catalano D, Szabo G. Acute binge drinking increases serum endotoxin and bacterial DNA levels in healthy individuals. PLoS One. 2014;9:e96864. https://doi.org/10.1371/journal.pone.0096864.

45. Hartmann P, et al. Deficiency of intestinal mucin-2 ameliorates experimental alcoholic liver disease in mice. Hepatology. 2013;58:108–19. https://doi.org/10.1002/hep.26321.

46. Rubio-Araiz A, et al. Disruption of blood-brain barrier integrity in postmortem alcoholic brain: preclinical evidence of TLR4 involvement from a binge-like drinking model. Addict Biol. 2017;22:1103–16. https://doi.org/10.1111/adb.12376.

47. Al-Sadi R, et al. Mechanism of interleukin-1beta induced-increase in mouse intestinal permeability in vivo. J Interf Cytokine Res. 2012;32:474–84. https://doi.org/10.1089/jir.2012.0031.

48. Al-Sadi R, Guo S, Ye D, Ma TY. TNF-alpha modulation of intestinal epithelial tight junction barrier is regulated by ERK1/2 activation of Elk-1. Am J Pathol. 2013;183:1871–84. https://doi.org/10.1016/j.ajpath.2013.09.001.

49. Al-Sadi R, et al. Interleukin-6 modulation of intestinal epithelial tight junction permeability is mediated by JNK pathway activation of claudin-2 gene. PLoS One. 2014;9:e85345. https://doi.org/10.1371/journal.pone.0085345.

50. Wang L, et al. Intestinal REG3 lectins protect against alcoholic steatohepatitis by reducing mucosa-associated microbiota and preventing bacterial translocation. Cell Host Microbe. 2016;19:227–39. https://doi.org/10.1016/j.chom.2016.01.003.

51. Grander, C. et al. Recovery of ethanol-induced Akkermansia muciniphila depletion ameliorates alcoholic liver disease. Gut. 2017. doi:https://doi.org/10.1136/gutjnl-2016-313432.

52. Hartmann P, et al. Modulation of the intestinal bile acid-FXR-FGF15 axis improves alcoholic liver disease in mice. Hepatology. 2017. https://doi.org/10.1002/hep.29676.

53. Rao RK. Acetaldehyde-induced barrier disruption and paracellular permeability in Caco-2 cell monolayer. Methods Mol Biol. 2008;447:171–83. https://doi.org/10.1007/978-1-59745-242-7_13.

54. Banan A, et al. NF-kappaB activation as a key mechanism in ethanol-induced disruption of the F-actin cytoskeleton and monolayer barrier integrity in intestinal epithelium. Alcohol. 2007;41:447–60. https://doi.org/10.1016/j.alcohol.2007.07.003.

13

The IFN-γ/PD-L1 axis between T cells and tumor microenvironment: hints for glioma anti-PD-1/PD-L1 therapy

Jiawen Qian[1,2†], Chen Wang[1,2†], Bo Wang[1,2], Jiao Yang[3], Yuedi Wang[1,2], Feifei Luo[2], Junying Xu[1,2], Chujun Zhao[4], Ronghua Liu[1] and Yiwei Chu[1,2*] (iD)

Abstract

Background: PD-L1 is an immune inhibitory receptor ligand that leads to T cell dysfunction and apoptosis by binding to its receptor PD-1, which works in braking inflammatory response and conspiring tumor immune evasion. However, in gliomas, the cause of PD-L1 expression in the tumor microenvironment is not yet clear. Besides, auxiliary biomarkers are urgently needed for screening possible responsive glioma patients for anti-PD-1/PD-L1 therapies.

Methods: The distribution of tumor-infiltrating T cells and PD-L1 expression was analyzed via immunofluorescence in orthotopic murine glioma model. The expression of PD-L1 in immune cell populations was detected by flow cytometry. Data excavated from TCGA LGG/GBM datasets and the Ivy Glioblastoma Atlas Project was used for in silico analysis of the correlation among genes and survival.

Results: The distribution of tumor-infiltrating T cells and PD-L1 expression, which parallels in murine orthotopic glioma model and human glioma microdissections, was interrelated. The IFN-γ level was positively correlated with PD-L1 expression in murine glioma. Further, IFN-γ induces PD-L1 expression on primary cultured microglia, bone marrow-derived macrophages, and GL261 glioma cells in vitro. Seven IFN-γ-induced genes, namely *GBP5*, *ICAM1*, *CAMK2D*, *IRF1*, *SOCS3*, *CD44*, and *CCL2*, were selected to calculate as substitute indicator for IFN-γ level. By combining the relative expression of the listed IFN-γ-induced genes, IFN-γ score was positively correlated with PD-L1 expression in different anatomic structures of human glioma and in glioma of different malignancies.

Conclusion: Our study identified the distribution of tumor-infiltrating T cells and PD-L1 expression in murine glioma model and human glioma samples. And we found that IFN-γ is an important cause of PD-L1 expression in the glioma microenvironment. Further, we proposed IFN-γ score aggregated from the expressions of the listed IFN-γ-induced genes as a complementary prognostic indicator for anti-PD-1/PD-L1 therapy.

Keywords: PD-L1, Immune checkpoint, IFN-γ, Glioma, Immune evasion

Background

Gliomas, characterized by immune evasive hallmarks, are the major primary tumors in the central nervous system (CNS) [1]. The immune microenvironment of glioma is a complex neuroinflammatory network that involves both positive and negative immune regulation [2]. T cells, the main executors in the anti-tumor immune response, are suppressed by various mechanisms at the tumor site [3–6], among which PD-1/PD-L1 axis-mediated functional inhibition plays a key role. PD-L1 is an immune inhibitory receptor ligand expressed on many types of cancer cells, such as melanomas, lymphomas, lung cancers, prostate cancers, and gliomas [7]. By binding to its receptor PD-1 expressed on the surface of activated T cells, PD-L1 leads to T cell dysfunction and apoptosis [8, 9]. This facilitates the

---
* Correspondence: yiweichu@fudan.edu.cn
†Jiawen Qian and Chen Wang contributed equally to this work.
[1]Department of Immunology, School of Basic Medical Sciences, and Institute of Biomedical Sciences, Fudan University, No. 138, Yi Xue Yuan Rd., Mail Box 226, Shanghai 200032, People's Republic of China
[2]Biotherapy Research Center, Fudan University, Shanghai 200032, China
Full list of author information is available at the end of the article

immunosuppressive microenvironment and tumor progression. Previously, studies have revealed that PD-L1 upregulation depended on IFN-γ-secreting CD8$^+$ lymphocytes [10]. IFN-γ binds with receptor and subsequently activates JAK/STAT signaling pathway, which leads to the downstream expression and activation of IRF-1, further inducing PD-L1 expression on tumor cells [11]. However, the driving factors of PD-L1 expression on various cells in the glioma microenvironment remain to be investigated.

Emerging evidence implies that PD-1/PD-L1 is a promising target to reverse the immune evasion of glioma [12]. Nduom et al. [13] measured PD-L1 expression in 94 patients and found that PD-L1 was a negative prognostic indicator for glioblastoma (GBM). Wang et al. [14] analyzed 976 glioma samples with transcriptome data and concluded that PD-L1 expression was positively correlated with the WHO classification of glioma. While abundant clinical studies on anti-PD-1/PD-L1 antibody specific to gliomas are in progress, the results remain unclear. Based on completed clinical trials of anti-PD-1/PD-L1 therapy targeting other tumors, nevertheless, screening for appropriate patients is crucial for favorable prognosis [15]. Although PD-L1 immunohistochemistry (IHC) has been approved by the FDA as the only predictive companion test for cancer immunotherapy such as pembrolizumab in non-small cell lung cancer patients, supplementary clinical indicators are urgently needed considering the high false negative rate [16]. Until now, biomarkers identifying possible responsive glioma patients have not been defined.

In this study, we investigated the distribution of T cells and PD-L1 expression on murine orthotopic glioma model and validated the results in human glioma samples from databases of the Cancer Genome Atlas (TCGA) and the Ivy Glioblastoma Atlas Project. We found that the distribution of PD-L1 in glioma coincides with morphologically apoptotic T cells and that IFN-γ induced PD-L1 expression on primary cultured microglia, bone marrow-derived macrophages (BMDM), and GL261 tumor cells, suggesting IFN-γ derived from tumor-infiltrating T cells may be the lead to induced PD-L1 expression in the microenvironment. We also found that, apart from the tumor cells previously reported, activated microglia and peripheral-derived macrophages in the microenvironment also present significant upregulation of PD-L1. Considering the importance of IFN-γ in inducing PD-L1 in the glioma microenvironment, it is assumed as a supplementary indicator to predict the expression of PD-L1. However, traditional IHC or RNA seq methods are insufficient to accurately measure the IFN-γ level in tumor samples. Here, we proposed IFN-γ score, aggregated from the expressions of seven IFN-γ-induced genes, as an ancillary marker in screening for appropriate glioma patients.

Methods

Mice

C57BL/6 mice (6–8 weeks) were purchased from Shanghai Slac Laboratory Animal Co., Ltd. (Shanghai, China). Mice were maintained under the specific pathogen-free condition and housed in the Animal Facility of Fudan University (Shanghai, China) according to the Guidelines for the Care and Use of Laboratory Animals (No. 55 issued by the Ministry of Health, People's Republic of China, on January 25, 1998), as administered by the Institutional Animal Care and Use Committee (IACUC) of Fudan University.

GL261 murine glioma model

GL261 murine glioma cell line was kindly provided by Dr. Liangfu Zhou (Huashan Hospital, Shanghai, China). GL261 was cultured in DMEM/F12 (Thermo Fisher, USA) supplemented with 10% heat-inactivated FBS (Thermo Fisher, USA), 2 mM glutamine (Thermo Fisher, USA), 100 U/ml penicillin (Thermo Fisher, USA), and 100 μg/ml streptomycin (Thermo Fisher, USA). Cells were maintained in the incubator at 37 °C in a humidified 5%CO_2/95% atmosphere with routine checks for mycoplasma contamination every 3 months. For tumor inoculation, anesthetized mice were immobilized and mounted onto a stereotactic head holder in the flat-skull position. The skin of the skull was dissected in the midline by a scalpel. The skull was carefully drilled with a 20-gauge needle tip (ML + 2.0; RC + 1.0 mm). Then, a microliter Hamilton syringe was inserted to a depth of 3 mm and retracted to a depth of 2.5 mm from the dural surface. Five microliters (2×10^4 cells/μl) of cell suspension or PBS was slowly injected in 2 min. The needle was then slowly taken out from the injection canal, and the skin was sutured. Terminal stage of GL261 murine glioma model was defined by agonal symptoms such as poor grooming, lethargy, weight loss, or seizures.

Primary adult microglia culture

Microglia were prepared from 6- to 8-week-old mice as described previously [17]. Briefly, the brains were dissected with the cerebella and olfactory bulbs taken off. The tissue was triturated mechanically and washed with PBS by centrifuging for 7 min at 500g, 4 °C. The supernatant was discarded, and pellets were re-suspended in 37% Percoll. Percoll gradients (70%/37%/30%/0%) were prepared and centrifuged for 5 min at 500g, 18 °C (low acceleration, brake off). Mononuclear cells were collected at 70%/37% Percoll interface. Microglia were enriched by CD11b microbeads (BD Bioscience, USA) according to the manufacturer's specification and harvested for purity check and further tests. Isolated microglia were plated onto 24-well plates (1×10^5 cells per well) and cultured in basic medium with additional 5 ng/ml recombination TGF-β1 (Miltenyi, Germany) and 10 ng/ml Recombinant Mouse M-CSF Protein (R&D, USA). Half of the medium was changed every 3 days, for a total of 10–14 days.

For T cell co-culture assay, adult microglia were plated onto 96-well plates at a density of 1×10^5 cells per well. Half of the medium was changed every 3 days, for a total of 7 days. On day 8, microglia were treated with or without 20% GCM for 24 h. The CD4$^+$ T Cell Isolation Kit (Miltenyi, Germany) was used for purification of CD4$^+$ T cells from the spleen of OT II mice. CD4$^+$ T cells were stained with CFSE dye (Invitrogen, USA) following the manufacturer's instructions. The microglia were washed with PBS for three times and then co-cultured with CD4$^+$ T cells (4×10^5 cells per well) for 4 days supplied with 0.1 μM OVA323–339 peptides (Sigma-Aldrich, USA). After co-culture, both microglia and T cells were determined by flow cytometric analysis.

Immunofluorescence
For immunofluorescence, sections were thawed and dried at room temperature and rinsed in PBS. For fixation, cells were washed with PBS and followed by 4% PFA for 5 min. Samples were permeabilized with 0.25% Triton X-100 for 15 min and blocked in blocking buffer containing 10% donkey serum for 2 h at room temperature or overnight at 4 °C. Then, samples were incubated with indicated primary antibodies (Additional file 1: Table S2) overnight at 4 °C. Samples were then washed with PBS and incubated with the appropriate fluorophore-conjugated secondary antibodies, namely Alexafloure-488, 594 (Thermo Fisher, USA) and Cy3 (JacksonImmunoResearch Laboratory, USA), at a dilution of 1:500 in 1% BSA for 1 h at room temperature. 4′, 6-Diamidino-2-phenylindole (DAPI) was used as a counterstain. Images were acquired by a fluorescence microscope Olympus IX73 (Olympus, Japan). Appropriate gain and black level settings were determined by control tissues stained with secondary antibodies. Analyses of images were performed using ImageJ software (NIH, USA). Quantitative analysis was performed with ImageJ to determine the T cell counts and mean intensity of PD-L1. For CD4$^+$ cell or CD8$^+$ cell counts, data were collected from five random fields for each region per mouse, $n = 4$. For mean intensity of PD-L1, data were collected from at least three and up to seven random fields for each region per mouse, $n = 5$.

FACS analyses
For fluorescence-activated cell sorting (FACS) analysis of brain tumor-infiltrating immune cells, mice were euthanized at the defined endpoint. Mononuclear cells in the brains were isolated as previously described and stained afterward with the respective antibodies for FACS analysis. For flow cytometry, cells were counted and incubated with Fc blocker (eBiosciences, USA) for 30 min,

followed by another 30-min incubation with conjugated antibodies for extracellular markers. For intracellular cytokine detection, cells were stimulated in vitro with Cell Stimulation Cocktail (eBiosciences, USA) for 5 h at 37 °C before FACS analysis. After stimulation, cells were stained for surface markers and cytokines with Intracellular Fixation and Permeabilization Buffer Set (eBiosciences, USA). All antibodies used for these experiments were listed in Additional file 1: Table S2. Proper isotype controls and compensation controls were performed in parallel. BD Biosciences Canto II (BD Biosciences, USA) was used for flow cytometry. FlowJo software (Tree Star, USA) was used for FACS data analysis.

Quantitative real-time PCR
Total RNA was isolated with RNAiso (Takara, Japan) following the manufacturer's protocol and reversely transcribed using PrimeScript™ RT reagent Kit with gDNA Eraser (Perfect Real Time) (Takara, Japan). Gene expression was detected using SYBR® Premix Ex TaqTM II (Tli RNaseH Plus) Kit (Takara, Japan). All RT-PCR amplifications were performed in triplicates in a 20-μl reaction volume with the indicated primer pairs. Primer sequences were listed in Additional file 2: Table S1. RT-PCRs were performed using 7500 Fast Real-Time PCR System (Applied Biosystems, USA). The amount of target mRNA was normalized to the expression level of β-actin generated from the same sample and subsequently to controls. Relative expression was calculated as $2^{-\Delta Ct}$.

IFN-γ score calculation and clinical data analysis
Firstly, 34 genes were sorted out by filtering genes from GO term: response to interferon-gamma (accession GO: 0034341, organism: *Homo sapiens*) with genes that were positively correlated with PD-L1 expression ($p < 0.05$; $r > 0.5$) from the TCGA lower grade glioma (LGG)/GBM datasets. Then, further crossing 34 genes with 840 genes that were positively correlated with PD-L1 expression ($p < 0.05$; $r > 0.3$) from the Ivy Glioblastoma Atlas Project, 7 genes were eventually sorted out, namely *GBP5*, *ICAM1*, *CAMK2D*, *IRF1*, *SOCS3*, *CD44*, and *CCL2*. Combining the relative expression levels of the sorted seven genes, IFN-γ score was calculated as a substitute indicator for IFN-γ level. Myeloid cell-related genes (*CD14*, *CD33*, *CD36*, *CD68*, *CX3CR1*, *ENG*, *ITGAL*, and *ITGAM*) were used to calculate myeloid cell score. T cell-related genes (*CD2*, *CD3D*, *CD3E*, *CD3G*, *CD4*, *CD8A*, *CD8B*, *CD28*, *CCR7*, and *IL2RA*) were used to calculate T cell score. The median value of IFN-γ score was used as the cutoff to divide patients with high IFN-γ score and patients with low IFN-γ score.

Data presentation and statistical analysis

GraphPad Prism 6.0 (GraphPad Software Inc., USA) was used for all data analysis. Parametric data were presented as mean ± standard error of the mean (SEM). Differences between two groups were analyzed using Student's unpaired t test. Analysis of variance (ANOVA) was used to compare multiple groups, and Pearson's correlation coefficient was used to analyze the correlation of the expression levels of genes. Statistical significance was determined at $p < 0.05$ in all cases.

Results

PD-1 expression on T cells was upregulated during glioma progression

We investigated the expression of PD-1 in tumor-infiltrating T cells during tumor progression in GL261 glioma orthotopic murine glioma model, the survival time of which is around 30 days [18]. Flow cytometry analysis of glioma-infiltrating immune cells showed that PD-1 expression on both CD4$^+$ and CD8$^+$ T cells gradually increased as tumor progressed (Fig. 1a–d), and non-inoculated brain was used as normal tissue. PD-1 was highly expressed on tumor-infiltrating T cells, and annexin V labeling revealed PD-1 expression was positively correlated with apoptosis of T cells, while the corresponding peripheral blood-derived T cells presented low PD-1 expression and no tendency to apoptosis (Fig. 1e–h). Besides, according to immunofluorescence, tumor-infiltrating T cells presented typical apoptotic morphology, such as reduced size compared with non-apoptotic CD8$^+$ T cells in meningeal vessels. Moreover, there were apoptotic bodies bounded by CD8$^+$ membrane and phagocytized by neighboring Iba1$^+$ microglia/macrophages. T cells accumulated at the meninges were in typical T cell shape and morphologically normal (Fig. 1i). The above suggests that upregulated PD-1 expression on T cells is related to its apoptosis at the glioma tumor site and the tumor microenvironment causes PD-1 induction in the T cells.

The distributions of tumor-infiltrating T cells and PD-L1 in the glioma microenvironment were interrelated

We then analyzed the distribution of tumor-infiltrating T cells. According to the density and morphological characteristics of Iba1$^+$ myeloid cells, the tumor area is divided into four parts. They are normal tissue (N), where microglia were of low density and in a typical ramified shape with small soma; tumor rim (TR), where microglia were of increased density with thicker branches and enlarged soma; invasive margin (IM), where a large number of microglia gathered at the leading edge of tumor invasion; and intratumoral region (IT), where Iba1$^+$ myeloid cells were typically amebiform (Fig. 2a). Immunofluorescence analysis of T cell density

in each tumor area indicated that IM and IT were the major infiltrating areas of T cells (Fig. 2b, c). While T cells of high density in the IM area were morphologically activated, those in the IT area were morphologically apoptotic. Besides, many CD4$^+$ or CD8$^+$ apoptotic bodies can be recognized in the IT area (Figs. 1i and 2b). In accordance with the apoptotic status of T cells in the IT area, PD-L1 expression was mainly found in the same IT area, especially around the necrotic tissue (Fig. 2d). Immunofluorescence analysis of PD-L1 intensity in each tumor area also indicated that IM and IT showed comparatively high PD-L1 expression, while N and TR had almost no expression of PD-L1 (Additional file 3: Figure S1A, B). Together, tumor-infiltrating T cells and PD-L1 presented unique distribution patterns in the tumor microenvironment. Different status of T cells can be found in tumor areas with high T cell density, which agrees with the expression of PD-L1 in the corresponding area. We speculate that, although successfully infiltrated in the tumor microenvironment, T cells are soon rendered inactive and even apoptotic, because of the upregulated PD-1 and its binding with high expression of PD-L1 in the certain tumor area.

Previous studies mainly focused on the expression of PD-L1 on tumor cells and its role in CTL inhibition, and PD-L1 expression on APCs and its potential role in the dysfunction of CD4$^+$ T cells remain neglected. Besides, our previous work demonstrated that most of the brain resident APCs, Iba1$^+$ microglia, were mainly presented in the IM and IT regions [17]. Immunofluorescence assay manifested likewise that Iba1$^+$ myeloid cells highly expressed PD-L1 in the IT area (Fig. 2e).

PD-L1 expression was found on glioma-infiltrating macrophages and microglia

We next analyzed the expression of PD-L1 in the major immune cell populations in the glioma microenvironment. We found that, compared with the CD45^{hi}CD11-b$^{lo/-}$ subsets and CD45^{lo}CD11b^{hi} subsets, PD-L1 was highly expressed in a population of CD45^{hi}CD11b^{hi} myeloid cells, the majority of which were activated microglia and peripheral-derived monocytes/macrophages (Fig. 3a, b). Together, PD-L1 is highly expressed in activated microglia and infiltrating myeloid cells, which might also account for T cell dysfunction and apoptosis.

IFN-γ correlated with upregulation of PD-L1 in the glioma microenvironment

The areas with high PD-L1 expression had simultaneously a large number of infiltrating T cells. It is known that IFN-γ induces PD-L1 expression on many cell types including glioma cell lines in vitro [19, 20]. We stimulated primary cultured microglia, BMDM, and GL261 tumor cells with IFN-γ in vitro, and flow cytometry

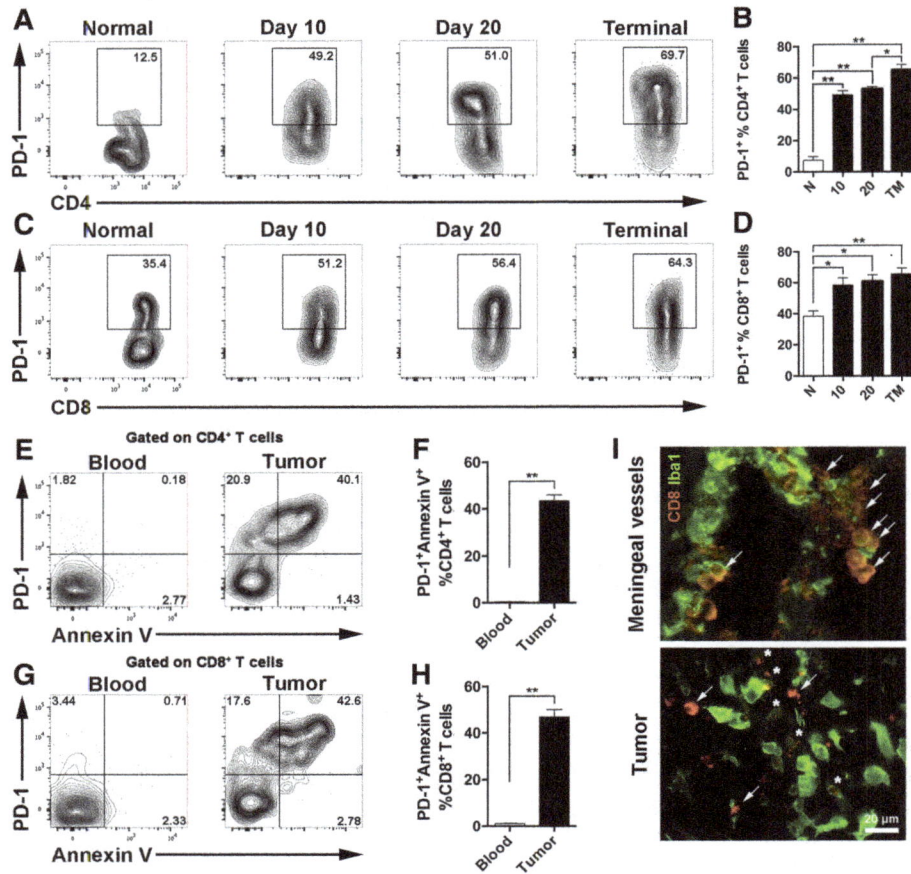

Fig. 1 PD-1 expression on T cells was upregulated during glioma progression that correlate with apoptosis. **a–d** Flow cytometry analysis of PD-1 expression on glioma-infiltrating T cells at indicated time points. Representative data of the PD-1 expression of CD4$^+$ T cells (**a**) and CD8$^+$ T cells (**c**) at the indicated time point and the statistical summary for CD4$^+$ T cells (**b**) and CD8$^+$ T cells (**d**), $n = 3–4$. N, normal brain; 10, 10 days after tumor inoculation; 20, 20 days after tumor inoculation; TM, terminal stage. **e–h** Flow cytometry analysis of T cell apoptosis by annexin V. Representative data of the apoptosis level of CD4$^+$ T cells (**e**) and CD8$^+$ T cells (**g**) from the peripheral blood and glioma tissue. The statistical summary for CD4$^+$ T cells (**f**) and CD8$^+$ T cells (**h**), $n = 12$. **i** Representative staining for Iba1 (green) and CD8 (red) in tumor-bearing brain (day 20). Arrow, morphologically intact T cells; asterisk, disintegrated T cells. Scale bar, 20 μm. One-way ANOVA was performed in **b** and **d**. Unpaired Student's t test was performed in **f** and **h**. *$p < 0.05$; **$p < 0.01$. All values are shown as mean ± SEM

analysis showed dramatic upregulation of PD-L1 on all three types of cells (Fig. 3c, d). Through microglia-mediated T cell proliferation activation experiments, we found that the PD-L1 expression of microglia significantly upregulated in the OVA$_{323–339}$- and GCM/OVA$_{323–339}$-treated groups (Fig. 3e). Notably, regardless of the level of T cell proliferation, as long as T cells were activated, they could significantly upregulate PD-L1 expression in antigen-presenting cells. The above results suggest that IFN-γ plays a major role in PD-L1 expression in the glioma microenvironment. Based on the flow cytometry analysis that the IFN-γ-secreting cells in GL261 tumors were T cells and CD45^{hi} CD4$^-$ CD8$^-$ NK subsets (Fig. 3f), we speculate that T cells and NK cells are the major source of IFN-γ in the tumor microenvironment.

Distribution pattern of tumor-infiltrating T cells and PD-L1 in human glioma samples

Similar distribution patterns of T cells and PD-L1 expression were found in human glioma samples as well, based on the data from the Ivy Glioblastoma Atlas Project (Fig. 4a). According to the expression level of T cell-related genes, T cells are mainly located in the cellular tumor (CT) area and perinecrotic zone (CTpnz) in human glioma samples (Fig. 4b), which were parallel to the IM and IT area in the murine model. PD-L1 expression in human glioma samples, on the other hand, was found mainly at the region of CTpnz and pseudo palisading cells around necrosis (CTpan) (Fig. 4c), which were equivalent to the area around the necrotic tissue. These data confirm that the expression pattern of PD-L1 and T cells in human samples are likewise consistent with those in the

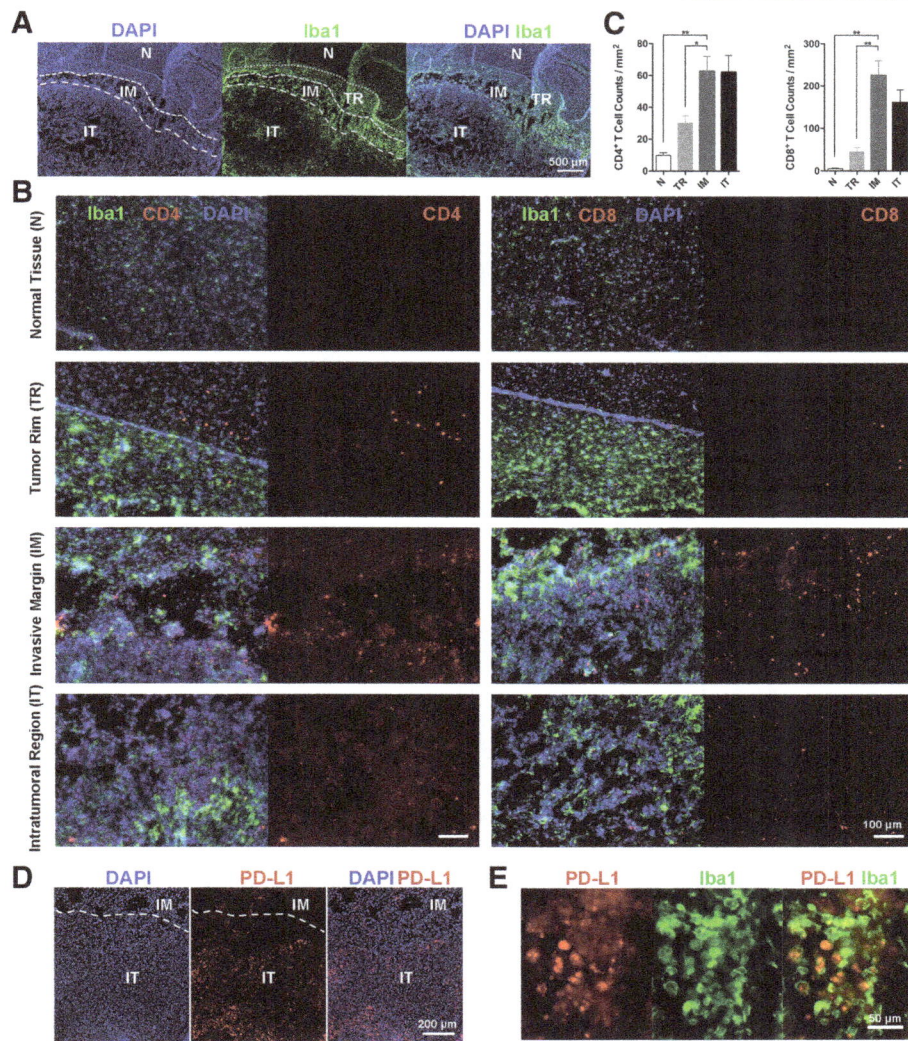

Fig. 2 The distribution of tumor-infiltrating T cells and PD-L1 in murine glioma model. **a** Murine glioma is divided into four parts according to the density and morphological characteristics of Iba1+ myeloid cells. Representative staining for Iba1 (green) and DAPI (blue) in the tumor-bearing brain (day 20). N, normal tissue; TR, tumor rim; IM, invasive margin; IT, intratumoral region. Scale bar, 500 μm. **b** Representative staining for Iba1 (green), CD4 (red) or CD8 (red), and DAPI (blue) in the tumor-bearing brain (day 20); different regions of the tumor-bearing brain were shown. Scale bar, 100 μm. **c** CD4$^+$ cell or CD8$^+$ cell counts per field were calculated. Data were collected from five random fields for each region per mouse, $n = 4$. One-way ANOVA was performed. *$p < 0.05$; **$p < 0.01$. All values are shown as mean ± SEM. **d** Representative staining for PD-L1 (red) and DAPI (blue) in the tumor-bearing brain (day 20). Scale bar, 200 μm. **e** Representative staining for Iba1 (green) and PD-L1 (red) in the IT area of tumor-bearing brain (day 20). Scale bar, 50 μm

murine glioma model, supporting the correlation between PD-1/PD-L1 axis and glioma-infiltrating T cell apoptosis. In addition, according to the database of the Ivy Glioblastoma Atlas Project, the distribution of PD-L1 was consistent with the distribution of the myeloid gene markers such as *ITGAM*, *CD14*, and *CD68* (Fig. 4c, d). Moreover, T cell score and myeloid cell score were positively correlated in human glioma samples (Fig. 4e).

IFN-γ-induced genes were positively correlated with progression of glioma and PD-L1 expression

While anti-PD-1/PD-L1 immune checkpoint blockade therapy serves as a promising glioma treatment with good prospect, it is still controversial to use the expression level of PD-L1 as a prognostic indicator for GBM. Certain limitations exist if PD-L1 is used alone as the indicator to screen patients suitable for PD-1/PD-L1 antibody treatment. Considering the apparent heterogeneity

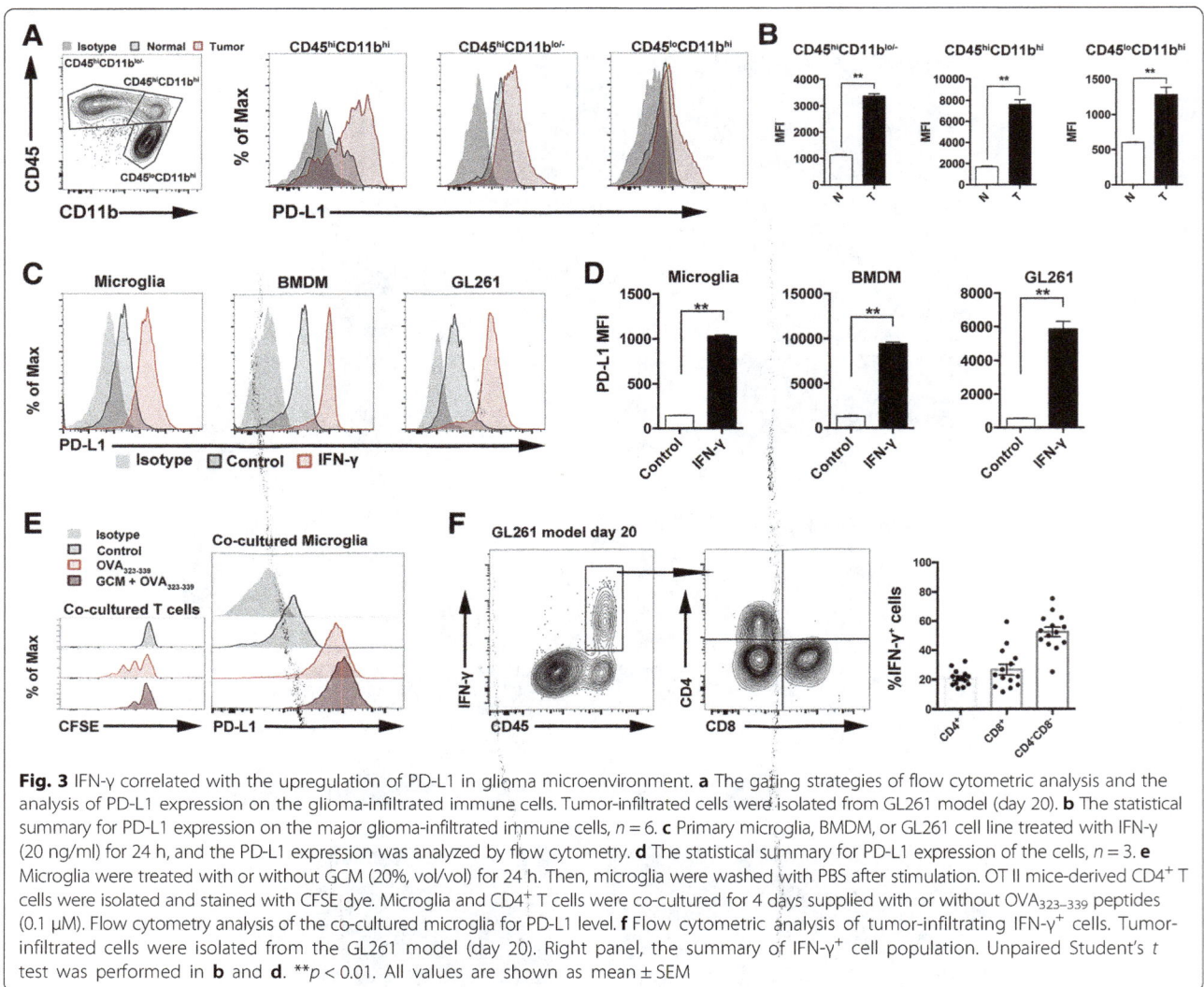

Fig. 3 IFN-γ correlated with the upregulation of PD-L1 in glioma microenvironment. **a** The gating strategies of flow cytometric analysis and the analysis of PD-L1 expression on the glioma-infiltrated immune cells. Tumor-infiltrated cells were isolated from GL261 model (day 20). **b** The statistical summary for PD-L1 expression on the major glioma-infiltrated immune cells, $n = 6$. **c** Primary microglia, BMDM, or GL261 cell line treated with IFN-γ (20 ng/ml) for 24 h, and the PD-L1 expression was analyzed by flow cytometry. **d** The statistical summary for PD-L1 expression of the cells, $n = 3$. **e** Microglia were treated with or without GCM (20%, vol/vol) for 24 h. Then, microglia were washed with PBS after stimulation. OT II mice-derived CD4$^+$ T cells were isolated and stained with CFSE dye. Microglia and CD4$^+$ T cells were co-cultured for 4 days supplied with or without OVA$_{323-339}$ peptides (0.1 μM). Flow cytometry analysis of the co-cultured microglia for PD-L1 level. **f** Flow cytometric analysis of tumor-infiltrating IFN-γ$^+$ cells. Tumor-infiltrated cells were isolated from the GL261 model (day 20). Right panel, the summary of IFN-γ$^+$ cell population. Unpaired Student's t test was performed in **b** and **d**. **$^{**}p < 0.01$. All values are shown as mean ± SEM

of PD-L1 distribution, tumor deemed PD-L1 negative might actually be PD-L1 positive at another biopsy site. A single slide from a single biopsy site is obviously a lack of representativeness. IFN-γ, correlated with upregulation of PD-L1, acts as an efficient cytokine and is expressed by only a few activated lymphocytes in the tumor, making it suitable for prognostic indicator. However, traditional IHC or RNA seq methods are insufficient to accurately measure the IFN-γ level in tumor samples. Therefore, we proposed IFN-γ score as a synergistic marker that could be used to predict PD-L1 expression in glioma samples.

To find the substitute indicator for IFN-γ level, we looked through the IFN-γ-induced genes. A total of 34 genes were sorted out by filtering 198 genes from GO term: response to interferon-gamma (accession GO: 0034341, organism: *Homo sapiens*) with 356 genes that were positively correlated with PD-L1 expression

($p < 0.05$; $r > 0.5$) from the TCGA lower grade glioma (LGG)/GBM datasets. Further crossing these 34 genes with 840 genes that were positively correlated with PD-L1 expression ($p < 0.05$; $r > 0.3$) from the Ivy Glioblastoma Atlas Project, 7 genes were eventually sorted out, namely *GBP5, ICAM1, CAMK2D, IRF1, SOCS3, CD44*, and *CCL2* (Fig. 5a). Based on the TCGA LGG/GBM datasets, the expression of each listed gene is positively correlated with the malignancy degree of glioma (Additional file 4: Figure S2A) and negatively with the survival of patients (Additional file 4: Figure S2B). By crossing these 7 genes with 133 genes from GO term: response to interferon-gamma (accession GO: 0034341, organism: *Mus musculus*), *Gbp5, Irf1*, and *Ccl2* were selected for further verification in the murine glioma model (Fig. 5a). According to qPCR, the relative expression of these three genes were low in the normal mice and increased as glioma progressed, which agreed with the

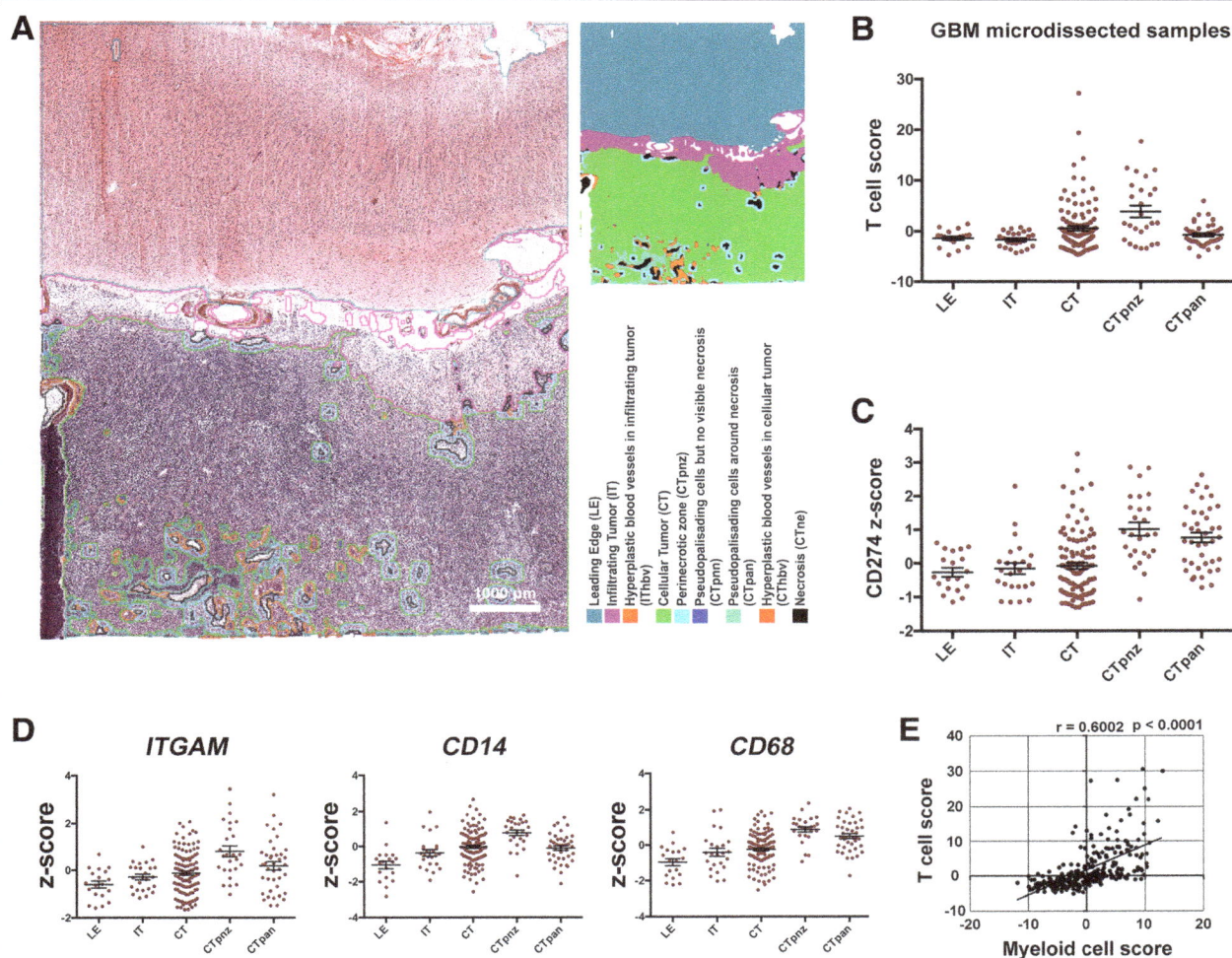

Fig. 4 Distribution pattern of tumor-infiltrating T cells and PD-L1 in human glioma samples. **a** Tumor feature annotation of human glioma sample in the Ivy Glioblastoma Atlas Project. Scale bar, 1000 μm. Image credit: Allen Institute. T cell score (**b**) and PD-L1 expression (**c**) in different parts of human glioma samples, n = 19–111. LE, leading edge; IT, infiltrating tumor; CT, cellular tumor; CTpnz, perinecrotic zone; CTpan, pseudopalisading cells around necrosis. **d** The expression of myeloid cell signature genes in different parts of human glioma samples according to the Ivy Glioblastoma Atlas Project, n = 19–111. **e** Correlation analysis between T cell score and myeloid cell score in human glioma samples. The data were derived from the Ivy Glioblastoma Atlas Project. Pearson's correlation coefficient was performed

relative expression of *Cd274* (PD-L1) and *Ifng* (Fig. 5b). Moreover, the expression of *Cd274* was well correlated with the respective expression of *Ifng*, *Irf1*, *Gbp5*, and *Ccl2* (Fig. 5c), demonstrating that selected IFN-γ-induced genes serve as feasible substitute indicators for IFN-γ level and thus might synergistically indicate the prognosis of glioma.

IFN-γ score: a candidate for prognostic indicator of glioma

Combining the relative expression levels of the seven sorted genes, IFN-γ score was calculated as substitute indicator for IFN-γ level. Based on TCGA LGG/GBM datasets, the IFN-γ score increased along with the malignancy degree of glioma, reaching an extremely high value in GBM (Fig. 6a; Additional file 4: Figure S2A).

The IFN-γ score presented a similar pattern as the expression levels of PD-L1 in both primary and non-primary glioma of various malignancies (Fig. 6b, c). IFN-γ score was positively correlated with the expression of PD-L1 in different types of glioma samples (Fig. 6d). Positive correlation of IFN-γ score and the expression of PD-L1 was also found in different anatomic structures of glioma, based on the Ivy Glioblastoma Atlas Project database (Fig. 6e). In addition, IFN-γ score was negatively correlated with the survival of glioma patients (Fig. 6f; Additional file 4: Figure S2B). All of the above confirmed the feasibility of IFN-γ score as complementary indicator for prognosis of glioma patients.

In conclusion, tumor-infiltrating T cells are initially activated and upregulate the expression of PD-1. IFN-γ,

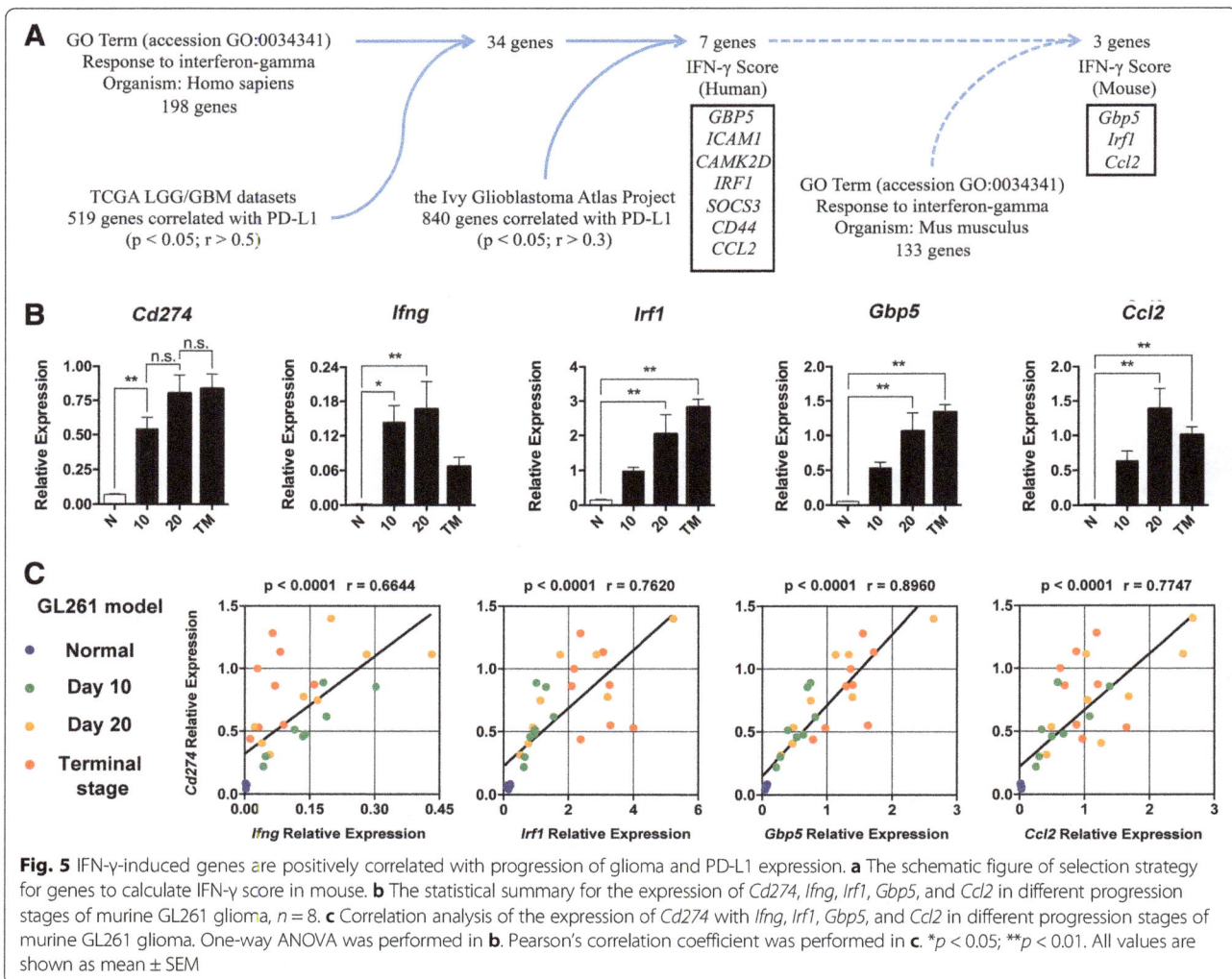

Fig. 5 IFN-γ-induced genes are positively correlated with progression of glioma and PD-L1 expression. **a** The schematic figure of selection strategy for genes to calculate IFN-γ score in mouse. **b** The statistical summary for the expression of *Cd274*, *Ifng*, *Irf1*, *Gbp5*, and *Ccl2* in different progression stages of murine GL261 glioma, $n = 8$. **c** Correlation analysis of the expression of *Cd274* with *Ifng*, *Irf1*, *Gbp5*, and *Ccl2* in different progression stages of murine GL261 glioma. One-way ANOVA was performed in **b**. Pearson's correlation coefficient was performed in **c**. *$p < 0.05$; **$p < 0.01$. All values are shown as mean ± SEM

secreted by activated T cells and possibly NK cells, induces the expression of PD-L1 not only on tumor cells but also on microglia and peripheral infiltrating immune cells. Through PD-L1/PD-1 axis, tumor-infiltrating T cells are rendered dysfunctional and apoptotic. Here, we propose IFN-γ score aggregated from seven IFN-γ-induced genes, namely *GBP5*, *ICAM1*, *CAMK2D*, *IRF1*, *SOCS3*, *CD44*, and *CCL2*, as auxiliary prognostic indicator for screening suitable patients for anti-PD-1/PD-L1 therapy (Fig. 7).

Discussion

Our study identified the distribution of PD-L1 in gliomas and that, apart from tumor cells in the tumor microenvironment, significantly increased PD-L1 expression was also spotted on activated microglia and peripheral-derived myeloid cells. Besides, we provided some evidence that IFN-γ played an important role in inducing the expression of PD-L1 in gliomas. IFN-γ score, aggregated from expression of IFN-γ downstream

genes as a substitute for the abundance of IFN-γ, is expected to serve as an auxiliary prognostic indicator for screening potential PD-1/PD-L1 antibody drug-applicable glioma patients.

Previous studies have focused on the mechanisms of PD-L1 expression in tumor cells, which include tumor endogenous proto-oncogenic signal, such as abnormal PI3K/Akt signaling pathway [21], and adaptive immune resistance, specifically the magnified negative feedback of the immune system that originally prevents over-activated immune cells from damaging the tissue [22, 23]. In gliomas, the latter mechanism may play a greater role in the expression of PD-L1 in the microenvironment. T cells are activated in the local region of tumor and thus secrete IFN-γ [24–26], which can subsequently induce upregulation of PD-L1 in tumor cells and immune cells in the microenvironment [11, 27], thereby inhibiting tumor eradication led by T cells. Notably, IFN-γ in the tumor microenvironment comes not only from T cells but also from NK cells. The vicious

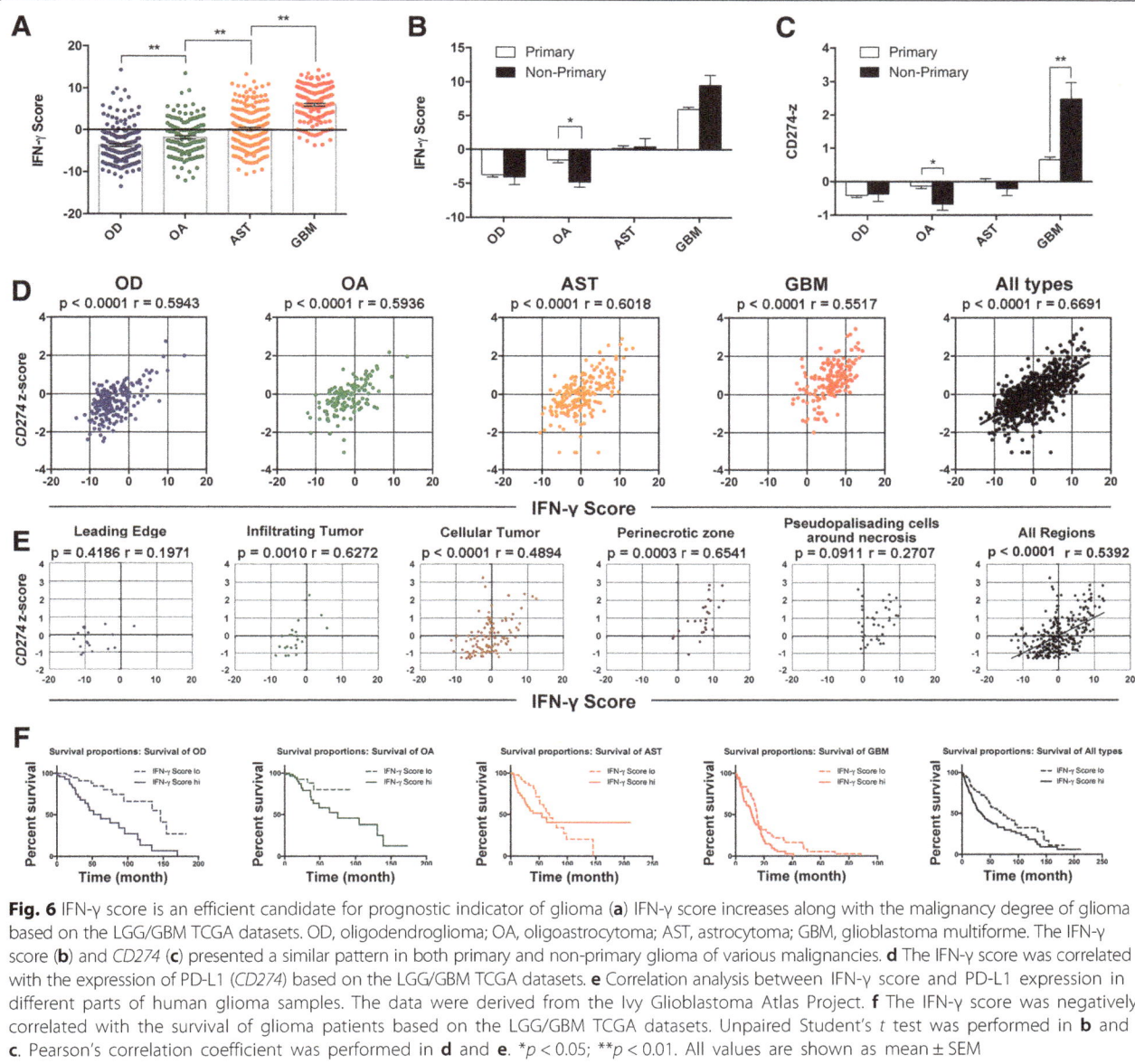

Fig. 6 IFN-γ score is an efficient candidate for prognostic indicator of glioma (**a**) IFN-γ score increases along with the malignancy degree of glioma based on the LGG/GBM TCGA datasets. OD, oligodendroglioma; OA, oligoastrocytoma; AST, astrocytoma; GBM, glioblastoma multiforme. The IFN-γ score (**b**) and *CD274* (**c**) presented a similar pattern in both primary and non-primary glioma of various malignancies. **d** The IFN-γ score was correlated with the expression of PD-L1 (*CD274*) based on the LGG/GBM TCGA datasets. **e** Correlation analysis between IFN-γ score and PD-L1 expression in different parts of human glioma samples. The data were derived from the Ivy Glioblastoma Atlas Project. **f** The IFN-γ score was negatively correlated with the survival of glioma patients based on the LGG/GBM TCGA datasets. Unpaired Student's *t* test was performed in **b** and **c**. Pearson's correlation coefficient was performed in **d** and **e**. *$p < 0.05$; **$p < 0.01$. All values are shown as mean ± SEM

effect of this negative feedback may be more pronounced in the CNS. The microglia, astrocytes, neurons, and epithelial cells in the CNS can be induced by IFN-γ and upregulate PD-L1 expression [28–30], which may exacerbate T cell dysfunction and apoptosis in gliomas. Such IFN-γ/PD-L1 axis-mediated immune suppression that also exists in the normal tissue inadvertently promotes glioma immune escape.

In the GL261 glioma model, we found that the expression of PD-1 was elevated in both CD4$^+$ and CD8$^+$ T cells. Previous studies have revealed that PD-L1 expressed by tumor cells suppresses cytotoxic activity of tumor-infiltrating CTLs [31–33]. In addition, we found that glioma-infiltrated antigen-presenting cells (microglia

and peripheral-derived macrophages) overexpressed PD-L1. The abovementioned suggests the importance of PD-1/PD-L1 axis on the functional inhibition of CD4$^+$ cells in glioma. It is indicated that the adaptive immune resistance not only occurs as the inhibition of CTL-mediated tumoricidal activity, but also as the activation of CD4$^+$ helper T cells in tumors, thus fundamentally affecting the entire tumor-immune microenvironment networks and disrupting the formation of anti-tumor immune microenvironments.

In the study, we proposed IFN-γ score as a complementary predictive biomarker, which is aggregated from the expression of seven selected genes. IRF1, directly participating in the regulation of PD-L1 expression, is

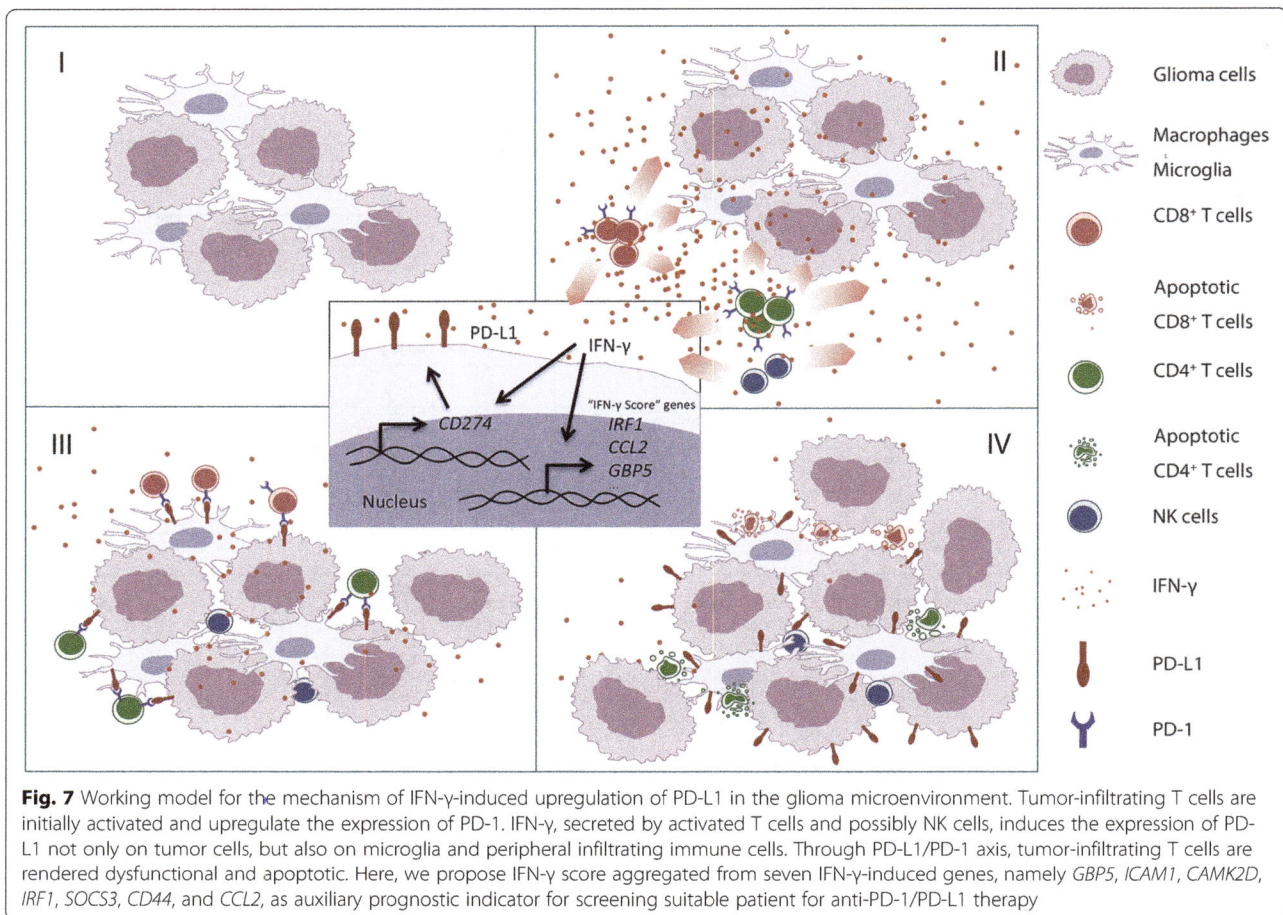

Fig. 7 Working model for the mechanism of IFN-γ-induced upregulation of PD-L1 in the glioma microenvironment. Tumor-infiltrating T cells are initially activated and upregulate the expression of PD-1. IFN-γ, secreted by activated T cells and possibly NK cells, induces the expression of PD-L1 not only on tumor cells, but also on microglia and peripheral infiltrating immune cells. Through PD-L1/PD-1 axis, tumor-infiltrating T cells are rendered dysfunctional and apoptotic. Here, we propose IFN-γ score aggregated from seven IFN-γ-induced genes, namely *GBP5*, *ICAM1*, *CAMK2D*, *IRF1*, *SOCS3*, *CD44*, and *CCL2*, as auxiliary prognostic indicator for screening suitable patient for anti-PD-1/PD-L1 therapy

essential in the constitutive and IFN-γ-induced expression of PD-L1 in various cancer cells [34–36]. A recent study confirmed that PD-L1 expression in melanoma cells is mainly regulated by the IFN-γ receptor signaling pathway which subsequently converged to the binding of IRF1 with the PD-L1 promoter [11]. Upregulation of GBP5 has been recognized in colon cancer [37]. In gastric cancer, positive correlation between immune cell infiltration and stromal and epithelial GBP5 expression has been reported [38]. A previous study demonstrated the role of GBP protein in the formation of inflammasome complex as well as its anti-inflammatory and autoimmunity-controlling effect [39], yet the specific function of the GBP protein family remains to be discovered. SOCS3, promoted by IFN-γ downstream genes STAT1 or STAT3 [40, 41], is known as a negative regulator of cytokine signaling and participant in control of CNS immunity [42, 43]. CCL2 is the key chemokine that recruits myeloid-derived cells to the tumor microenvironment in glioma [44]. According to previous studies, peripherally derived myeloid cells usually perform immunosuppressive functions in gliomas [45–47]. Besides, the expression levels of all seven genes were negatively correlated with the survival of glioma patients. All the evidence indicated that the expression of PD-L1 and other immune inhibitory mechanisms in the glioma microenvironment might serve as negative feedback mechanisms that followed, rather than preceded, T cell activation and IFN-γ secretion.

Conclusions

Our study proposed a possibility that the expression of PD-L1 in the glioma microenvironment is intrinsically driven by the immune system and implies that anti-PD-1/PD-L1 therapy might be preferentially beneficial for patients with high IFN-γ score. More importance should be attached to the screening of potentially responsive patients. Further investigation is required to examine the IFN-γ score and the response to anti-PD-1/PD-L1 therapy in clinical trials.

Additional files

Additional file 1: Table S2. Technical specifications of antibodies used in our study. (DOC 46 kb)

Additional file 2: Table S1. Primer sequences for qPCR used in the study. (DOC 31 kb)

Additional file 3: Figure S1. Distribution of PD-L1 in the murine glioma model. (A) Representative staining for PD-L1 (red) and DAPI (blue) in the tumor-bearing brain (day 20); different regions of the tumor-bearing brain were shown. Scale bar, 100 μm. (B) PD-L1 intensity of different regions was calculated. Data were collected from four to seven randomly selected areas for each corresponding region per mouse, $n = 3$. One-way ANOVA was performed. *, $p < 0.05$; **, $p < 0.01$. All values are shown as mean ± SEM. (DOC 609 kb)

Additional file 4: Figure S2. IFN-γ score is an efficient candidate for prognostic indicator of glioma. (A) The expression of PD-L1 and other IFN-γ-induced genes increases along with the malignancy degree of glioma based on the LGG/GBM TCGA datasets. OD, oligodendroglioma; OA, oligoastrocytoma; AST, astrocytoma; GBM, glioblastoma multiforme. (B) The expression of PD-L1 and other IFN-γ-induced genes was negatively correlated with the survival of glioma patients based on the LGG/GBM TCGA datasets. (DOC 1515 kb)

Abbreviations

BMDM: Bone marrow-derived macrophages; CNS: Central nervous system; CT: Cellular tumor; CTpan: Pseudopalisading cells around necrosis; CTpnz: Perinecrotic zone; FACS: Fluorescence-activated cell sorting; GBM: Glioblastoma; IHC: Immunohistochemistry; IM: Invasive margin; IT: Intratumoral region; LGG: Lower grade glioma; N: Normal tissue; TCGA: The Cancer Genome Atlas; TR: Tumor rim

Funding

This work was supported by the National Natural Science Foundation of China (31570892, 31770992, 81730045, and 91527305) and the Science and Technology Commission of Shanghai Municipality (15JC1401200).

Authors' contributions

JQ and YC designed the experiments. JQ, CW, BW, and JY conducted the studies. YW, FL, and JX assisted with the experiments. JQ and CZ conducted the in silico analysis. RL provided intellectual input. YC supervised the study. JQ, CW, and YC interpreted the data and wrote the manuscript. All authors read and approved the final manuscript.

Competing interests

The authors declare that they have no competing interests.

Author details

[1]Department of Immunology, School of Basic Medical Sciences, and Institute of Biomedical Sciences, Fudan University, No. 138, Yi Xue Yuan Rd., Mail Box 226, Shanghai 200032, People's Republic of China. [2]Biotherapy Research Center, Fudan University, Shanghai 200032, China. [3]Jiangsu Key Lab of Medical Optics, Suzhou Institute of Biomedical Engineering and Technology, Chinese Academy of Sciences, Suzhou 215000, China. [4]Northfield Mount Hermon School, Mount Hermon, MA 01354, USA.

References

1. Louis DN, Perry A, Reifenberger G, et al. The 2016 World Health Organization Classification of tumors of the central nervous system: a summary. Acta Neuropathol. 2016;131(6):803–20.
2. Gieryng A, Pszczolkowska D, Walentynowicz KA, et al. Immune microenvironment of gliomas. Lab Invest. 2017;97(5):498–518.
3. Walunas TL, Bakker CY, Bluestone JA. CTLA-4 ligation blocks CD28-dependent T cell activation. J Exp Med. 1996;183(6):2541–50.
4. Curiel TJ, Coukos G, Zou L, et al. Specific recruitment of regulatory T cells in ovarian carcinoma fosters immune privilege and predicts reduced survival. Nat Med. 2004;10(9):942–9.
5. Gabrilovich DI, Nagaraj S. Myeloid-derived suppressor cells as regulators of the immune system. Nat Rev Immunol. 2009;9(3):162–74.
6. Lob S, Konigsrainer A, Rammensee HG, et al. Inhibitors of indoleamine-2,3-dioxygenase for cancer therapy: can we see the wood for the trees? Nat Rev Cancer. 2009;9(6):445–52.
7. Alsaab HO, Sau S, Alzhrani R, et al. PD-1 and PD-L1 checkpoint signaling inhibition for cancer immunotherapy: mechanism, combinations, and clinical outcome. Front Pharmacol. 2017;8:561.
8. Keir ME, Butte MJ, Freeman GJ, et al. PD-1 and its ligands in tolerance and immunity. Annu Rev Immunol. 2008;26:677–704.
9. Freeman GJ, Long AJ, Iwai Y, et al. Engagement of the PD-1 immunoinhibitory receptor by a novel B7 family member leads to negative regulation of lymphocyte activation. J Exp Med. 2000;192(7):1027–34.
10. Spranger S, Spaapen RM, Zha Y, et al. Up-regulation of PD-L1, IDO, and T(regs) in the melanoma tumor microenvironment is driven by CD8(+) T cells. Sci Transl Med. 2013;5(200):200ra116.
11. Garcia-Diaz A, Shin DS, Moreno BH, et al. Interferon receptor signaling pathways regulating PD-L1 and PD-L2 expression. Cell Rep. 2017;19(6):1189–201.
12. Xue S, Hu M, Iyer V, et al. Blocking the PD-1/PD-L1 pathway in glioma: a potential new treatment strategy. J Hematol Oncol. 2017;10(1):81.
13. Nduom EK, Wei J, Yaghi NK, et al. PD-L1 expression and prognostic impact in glioblastoma. Neuro-Oncology. 2016;18(2):195–205.
14. Wang Z, Zhang C, Liu X, et al. Molecular and clinical characterization of PD-L1 expression at transcriptional level via 976 samples of brain glioma. Oncoimmunology. 2016;5(11):e1196310.
15. Balar AV, Castellano D, O'Donnell PH, et al. First-line pembrolizumab in cisplatin-ineligible patients with locally advanced and unresectable or metastatic urothelial cancer (KEYNOTE-052): a multicentre, single-arm, phase 2 study. Lancet Oncol. 2017;18(11):1483–92.
16. Leonardi GC, Gainor JF, Altan M, et al. Safety of programmed death-1 pathway inhibitors among patients with non-small-cell lung cancer and preexisting autoimmune disorders. J Clin Oncol. 2018;36(19):1905–12.
17. Qian J, Luo F, Yang J, et al. TLR2 promotes glioma immune evasion by downregulating MHC class II molecules in microglia. Cancer Immunol Res. 2018;6(10):1220–33.
18. Maes W, van Gool SW. Experimental immunotherapy for malignant glioma: lessons from two decades of research in the GL261 model. Cancer Immunol Immunother. 2011;60(2):153–60.
19. Waeckerle-Men Y, Starke A, Wuthrich RP. PD-L1 partially protects renal tubular epithelial cells from the attack of CD8+ cytotoxic T cells. Nephrol Dial Transplant. 2007;22(6):1527–36.
20. Muhlbauer M, Fleck M, Schutz C, et al. PD-L1 is induced in hepatocytes by viral infection and by interferon-alpha and -gamma and mediates T cell apoptosis. J Hepatol. 2006;45(4):520–8.
21. Parsa AT, Waldron JS, Panner A, et al. Loss of tumor suppressor PTEN function increases B7-H1 expression and immunoresistance in glioma. Nat Med. 2007;13(1):84–8.
22. Tumeh PC, Harview CL, Yearley JH, et al. PD-1 blockade induces responses by inhibiting adaptive immune resistance. Nature. 2014;515(7528):568–71.
23. Sharma P, Hu-Lieskovan S, Wargo JA, et al. Primary, adaptive, and acquired resistance to cancer immunotherapy. Cell. 2017;168(4):707–23.
24. Yoneda Y, Yoshida R. The role of T cells in allografted tumor rejection: IFN-gamma released from T cells is essential for induction of effector macrophages in the rejection site. J Immunol. 1998;160(12):6012–7.
25. Bohm W, Thoma S, Leithauser F, et al. T cell-mediated, IFN-gamma-facilitated rejection of murine B16 melanomas. J Immunol. 1998;161(2):897–908.
26. Lauwerys BR, Garot N, Renauld JC, et al. Cytokine production and killer activity of NK/T-NK cells derived with IL-2, IL-15, or the combination of IL-12 and IL-18. J Immunol. 2000;165(4):1847–53.
27. Abiko K, Matsumura N, Hamanishi J, et al. IFN-gamma from lymphocytes induces PD-L1 expression and promotes progression of ovarian cancer. Br J Cancer. 2015;112(9):1501–9.
28. Schachtele SJ, Hu S, Sheng WS, et al. Glial cells suppress postencephalitic CD8+ T lymphocytes through PD-L1. Glia. 2014;62(10):1582–94.
29. Liu Y, Carlsson R, Ambjorn M, et al. PD-L1 expression by neurons nearby tumors indicates better prognosis in glioblastoma patients. J Neurosci. 2013;33(35):14231–45.

30. Rodig N, Ryan T, Allen JA, et al. Endothelial expression of PD-L1 and PD-L2 down-regulates CD8+ T cell activation and cytolysis. Eur J Immunol. 2003; 33(11):3117–26.

31. Iwai Y, Ishida M, Tanaka Y, et al. Involvement of PD-L1 on tumor cells in the escape from host immune system and tumor immunotherapy by PD-L1 blockade. Proc Natl Acad Sci U S A. 2002;99(19):12293–7.

32. Hirano F, Kaneko K, Tamura H, et al. Blockade of B7-H1 and PD-1 by monoclonal antibodies potentiates cancer therapeutic immunity. Cancer Res. 2005;65(3):1089–96.

33. Abiko K, Mandai M, Hamanishi J, et al. PD-L1 on tumor cells is induced in ascites and promotes peritoneal dissemination of ovarian cancer through CTL dysfunction. Clin Cancer Res. 2013;19(6):1363–74.

34. Sato H, Niimi A, Yasuhara T, et al. DNA double-strand break repair pathway regulates PD-L1 expression in cancer cells. Nat Commun. 2017;8(1):1751.

35. Li N, Wang J, Zhang N, et al. Cross-talk between TNF-alpha and IFN-gamma signaling in induction of B7-H1 expression in hepatocellular carcinoma cells. Cancer Immunol Immunother. 2018;67(2):271–83.

36. Lai Q, Wang H, Li A, et al. Decitibine improve the efficiency of anti-PD-1 therapy via activating the response to IFN/PD-L1 signal of lung cancer cells. Oncogene. 2018;37(17):2302–12.

37. Friedman K, Brodsky AS, Lu S, et al. Medullary carcinoma of the colon: a distinct morphology reveals a distinctive immunoregulatory microenvironment. Mod Pathol. 2016;29(5):528–41.

38. Blakely AM, Matoso A, Patil PA, et al. Role of immune microenvironment in gastrointestinal stromal tumours. Histopathology. 2018;72(3):405–13.

39. Shenoy AR, Wellington DA, Kumar P, et al. GBP5 promotes NLRP3 inflammasome assembly and immunity in mammals. Science. 2012; 336(6080):481–5.

40. Kershaw NJ, Murphy JM, Liau NP, et al. SOCS3 binds specific receptor-JAK complexes to control cytokine signaling by direct kinase inhibition. Nat Struct Mol Biol. 2013;20(4):469–76.

41. Babon JJ, Kershaw NJ, Murphy JM, et al. Suppression of cytokine signaling by SOCS3: characterization of the mode of inhibition and the basis of its specificity. Immunity. 2012;36(2):239–50.

42. Cao L, Wang Z, Wan W. Suppressor of cytokine signaling 3: emerging role linking central insulin resistance and Alzheimer's disease. Front Neurosci. 2018;12:417.

43. Iwahara N, Hisahara S, Kawamata J, et al. Role of suppressor of cytokine signaling 3 (SOCS3) in altering activated microglia phenotype in APPswe/PS1dE9 mice. J Alzheimers Dis. 2017;55(3):1235–47.

44. Chang AL, Miska J, Wainwright DA, et al. CCL2 produced by the glioma microenvironment is essential for the recruitment of regulatory T cells and myeloid-derived suppressor cells. Cancer Res. 2016;76(19):5671–82.

45. Antonios JP, Soto H, Everson RG, et al. Immunosuppressive tumor-infiltrating myeloid cells mediate adaptive immune resistance via a PD-1/PD-L1 mechanism in glioblastoma. Neuro-Oncology. 2017;19(6):796–807.

46. Yao Y, Ye H, Qi Z, et al. B7-H4(B7x)-mediated cross-talk between glioma-initiating cells and macrophages via the IL6/JAK/STAT3 pathway lead to poor prognosis in glioma patients. Clin Cancer Res. 2016;22(11):2778–90.

47. Kohanbash G, McKaveney K, Sakaki M, et al. GM-CSF promotes the immunosuppressive activity of glioma-infiltrating myeloid cells through interleukin-4 receptor-alpha. Cancer Res. 2013;73(21):6413–23.

14

CSF sTREM2 in delirium—relation to Alzheimer's disease CSF biomarkers Aβ42, t-tau and p-tau

Kristi Henjum[1*], Else Quist-Paulsen[2,3], Henrik Zetterberg[4,5,6,7], Kaj Blennow[4,5], Lars N. G. Nilsson[1†] and Leiv Otto Watne[8,9†]

Abstract

Background: Delirium and dementia share symptoms of cognitive dysfunctions, and mechanisms of neuroinflammation appear involved in both conditions. Triggering receptor expressed on myeloid cells 2 (*TREM2*) is linked to dementia and neurodegenerative disease. It encodes expression of an innate immune receptor in the brain expressed by microglia. The level of the soluble fragment of TREM2 (sTREM2) is reported to increase in the cerebrospinal fluid (CSF) already in prodromal and asymptomatic Alzheimer's disease.

Methods: We analyzed the level of CSF sTREM2 in relation to delirium and dementia. The study included patients with or without pre-existing dementia who underwent acute hip fracture surgery ($n = 120$), and some of the patients developed delirium ($n = 65$). A medical delirium cohort ($n = 26$) was also examined. ELISA was used to determine the level of sTREM2 in CSF.

Results: Delirium was associated with a higher level of CSF sTREM2 only among those without pre-existing dementia ($p = 0.046$, $n = 15$, $n = 44$), particularly among patients developing delirium after CSF sampling ($p = 0.02$, $n = 7$, $n = 44$). Between patients with dementia, there was no group difference, but the CSF sTREM2 level increased with waiting time for surgery ($r_S = 0.39$, $p = 0.002$, $n = 60$) and correlated well with the CSF Alzheimer's disease biomarkers, Aβ42, and t-tau/p-tau ($r_S = 0.40$, $p = 0.002$, $r_S = 0.46$, $p < 0.001$/ $r_S = 0.49$, $p < 0.001$, $n = 60$). Among patients with dementia, the level of Aβ38 and Aβ40 also correlated positively with sTREM2 in CSF (Aβ38$_{MSD}r_S = 0.44$, $p = 0.001$; Aβ40$_{MSD}r_S = 0.48$, $p < 0.001$; Aβ42$_{MSD}r_S = 0.43$, $p < 0.001$, $n = 60$).

Conclusion: The findings reinforce the involvement of neuroinflammation in delirium, yet with separate responses in patients with or without pre-existing dementia. Our findings support the concept of primed microglia in neurodegenerative disease and central immune activation after a peripheral trauma in such patients. A CSF biomarker panel of neuroinflammation might be valuable to prevent delirium by identifying patients at risk.

Keywords: Delirium, Dementia, Alzheimer's disease, CSF biomarkers, Soluble TREM2

Background

Delirium is an acute state of confusion with fluctuating symptoms of disturbed attention and cognition commonly precipitated by stress, such as surgery, in frail patients [1]. Besides unpleasant while ongoing, a delirium carries the risk of increased mortality and long-term

* Correspondence: kristi.henjum@medisin.uio.no
†Lars N. G. Nilsson and Leiv Otto Watne contributed equally to this work.
[1]Department of Pharmacology, Institute of Clinical Medicine, University of Oslo and Oslo University Hospital, P.O. box 1057 Blindern, 0316 Oslo, Norway
Full list of author information is available at the end of the article

sequela of cognitive functions [2]. Although much is unknown, the delirium pathogenesis is thought to involve disturbed neurotransmission and/or induced inflammation with microglial activation [3]. The neuroinflammatory hypothesis suggest that delirium symptoms arise as central immunity is activated by initial peripheral inflammation that convey to the brain [4, 5].

While delirium increases the risk of dementia, dementia is also a delirium risk factor [6–8]. The most common cause of dementia is Alzheimer's disease (AD), a neurodegenerative disorder with pathological hallmarks amyloid plaques and neurofibrillary tangles [9]. Already at a preclinical stage with evident neuropathology is AD found to increase the risk of delirium [10, 11]. Neuroinflammation with microglial activation and astrogliosis also plays a role in AD [12]. Thus, delirium and dementia etiology are intertwined with shared pathogenic mechanisms such as microglial activation and other facets of neuroinflammation [13].

Microglia, the resident immune cells of the brain, express the innate immune receptor triggering receptor expressed on myeloid cells 2 (TREM2) [14]. Variants of *TREM2* are known as dementia risk factors [15–17] linking *TREM2* to age-related neurodegeneration. The transmembrane TREM2 receptor undergoes ectodomain shedding releasing soluble TREM2 (sTREM2) [18] (Fig. 1a). In the cerebrospinal fluid (CSF) of AD patients, sTREM2 is reported increased [19, 20]. An even higher level is observed at the prodromal mild cognitive impairment (MCI) stage of AD [21]. Moreover, the level of CSF sTREM2 correlates positively with the core CSF biomarkers amyloid beta 1–42 (Aβ42), total-tau (t-tau), and phosphorylated-tau (p-tau) in asymptomatic patients, which further suggests an early involvement of reactive microgliosis [22, 23].

In the present study, we analyzed the CSF sTREM2 level in patients with or without pre-existing dementia. The patients all suffered a hip fracture with subsequent hospital admission and surgery that for some led to delirium, and we evaluated CSF sTREM2 as a putative biomarker of delirium. Given the abovementioned biomarker correlations in AD, we also examined the relation between CSF sTREM2 and AD core biomarkers, CSF Aβ42, t-tau, and p-tau. For the potential influence of a peripheral trauma, we investigated how the CSF sTREM2 level related to time after hip fracture. We also included a patient group with delirium associated with a medical condition to evaluate potential similarities and dissimilarities to hip fracture-triggered delirium.

Methods

Hip fracture cohort

The hip fracture patients, which were recruited from the Oslo Orthogeriatric trial (OOT), were admitted to the Oslo University Hospital Ullevål (OUS, Ullevål) between September 2009 and January 2012 [24, 25]. Delirium was assessed using the Confusion Assessment Method (CAM) [26] by the study physician or a study nurse. Delirium was assessed daily preoperatively and until the fifth postoperative day or in case of delirium until discharge. Pre-fracture dementia status was decided by consensus and based on the International Classification of Diseases – 10 (ICD-10) criteria for dementia by an expert panel as previously described [25].

The hip fracture patients ($n = 120$) were grouped both according to delirium and dementia status into either of the following groups (see Fig. 1a and Table 1)

1. No delirium during the hospital stay (no delirium) ($n = 54$)
   a. No delirium, and without pre-fracture dementia ($n = 44$)
   b. No delirium, but pre-fracture dementia ($n = 10$)
2. Delirium during the hospital stay (delirium) ($n = 65$)
   a. Delirium, but without pre-fracture dementia ($n = 15$)
   b. Delirium with pre-fracture to dementia ($n = 50$)

Delirium patients included prevalent delirium (those that developed delirium preoperatively; $n = 41$) and incident delirium (postoperative delirium in those free from delirium before surgery; $n = 21$). The sub-classification of delirium onset was applied for delirium onset analyses.

Medical delirium cohort

The medical delirium cohort was recruited from a prospective study at the same hospital in which 244 patients who underwent lumbar puncture (LP) due to suspicion of acute central nervous system (CNS) infection were included. Patients were included between January 2014 and December 2015. The patients included in the current study ($n = 26$) were those in which a CNS infection was ruled out and delirium triggered by another medical condition was considered the most likely explanation for the acute cognitive symptoms. Pneumonia and urinary tract infection were the most frequent diagnoses in this group. All patients had encephalopathy at the time of the LP. Delirium was assessed either by the study physician with CAM, or by clinical evaluation of treating physician in the medical ward. Dementia status was set from the hospital records. These delirium patients formed a separate group labeled "medical delirium" afflicted by delirium with another precipitating factor than the hip fracture patients.

CSF sampling, handling, and storage

In the hip fracture cohort, CSF was collected in connection with the orthopedic surgery at the onset of spinal anesthesia before administrating the anesthetic agents. CSF of patients with medical delirium was obtained during the diagnostic lumbar puncture (LP) at a median of 1 day after CNS symptoms developed. CSF was collected in polypropylene tubes and centrifuged as soon as possible, and supernatant aliquots were stored in polypropylene tubes at −80 °C [27].

Table 1 Characteristics of the hip fracture and medical delirium patients

	Hip fracture cohort					Medical delirium
	All	No delirium	Delirium			
			All	Incident	Prevalent	Medical
PATIENTS *WITHOUT* DEMENTIA						
N	59	44	15	7	8	17
Age (years)	84 (10)	84 (16)	85 (7)	86 (11)	85 (7)	66 (16)
Gender						
Male	17	11	6	3	3	10
Female	42	33	9	4	5	7
Time to surgery (h)*	23 (17)	23 (17)	27 (15)	22 (19)	30 (14)	–
CSF sTREM2 ng/ml	7.8 (5.7)	7.4 (5)	11.1(11)	11.6 (5)	7.8 (15)	5.6 (8)
CSF biomarkers						
N	57	44	13	5	8	
CSF Aβ42 (pg/ml)	446 (367)	479 (414)	283 (224)	283 (232)	295 (253)	–
CSF t-tau (pg/ml)	369 (276)	356 (198)	564 (638)	564 (369)	587 (795)	–
CSF p-tau (pg/ml)	57(35)	54 (33)	78 (68)	78 (19)	88 (89)	–
CSF Aβ42 cut-off (< 530 pg/ml)						
Below	37	26	11	4	7	–
Above	20	18	2	1	1	–
CSF p-tau cut-off (≥ 60 pg/ml)						
Above	26	17	9	4	5	–
Below	31	27	4	1	3	–
CSF t-tau cut-off (> 350 pg/ml)						
Above	32	23	9	5	4	–
Below	25	21	4	–	4	–
PATIENTS *WITH* DEMENTIA						
N	61	10	50	13	33	9
Age (years)	86 (9)	86.5 (17)	85(9)	87 (8)	85 (8)	71(23)
Gender						
Male	16	1	15	5	8	6
Female	45	9	35	8	25	3
Time to surgery (h)*	26 (28)	27 (16)	26(31)	18(19)	38 (24)	–
CSF sTREM2 ng/ml	7.0 (7.8)	9.2 (16)	7.3 (7)	6.1 (10)	8.5 (8)	6.9(6.7)
CSF biomarkers, N	60	9	50	13	33	
CSF Aβ42 (pg/ml)	265 (166)	317 (290)	258 (172)	268 (219)	269 (174)	–
CSF t-tau (pg/ml)	408 (379)	441 (503)	408 (366)	385 (293)	407 (329)	–
CSF p-tau (pg/ml	55 (41)	58 (57)	55 (35)	55 (47)	55 (31)	–
CSF Aβ42 cut-off (< 530 pg/ml)						
Below	55	7	47	11	1	–
Above	5	2	3	2	32	–
CSF p-tau cut-off (≥ 60 pg/ml)						
Above	24	4	20	5	13	–
Below	36	5	30	8	20	–
CSF t-tau cut-off (> 350 pg/ml)						
Above	38	5	33	8	22	–
Below	22	4	17	5	11	–

Data are presented as median and interquartile range (IQR), waiting time for surgery. Aβ42, amyloid beta 1–42; t-tau, total-tau; p-tau, phosphorylated tau; sTREM2, soluble triggering receptor expressed on myeloid cells
*Time to surgery, hours from hospital admission to surgery (onset of anesthesia) and CSF sampling

CSF sTREM2 measurements

CSF sTREM2 was assayed by a sensitive TREM2 enzyme-linked immunosorbent assay (ELISA) as previously described [22]. Briefly, plates were incubated with an anti-humanTREM2 polyclonal capture antibody overnight at 4 °C (AF1828, R&D Systems, Minneapolis, MN, USA) and TREM2 detected by a mouse anti-human TREM2 monoclonal HRP-conjugated antibody (1 h incubation at room temperature (RT);SEK11084, Sino Biologics, Beijing, China). Samples were assayed in duplicates (2 h incubation at RT) with known cohort (hip fracture or medical), but with the clinical identity unknown to the operator. Samples with extreme values were assayed again, including the same and an increased sample dilution to verify measurements in the repeated assay. Two internal standard (CSF) samples were included in each assay to assess interday variability and used to adjust the medical delirium cohort which was assayed separately from the hip fracture cohort, with a final CV < 10% across assays.

CSF Aβ, t-tau, and p-tau measurements

CSF levels of t-tau, p-tau, and Aβ42 were quantified with commercially available ELISAs; Innotest® hTau Ag, Innotest® phoshoTau (181P), and Innotest® β-amyloid 1–42 as previously described [28–30] (Fujirebio Europe, Gent, Belgium). CSF Aβ peptide levels were determined with CSF $Aβ_{1-38}$ (Aβ38), $Aβ_{1-40}$ (Aβ40), and $Aβ_{1-42}$ (Aβ42) MSD Triplex assay (Meso Scale Discovery, Rockwilly, MA, USA). All these analyses were performed at the Clinical Neurochemistry Laboratory at Sahlgrenska University Hopsital, Mölndal, Sweden. CSF cut-off for pathological level was < 530 pg/ml (Aβ42 +/−), ≥ 60 pg/ml (p-tau+/−), and > 350 pg/ml (t-tau +/−) [31].

Statistical analyses

Analyses were performed by parametric or non-parametric statistics as appropriate depending on the data distribution. Data distribution was assessed by histogram, probability-probability (P-P), and quantile-quantile (Q-Q) plots. As CSF sTREM2 raw data were skewed, continuous data are reported by median (interquartile range (IQR)) and group differences analyzed by Mann-Whitney or Kruskal-Wallis test. p values of group comparisons were obtained by Mann-Whitney test, unless otherwise reported. The correlation analyses are reported by Spearman's rho correlation coefficient (r_s).

Multiple linear regression was used for analyses with multiple predictor variables. For stepwise multiple linear regression, predictors were included based on significance in univariate analyses and biological grounds, including predictors with highest assumed degree of explained variability first. The data transformation by the natural logarithm (ln) (ln(CSF sTREM2 ng/ml)

approximated a normal distribution and was therefore applied for analyses requiring parametric tests (linear regressions). Standardized residuals in linear regressions met the criteria of normal distribution. In regression analyses with delirium, no delirium was coded as 0 and delirium as 1. In linear regressions with delirium onset; no delirium was coded as 0, incident delirium as 1, and prevalent delirium as 2.

All hypotheses were two-sided and the reported p values are therefore two-tailed. The significance level was set at $p < 0.05$. Statistical analyses were performed by the Statistical Package for Social Sciences (SPSS, versions 24 and 25; IBM, Armonk, NY, USA). Graphical illustrations were created with GraphPad Prism (version 7.04 Graph Pad Software, La Jolla, CA, USA).

Results

Increased CSF sTREM2 with delirium in hip fracture patients without pre-existing dementia

The patients studied did or did not develop delirium during hospitalization after a hip fracture requiring acute surgery. Around half of the patients included were demented before the accident, and a large proportion of those demented patients developed delirium after the hip fracture (≈ 80%; study setup in Fig. 1a). All the patients displayed an advanced age irrespective of dementia diagnosis (median age 85 years). The gender distribution was similar between groups (Table 1). Gender did not influence the CSF sTREM2 level and was therefore not included in the further analyses (data not shown).

Initial analyses of the CSF sTREM2 level showed a considerable intragroup variability, both among patients with and without delirium, with no separation between these two groups ($p = 0.25$, CSF sTREM2: 7.7(7.9) versus 7.4(5.4) ng/ml, $n = 65$, $n = 54$; Fig. 1b). Neuropathology of several dementia disorders involves microglial activation, and the underlying pathogenic processes may be different in delirium superimposed on dementia as compared to delirium in the absence of pre-existing dementia. Interestingly when stratifying patients according to pre-fracture dementia, an increased CSF sTREM2 level was only associated with delirium among those patients who were not demented before the hip fracture ($p = 0.046$, CSF sTREM2: 11.1(11.0) versus 7.4(5.0) ng/ml, $n = 15$, $n = 44$). In contrast, among patients with a pre-existing dementia, the CSF sTREM2 level did not differ between those patients who did or did not develop delirium ($p = 0.94$, $n = 50$, $n = 10$; Fig. 1c and Table 1).

CSF sTREM2 in relation to onset of delirium in hip fracture patients

During delirium, microglial reactivity may be transient and CSF sTREM2 levels may therefore fluctuate in a manner

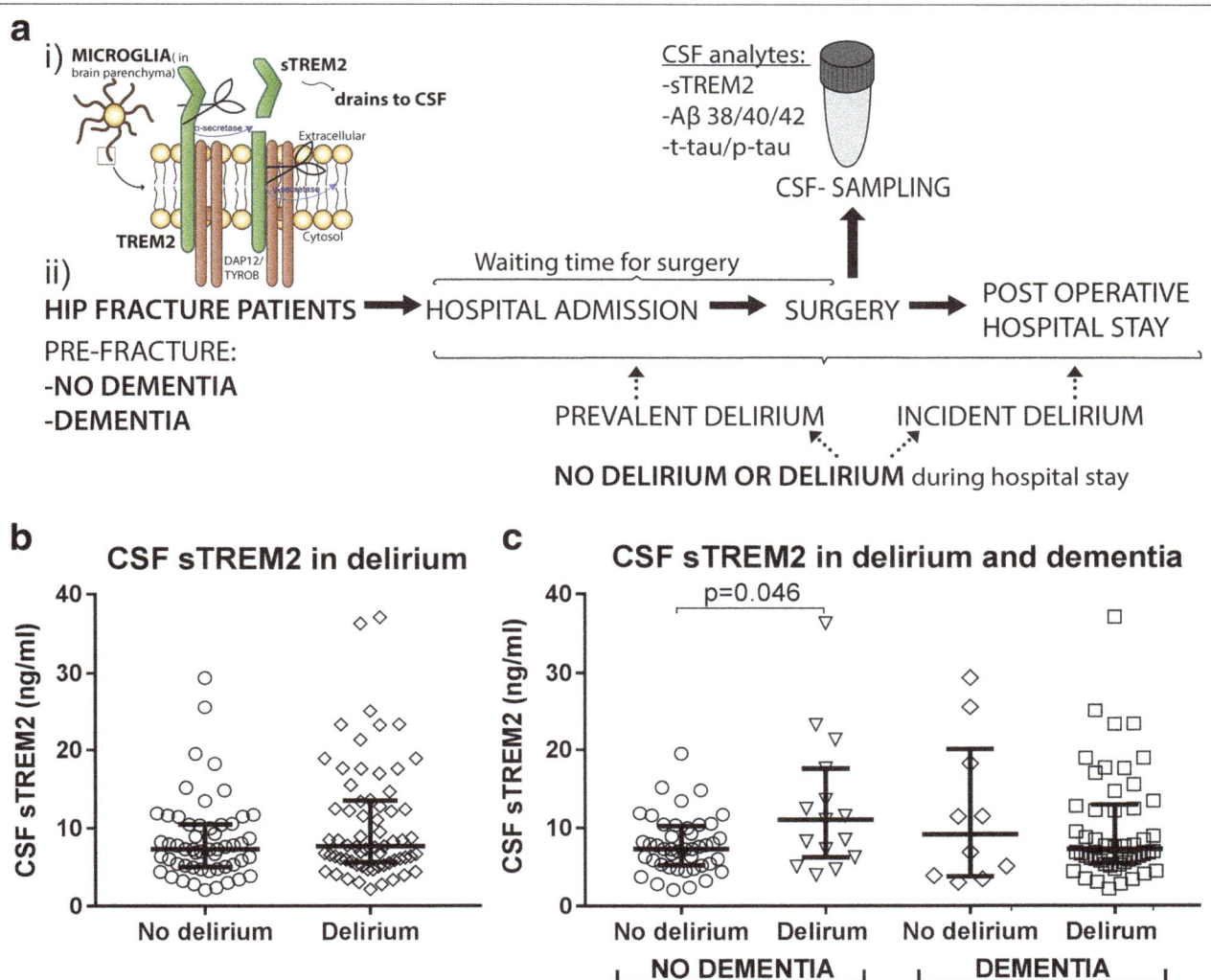

Fig. 1 CSF sTREM2 in patients hospitalized by a hip fracture. **a** A fragment of the microglial receptor TREM2 and sTREM2, released after ectodomain shedding, drains to the CSF. Sampling and time line of hip fracture patients admitted to the hospital where some of them developed delirium. **b** CSF sTREM2 level did not discriminate patients not developing delirium from patients developing delirium during hospitalization for an acute hip fracture surgery ($p = 0.25$, $n = 54$, $n = 65$). **c** Stratification and separate analyses of patients with and without pre-existing dementia showed significantly higher CSF sTREM2 level in delirium of patients without pre-existing dementia ($p = 0.046$, $n = 15$, $n = 44$). Dementia patients with and without delirium had a similar CSF sTREM2 level ($p = 0.94$, $n = 10$, $n = 50$). Two tailed p values were obtained by Mann-Whitney test, while larger and smaller lines represent the median and interquartile range respectively. CSF: cerebrospinal fluid, sTREM2: soluble TREM2

not directly related to clinical symptoms. To investigate possible changes in CSF sTREM2 with delirium progression, we stratified the delirium patients by onset of delirium relative to time of surgery when CSF was sampled (see Fig. 1a). Patients with pre-operational delirium were classified as having prevalent delirium, while those with post-operational delirium were categorized as having incident delirium. Among patients without pre-existing dementia, the incident delirium group showed an increased CSF sTREM2 level as compared to patients not developing delirium ($p = 0.02$, CSF sTREM2: 11.6 (5.0) versus 7.4 (5.0) ng/ml, $n = 7$, $n = 44$). The patients with prevalent delirium displayed a large variability in CSF sTREM2 and did not differ statistically neither from the unaffected patient group nor from the group having incident delirium ($p = 0.46$, $p = 0.45$, $n = 8$, $n = 44$, $n = 7$). When likewise stratifying patients with pre-existing dementia into subgroups of onset of delirium, the CSF sTREM2 level did not differ between the three groups ($p = 0.62$, Kruskal-Wallis test, Fig. 2 and Table 1).

CSF sTREM2 in relation to waiting time for surgery among hip fracture patients

A peripheral insult, such as a hip fracture, may trigger a central immune response [32]. The CSF sTREM2 level correlated positively to waiting time for surgery after hospital admission (waiting time for surgery (h); $r_S = 0.23$, $p = 0.01$,

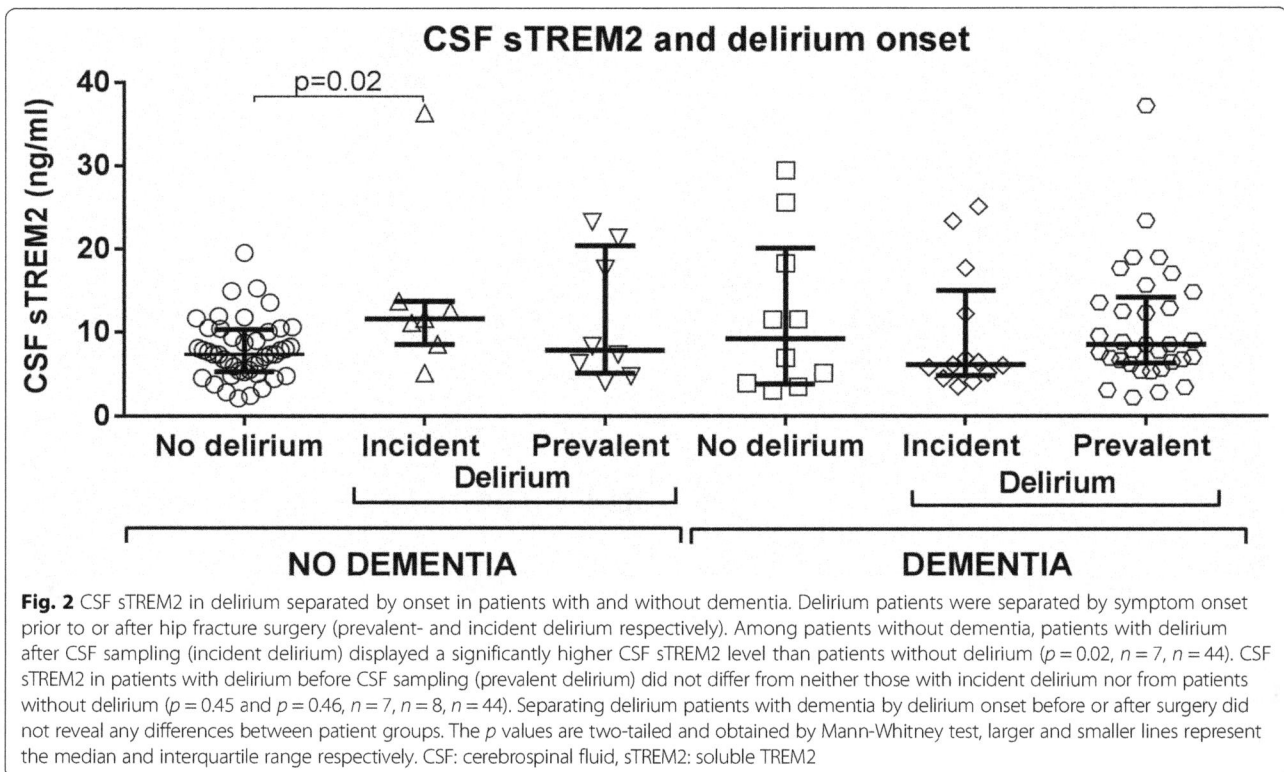

Fig. 2 CSF sTREM2 in delirium separated by onset in patients with and without dementia. Delirium patients were separated by symptom onset prior to or after hip fracture surgery (prevalent- and incident delirium respectively). Among patients without dementia, patients with delirium after CSF sampling (incident delirium) displayed a significantly higher CSF sTREM2 level than patients without delirium ($p = 0.02$, $n = 7$, $n = 44$). CSF sTREM2 in patients with delirium before CSF sampling (prevalent delirium) did not differ from neither those with incident delirium nor from patients without delirium ($p = 0.45$ and $p = 0.46$, $n = 7$, $n = 8$, $n = 44$). Separating delirium patients with dementia by delirium onset before or after surgery did not reveal any differences between patient groups. The p values are two-tailed and obtained by Mann-Whitney test, larger and smaller lines represent the median and interquartile range respectively. CSF: cerebrospinal fluid, sTREM2: soluble TREM2

$n = 119$). The positive correlation in all patients was presumably due to a stronger positive relationship between CSF sTREM2 and waiting time for surgery among patients with pre-existing dementia, which remained when demented patients not developing delirium were excluded ($r_S = 0.39$, $p = 0.002$, $n = 60$; $r_S = 0.40$, $p = 0.005$, $n = 49$, Fig. 3 and Table 2).

Having found CSF sTREM2 to relate positively to surgery waiting time among patients with pre-existing dementia, we were concerned that this masked an effect of delirium on CSF TREM2 in our previous analyses of patients with pre-existing dementia. We adjusted for surgery waiting time, but delirium did still not affect the CSF TREM2 level in this group of demented patients (multiple linear regression bivariate model; waiting time for surgery (h): $\beta 1 = 0.007$, $p = 0.02$, delirium: $\beta 2 = -0.12$, $p = 0.60$, $n = 59$, Table 3). The same analyses of delirium patients with pre-existing dementia sub-grouped relative to delirium onset (incident or prevalent delirium) reiterated that surgery waiting time, but not delirium onset, influenced the CSF TREM2 level (data not shown).

CSF sTREM2 in relation to age among hip fracture patients

The study group was of an advanced age (median of 85 years), and CSF sTREM2 did not relate to patient age

($r_S = 0.09$, $p = 0.32$, $n = 120$, Additional file 1: Figure S1). Morbidity or comorbidity might have masked an effect of aging on CSF sTREM2 that we observed in a cohort with a wider age distribution [22]. However, CSF sTREM2 did still not relate to age when restricting the analysis to the patient group having neither pre-existing dementia nor delirium ($r_S = 0.12$, $p = 0.43$, $n = 44$; Additional file 1: Figure S1A and Table 2). The four study groups of the hip fracture cohort, patients with or without delirium and with or without pre-existing dementia, were age-matched when assessing median age. However, the patient group having neither pre-existing dementia nor delirium had a greater proportion of relatively young individuals than the other groups. Neuroinflammation is a feature of aging, and we wanted to ensure that the age distribution did not infer with our analyses. We approached this by adjusting for age and analyzing data with multiple linear regression models. CSF sTREM2 remained significantly increased with delirium in age-adjusted analyses of patients without dementia ($p < 0.05$, ln(CSFsTREM2); univariate model: delirium $\beta 1 = 0.40$, $p = 0.01$; with a bivariate model: delirium $\beta 1 = 0.35$ $p = 0.03$; age $\beta 2 = 0.01$, $p = 0.22$, $n = 59$). This finding reiterated when reanalyzing the effect of incident delirium among patients without dementia (ln(CSFsTREM2): incident delirium $\beta 1 = 0.52$, $p = 0.01$; a bivariate model: incident delirium $\beta 1 = 0.47$, $p = 0.03$; age $\beta 2 = 0.01$, $p = 0.26$, $n = 51$, Table 3).

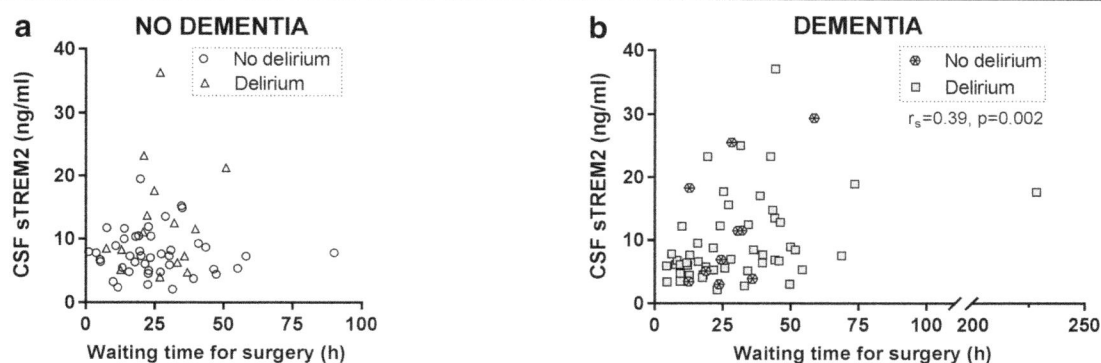

Fig. 3 Time-dependent influence of waiting time for hip fracture surgery the CSF sTREM2. CSF was sampled immediately before surgery started. **a** Among patients without dementia, there was no correlation between the CSF sTREM2 level and waiting time for surgery from hospital admission (hours; waiting time for surgery). **b** In contrast, among dementia cases, the CSF sTREM2 level increased with time from hospital admission until surgery with a positive correlation coefficient (r_s). The correlations are calculated for all patients with or without pre-existing dementia respectively, but patients with and without delirium are indicated by separate symbols. CSF: cerebrospinal fluid, sTREM2: soluble TREM2. r_s: Spearman's rho

CSF sTREM2 in relation to amyloid-β metabolism and plaque sequestration in hip fracture patients

In several reports, CSF sTREM2 level relates to CSF core biomarkers of Alzheimer's disease Aβ42, t-tau, and p-tau [19, 21, 22]. We hypothesized observing such relations in the present study, with the comorbidities delirium or pre-existing dementia acting as possible confounders. First the relations were analyzed in all patients, then patients were stratified by dementia status and finally by delirium. After stratification by both factors, only two patient groups, those neither having pre-existing dementia nor delirium ($n = 44$) and those being afflicted by both conditions simultaneously ($n = 50$) were of a sufficient group size to merit further statistical analyses (Table 1).

Reduced CSF Aβ42 is assumed to reflect parenchymal Aβ sequestration by plaques in AD brain. CSF sTREM2 and CSF Aβ42 related positively in the entire hip fracture cohort ($r_S = 0.22$, $p = 0.02$, $n = 117$). When stratifying study subjects by pre-existing dementia status, CSF sTREM2 and CSF Aβ42 did not correlate in patients without pre-existing dementia, not even after excluding patients with delirium. In contrast, there was a strong positive relation between CSF sTREM2 and CSF Aβ42 of patients with pre-existing dementia which grew stronger when demented patients without delirium were excluded from the analysis ($r_S = 0.40$, $p = 0.002$, $n = 60$; $r_S = 0.53$, $p < 0.001$, $n = 50$, Fig. 4 and Table 2).

How prone an Aβ peptide is to form amyloid fibrils and be sequestered by a pre-existing Aβ deposit in the brain

Table 2 CSF sTREM2 Spearman's Rho correlations in the hip fracture cohort

	PATIENTS *WITHOUT* DEMENTIA						PATIENTS *WITH* DEMENTIA					
	All		No delirium		Delirium		All		No delirium		Delirium	
N	59		44		15		61 (60)		10		50	
	Rho	p	Rho	p	Rho	p	Rho	p	Rho	p	Rho	p
Age	0.21	0.12	0.12	0.43	0.23	0.40	0.00	0.98	0.16	0.66	-0.05	0.74
Time to surgery (hours) *	0.01	0.93	-0.03	0.83	0.06	0.84	0.39	0.002	0.43	0.21	0.40	0.005
CSF Biomarkers												
N	57		44		13		60		9		50	
	Rho	p	Rho	p	Rho	p	Rho	p	Rho	p	Rho	p
CSF Aβ42 (pg/ml)	0.11	0.40	0.20	0.18	0.31	0.30	0.40	0.002	0.02	0.97	0.53	<0.001
CSF Aβ38 (pg/ml) MSD	0.09	0.49	0.06	0.71	0.18	0.55	0.44	<0.001	0.40	0.29	0.45	0.001
CSF Aβ40 (pg/ml) MSD	0.14	0.32	0.12	0.44	0.23	0.45	0.48	<0.001	0.37	0.33	0.51	<0.001
CSF Aβ42 (pg/ml) MSD	0.09	0.52	0.24	0.12	-0.13	0.67	0.43	0.001	0.15	0.70	0.53	<0.001
CSF t-tau (pg/ml)	0.14	0.28	-0.04	0.82	0.20	0.51	0.46	<0.001	0.83	0.005	0.34	0.016
CSF p-tau (pg/ml)	0.12	0.38	-0.02	0.90	0.23	0.46	0.49	<0.001	0.77	0.016	0.37	0.008

Aβ42, amyloid beta 1–42; t-tau, total-tau; p-tau, phosphorylated tau; sTREM2, soluble triggering receptor expressed on myeloid cells
*Time to surgery, hours from hospital admission to surgery (onset of anesthesia) and CSF sampling

Table 3 Influence of multiple predictors on CSF sTREM2[a] analyzed by multiple linear regression

Patient group	Analysis	Predictor β	p	n
Dementia	Delirium adjusted by waiting time for surgery			59
	Waiting time for surgery (β1)	0.007	0.02	
	Delirium (β2)	-0.12	0.60	
No dementia	Delirium (at any time)			59
	Delirium (univariate)	0.40	0.01	
	Delirium (adjusted) (β1)	0.35	0.03	
	Age (β2)	0.01	0.22	
	Delirium onset: incident delirium			51
	Incident delirium (univariate)	0.52	0.01	
	Incident delirium (β1)	0.47	0.03	
	Age (β2)	0.01	0.26	
Dementia	AD pathological CSF-biomarkers, age and delirium			59
	p-tau (β1)	0.01	<0.001	
	Aβ42 (β2)	0.002	0.002	
	Age (β3)	0.0001	0.91	
	Delirium (β4)	- 0.03	0.86	
No dementia	AD pathological CSF-biomarkers, age and delirium			57
	Delirium (β1)	0.47	0.02	
	p-tau (β2)	0.0000	0.97	
	Aβ42 (β3)	0.0000	0.16	
	Age (β4)	0.013	0.13	
No dementia	Incident (hip fracture) and medical delirium age adjusted			24
	Incident delirium (univariate)	0.62	0.05	
	Incident delirium (β1)	0.27	0.48	
	Age (β2)	0.02	0.15	

[a]*Linear regression with the dependent variable ln (sTREM2ng/ml). Aβ42; amyloid beta 1-42, t-tau; total-tau; p-tau; phosphorylated tau, sTREM2; soluble triggering receptor expressed on myeloid cells*

heavily depends on the C-terminal extension. Indeed, in clinical studies, only the level of hydrophobic Aβ peptides extending to position 42 decrease in CSF when Aβ deposits begin to form in brain [33]. Thus, an increased CSF level of a C-terminal truncated Aβ peptide, e.g., CSF $Aβ_{1-38}$ likely reflect Aβ-monomer metabolism (production or catabolism). Here, we related analyses of CSF Aβ38, Aβ40, and Aβ42 MSD ELISA levels to CSF sTREM2. Our intent was to distinguish if a putative relation between CSF sTREM2 and CSF Aβ42 was linked to Aβ-metabolism or Aβ-plaque sequestration. The MSD analyses outcome was reminiscent to the Innotest Aβ42 analysis, with CSF sTREM2 and CSF Aβ relating positively to all three Aβ peptides ($Aβ38_{MSD}$, $Aβ40_{MSD}$, and $Aβ42_{MSD}$). Upon stratification, the effect was prominent among patients with pre-existing dementia and even stronger when further excluding those patients who did not develop delirium ($Aβ38_{MSD}r_S =$

0.45, $p = 0.001$; $Aβ40_{MSD}r_S = 0.51$, $p < 0.001$; Aβ42MSD rS = 0.53, $p < 0.001$, $n = 50$; Additional file 1: Figure S2 and Table 2).

CSF sTREM2 in relation to CSF tau markers in hip fracture patients

CSF t-tau and p-tau concentrations are thought to reflect altered tau metabolism that relates to neurodegeneration and tangle formation in AD [34]. CSF sTREM2 related positively to both CSF t-tau and p-tau in the entire hip fracture patient cohort ($r_S = 0.32$, $p = 0.001$ for both, $n = 117$). Stratification by dementia status gave results reminiscent of the CSF Aβ-data, with strong correlations to CSF sTREM2 restricted to patients with pre-existing dementia (t-tau, $r_S = 0.46$, $p < 0.001$; p-tau, $r_S = 0.49$, $p < 0.001$, $n = 60$). The relation between CSF-TREM2 and tau markers remained but were weaker

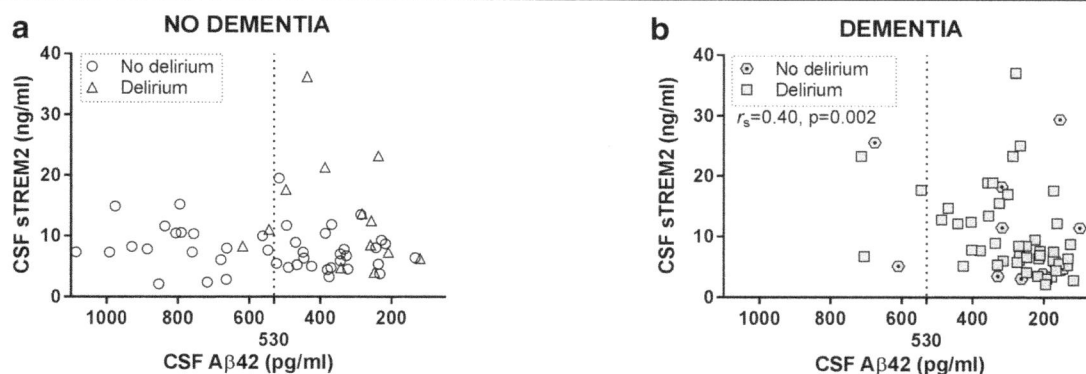

Fig. 4 Relation between the level of CSF biomarkers sTREM2 and Aβ42 in hip fracture patients. **a** Among patients without pre-existing dementia, there was no correlation between sTREM2 and Aβ42 in CSF, but (**b**) a positive relation in patients with dementia as indicated by a significant and positive correlation (r_s). The correlations are calculated for all patients with or without dementia respectively, but patients with and without delirium are indicated by separate symbols. The dotted lines show the pathological biomarker cut-off level (530 pg/ml). To present Figs. 4 and 5 in the same manner, the x-axes in Fig. 4 are reversed because a low level indicates Aβ pathology. CSF: cerebrospinal fluid, Aβ42: amyloid beta 1–42, sTREM2: soluble TREM2. r_s: Spearman's rho

when restricting the analyses to demented patients who also developed delirium (t-tau, $r_S = 0.34$, $p = 0.016$, $n = 50$ and p-tau, $r_S = 0.37$, $p = 0.008$, $n = 50$; Fig. 5, Table 2).

CSF sTREM2 and predictive ability of delirium, age, and AD CSF-biomarker level

Only among patients with pre-existing dementia did CSF sTREM2 relate positively to the three CSF AD core biomarkers (Aβ42, t-tau, and p-tau). Here in a separate examination, CSF Aβ42 and p-tau were included in multiple linear regressions to explore if AD core biomarkers together better explained the variability of CSF sTREM2. The biomarker CSF p-tau was chosen above t-tau since it is more AD-specific [35] and since previous analyses gave slightly higher correlation coefficients to CSF sTREM2. Such analyses enabled us to examine if effects of AD neuropathology, reflected by biomarkers CSF Aβ42 and CSF p-tau, masked an effect of delirium on CSF TREM2.

Again, the hip fracture patient cohort was stratified for pre-existing dementia. Variables included were delirium, age, CSF Aβ42, and CSF p-tau. In the patient group with pre-existing dementia, the AD CSF biomarkers were included as predictors before incorporating age and delirium in the analysis. CSF p-tau explained most variability as a sole predictor of CSF TREM2 level ($R = 0.50$). Including CSF Aβ42 as a second predictor increased the explained CSF sTREM2 level variability ($R = 0.61$), while age and delirium did not further increase predictive ability (ln(CSF sTREM2): CSF p-tau $\beta1 = 0.01$, $p < 0.001$; CSF Aβ42 $\beta2 = 0.002$, $p = 0.002$; age $\beta3 = 0.0001$, $p = 0.91$; delirium $\beta4 = -0.03$, $p = 0.86$; $n = 59$). Irrespective of the

number of predictors included, the effect size (β) remains essentially the same (Table 3).

The patient group without pre-existing dementia was examined in the same manner with multiple linear regressions. Delirium was included as the initial predictor before incorporating age and the AD core CSF biomarkers Aβ42 and p-tau. Delirium was the only significant predictor in this patient group ($R = 0.34$ as a single predictor). CSF AD core biomarkers did not have a significant impact and their inclusion and subsequent adjustment did not influence the effect size (β) of delirium (ln(CSF sTREM2): delirium $\beta1 = -0.47$, $p = 0.02$; CSF p-tau $\beta2 = 0.000$, $p = 0.97$; CSF Aβ42 $\beta3 = 0.000$, $p = 0.16$; age $\beta4 = 0.013$, $p = 0.13$, $n = 57$). This model suggest that patients without pre-existing dementia, but afflicted by a hip fracture and subsequent delirium would result in an increased CSF TREM2 level (≈ 1.5 ng/ml). This applied to conditions adjusted for interfering factors, age, or CSF biomarker levels indicating AD neuropathology (Table 3).

CSF sTREM2 and ratios of tau and amyloid CSF biomarkers

We then examined ratios of amyloid and tau CSF biomarkers, which are more discriminative than a single biomarker to the diagnosis and prognosis of AD [36, 37]. Biomarker ratios (t-tau/Aβ42 or p- tau/Aβ42) separated non-demented patients with or without delirium (Additional file 1: Table S1), consistent with a previous report [10]. There was no correlation between CSF sTREM2 and CSF t-tau/Aβ42 and p-tau/Aβ42 among those with dementia or without dementia (Additional file 1: Table S1 and Figure S3).

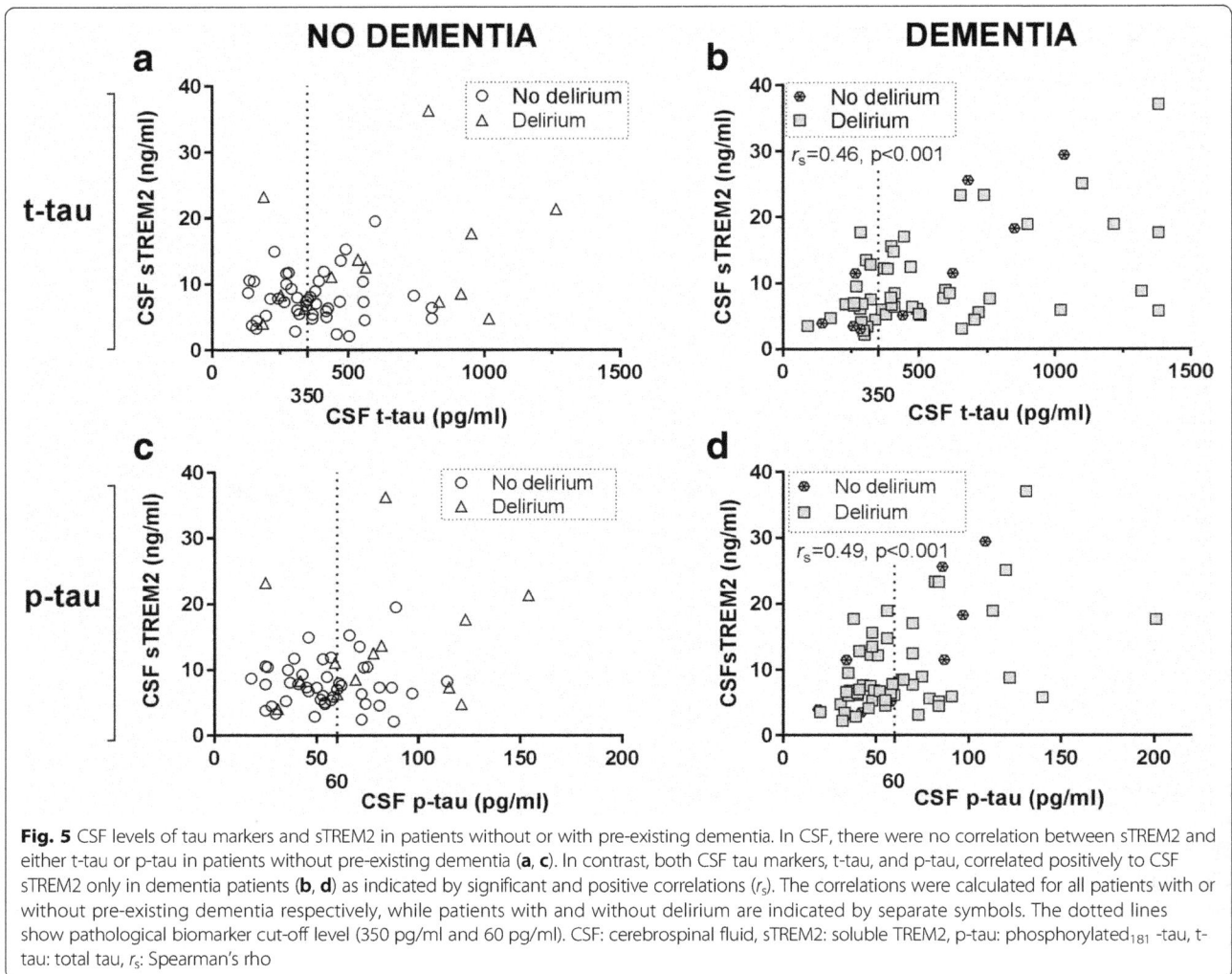

Fig. 5 CSF levels of tau markers and sTREM2 in patients without or with pre-existing dementia. In CSF, there were no correlation between sTREM2 and either t-tau or p-tau in patients without pre-existing dementia (**a, c**). In contrast, both CSF tau markers, t-tau, and p-tau, correlated positively to CSF sTREM2 only in dementia patients (**b, d**) as indicated by significant and positive correlations (r_s). The correlations were calculated for all patients with or without pre-existing dementia respectively, while patients with and without delirium are indicated by separate symbols. The dotted lines show pathological biomarker cut-off level (350 pg/ml and 60 pg/ml). CSF: cerebrospinal fluid, sTREM2: soluble TREM2, p-tau: phosphorylated$_{181}$-tau, t-tau: total tau, r_s: Spearman's rho

CSF sTREM2 level and AD neuropathology

AD is the major cause of dementia. To identify hip fracture patients with pre-existing dementia likely due to AD, we applied cut-off values for the CSF Aβ42 and CSF-tau [31]. Thus patients were stratified for having a CSF Aβ42-level above or below AD cut-off (Aβ−/Aβ+) and likewise tau-level (t-tau or p-tau) above or below AD cut-off (tau +/tau-) [38]. Most patients with pre-existing dementia were below CSF Aβ42 cut-off (≈ 90%), while fewer patients were above CSF-tau cut-off (≈ 40%, Table 1).

Among patients neither having delirium nor pre-existing dementia, CSF sTREM2 level did not differ between those who were above or below CSF-biomarker CSF Aβ42 level cut-off for AD ($p = 0.22$, $n = 26$ $n = 18$). Among patients without pre-existing dementia and a CSF Aβ42 level below cut-off, CSF sTREM2 was higher in those with subsequent delirium ($n = 11$) as compared to unaffected subjects ($n = 26$; $p = 0.048$). The analyses gave similar results as when all patients without pre-

existing dementia were included in the analyses ($p = 0.046$, Fig. 1c). Corresponding analyses for tau (t-tau or p-tau positive) yielded essentially the same results (data not shown). These analyses confirm multiple linear regression analyses of CSF Aβ42 and CSF tau markers not influencing the CSF sTREM2 level in patients without pre-existing dementia.

CSF sTREM2 in patients with medical delirium

We also included a group of delirium patients having delirium secondary to a medical condition with or without pre-existing dementia (medical delirium, $n = 26$, Table 1). There was a trend of a lower CSF sTREM2 level in patients with medical delirium as compared to those with delirium after a hip fracture ($p = 0.08$; CSF sTREM2 ng/ml: 6.1 (7.3) vs 7.7 (7.9), $n = 26$, $n = 65$, Figs. 1b and 6).

Restricting the analyses only to patients without pre-existing dementia, CSF sTREM2 was reduced in

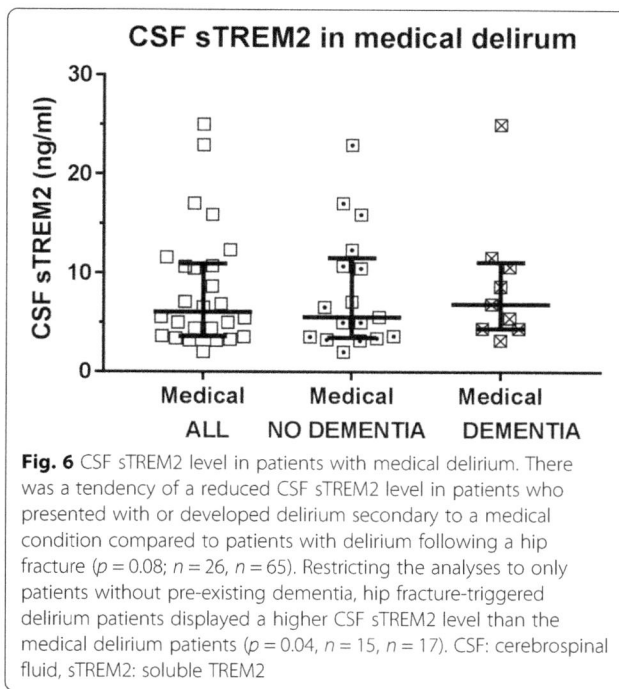

Fig. 6 CSF sTREM2 level in patients with medical delirium. There was a tendency of a reduced CSF sTREM2 level in patients who presented with or developed delirium secondary to a medical condition compared to patients with delirium following a hip fracture ($p = 0.08$; $n = 26$, $n = 65$). Restricting the analyses to only patients without pre-existing dementia, hip fracture-triggered delirium patients displayed a higher CSF sTREM2 level than the medical delirium patients ($p = 0.04$, $n = 15$, $n = 17$). CSF: cerebrospinal fluid, sTREM2: soluble TREM2

medical delirium as compared to patients with hip fracture triggered delirium ($p = 0.04$; $n = 17$, $n = 15$, Figs. 1 and 6; Table 1). Restricting the hip fracture cohort delirium patients to those with incident delirium CSF sTREM2 was lower, and close to significant ($p = 0.055$; $n = 7$, $n = 17$), but not when compared to those with prevalent delirium ($p = 0.18$, $n = 8$, $n = 17$; Figs. 2 and 6).

Analyzing only those with pre-existing dementia, CSF sTREM2 in patients with medical delirium did not statistically differ from hip fracture patients with delirium ($p = 0.56$, $n = 9$, $n = 50$; Fig. 1c and 6 and Table 1), nor when comparing to each subgroup.

CSF sTREM2 in medical delirium patients in relation to age and gender

Like in the hip fracture cohort, we found CSF sTREM2 not related to age neither when analyzing all medical delirium patients ($r_S = 0.23$, $p = 0.26$, $n = 26$) nor when restricting the analysis to patients without dementia ($r_S = 0.41$, $p = 0.11$, $n = 17$, Additional file 1: Figure S4). Patients admitted to the hospital with medical delirium were younger with a greater age range (66(16) years, Table 1) than the patients having a hip fracture accident. When adjusting for age, the level of CSF sTREM2 was not significantly higher in hip fracture triggered delirium relative to medical delirium. However, the group size is almost too small to allow statistical age adjustment with several covariates, and the loss of significance from

univariate analyses may be explained by additional noise from the added predictor (ln(CSFsTREM2) univariate model; delirium: $\beta1 = 0.62$, $p = 0.05$, and with a bivariate model and age included: delirium $\beta1 = 0.27$, $p = 0.48$, age $\beta2 = 0.02$, $p = 0.15$, $n = 24$).

Discussion

This is the first study to report on CSF sTREM2 level in delirium. Moreover, the study differs from previous investigations by analyzing CSF sTREM2 as a biomarker in a dementia population of an advanced age. Although we did not see an overall effect of delirium, analyzing patients with and without pre-existing dementia separately revealed a clear differential effect on CSF sTREM2 and interrelations to other biomarkers in these two populations. Delirium increased CSF sTREM2 only in patients without pre-existing dementia. TREM2 is a highly microglial-specific receptor, and ectodomain shedding of TREM2 releases sTREM2 that then presumably drains to CSF [18]. The level of sTREM2 in the brain reflects amyloid-induced microglial activation in transgenic mice with aging as judged by PET imaging [39]. Patient studies also suggest that microglial-derived CSF sTREM2 increases with a general glial-mediated immune response, e.g., a positive relation with the astroglial CSF-marker YKL-40 [19]. We therefore argue that increased sTREM2 in delirium without pre-existing dementia is due to central microglial activation. We speculate that CSF sTREM2 increases only in delirium patients without dementia because the pathogenic process is less complex and the inflammatory process will more clearly stand out in this patient group.

Increased CSF sTREM2 with delirium triggered by hip fracture was most prominent in incident delirium, i.e., in CSF sampled before the delirium syndrome was evident in non-demented patients. Medical delirium patients all suffered encephalopathy at the time of CSF sampling. Interestingly, patients with medically induced delirium displayed lower CSF sTREM2 relative to patients with hip fracture-triggered delirium. This effect was close to significant when compared to incident delirium patients alone. Thus, stratification of delirium-afflicted patients suggests that CSF sTREM2 increases transiently prior to delirium onset, but then declines. An early but transient glial response in delirium is supported by increased levels of other CSF biomarkers of immune responses in incident delirium, such as neopterin [40] and astroglia-derived S-100β [41]. Thus, CSF sTREM2 is a promising biomarker of microglial activation that is presumably more usable to detect transient responses, which is consistent with TREM2 having a rapid cell surface turnover (< 1 h) [42]. Longitudinal studies and continuous CSF sampling of delirium patients could confirm or refute this hypothesis, although it might be ethical challenging to conduct such a study with fragile patients.

In contrast, delirium did not alter the CSF sTREM2 level in patients with pre-existing dementia nor did dementia by itself affect CSF sTREM2. CSF sTREM2 is reported increased in younger and CSF biomarker-selected AD patients (mean ≈ 65–70 years) (e.g., [19, 20]). We speculate that superimposed dementia with Aβ deposits and tau inclusions continuously stimulating microglial activation diminish the effect of delirium on microglial response and sTREM2 release. Such proteinaceous neuropathology might also lead to an increased protein turnover preventing a raised interstitial sTREM2 level in demented patients. Importantly, as compared to many other CSF-dementia studies, the patients examined by us were markedly older (median ≈ 85 years) and not biomarker-selected and their dementia pathogenesis was likely more heterogeneous [43, 44]. Thus, comorbidities and advanced age could have diluted the direct link from AD neuropathology to enhanced sTREM2 release and CSF sTREM2.

The initial hip fracture trauma presumably activated peripheral immune responses in the patients. The neuroinflammatory hypothesis of delirium suggests that brain dysfunctions and clinical presentation are secondary to peripheral immune activation [4]. Dementia patients displaying increased CSF sTREM2 with waiting time for acute hip fracture surgery is consistent with this theory. That this only was evident among dementia patients also support the concept of primed more easily activated microglia in neurodegenerative disease compared to a healthy brain [45, 46].

Exploring relations between CSF biomarkers may provide better pathogenic understanding by hinting to simultaneously ongoing processes in the brain. CSF Aβ and t-tau/p-tau markers related positively to CSF sTREM2 only in dementia patients with delirium, possibly suggesting somewhat distinct biological processes of delirium with or without pre-existing dementia. CSF sTREM2 related positively to CSF Aβ42 in the demented patients, essentially all of which were below the CSF Aβ42 cut-off level. Clinical data suggest that Aβ42 is sequestered by senile plaques, long before symptom onset leading to a pronounced drop in CSF Aβ42. This low CSF Aβ42 level is then stable in the individual patient [47, 48]. Thus, a positive relation between CSF Aβ42 and CSF sTREM2 in demented patients does presumably not relate to the extent of amyloid deposition. Instead, it is more likely to reflect shared protein synthesis and metabolism of Aβ precursor protein (AβPP) and TREM2, an idea which is consistent with our findings of positive relations also to the shorter and far less plaque-sequestered C-terminal truncated peptides Aβ38 and

Aβ40 [49]. AβPP and TREM2 share common features of ectodomain shedding by ADAMs α-secretase and subsequent γ-secretase cleavage [18, 50–52], and although they are released by different cell types, one can speculate whether both play a role to similar physiological functions that involve neuronal-glial communication.

An expanding literature links Aβ production to neuronal and synaptic activity and biological rhythms, e.g., sleep-wakefulness [53, 54]. We speculate that delirium in dementia patients triggers neuronal network activation with concomitant enhanced release of Aβ peptides, t-tau/p-tau, and sTREM2; all reflected by a transiently increased CSF level. Interestingly, a recent study demonstrated with isotope labeling kinetics that increased CSF-tau in early AD reflects neuronal tau-synthesis and positively correlates with amyloid-PET, but not tau-PET [55]. Thus, CSF- t-tau/p-tau levels might also reflect neuronal activity associated with amyloid, and not simply axonal damage and tauopathy as previously thought. There are reports of neuronal network disturbances in Alzheimer's disease as well as delirium [56, 57]. Thus, our observations of positive CSF-biomarker associations only in demented patients might be due to the susceptibility of frail brains to neuronal network dysfunctions.

CSF sTREM2 and tau markers interrelated in several studies of AD cohorts, yet in different subpopulations [19, 20, 58]. CSF sTREM2 clearly increased in a cohort of suspected non-amyloid pathology (SNAP) patients having cognitive dysfunctions and only positive CSF-tau biomarkers indicating that elevated CSF sTREM2 can occur independent of amyloid pathology [58]. Indeed, inclusion of p-tau in linear regression analyses showed that p-tau was the best sole predictor. Including CSF Aβ42 as a second predictor better explained CSF sTREM2 variability in the dementia group, while incorporating variables age and delirium did not. Thus, in dementia patients, the existing neuropathology seemed to exceed any delirium effects again suggesting pathogenic differences of delirium with and without pre-existing dementia.

With aging, dementia does not well relate to Aβ pathology and tauopathy, presumably because of increased importance of cerebrovascular comorbidity [59]. The high median age and limited age distribution of the study cohort likely explain why CSF sTREM2 did not relate to age. There might also be a ceiling effect of CSF sTREM2 with aging, which would be worth further studying. CSF sTREM2 increases with aging in several studies that involved younger patient populations [20–22]. Indeed, there was a tendency of a positive correlation with aging among patients with medical delirium that included younger individuals.

Conclusion

The present biomarker analyses hint at the biological processes of delirium being dependent on pre-existing dementia with selectively increased CSF sTREM2 in delirium only in the absence of dementia. These preliminary findings need replication in independent patient cohorts and assays. Statistical power is a study limitation with small cohorts after stratification. CSF sampling aged frail patients in a confused state is practically and ethically difficult and the CSF material used is unique in size and composition. As judged by mutant TREM2-variants, both increased and decreased shedding can reflect reduced cell surface TREM2 and impaired gene function [51, 60]. Increased sTREM2 likely represents microglial activation but whether such central immune activation is beneficial or detrimental to brain functions remains unclear. Increased CSF sTREM2 prior to delirium could possibly serve as a delirium risk indicator, albeit not alone. An inflammatory CSF biomarker panel that includes sTREM2 might aid identification of at-risk patients with special care requirements in the postoperative care unit.

Additional file

Additional file 1: Figure S1. CSF sTREM2 and the relation to age in hip fracture patients. **Figure S2.** Triplex MSD measurements of CSF Aβ peptides in dementia patients. **Table S1.** CSF t-tau/Aβ42 and p-tau/Aβ42 ratios and correlations to CSF sTREM2 in the hip fracture cohort. **Figure S3.** CSF sTREM2 and the ratios of t-tau/Aβ42 and p-tau/Aβ42. **Figure S4.** CSF sTREM2 and age in medical delirium patients (PDF 4106 kb)

Abbreviations

AD: Alzheimer's disease; ADAMs: A disintegrin and metalloprotease; Aβ38: Amyloid beta 1–38; Aβ40: Amyloid beta 1–40; Aβ42: Amyloid beta 1–42; AβPP: Aβ precursor protein; CAM: Confusion Assessment Method; CNS: Central nervous system; CSF: Cerebrospinal fluid; ELISA: Enzyme-linked immunosorbent assay; In: Natural logarithm; LP: Lumbar puncture; MCI: Mild cognitive impairment; OUS: Oslo University Hospital; p-tau: Phosphorylated tau; sTREM2: Soluble TREM2; TREM2: Triggering receptor expressed on myeloid cells 2; t-tau: Total tau

Acknowledgements

Foremost, we would like to thank all patients included in the study. We would like to thank the staff at the Department of Orthopedic Surgery, Department of Anesthesiology, Department of Internal Medicine, and Department of Neurology, and from the Department of Infectious Diseases, we would like to thank the principal investigator of the CNS infection study Dr. Vidar Ormaasen and prof Dag Kvale who were responsible for the biobank at Oslo University Hospital. Kjetil Røysland at the Oslo Centre for Biostatistics and Epidemiology (OCBE) at UiO and Oslo University hospital (OUS) is greatly acknowledged for providing statistical advice. HZ is a Wallenberg Academy Fellow. KB holds the Torsten Söderberg Professorship in Medicine.

Funding

The work was funded by grants from University in Oslo (UiO), Anders Jahre's stiftelse, Norwegian National Health Organization and the South-Eastern Norway Regional Health Authorities, and Alzheimerfondet Civitan Foundation (Norway).

Authors' contributions

LOW designed and coordinated the study. LOW and EQP contributed to the data acquisition and gave clinical advice. KH assayed CSF sTREM2. HZ and KB were in charge of the Aβ peptides and tau measurements (ELISA and MSD). KH analyzed the data and interpreted these together with LOW and LNGN. KH drafted the manuscript and critically revised it together with LOW and LNGN. KH and LNGN wrote the final manuscript. All authors contributed with critical revision and approved the final manuscript.

Competing interests

LN, KH, LOW, and EQP declare that they have no competing interests. HZ has served at advisory boards for Eli Lilly, Roche Diagnostics and Wave, has received travel support from Teva and is a co-founder of Brain Biomarker Solutions in Gothenburg AB, a GU Ventures-based platform company at the University of Gothenburg. KB has served as a consultant or at advisory boards for Alzheon, BioArctic, Biogen, Eli Lilly, Fujirebio Europe, IBL International, Merck, Novartis, Pfizer, and Roche Diagnostics, and is a co-founder of Brain Biomarker Solutions in Gothenburg AB, a GU Venture-based platform company at the University of Gothenburg.

Author details

[1]Department of Pharmacology, Institute of Clinical Medicine, University of Oslo and Oslo University Hospital, P.O. box 1057 Blindern, 0316 Oslo, Norway. [2]Department of Infectious Diseases, Oslo University Hospital, Ullevaal Hospital, P.O. Box 4956 Nydalen, N-0450 Oslo, Norway. [3]Institute of Clinical Medicine, University of Oslo, P.O. Box 1171 Blindern, 0318 Oslo, Norway. [4]Department of Psychiatry and Neurochemistry, Institute of Neuroscience and Physiology, The Sahlgrenska Academy at University of Gothenburg, SE-431 80 Mölndal, Sweden. [5]Clinical Neurochemistry Laboratory, Sahlgrenska University Hospital, SE-431 80 Mölndal, Sweden. [6]Department of Degenerative Disease, UCL Institute of Neurology, Queen Square, Gower Street, London WC1E 6BT, UK. [7]UK Dementia Research Institute at UCL, Gower Street, London WC1E 6BT, UK. [8]Oslo Delirium Research Group, Department of Geriatric Medicine, Oslo University Hospital, PO box 4950 Nydalen, N-0424 Oslo, Norway. [9]Institute of Basic Medical Sciences, University of Oslo, Domus Medica, Sognsvannsveien 9, N-0372 Oslo, Norway.

References

1. Bruce AJ, Ritchie CW, Blizard R, Lai R, Raven P. The incidence of delirium associated with orthopedic surgery: a meta-analytic review. Int Psychogeriatr. 2007;19:197–214.
2. Davis DH, Muniz-Terrera G, Keage HA, Stephan BC, Fleming J, Ince PG, Matthews FE, Cunningham C, Ely EW, MacLullich AM, Brayne C. Association of delirium with cognitive decline in late life: a neuropathologic study of 3 population-based cohort studies. JAMA Psychiatry. 2017;74:244–51.
3. Cerejeira J, Lagarto L, Mukaetova-Ladinska EB. The immunology of delirium. Neuroimmunomodulation. 2014;21:72–8.
4. Cerejeira J, Firmino H, Vaz-Serra A, Mukaetova-Ladinska EB. The neuroinflammatory hypothesis of delirium. Acta Neuropathol. 2010;119:737–54.
5. van Gool WA, van de Beek D, Eikelenboom P. Systemic infection and delirium: when cytokines and acetylcholine collide. Lancet. 2010;375:773–5.
6. Davis DH, Muniz Terrera G, Keage H, Rahkonen T, Oinas M, Matthews FE, Cunningham C, Polvikoski T, Sulkava R, MacLullich AM, Brayne C. Delirium is a strong risk factor for dementia in the oldest-old: a population-based cohort study. Brain. 2012;135:2809–16.
7. Ahmed S, Leurent B, Sampson EL. Risk factors for incident delirium among older people in acute hospital medical units: a systematic review and meta-analysis. Age Ageing. 2014;43:326–33.
8. Krogseth M, Wyller TB, Engedal K, Juliebo V. Delirium is an important predictor of incident dementia among elderly hip fracture patients. Dement Geriatr Cogn Disord. 2011;31:63–70.
9. Duyckaerts C, Delatour B, Potier MC. Classification and basic pathology of Alzheimer disease. Acta Neuropathol. 2009;118:5–36.
10. Idland AV, Wyller TB, Stoen R, Eri LM, Frihagen F, Raeder J, Chaudhry FA, Hansson O, Zetterberg H, Blennow K, et al. Preclinical amyloid-beta and Axonal degeneration pathology in delirium. J Alzheimers Dis. 2017;55:371–9.
11. Cunningham EL, McGuinness B, McAuley DF, Toombs J, Mawhinney T, O'Brien S, Beverland D, Schott JM, Lunn MP, Zetterberg H, Passmore AP. CSF Beta-amyloid 1-42 concentration predicts delirium following elective

arthroplasty surgery in an observational cohort study. Ann Surg. 2018.

12. Heneka MT, Kummer MP, Latz E. Innate immune activation in neurodegenerative disease. Nat Rev Immunol. 2014;14:463–77.

13. Fong TG, Davis D, Growdon ME, Albuquerque A, Inouye SK. The interface between delirium and dementia in elderly adults. Lancet Neurol. 2015;14:823–32.

14. Hickman SE, Kingery ND, Ohsumi TK, Borowsky ML, Wang LC, Means TK, El KJ. The microglial sensome revealed by direct RNA sequencing. Nat Neurosci. 2013;16:1896–905.

15. Jonsson T, Stefansson H, Steinberg S, Jonsdottir I, Jonsson PV, Snaedal J, Bjornsson S, Huttenlocher J, Levey AI, Lah JJ, et al. Variant of TREM2 associated with the risk of Alzheimer's disease. N Engl J Med. 2013;368:107–16.

16. Guerreiro RJ, Lohmann E, Bras JM, Gibbs JR, Rohrer JD, Gurunlian N, Dursun B, Bilgic B, Hanagasi H, Gurvit H, et al. Using exome sequencing to reveal mutations in TREM2 presenting as a frontotemporal dementia-like syndrome without bone involvement. JAMA Neurol. 2013;70:78–84.

17. Guerreiro R, Wojtas A, Bras J, Carrasquillo M, Rogaeva E, Majounie E, Cruchaga C, Sassi C, Kauwe JS, Younkin S, et al. TREM2 variants in Alzheimer's disease. N Engl J Med. 2013;368:117–27.

18. Wunderlich P, Glebov K, Kemmerling N, Tien NT, Neumann H, Walter J. Sequential proteolytic processing of the triggering receptor expressed on myeloid cells-2 (TREM2) protein by ectodomain shedding and gamma-secretase-dependent intramembranous cleavage. J Biol Chem. 2013;288:33027–36.

19. Heslegrave A, Heywood W, Faterson R, Magdalinou N, Svensson J, Johansson P, Ohrfelt A, Blennow K, Hardy J, Schott J, et al. Increased cerebrospinal fluid soluble TREM2 concentration in Alzheimer's disease. Mol Neurodegener. 2016;11:3.

20. Piccio L, Deming Y, Del-Aguila JL, Ghezzi L, Holtzman DM, Fagan AM, Fenoglio C, Galimberti D, Borroni B, Cruchaga C. Cerebrospinal fluid soluble TREM2 is higher in Alzheimer disease and associated with mutation status. Acta Neuropathol. 2016;131:925–33.

21. Suarez-Calvet M, Kleinberger G, Araque Caballero MA, Brendel M, Rominger A, Alcolea D, Fortea J, Lleo A, Blesa R, Gispert JD, et al. sTREM2 cerebrospinal fluid levels are a potential biomarker for microglia activity in early-stage Alzheimer's disease and associate with neuronal injury markers. EMBO Mol Med. 2016;8:466–76.

22. Henjum K, Almdahl IS, Arskog V, Minthon L, Hansson O, Fladby T, Nilsson LN. Cerebrospinal fluid soluble TREM2 in aging and Alzheimer's disease. Alzheimers Res Ther. 2016;8:17.

23. Gispert JD, Suarez-Calvet M, Monte GC, Tucholka A, Falcon C, Rojas S, Rami L, Sanchez-Valle R, Llado A, Kleinberger G, et al. Cerebrospinal fluid sTREM2 levels are associated with gray matter volume increases and reduced diffusivity in early Alzheimer's disease. Alzheimers Dement. 2016;12:1259–72.

24. Wyller TB, Watne LO, Torbergsen A, Engedal K, Frihagen F, Juliebo V, Saltvedt I, Skovlund E, Raeder J, Conroy S. The effect of a pre- and post-operative orthogeriatric service on cognitive function in patients with hip fracture. The protocol of the Oslo Orthogeriatrics Trial. BMC Geriatr. 2012;12:36.

25. Watne LO, Torbergsen AC, Conroy S, Engedal K, Frihagen F, Hjorthaug GA, Juliebo V, Raeder J, Saltvedt , Skovlund E, Wyller TB. The effect of a pre- and postoperative orthogeriatric service on cognitive function in patients with hip fracture: randomized controlled trial (Oslo Orthogeriatric trial). BMC Med. 2014;12:63.

26. Inouye SK, van Dyck CH, Alessi CA, Balkin S, Siegal AP, Horwitz RI. Clarifying confusion: the confusion assessment method. A new method for detection of delirium. Ann Intern Med. 1990;113:941–8.

27. Watne LO, Hall RJ, Molden E, Raeder J, Frihagen F, MacLullich AM, Juliebo V, Nyman A, Meagher D, Wyller TB. Anticholinergic activity in cerebrospinal fluid and serum in individuals with hip fracture with and without delirium. J Am Geriatr Soc. 2014;62:94–102.

28. Vanderstichele H, Van KE, Hesse C, Davidsson P, Buyse MA, Andreasen N, Minthon L, Wallin A, Blennow K, Vanmechelen E. Standardization of measurement of beta-amyloid(1-42) in cerebrospinal fluid and plasma. Amyloid. 2000;7:245–58.

29. Vanmechelen E, Vanderstichele H, Davidsson P, Van KE, Van Der Perre B, Sjogren M, Andreasen N, Blennow K. Quantification of tau phosphorylated at threonine 181 in human cerebrospinal fluid: a sandwich ELISA with a synthetic phosphopeptide for standardization. Neurosci Lett. 2000;285:49–52.

30. Blennow K, Wallin A, Agren H, Spenger C, Siegfried J, Vanmechelen E. Tau protein in cerebrospinal fluid: a biochemical marker for axonal degeneration in Alzheimer disease? Mol Chem Neuropathol. 1995;26:231–45.

31. Hansson O, Zetterberg H, Buchhave P, Londos E, Blennow K, Minthon L. Association between CSF biomarkers and incipient Alzheimer's disease in patients with mild cognitive impairment: a follow-up study. Lancet Neurol. 2006;5:228–34.

32. Chavan SS, Pavlov VA, Tracey KJ. Mechanisms and therapeutic relevance of neuro-immune communication. Immunity. 2017;46:927–42.

33. Olsson B, Lautner R, Andreasson U, Ohrfelt A, Portelius E, Bjerke M, Holtta M, Rosen C, Olsson C, Strobel G, et al. CSF and blood biomarkers for the diagnosis of Alzheimer's disease: a systematic review and meta-analysis. Lancet Neurol. 2016;15:673–84.

34. Hampel H, Blennow K, Shaw LM, Hoessler YC, Zetterberg H, Trojanowski JQ. Total and phosphorylated tau protein as biological markers of Alzheimer's disease. Exp Gerontol. 2010;45:30–40.

35. Zetterberg H. Review: tau in biofluids - relation to pathology, imaging and clinical features. Neuropathol Appl Neurobiol. 2017;43:194–9.

36. Duits FH, Teunissen CE, Bouwman FH, Visser PJ, Mattsson N, Zetterberg H, Blennow K, Hansson O, Minthon L, Andreasen N, et al. The cerebrospinal fluid "Alzheimer profile": easily said, but what does it mean? Alzheimers Dement. 2014;10:713–723.e712.

37. Li G, Sokal I, Quinn JF, Leverenz JB, Brodey M, Schellenberg GD, Kaye JA, Raskind MA, Zhang J, Peskind ER, Montine TJ. CSF tau/Abeta42 ratio for increased risk of mild cognitive impairment: a follow-up study. Neurology. 2007;69:631–9.

38. Dubois B, Feldman HH, Jacova C, Hampel H, Molinuevo JL, Blennow K, DeKosky ST, Gauthier S, Selkoe D, Bateman R, et al. Advancing research diagnostic criteria for Alzheimer's disease: the IWG-2 criteria. Lancet Neurol. 2014;13:614–29.

39. Brendel M, Kleinberger G, Probst F, Jaworska A, Overhoff F, Blume T, Albert NL, Carlsen J, Lindner S, Gildehaus FJ, et al. Increase of TREM2 during aging of an Alzheimer's disease mouse model is paralleled by microglial activation and amyloidosis. Front Aging Neurosci. 2017;9:8.

40. Hall RJ, Watne LO, Idland AV, Raeder J, Frihagen F, MacLullich AM, Staff AC, Wyller TB, Fekkes D. Cerebrospinal fluid levels of neopterin are elevated in delirium after hip fracture. J Neuroinflammation. 2016;13:170.

41. Hov KR, Bolstad N, Idland AV, Zetterberg H, Blennow K, Chaudhry FA, Frihagen F, Raeder J, Wyller TB, Watne LO. Cerebrospinal fluid S100B and Alzheimer's disease biomarkers in hip fracture patients with delirium. Dement Geriatr Cogn Dis Extra. 2017;7:374–85.

42. Thornton P, Sevalle J, Deery MJ, Fraser G, Zhou Y, Stahl S, Franssen EH, Dodd RB, Qamar S, Gomez Perez-Nievas B, et al. TREM2 shedding by cleavage at the H157-S158 bond is accelerated for the Alzheimer's disease-associated H157Y variant. EMBO Mol Med. 2017;9:1366–78.

43. Savva GM, Wharton SB, Ince PG, Forster G, Matthews FE, Brayne C. Age, neuropathology, and dementia. N Engl J Med. 2009;360:2302–9.

44. Mattsson N, Rosen E, Hansson O, Andreasen N, Parnetti L, Jonsson M, Herukka SK, van der Flier WM, Blankenstein MA, Ewers M, et al. Age and diagnostic performance of Alzheimer disease CSF biomarkers. Neurology. 2012;78:468–76.

45. Cunningham C. Microglia and neurodegeneration: the role of systemic inflammation. Glia. 2013;61:71–90.

46. Cunningham C, Deacon RM, Chan K, Boche D, Rawlins JN, Perry VH. Neuropathologically distinct prion strains give rise to similar temporal profiles of behavioral deficits. Neurobiol Dis. 2005;18:258–69.

47. Andreasen N, Minthon L, Vanmechelen E, Vanderstichele H, Davidsson P, Winblad B, Blennow K. Cerebrospinal fluid tau and Abeta42 as predictors of development of Alzheimer's disease in patients with mild cognitive impairment. Neurosci Lett. 1999;273:5–8.

48. Buchhave P, Blennow K, Zetterberg H, Stomrud E, Londos E, Andreasen N, Minthon L, Hansson O. Longitudinal study of CSF biomarkers in patients with Alzheimer's disease. PLoS One. 2009;4:e6294.

49. Iwatsubo T, Mann DM, Odaka A, Suzuki N, Ihara Y. Amyloid beta protein (a beta) deposition: a beta 42(43) precedes a beta 40 in Down syndrome. Ann Neurol. 1995;37:294–9.

50. O'Brien RJ, Wong PC. Amyloid precursor protein processing and Alzheimer's disease. Annu Rev Neurosci. 2011;34:185–204.

51. Kleinberger G, Yamanishi Y, Suarez-Calvet M, Czirr E, Lohmann E, Cuyvers E, Struyfs H, Pettkus N, Wenninger-Weinzierl A, Mazaheri F, et al. TREM2 mutations implicated in neurodegeneration impair cell surface transport and phagocytosis. Sci Transl Med. 2014;6:243ra286.

52. Song WM, Joshita S, Zhou Y, Ulland TK, Gilfillan S, Colonna M. Humanized TREM2 mice reveal microglia-intrinsic and -extrinsic effects of R47H polymorphism. J Exp Med. 2018;215:745–60.

53. Bero AW, Yan P, Roh JH, Cirrito JR, Stewart FR, Raichle ME, Lee JM, Holtzman DM. Neuronal activity regulates the regional vulnerability to amyloid-beta deposition. Nat Neurosci. 2011;14:750–6.

54. Ju YE, Lucey BP, Holtzman DM. Sleep and Alzheimer disease pathology--a bidirectional relationship. Nat Rev Neurol. 2014;10:115–9.

55. Sato C, Barthelemy NR, Mawuenyega KG, Patterson BW, Gordon BA, Jockel-Balsarotti J, Sullivan M, Crisp MJ, Kasten T, Kirmess KM, et al. Tau kinetics in neurons and the human central nervous system. Neuron. 2018;97:1284–1298.e1287.

56. Choi SH, Lee H, Chung TS, Park KM, Jung YC, Kim SI, Kim JJ. Neural network functional connectivity during and after an episode of delirium. Am J Psychiatry. 2012;169:498–507.

57. Rombouts SA, Barkhof F, Goekoop R, Stam CJ, Scheltens P. Altered resting state networks in mild cognitive impairment and mild Alzheimer's disease: an fMRI study. Hum Brain Mapp. 2005;26:231–9.

58. Suarez-Calvet M, Araque Caballero MA, Kleinberger G, Bateman RJ, Fagan AM, Morris JC, Levin J, Danek A, Ewers M, Haass C, Dominantly Inherited Alzheimer N. Early changes in CSF sTREM2 in dominantly inherited Alzheimer's disease occur after amyloid deposition and neuronal injury. Sci Transl Med. 2016;8:369ra178.

59. Snowdon DA, Greiner LH, Mortimer JA, Riley KP, Greiner PA, Markesbery WR. Brain infarction and the clinical expression of Alzheimer disease. The Nun Study. JAMA. 1997;277:813–7.

60. Schlepckow K, Kleinberger G, Fukumori A, Feederle R, Lichtenthaler SF, Steiner H, Haass C. An Alzheimer-associated TREM2 variant occurs at the ADAM cleavage site and affects shedding and phagocytic function. EMBO Mol Med. 2017;9:1356–65.

15

A central role for glial CCR5 in directing the neuropathological interactions of HIV-1 Tat and opiates

Sarah Kim[1], Yun Kyung Hahn[1], Elizabeth M Podhaizer[2], Virginia D McLane[2], Shiping Zou[1,4], Kurt F Hauser[1,2,3] and Pamela E Knapp[1,2,3]*

Abstract

Background: The collective cognitive and motor deficits known as HIV-associated neurocognitive disorders (HAND) remain high even among HIV+ individuals whose antiretroviral therapy is optimized. HAND is worsened in the context of opiate abuse. The mechanism of exacerbation remains unclear but likely involves chronic immune activation of glial cells resulting from persistent, low-level exposure to the virus and viral proteins. We tested whether signaling through C-C chemokine receptor type 5 (CCR5) contributes to neurotoxic interactions between HIV-1 transactivator of transcription (Tat) and opiates and explored potential mechanisms.

Methods: Neuronal survival was tracked in neuronal and glial co-cultures over 72 h of treatment with HIV-1 Tat ± morphine using cells from CCR5-deficient and wild-type mice exposed to the CCR5 antagonist maraviroc or exogenously-added BDNF (analyzed by repeated measures ANOVA). Intracellular calcium changes in response to Tat ± morphine ± maraviroc were assessed by ratiometric Fura-2 imaging (analyzed by repeated measures ANOVA). Release of brain-derived neurotrophic factor (BDNF) and its precursor proBDNF from CCR5-deficient and wild-type glia was measured by ELISA (analyzed by two-way ANOVA). Levels of CCR5 and μ-opioid receptor (MOR) were measured by immunoblotting (analyzed by Student's t test).

Results: HIV-1 Tat induces neurotoxicity, which is greatly exacerbated by morphine in wild-type cultures expressing CCR5. Loss of CCR5 from glia (but not neurons) eliminated neurotoxicity due to Tat and morphine interactions. Unexpectedly, when CCR5 was lost from glia, morphine appeared to entirely protect neurons from Tat-induced toxicity. Maraviroc pre-treatment similarly eliminated neurotoxicity and attenuated neuronal increases in $[Ca^{2+}]_i$ caused by Tat ± morphine. proBDNF/BDNF ratios were increased in conditioned media from Tat ± morphine-treated wild-type glia compared to CCR5-deficient glia. Exogenous BDNF treatments mimicked the pro-survival effect of glial CCR5 deficiency against Tat ± morphine.

Conclusions: Our results suggest a critical role for glial CCR5 in mediating neurotoxic effects of HIV-1 Tat and morphine interactions on neurons. A shift in the proBDNF/BDNF ratio that favors neurotrophic support may occur when glial CCR5 signaling is blocked. Some neuroprotection occurred only in the presence of morphine, suggesting that loss of CCR5 may fundamentally change signaling through the MOR in glia.

Keywords: Human immunodeficiency virus, Morphine, C-C chemokine receptor 5, Maraviroc, Brain-derived neurotrophic factor, NeuroHIV

* Correspondence: pamela.knapp@vcuhealth.org
[1]Department of Anatomy and Neurobiology, Virginia Commonwealth University School of Medicine, 1217 E. Marshall St, Richmond, VA 23298-0709, USA
[2]Department of Pharmacology and Toxicology, Virginia Commonwealth University, Richmond, VA 23298, USA
Full list of author information is available at the end of the article

Background

Human immunodeficiency virus type 1 (HIV-1) remains a global epidemic [1]. Despite significant antiretroviral suppression of HIV-1 propagation in the periphery, limited penetration of combination antiretroviral therapy (cART) drugs through the blood-brain barrier [2, 3] as well as the early viral integration into the host genome cultivates a reservoir in which low levels of viral replication can be sustained in the central nervous system (CNS) [4–6]. Thus, HIV-1+ individuals are especially vulnerable to CNS injury, which afflicts as many as 50% of this population [7–9]. The neurological consequences of HIV-1 infection are known collectively as HIV-associated neurocognitive disorders (HAND). HAND presents as a spectrum of deficits ranging from mild or asymptomatic cognitive disorders to severe, HIV-associated dementia and includes a variety of cognitive, behavioral, and/or motor symptoms [10]. Postmortem findings in HIV-infected individuals, even those effectively treated with cART, often include signs of prominent CNS inflammation, such as increased numbers and/or activation of microglia and astroglia, perivascular inflammation, and leukocytic infiltration resulting in marked neuronal degeneration [11–13]. Notably, neuronal injury and alterations in signaling are not accompanied by direct viral infection of neurons [14–16]. Instead, microglia and macrophages are the major source of productive viral infection in the CNS [17–19]. Small numbers of astrocytes are infected and can produce toxic proteins that injure bystander neurons, but they have not been reliably shown to produce virus [20, 21]. These combined findings highlight the importance of glial impact on neurons, which is normally critical in maintaining proper neuronal activity and survival and suggests a mode of indirect injury that is a consequence of the innate CNS immune response to HIV.

HIV-1 infection and injection drug use are interlinked epidemics, due in large part to needle sharing and increased risky sexual behavior. Because heroin (diacetyl morphine) is widely abused and its active metabolite, morphine, is an opiate prescribed for pain syndromes experienced by HIV patients, we and others are interested in neurological interactions of HIV-1 and heroin/morphine. The comorbid effects of HIV and opiates are not trivial. HIV+ individuals who also abuse opiates demonstrate more severe neuropathology than those who do not, and these findings can translate to exacerbated and accelerated HAND [22–25]. The actions of morphine in this context occur primarily through the activation of μ-opioid receptors (MORs) expressed on glial cells. MOR activation results in the potentiation of HIV-induced release of pro-inflammatory factors (e.g., TNFα, IL-1β, IL-6, CCL5, and CCL2), as well as oxidative and

nitrosative stress, mitochondrial dysregulation, elevated intracellular calcium levels, and excess extracellular glutamate (via restriction of astroglial glutamate uptake), all of which promote neurotoxicity [26–30]. Dysregulated release of inflammatory factors upon chronic exposure to viral proteins may recruit and activate more immune cells, propagating a cycle of increasing inflammation with significant downstream neuronal consequences.

One receptor vulnerable to the aforementioned dysregulation by HIV infection is C-C chemokine receptor 5 (CCR5). CCR5 is widely expressed on T lymphocytes, macrophages, microglia, and dendritic cells and plays a critical role in inducing migration of immune cells to sites of infection and injury in response to elevated levels of certain C-C-chemokine ligands (MIP-1α/CCL3, MIP-1β/CCL4, CCL5/RANTES) [31]. CCR5 and its ligands are upregulated during HIV infection, leading to excess activation of CCR5-expressing cells, including CNS microglia and astrocytes [32, 33]. A homozygous deletion of 32 base pairs in the CCR5 gene prevents its expression on the cell surface and confers improved but not absolute immunity to infection with R5-tropic strains of HIV-1 [34]. Individuals carrying the allele show slowed disease progression upon infection with HIV and less cognitive impairment [35–38]. Furthermore, maraviroc, a CCR5 antagonist with relatively high CNS penetrance [39], reduces microglial activation in the simian immunodeficiency virus-infected model to uninfected control levels and reduces the expression of several pro-inflammatory factors [40]. cART regimens that are supplemented with maraviroc improve the neurocognitive status of HIV+ patients and reduce CSF levels of TNFα [41, 42]. Morphine can alter CCR5 expression by monocytes and activated T cells, contributing to increased viral entry and replication, and excess CNS immune activation [43, 44]. We previously demonstrated that loss of CCL5, a CCR5 ligand, prevented widespread glial activation and reduced levels of another inflammatory ligand (CCL2), suggesting CCL5 may be an upstream activating signal that promotes the expansion of downstream pro-inflammatory responses [45]. The present studies investigate whether interrupting CCR5 signaling may protect neurons against the comorbid effects of HIV-1 and opiate exposure, apart from any effect of blocking HIV entry. We demonstrate using mixed glial-neuronal co-cultures that morphine potentiates Tat-induced neuronal death and that a loss of CCR5 expression on glial cells rescues neurons from such enhanced neurotoxicity. Surprisingly, morphine completely protected against Tat neurotoxicity in cultures with CCR5-null glia even though Tat by itself was still toxic. Levels of brain-derived neurotrophic factor (BDNF) are reduced in HIV+ individuals and by glycoprotein 120 (gp120), an HIV-1 envelope protein with neurotoxic properties [46, 47]. We found that the ratio of neurotrophic BDNF to its neurotoxic precursor (proBDNF) was altered in CCR5-null glia exposed to Tat and morphine co-treatment such that the environment favored neuronal support. BDNF also rescued neurons from Tat + morphine neurotoxicity in a manner similar to the loss of glial CCR5 expression. Overall, we postulate that CCL5/CCR5 signaling is a point of convergence for opiate-Tat interactions within the inflammatory milieu of the HIV-infected CNS. Blocking CCR5 appears to enhance neuroprotection, perhaps by increasing BDNF-related neuroprotection. Inactivation or loss of CCR5 may also change heterologous interactions between MOR and CCR5 related to toxicity and protection.

Methods

Experiments were conducted in compliance with procedures reviewed and approved by the Virginia Commonwealth University Institutional Animal Care and Use Committee.

CCR5-null mice

Transgenic mice in which there has been a loss in CCR5 expression were obtained from Jackson Labs (Bar Harbor, ME) and maintained as homozygous breeding trios. Briefly, the insertion of a neomycin resistance gene to replace the single coding exon has resulted in the constitutive loss of CCR5 expression. To confirm the loss of CCR5, tail snips and harvested glial cells were digested and DNA was isolated as per the instructions of the manufacturer (KAPA Mouse Genotyping; KAPA Biosystems; Wilmington, MA). Primer sets designed to identify the neomycin resistance gene as well as the CCR5 coding exon were obtained from Jackson Labs. Polymerase chain reaction was carried out to confirm the presence of the neomycin resistance gene and the absence of the CCR5 sequence (Fig. 1a). Because the

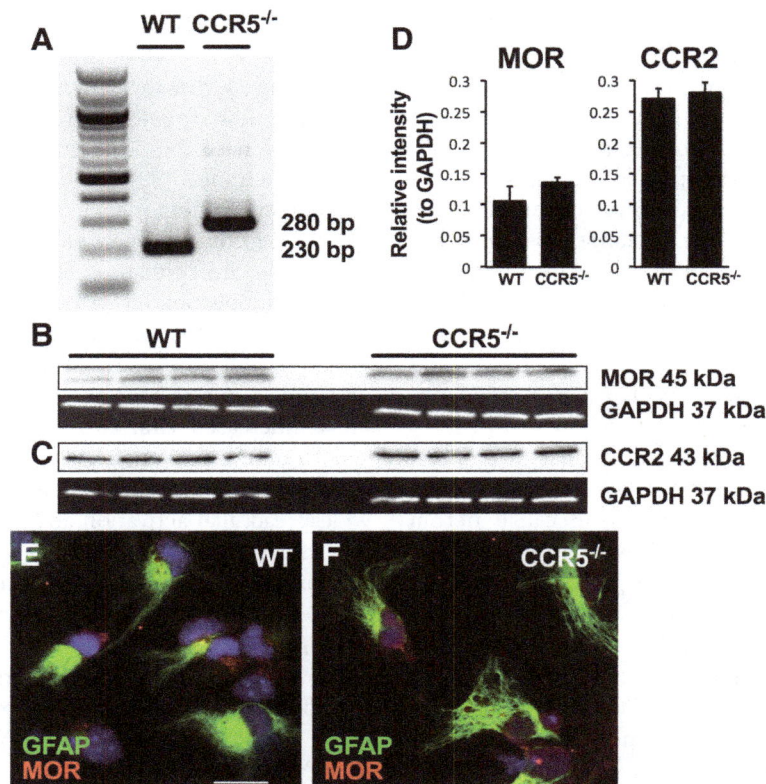

Fig. 1 Expression of MOR and CCR2 are not altered in cell cultures derived from CCR5-null mice. **a** The CCR5 knockout was verified by the presence of a 280-bp band that represents the neomycin resistance gene insertion into the single coding exon of the receptor. A 230-bp band indicates the presence of the CCR5 receptor in wild-type mice. A 100-bp ladder is shown for reference. **b, c** MOR and CCR2 protein levels were assessed in both wild-type and CCR5-deficient glia and normalized against GAPDH. **d** Statistical comparison (two-tailed Student's t test) demonstrated no significant difference between genotypes in levels of either receptor. **e, f** Immunocytochemistry of wild-type (**e**) and knockout (**f**) glia show similar expression of MOR (red) in GFAP+ (green) astrocytes. Astrocyte morphology varies widely in the cultures. MOR appears as a punctate distribution along the cell surfaces as well as in cytoplasmic areas. Scale bar = 20 μM

knockout is global, CCR5-deficient glia or neurons are reconstituted into co-cultures with wild-type neurons or glia, respectively, to study effects of mutations in a single cell type. Mice of the C57Bl6/J background strain were used as wild-type controls. The CCR5-null mice displayed no overt signs of illness or problems during development, and litters occur in a similar frequency and size as the C57Bl6/J strain.

Primary co-cultures of mixed glia and striatal neurons

Mixed glial cultures (approximately 90% astroglia, 8% microglia, and 2% glial progenitors/incipient oligodendroglia [30]) were obtained from C57Bl6/J or CCR5-deficient pups at 0–1 day postnatal. Whole brains were dissected, minced, and incubated with trypsin (2.5 mg/ml) and DNase (0.015 mg/ml) in Dulbecco's modified Eagle's medium (Invitrogen, Carlsbad, CA; 30 min, 37 °C). Tissue was resuspended in medium containing 10% fetal bovine serum (Hyclone, Logan, UT), triturated, and filtered twice through 100 μm and 40 μm pore nylon mesh, then plated onto poly-L-Lysine-coated (Sigma-Aldrich, St Louis, MO; 0.5 mg/ml) 24-well plates at a density of 75×10^3 cell/well. Glia reached confluency after 7–8 days, after which neurons were plated onto their surface.

Neurons were cultured from striata dissected from C57Bl6/J or CCR5-deficient mice at gestational days 15–17. Tissue was incubated (30 min, 37 °C) with trypsin (2.5 mg/ml) and DNase (0.015 mg/ml) in neurobasal medium (Invitrogen), supplemented with B-27 (Invitrogen), L-glutamine (9.5 mM; Invitrogen), glutamate (25 μM; Sigma), and antibiotic/antimycotic solution containing penicillin, streptomycin, and amphotericin B (Invitrogen). After centrifugation, the tissue was triturated and filtered twice through a 70 μm pore nylon mesh to achieve a single-cell suspension. The cells were then plated on top of a bed of confluent glia at 25×10^3 cells/well, and the co-cultures were grown for another 7–8 days in the supplemented neurobasal medium. At this point, the neurons were relatively mature, as previously assessed by the expression of microtubule-associated protein 2 and an array of receptors such as NMDA-R and, importantly, the opiate receptors. Mature neurons also take on a distinct morphology compared to neural progenitor cells, possessing a larger cell body with a prominent nucleus and established axonal and dendritic processes.

Repeated measures assessment

Each plate was maintained in a temperature-controlled, CO_2-regulated chamber (37 °C, 5% CO_2) in a heat insert MXX holder (PeCon Instruments, Erbach, Germany) and placed on the scanning stage of a Zeiss Axio Observer Z1 inverted microscope (Carl Zeiss, Inc., Thornwood,

NY). Five to ten non-overlapping fields, each containing five to ten striatal neurons, were selected from each well based on distinctive neuronal morphology, including features listed in the previous section. Time-lapse images of the selected fields were recorded in 1-h intervals for 72 h using an automated, computer-controlled stage encoder and Axiovision 4.6 software (Carl Zeiss, Inc.). Pre-selected neurons were followed over the 72-h time course and assessed for survival in each hourly image. Neuronal death was determined through morphological criteria, including neurite disintegration, loss of phase brightness, and involution or complete fragmentation of the cell body, all of which were present in each cell counted for analysis (Fig. 2). The number of viable neurons was binned into 4-h intervals for analysis (see the "Statistical Methods" section).

Intracellular calcium assessment

Co-cultures of mixed glia and neurons were prepared on 12-well glass-bottom MatTek (Ashland, MA) plates for calcium imaging. Cells were loaded with 1-μM Fura-2 AM (Invitrogen, Carlsbad, CA) suspended in DMSO for 30 min then washed. This concentration was optimized for minimal astrocyte loading to reduce background signals. The plate was incubated for 30 min in a temperature- and CO_2-regulated chamber (37 °C, 5% CO_2) to ensure de-esterification of the acetoxy methylester (AM) group. On a computer-controlled stage embedded in a Zeiss Axio Observer Z1 microscope, two 20X fields containing five to ten neurons were identified in each well and imaged using Zeiss Zen software (Carl Zeiss Microscopy, LLC, Thornwood, NY). Cells were treated with Tat ± morphine ± maraviroc, and a series of fluorescent images of the same neurons (excitation at 340 and 380 nm, emission at 510 nm) was taken every 15 min for 1 h. Two regions of interest (ROIs; each 15–20 pixels), positioned to avoid both the nucleus and margins of the cell, were selected within the scant cytoplasm of all neurons. ROIs were selected in neurons based on Fura-2 loading but prior to ratiometric imaging.

HIV-1 Tat and drug treatments

Cultures were treated with Tat_{1-86} Clade IIIB (1.2 ng/μl; ImmunoDiagnostics, Woburn, MA), morphine sulfate (500 nM; NIDA Drug Supply System), the broad-spectrum opioid receptor antagonist naloxone (1.5 μM; Sigma), or maraviroc (50 nM; BOC Sciences, Shirley, NY), a small molecule, allosteric inhibitor of CCR5, as well as a number of drug combinations. Tat and morphine were added concurrently; naloxone and maraviroc were given 1 h prior to Tat and morphine treatments. To explore compensatory repercussions of a constitutive knockout, we compared maraviroc treatments to CCR5-

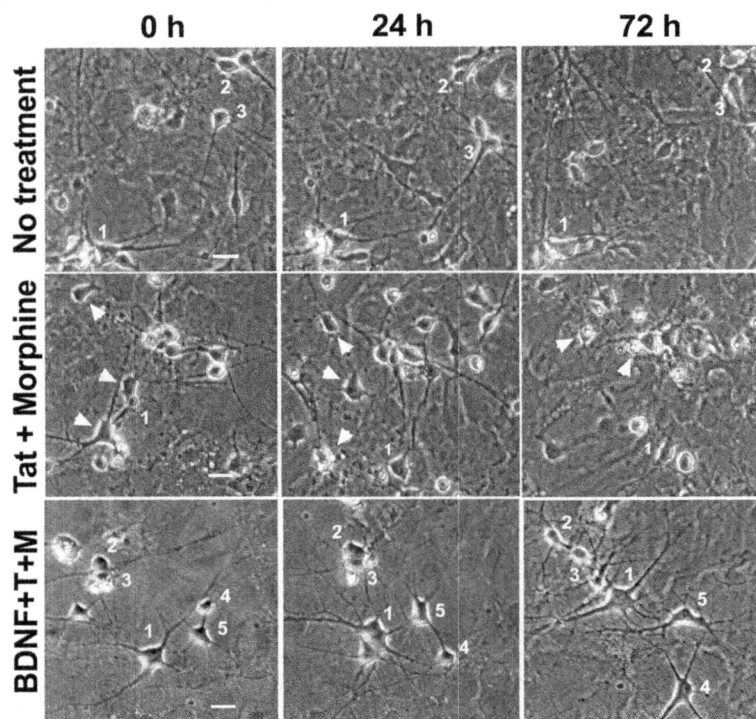

Fig. 2 Representative time-lapse images track neuronal fate. Time-lapse images of co-cultures of wild-type neurons and glia were taken every hour to track neuron survival. The fate of individual neurons can be tracked over time by following the labeled number in the image. Neurons were pre-selected in the image taken at 0 h and followed for the duration of the experiment or until time of death. Death was determined using a set of rigorous morphological criteria including loss of phase brightness, fragmentation of neurites, and collapse of the cell soma (white arrowheads). Representative images from three treatment groups (no treatment, Tat + morphine, BDNF + Tat + morphine) are shown here. Wells receiving no treatment typically showed 85–90% survival rates. Data in Figs. 3 and 6 show that Tat + morphine treatment results in a higher frequency of neuron death by 72 h, and BDNF rescues neurons from the death induced by Tat + morphine treatment. Scale bars for each set of panels = 20 µM

deficient cultures in two different paradigms. In short-term experiments, maraviroc was added immediately prior to the start of the time-lapse imaging. In long-term experiments, maraviroc was added to the media for the duration of the co-culture maturation and imaging period (approximately 2 weeks) and refreshed every 2–3 days. The Tat concentration was chosen based on prior studies that similarly showed neuron death within the 72-h period [30]. Morphine, naloxone, and maraviroc concentrations were based on previous studies from this lab and chosen to produce full receptor occupancy or antagonism. BDNF (50 ng/ml) was purchased through Sigma-Aldrich.

ELISA

C57 wild-type or CCR5-deficient glia were matured for 7–8 d and then treated with Tat and/or morphine for 6 or 24 h. Media was harvested and immediately stored in – 80 °C. The conditioned media were assessed for BDNF (Abcam, Cambridge, UK) and proBDNF (Biosensis, Thebarton, Australia) by ELISA according to manufacturers' instructions. 3,3′,5,5′-tetramethylbenzidine substrate

was added for color development, and plates were read at 450 nm on a SpectraMax M2 microplate reader (Molecular Devices, San Jose, CA) immediately after terminating the reaction, then analyzed using SoftPro Max 1.6 software. BDNF and proBDNF levels were determined based on a standard curve.

Immunoblotting

CCR2 and MOR proteins were assessed in cultured wild-type C57 and CCR5-knockout glial cells. Cells were harvested in lysis buffer containing 1× Tris-buffered saline (TBS), 1% NP-40, 1% Triton X-100, 1 mM PMSF, 10% glycerol, and Halt Protease Inhibitor Cocktail (Thermo Fisher Scientific, Waltham, MA), centrifuged (15 min, 40,000 rpm) and stored at – 80 °C until use. Protein concentration of each sample was measured using the BCA protein assay (Thermo Fisher Scientific). Forty µg of protein lysates were loaded into each well of a 4–20% Tris-HCl Ready Gel (Bio-Rad Laboratories, Hercules, CA) along with Precision Plus Protein Dual Color Standards (Bio-Rad; MW range 10–250 kDa) to visualize protein transfer and determine molecular weight. Proteins were transferred to PVDF membranes (Bio-Rad). Antibodies to CCR2 (1:1000, Abcam), MOR (1:1000, Antibodies Incorporated), and GAPDH (1:2000, Abcam) were used to probe the blots. Fluorescent secondary antibodies were then visualized on a ChemiDoc Gel Imaging system and analyzed with Bio-Rad Image Lab Software 5.2.1. CCR2 and MOR values were normalized to GAPDH.

Immunocytochemistry

Wild-type and CCR5-deficient glial cultures were grown to confluence on glass coverslips, fixed in 4% paraformaldehyde and permeabilized (0.1% Triton X-100, 1% normal goat serum) for 15 min. After blocking for 1 h (1% normal goat serum, 0.1% BSA), primary antibodies to GFAP (1:1000, Millipore) and MOR (1:500, Antibodies Incorporated, Davis, CA) were used to label astrocytes and MOR, after which nuclei were identified by the Hoechst 33342 stain (1:20,000). Coverslips were mounted on glass microscope slides with Prolong Gold anti-fade reagent (Invitrogen).

Statistical methods

Time-lapse studies tracking neuron survival were analyzed by repeated measures ANOVA (Graph Pad Prism 7). The number of viable neurons was binned into 4-h intervals and analyzed to compare treatment effects. Bonferroni's post hoc test was used to determine group differences following confirmation of main effects. Findings are presented as a mean percentage of viable neurons relative to the total number of pre-selected neurons. Intracellular calcium levels were calculated as a percent of control, defined as untreated neurons measured at baseline. Mean effects of Tat ± morphine ± maraviroc on $[Ca^{2+}]_i$ in individual neurons were analyzed at 15-min intervals up to 1 h using repeated measures ANOVA with Duncan's post hoc testing (Statistica 13.2, Dell Inc., Tulsa, OK). ELISA results were analyzed using two-way ANOVA followed by Fisher's PLSD post hoc testing to assess individual group differences. Protein expression levels of MOR and CCR2 were statistically compared using a two-tailed Student's t test. An alpha level of $p \leq 0.05$ was considered significant for all tests. Data are expressed as mean values ± standard error of the mean (SEM).

Results

Characterization of CCR5, MOR, and CCR2 expression in wild-type and CCR5-deficient cultures

DNA and protein analysis were used to characterize expression of CCR5, MOR, and CCR2 in both wild-type and CCR5-deficient mixed glial cultures. We first confirmed that cultures derived from CCR5-null transgenic mice did not express CCR5 using PCR (Fig. 1a). Western

blots showed that MOR protein levels did not differ between wild-type and CCR5-null glial cultures when MOR expression was examined as a fraction of GAPDH (Fig. 1b, d). Immunocytochemical labeling of astrocytes expressing both GFAP and MOR demonstrates similar morphological distribution of MOR irrespective of CCR5 expression, namely, both cytoplasmic and more superficial punctate distribution near the cell body and along processes (Fig. 1e, f). Because of the constitutive loss of CCR5 in the transgenic mice, expression of a closely related chemokine receptor, CCR2, was examined to investigate the possibility of compensatory co-regulation. Western blot analysis showed no differences in CCR2 expression across several samples ($n = 4$) of wild-type and CCR5-null glia (Fig. 1c, d). Relative intensities for both CCR2 and MOR were quantified (Fig. 1d) and analyzed using a two-tailed Student's t test.

Enhanced HIV-1 Tat and opiate neurotoxicity reversed by loss of glial CCR5

In order to investigate the role of CCR5 in mediating the neurotoxic interactions between Tat and morphine, we established a series of co-cultures in which the glia, neurons, or both lacked CCR5. Representative images shown in Fig. 2 illustrate the fate of selected neurons when tracked over the 72-h trial. Using C57Bl6/J wild-type co-cultures, we confirmed that Tat is neurotoxic and that interactions with morphine enhanced Tat-induced toxicity over a 72-h period [30] (Fig. 3a). These effects appear to be mediated by opioid receptors, most likely MOR, since pre-treatment with the broad-spectrum opioid receptor antagonist naloxone eliminated Tat and morphine interactions. In cultures where glia did not express CCR5, exposure to Tat by itself still led to significant levels of neurotoxicity (Fig. 3b). However, the presence of morphine had unexpected effects. When CCR5 was absent from glia, the neurons were protected from Tat and morphine interactions as hypothesized. Surprisingly, in the presence of morphine, the neurotoxic effects of Tat were completely abolished, since neurons in the Tat and morphine co-exposure group showed no additional losses compared to controls. Naloxone pre-treatment blocked the ability of morphine to exacerbate neuronal losses following Tat exposure (compare Fig. 3a, b). Importantly, naloxone also reversed the unexpected protective effects of morphine in CCR5-deficient glial cultures co-exposed to Tat. The paradoxical effect of morphine to protect against Tat neurotoxicity CCR5-deficient conditions thus appears to be mediated through actions mediated by opioid receptors. These effects were presumed specific for glial loss of CCR5, as cultures with CCR5-deficient neurons, but with CCR5-expressing glia, exhibited levels of neuronal death similar to those seen in wild-type co-cultures

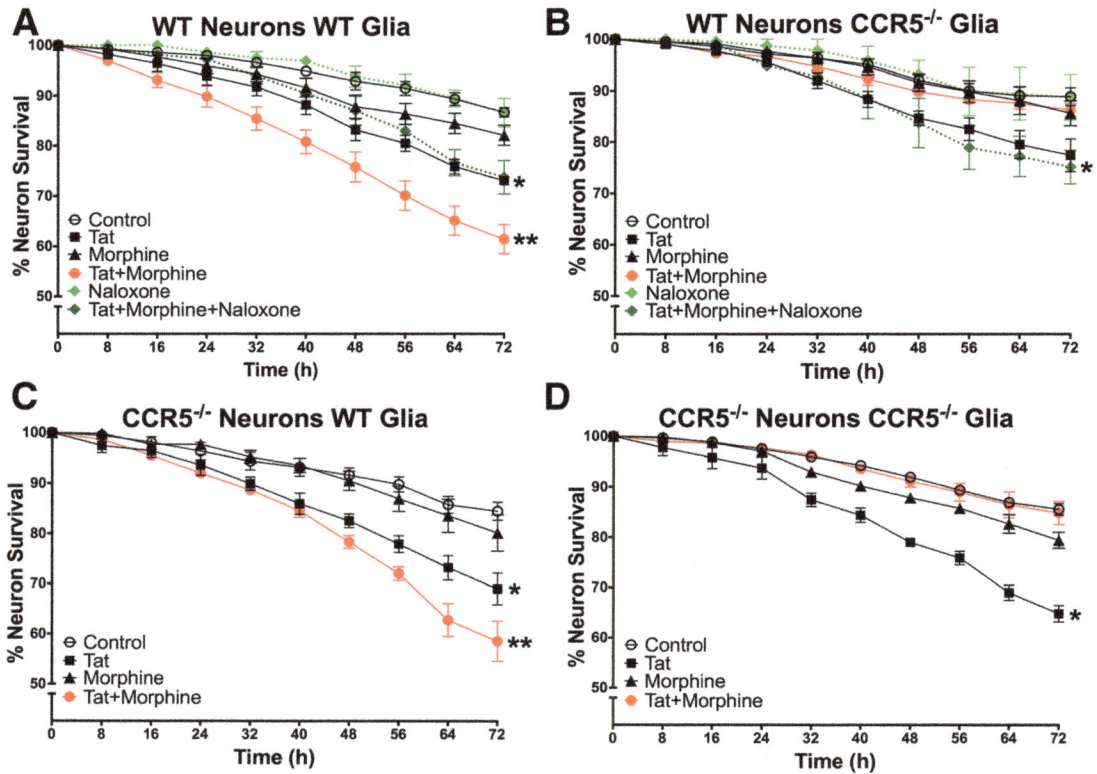

Fig. 3 Neurotoxic effects of HIV-1 Tat and morphine are reversed by loss of glial CCR5. **a** In C57Bl6/J wild-type co-cultures, Tat is neurotoxic (*$p = 0.001$ vs control), and co-exposure to morphine enhanced Tat-induced toxicity over a 72-h period (**$p < 0.001$ vs control, $p < 0.05$ vs Tat). This interaction was blocked by pretreatment with naloxone, a broad-spectrum opioid receptor antagonist. Naloxone or morphine by themselves had no effect on neuronal survival ($n = 4$–8). **b**–**d** To explore the role of CCR5 in mediating neurotoxic interactions between Tat and morphine, co-cultures in which glia, neurons, or both were deficient in CCR5 were established. **b** In co-cultures where glia are CCR5-null but neurons are wild-type, exposure to Tat by itself still led to significant neurotoxicity (*$p < 0.001$ vs control); however, the morphine-enhanced neurotoxicity seen in wild-type cultures was eliminated. In fact, morphine co-treatment entirely abolished Tat toxic effects, restoring neuronal survival to control levels. Pre-treatment with naloxone re-established Tat toxicity, suggesting that actions at the μ-opioid receptor mediate this neuroprotection ($n = 4$–8). **c** In co-cultures where neurons are CCR5-null but glia are wild-type, the survival curves are similar to wild-type co-cultures ($n = 5$). **d** In co-cultures between CCR5-deficient glia and neurons, the survival curves are similar to co-cultures where only glia were CCR5-deficient ($n = 5$). Overall, the results from the CCR5-deficient co-cultures suggest an important role for glial CCR5 in the neurotoxic interactions of HIV-1 Tat and opiates that act at the MOR

exposed to Tat ± morphine (Fig. 3c). Importantly, there was no effect of morphine alone on neuronal survival in any combination of the co-cultured cells. Lastly, co-cultures in which both neurons and glia were CCR5-deficient showed survival curves similar to those in which glia alone were CCR5-deficient (Fig. 3d). Overall, these results suggest an important role for CCR5-expressing glia, as well as the importance of CCR5 and MOR interactions, in mediating the neurotoxic interactions of HIV-1 Tat and opiates.

Constitutive CCR5 loss affects neuronal survival differently than short-term CCR5 blockade

Long-term, constitutive knockout of CCR5 might result in compensatory changes during development that alter

neuronal sensitivity to Tat or morphine. To explore this hypothesis, we used a paradigm where the length of CCR5 blockade was controlled using the CCR5 antagonist maraviroc (Fig. 4). Here we show that a relatively long-term, 2-week incubation with maraviroc (LT-MVC) mimicked the effects on neuron survival seen in co-cultures with CCR5-deficient glia. That is, morphine–Tat interactions that enhance neurotoxicity were negated, and morphine additionally protected completely against Tat neurotoxicity. However, shorter-term exposure to maraviroc, starting immediately before Tat and morphine were co-administered (ST-MVC), had much more limited effects. Short-term maraviroc treatment reduced the interactive effects of Tat and morphine; however, it did not reduce the neurotoxicity of Tat itself irrespective of whether morphine was present.

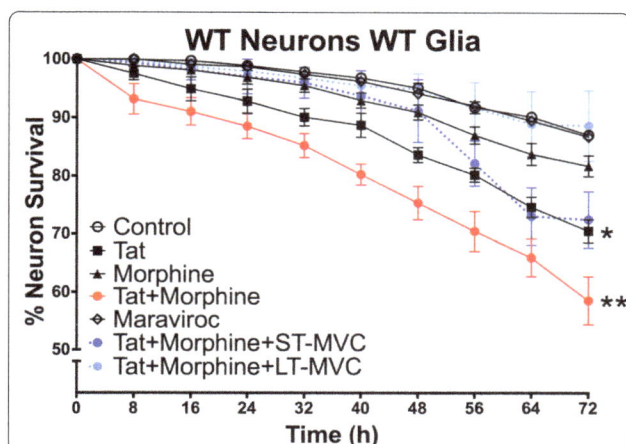

Fig. 4 Constitutive CCR5 loss affects neuron survival differently than short-term CCR5 blockade. Maraviroc was applied to the co-culture to compare the effects of a CCR5 antagonist to a genetic knockout. Maraviroc was applied in two different paradigms that permitted us to manipulate the time period of CCR5 loss. The first was a short-term pre-treatment immediately before adding Tat and/or morphine (ST-MVC; $n = 4$); in this paradigm, maraviroc was on the cultures for a period of 72 h, during the time of Tat and morphine treatments. The second was a longer-term exposure starting 3 days after glia were plated and continuing for the entire 2-week duration of the experiment with replacement of the media every 48 h (LT-MVC; $n = 4$). The Tat + morphine + LT-MVC survival curve matched that of cultures with CCR5-deficient glia. The Tat + morphine + ST-MVC eliminated the morphine–Tat interaction and only showed a trend towards eliminating Tat toxicity ($p = 0.08$ vs control). This set of studies suggests that compensatory effects occur over time with CCR5, which dramatically alter morphine–Tat interaction and neurotoxicity

Maraviroc protects against acute increases in neuronal $[Ca^{2+}]_i$

Disruptions in calcium homeostasis are a common response to neurotoxic signals. As an indicator of how maraviroc affected neuronal function, we performed ratiometric imaging with Fura-2 to assess changes in the $[Ca^{2+}]_i$ level of individual neurons over a 60-min period of treatment with Tat ± morphine ± maraviroc. Tat ± morphine treatments significantly increased $[Ca^{2+}]_i$ by 15 min, and this was maintained for the duration of the trial (Fig. 5). Importantly, even at this early time point, co-exposure to maraviroc blocked the changes, suggesting that reduced CCR5 signaling had the effect of maintaining normal $[Ca^{2+}]_i$ levels and stabilizing neuronal function.

BDNF protects against Tat toxicity and HIV-1 Tat and morphine interactions

BDNF was applied to co-cultures to see if it would promote the survival of striatal neurons co-exposed to Tat + morphine. Co-cultures of wild-type neurons and glia were treated with BDNF concurrently with combined Tat and morphine for 72 h. Time-lapse analysis demonstrated that exogenous BDNF was partially protective against the neurotoxic effects of Tat alone, which was not the case for CCR5 deficiency. However, similar to CCR5 deficiency, BDNF reversed the combined neurotoxic effects of Tat + morphine (Fig. 6). BDNF alone at this concentration did not increase the survival of neurons in untreated, wild-type cultures; survival of both was over 90%.

Loss of glial CCR5 expression produces a shift in proBDNF/BDNF levels

Based on our prior studies demonstrating significant but reversible reduction in glial production of mBDNF after exposure to HIV-infected supernatant ± morphine [48], as well as other studies where HIV-1 gp120 altered BDNF processing [47], we analyzed levels of both mBDNF and its precursor, proBDNF, which binds p75NTR to activate cell death pathways. We also compared changes in their ratios. Wild-type and CCR5-deficient glial cultures were treated with Tat (Fig. 7a), morphine (Fig. 7b), or concurrent Tat and morphine (Fig. 7c) and harvested at 6- and 24-h time points for protein analysis. After Tat treatment, mBDNF levels measured by ELISA were unchanged from levels in media in untreated control cultures at both 6 h and 24 h (Fig. 7a (i, iv)). Tat by itself significantly reduced proBDNF in wild-type cultures versus control cultures at 6 h, with a strong trend towards reduction in both wild-type and CCR5-deficient cultures at 24 h (Fig. 7a (ii, v)). Morphine by itself reduced only proBDNF and only in CCR5-deficient cultures (Fig. 7b (ii, v)). The combination of Tat and morphine showed a strong trend to reduce mBDNF in wild-type cultures at 6 h (Fig. 7c (i)) and was the only treatment to affect mBDNF. The ratio of proBDNF to mBDNF has been used as one index of relative neurotrophic support [47]. CCR5 deficiency strongly reduced this ratio by over twofold at 6 h in cells treated with Tat and morphine (Fig. 7c (iii)), and the protection of neurons in the CCR5-deficient glial environment may reflect the relative increase in mBDNF. A similar trend noted at 24 h was noted ($p = 0.17$) (Fig. 7c (vi)). The only other significant change in this ratio was a much smaller, but still significant, decrease in CCR5-deficient cultures treated with Tat (Fig. 7a (vi)).

Discussion

Mild-to-moderate HAND still occurs in roughly 50% of HIV-infected individuals who receive typical antiretroviral therapy, in part due to relatively low penetration of cART drugs through the blood-brain barrier but also due to the extended lifespan afforded by long-term

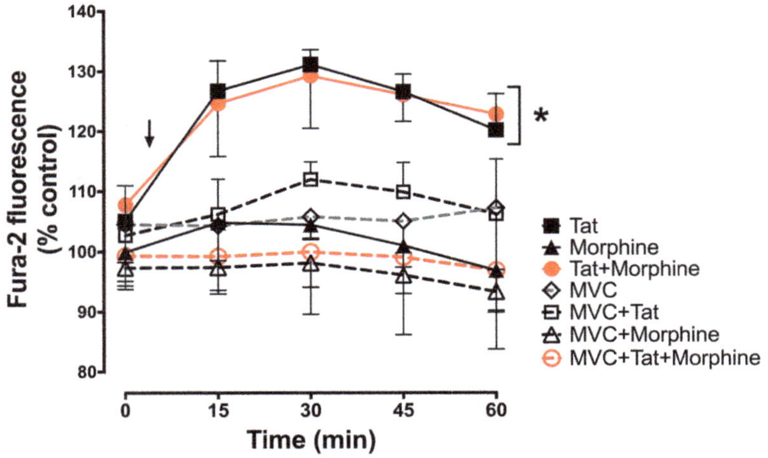

Fig. 5 Maraviroc reduces Tat-mediated increases in $[Ca^{2+}]_i$. Intracellular calcium levels were assessed in neuron-glia co-cultures by ratiometric imaging of Fura-2. A series of images were taken every 15 min for 1 h to track the response of individual neurons. Initial $[Ca^{2+}]_i$ measurements were taken prior to any treatment at the 0-min time point. Tat and/or morphine treatments were applied 10 min prior to the second reading (marked by arrow). There were significant effects for both time ($p = 0.001$) and treatment ($p = 0.009$) when assessed by repeated measures ANOVA. Treatment with Tat or Tat + morphine (marked by asterisk) led to significant increases in $[Ca^{2+}]_i$, as indicated by increased F340/F380 ratios. Pre-treatment with maraviroc blocked the Tat + morphine-induced increase ($p = 0.008$; Duncan's post hoc test) as well as the Tat-mediated response ($p = 0.054$). Morphine and maraviroc alone did not significantly alter $[Ca^{2+}]_i$. Results are presented as percent of the control F340/F380 ratios for each concurrent time point ($n = 3$ independent experiments)

cART treatment. Even in patients where viral replication is undetectable, the release of toxins such as HIV-1 Tat, an early viral protein required for the transactivation of HIV transcription, can persist. While Tat may have direct excitotoxic effects on neurons, particularly well-

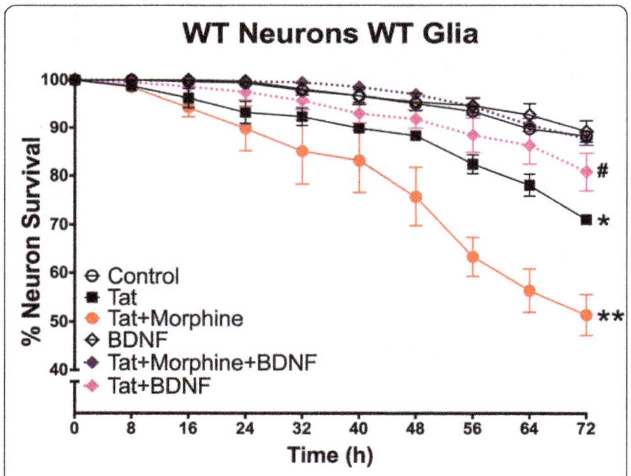

Fig. 6 Exogenous BDNF protects against Tat + morphine treatment. Wild-type, mixed glial-neuronal co-cultures were treated with BDNF in conjunction with Tat or Tat + morphine co-treatment (represented by dotted survival curves). Tat alone was toxic compared to no treatment (*$p < 0.05$), and Tat + morphine co-treatment was significantly more toxic than Tat treatment alone (**$p < 0.0001$). BDNF applied for 72 h was entirely protective against Tat and morphine co-exposure, reducing toxicity to control levels ($n = 4$). BDNF was partially protective against Tat alone. Survival of neurons treated with Tat + BDNF was not significantly different from either controls or cultures treated with Tat alone (#) ($n = 4$)

documented in purified neuronal cultures [30, 49], it also fosters an environment of chronic inflammation through effects on astroglia and microglia. This may result in indirect neurotoxicity through the production of reactive oxygen and nitrosative species and via the release of proinflammatory chemokines and cytokines [50–52], triggering a cascade of inflammatory events that is ultimately damaging to neurons. Furthermore, Tat is present in measurable levels circulating in the blood and CSF of HIV patients [53, 54], suggesting that it is a clinically relevant surrogate for some aspects of HIV neuropathogenesis, especially in virally suppressed patients.

CCR5 is a chemokine receptor that also functions as a major co-receptor for HIV entry. It is normally expressed at low levels by glia throughout the CNS, but this expression can be upregulated by HIV-1 and by Tat [55]. CCR5 expression can also be upregulated in an additive or interactive manner with co-exposure to Tat and the preferential MOR agonist morphine [56]. We have been interested in understanding the role of the CCL5-CCR5 axis in mediating HIV and Tat-induced inflammation and neurotoxicity, with a special interest in whether moderating this chemokine system might be useful in reducing neurotoxic interactions between HIV-1 Tat and opiate exposure. We showed that intrastriatal delivery of Tat caused a local inflammation, characterized by astroglial expression of CCL2 (MCP-1) and 3-nitrotyrosine expression in microglia that was exacerbated by co-administering time-release, subcutaneous morphine pellet implants. Microglial 3-nitrotyrosine and astroglial expression of CCL2

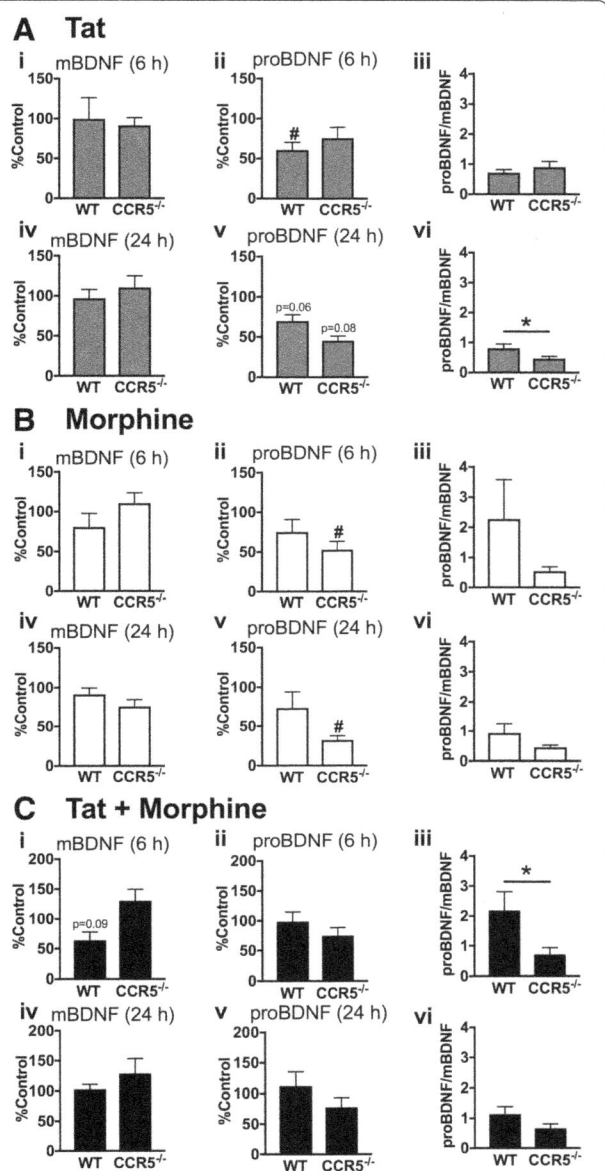

Fig. 7 Loss of glial CCR5 expression produces a shift in proBDNF/mBDNF levels. mBDNF and proBDNF levels were analyzed in conditioned media from wild-type or CCR5-deficient glia treated with Tat and/or morphine after 6 and 24 h to determine if the levels of proBDNF and mBDNF and their ratios were altered ($n = 7–8$). **a** Tat significantly reduced proBDNF in wild-type cultures compared to untreated control levels at 6 h (ii) with similar trends in both genotypes at 24 h (v). The ratio of proBDNF/mBDNF was significantly higher in wild-type cells at 24 h, suggesting reduced neuronal support (vi). **b** Morphine significantly decreased proBDNF in CCR5-deficient glia at both 6 and 24 h compared to control levels (ii, v). These decreases in proBDNF did not significantly alter the proBDNF/ mBDNF ratios (iii, vi). **c** Tat + morphine treatment did not significantly alter mBDNF and proBDNF levels in glia of either genotype, although there was a strong trend to decrease mBDNF in wild-type cultures at 6 h (i). Nevertheless the treatment very significantly decreased the proBDNF/ mBDNF ratio at 6 h (iii), suggesting enhanced protection with CCR5 deficiency. A slight trend towards this shift continued at 24 h (vi; $p = 0.17$). #$p < 0.05$ vs control; *$p < 0.05$ for all figures

were not seen in a CCL5 (RANTES)-deficient mouse, strongly implicating CCL5-to-CCR5 signaling in the amplification of astroglial CCL2 production and resultant macrophage/microglial activation and recruitment [45]. In a related study, we also showed that pretreating Tat-inducible transgenic mice with maraviroc attenuated the withdrawal-mediated increase in levels of many of the cytokines that occurred in mice co-exposed to Tat and morphine and restored antinociceptive properties of morphine that were attenuated by Tat [57]. CCR5 loss is also protective against other HIV proteins, including gp120 [58], as assessed by reduced neuronal damage and microglial activation.

The present studies used both genetic (glia and neurons derived from a constitutive, CCR5-deficient mouse) and pharmacologic (CCR5 blocker maraviroc) approaches to demonstrate that CCR5 is directly involved in HIV neuropathogenic mechanisms irrespective of viral titers. That CCR5 plays a role in the inflammatory processes associated with many disease states, such as cerebral ischemia and reperfusion injury, and neuropathic pain is well-established [59, 60]. In HIV, the role of CCR5 in neurologic outcomes is more difficult to assign since CCR5 is a major co-factor for the infection process. A naturally occurring, 32 base-pair deletion in the CCR5 gene produces a nonfunctional protein, effectively rendering a knockout of the receptor. HIV+ individuals who possess one copy of this mutation show slower progression to AIDS and a reduced occurrence of HAND than those without the mutation [36, 37]. Studies in which maraviroc supplemented the antiretroviral therapy regimen in virally suppressed patients led to improvements in cognition [41, 61]. However, due to the role of CCR5 as a co-receptor for HIV entry, it is unclear if the reduced prevalence of HAND in this population is due to decreased inflammation or decreased progression of infection. In this study, we isolated the inflammatory effects of HIV-1 Tat without the confounding effects of viral infection and replication in monocytes and microglia. Since our paradigm is non-infectious, the findings establish that blocking CCR5 activity can significantly improve neuronal outcomes by mechanisms not involving reduced HIV infection.

As we hypothesized, when CCR5 was deleted from glia in mixed glial cultures, co-cultured neurons were protected against the enhanced degree of toxicity resulting from co-exposure to Tat and morphine. Surprisingly, when CCR5 was absent from glia, morphine appeared to entirely protect co-cultured neurons from the effects of Tat (Fig. 3b). These findings were further explored and confirmed in an alternative, pharmacological approach utilizing maraviroc to control the length of CCR5 blockade. When maraviroc was given to more mature co-cultures concurrent with Tat ± morphine treatments for 72 h, protection was seen against the interactive effects of Tat and morphine co-exposure. In co-cultures incubated with maraviroc for their entire developmental period in vitro, to mimic a constitutive knockout, neurons were additionally protected from Tat-induced toxicity when morphine was present (Fig. 4). Maraviroc may thus afford additional neuroprotection to individuals exposed to opioids, depending on timing and duration of maraviroc therapy. Notably, maraviroc blocked the increase in neuronal $[Ca^{2+}]_i$ seen at acute time points after exposure to Tat ± morphine (Fig. 5), suggesting that early events leading to neuronal dysfunction may be CCR5-dependent and reversible. Naloxone pretreatment revealed that both the predicted and unexpected protective effects of morphine were mediated by opioid receptors.

We explored a potential mechanism for the aforementioned protective effects against both Tat and Tat + morphine. BDNF, a neurotrophin that modulates development and survival of young neurons and is important in establishing and maintaining normal synaptic connectivity, has surfaced as a potential therapeutic target in HAND. Both microglia and astrocytes can be a major source of released BDNF [62, 63]. The mature form of BDNF (mBDNF) preferentially binds TrkB, through which it initiates PI3K and MAPK signaling pathways in neurons, as well as NF-κB-mediated activation of transcription factors [64, 65]. proBDNF binds the alternative p75NTR to initiate pro-apoptotic cascades [66]. Levels of mBDNF are reportedly reduced in HIV+ individuals and also modulated by drugs of abuse [47, 67, 68]. For example, morphine exposures in vivo appear to increase the extracellular protease tissue plasminogen activator, thus increasing cleavage of proBDNF to mBDNF. Withdrawal from morphine had the opposite effect [69]. Intracellular conversion of proBDNF to mBDNF in neurons is reduced by the HIV surface envelope protein gp120, which reduces levels of the intracellular protease furin [47]. Exogenous mBDNF can rescue neurons exposed to gp120 both in vivo and in vitro [70, 71], likely involving downregulation of CXCR4. In a prior study involving glia exposed to HIV-infective supernatant ± morphine, mBDNF levels, but not glial-derived neurotrophic factor (GDNF) levels, were significantly decreased. This reduction was reversed upon removal of HIV treatment [48]. The relatively higher proBDNF/mBDNF ratio measured in the medium of wild-type versus CCR5-null glial cultures exposed to Tat and morphine (Fig. 7c (iii)) is in line with the outcomes above since neurons co-cultured with CCR5-null glia were protected. We measured significant differences in proBDNF/mBDNF ratios at 6 h with trends at 24 h. These time points reflect prior studies that have demonstrated transient increases in BDNF mRNA and protein

levels. For instance, response to cortical injury in rats involves an increase in BDNF mRNA from 1 h that begins to decline after 24 h [72, 73]. gp120 also leads to early changes in BDNF and proBDNF release from cerebellar or cortical neurons, from 1 h post-treatment [47]. As demonstrated by the persistently high percentage of neuronal survival in BDNF-treated co-cultures (Fig. 4), these rapid, transient neuroprotective signals may result in long-lasting effects even in the face of a complex milieu of secondary and tertiary factors by 72 h of treatment exposure. Activation of p75NTR, for instance, in multiple cell types has elucidated a role in immune response regulation. Injury to retinal ganglion neurons leads to the upregulation of p75NTR of nearby Müller glial cells, which can activate downstream cytokine production that is thought to eventually lead to the damage and demise of bystander neurons [74]. Our findings are further supported in other models of neuronal injury such as cerebral ischemia, in which the loss of CCR5 reduces long-term inflammatory injury, potentially through increases in BDNF levels [60, 75]. However, while we demonstrated that Tat and/or morphine treatment led to specific changes in mBDNF and proBDNF levels, shifts in p75NTR and TrkB levels may add a degree of complexity in determining the fate of the neurons, as receptor expression is responsive to injury in a time- and cell-dependent manner [76–78].

Opiates and HIV have historically been interlinked epidemics, and injection drug use carries an increased risk of contracting HIV. Moreover, opiates are used to manage HIV-related pain syndromes, which may impact HAND symptoms in virally suppressed individuals. Cooperative effects between HIV and opiates that increase CNS inflammation are well-documented, and many involve the HIV co-receptor CCR5. For example, opiates modulate CCR5 expression in a number of CNS and immune cells, including microglia [56], astrocytes [79], and peripheral monocytes [43], and can thereby increase rates of HIV infection as well as pro-inflammatory products and immune cell recruitment. The analgesic properties of MOR activation are also reduced when there is an abundance of CCR5 ligands [80]. MOR function is also altered by Tat exposure, which lowers morphine efficacy through decreased G-protein activation [81]. Reduced MOR signaling would tend to increase the amounts of opiates used by HIV-infected individuals for effective analgesia or for illicit effects.

In earlier studies, wild-type neurons co-cultured with MOR-deficient glia were completely protected against the exaggerated neurotoxic effects of co-exposure to Tat + morphine. These result were consistent with findings that the selective MOR antagonist β-funaltrexamine prevented morphine from exacerbating Tat-induced increases in proinflammatory cytokine transcripts in astroglia [27]. Surprisingly, morphine also afforded neuroprotection against Tat [30]. Given that the present results show strikingly similar protective effects in the absence of glial CCR5 (Fig. 3b), a possible interaction between CCR5 and MOR signaling that modulates neuroprotection seems likely. Some interactions between opiates and CCR5 are likely to involve the heterologous interactions that can occur between G-protein-coupled receptors (GPCRs) and that have been shown for MOR and CCR5 [82, 83]. Heterologous desensitization may explain a reduced chemotactic effect of CCR5 by pretreatment with MOR agonists [80]. Recently, synthetic, bivalent ligands composed of maraviroc and naltrexone that target the proposed CCR5-MOR heteromers/oligomers have shown that such interactions may occur in a cell type-specific manner [84–86]. The inability to form MOR-CCR5 heterodimers in CCR5-null (or MOR-null) glia may alter the cellular response to concurrent morphine exposure, contributing to neuroprotection. Although such a response might additionally involve contributions from κ-(KOR) or δ-(DOR) opioid receptors, morphine has lower affinity at KOR or DOR (than MOR). Prior studies also indicate that MOR is largely responsible for the morphine and Tat-induced inflammation and bystander neurotoxicity that is mediated by glia [28, 30].

This study establishes a role of glial CCR5, unrelated to infective processes, in mediating neurotoxicity due to HIV-1 Tat and the interactive effects of Tat and morphine. The differential toxic versus protective effects of morphine in the presence or absence of CCR5 hint at complex relationships that may involve heterologous interactions between CCR5 and MOR. Other results infer a role for BDNF, and perhaps an altered balance between proBDNF and mBDNF levels, in some aspects of the protection. These studies are particularly pertinent to HIV+ individuals who are virally suppressed, yet still develop mild neurocognitive deficits via ongoing, low levels of neuroinflammation in the CNS that involve CCR5 activation.

Conclusion

HIV antiretroviral therapy has been successful in limiting AIDS-related complications, but neurocognitive deficits due to the inflammation driven by early CNS viral penetration persist in up to 50% of HIV-infected individuals. Opiate exposure, which is common in the HIV+ population, worsens the severity of HAND. The cellular mechanism(s) that exacerbate inflammation and CNS disease remain largely unexplained. We tested the hypothesis that the CCL5-CCR5 axis plays a pivotal role in opiate exacerbation of HIV deficits using both genetic and pharmacological approaches. Loss of glial, but not neuronal, CCR5 protected striatal neurons from HIV-1 Tat and morphine co-exposure. Importantly, loss of CCR5 not only blocked the interactive effects of Tat and morphine, but also reversed the Tat toxicity seen in the cultures as long as morphine was present. These findings were confirmed with both long- and short-term exposure to the CCR5 antagonist maraviroc. We measured a shift in the ratio of proBDNF/mBDNF released from CCR5-deficient glia that favored neuroprotection, and exogenous BDNF protected neurons from HIV-1 Tat and morphine exposure in a manner that mirrored the effects of CCR5 deficiency. Our findings suggest that CCR5 is involved in processes that impact neuronal survival and function unrelated to its important role in HIV infection, at least partly by altering the balance between proBDNF and mBDNF levels. The differential toxicity of morphine/opioids in the presence or absence of CCR5 also hints at complex relationships between CCR5 and MOR that may involve heterologous interactions. Our findings are pertinent in terms of understanding and treating HIV+ individuals who develop neurocognitive deficits even though their peripheral viremia is well-controlled.

Abbreviations

$[Ca^{2+}]_i$: Intracellular calcium concentration; ANOVA: Analysis of variance; BDNF: Brain-derived neurotrophic factor; cART: Combined antiretroviral therapy; CCL2: C-C chemokine ligand 2; CCR5: C-C chemokine receptor 5; CNS: Central nervous system; DOR: δ-opioid receptor; ELISA: Enzyme-linked immunosorbent assay; GDNF: Glial-derived neurotrophic factor; Gp120: Glycoprotein 120; GPCR: G-protein-coupled receptor; HAND: HIV-associated neurocognitive disorders; HIV: Human immunodeficiency virus; KOR: κ-opioid receptor; MAPK: Mitogen-activated protein kinase; MOR: μ-opioid receptor; NF-B: Nuclear factor kappa-light-chain-enhancer of activated B cells; NTR: Neurotrophin receptor; PI3K: Phosphoinositide 3-kinase; ROI: Region of interest; Tat: HIV-1 transactivator of transcription; tPA: Tissue plasminogen activator; TrkB: Tyrosine receptor kinase B

Funding

This work was supported by the NIH (R01 DA034231 to PEK and KFH, F30 DA044875 to SK, K02DA027374 to KFH). The sponsors were not involved in the design of the study; the collection, analysis, and interpretation of the data, the writing of the manuscript; nor the decision to submit for publication.

Authors' contributions

PEK and KFH designed the research project and PEK supervised the work. SK conducted all experiments presented in the main body of the text and contributed to the design of the study. EMP conducted preliminary studies and contributed to manuscript revisions. YKH, SZ, and VDM were involved in developing the immunoblot/ELISA, time-lapse imaging/analysis, and intracellular calcium assessment methods, respectively, and also contributed to manuscript revisions. SK and PEK wrote the manuscript. PEK, KFH, and SK secured funding for this project. All authors read and approved the final manuscript.

Competing interests
The authors declare that they have no competing interests.

Author details
[1]Department of Anatomy and Neurobiology, Virginia Commonwealth University School of Medicine, 1217 E. Marshall St, Richmond, VA 23298-0709, USA. [2]Department of Pharmacology and Toxicology, Virginia Commonwealth University, Richmond, VA 23298, USA. [3]Institute for Drug and Alcohol Studies, Virginia Commonwealth University, Richmond, VA 23298, USA. [4]Present Address: BioLegend, Inc., 210 Rustcraft Rd., Dedham, MA 02026, USA.

References
1. UNAIDS. http://www.unaids.org/en/resources/fact-sheet. Accessed on 10 Jan 2018.
2. Yazdanian M. Blood-brain barrier properties of human immunodeficiency virus antiretrovirals. J Pharm Sci. 1999;88:950–4.
3. Powderly WG. Current approaches to treatment for HIV-1 infection. J Neuro-Oncol. 2000;6(Suppl 1):S8–s13.
4. Resnick L, Berger JR, Shapshak P, Tourtellotte WW. Early penetration of the blood-brain-barrier by HIV. Neurology. 1988;38:9–14.
5. Sturdevant CB, Joseph SB, Schnell G, Price RW, Swanstrom R, Spudich S. Compartmentalized replication of R5 T cell-tropic HIV-1 in the central nervous system early in the course of infection. PLoS Pathog. 2015; 11:e1004720.
6. Xiao Q, Li J, Yu Q, Bao R, Liu J, Liu H, Zhou L, Xian Q, Wang Y, Cheng-Mayer C, et al. Distinct compartmentalization in the CNS of SHIVKU-1-infected Chinese rhesus macaque is associated with severe neuropathology. J Acquir Immune Defic Syndr. 2015;70:e168–71.
7. Bednar MM, Sturdevant CB, Tompkins LA, Arrildt KT, Dukhovlinova E, Kincer LP, Swanstrom R. Compartmentalization, viral evolution, and viral latency of HIV in the CNS. Curr HIV/AIDS Rep. 2015;12:262–71.
8. Heaton RK, Clifford DB, Franklin DR Jr, Woods SP, Ake C, Vaida F, Ellis RJ, Letendre SL, Marcotte TD, Atkinson JH, et al. HIV-associated neurocognitive disorders persist in the era of potent antiretroviral therapy: CHARTER study. Neurology. 2010;75:2087–96.
9. Maschke M, Kastrup O, Esser S, Ross B, Hengge U, Hufnagel A. Incidence and prevalence of neurological disorders associated with HIV since the introduction of highly active antiretroviral therapy (HAART). J Neurol Neurosurg Psychiatry. 2000;69:376–80.
10. Sacktor N, McDermott MP, Marder K, Schifitto G, Selnes OA, McArthur JC, Stern Y, Albert S, Palumbo D, Kieburtz K, et al. HIV-associated cognitive impairment before and after the advent of combination therapy. J Neuro-Oncol. 2002;8:136–42.
11. Antinori A, Arendt G, Becker JT, Brew BJ, Byrd DA, Cherner M, Clifford DB, Cinque P, Epstein LG, Goodkin K, et al. Updated research nosology for HIV-associated neurocognitive disorders. Neurology. 2007;69:1789–99.
12. Bell JE. An update on the neuropathology of HIV in the HAART era. Histopathology. 2004;45:549–59.
13. Everall I, Vaida F, Khanlou N, Lazzaretto D, Achim C, Letendre S, Moore D, Ellis R, Cherner M, Gelman B, et al. Cliniconeuropathologic correlates of human immunodeficiency virus in the era of antiretroviral therapy. J Neuro-Oncol. 2009;15:360–70.
14. An SF, Groves M, Giometto B, Beckett AA, Scaravilli F. Detection and localisation of HIV-1 DNA and RNA in fixed adult AIDS brain by polymerase chain reaction/in situ hybridisation technique. Acta Neuropathol. 1999;98:481–7.
15. Takahashi K, Wesselingh SL, Griffin DE, McArthur JC, Johnson RT, Glass JD. Localization of HIV-1 in human brain using polymerase chain reaction/in situ hybridization and immunocytochemistry. Ann Neurol. 1996;39:705–11.
16. Wiley CA, Schrier RD, Nelson JA, Lampert PW, Oldstone MB. Cellular localization of human immunodeficiency virus infection within the brains of acquired immune deficiency syndrome patients. Proc Natl Acad Sci U S A. 1986;83:7089–93.
17. Cosenza MA, Zhao ML, Si Q, Lee SC. Human brain parenchymal microglia express CD14 and CD45 and are productively infected by HIV-1 in HIV-1 encephalitis. Brain Pathol. 2002;12:442–55.
18. Kramer-Hammerle S, Rothenaigner I, Wolff H, Bell JE, Brack-Werner R. Cells of the central nervous system as targets and reservoirs of the human immunodeficiency virus. Virus Res. 2005;111:194–213.
19. Williams KC, Hickey WF. Central nervous system damage, monocytes and macrophages, and neurological disorders in AIDS. Annu Rev Neurosci. 2002; 25:537–62.
20. Churchill MJ, Wesselingh SL, Cowley D, Pardo CA, McArthur JC, Brew BJ, Gorry PR. Extensive astrocyte infection is prominent in human immunodeficiency virus-associated dementia. Ann Neurol. 2009;66:253–8.
21. Bagasra O, Lavi E, Bobroski L, Khalili K, Pestaner JP, Tawadros R, Pomerantz RJ. Cellular reservoirs of HIV-1 in the central nervous system of infected individuals: identification by the combination of in situ polymerase chain reaction and immunohistochemistry. AIDS. 1996;10:573–85.
22. Anthony IC, Arango JC, Stephens B, Simmonds P, Bell JE. The effects of illicit drugs on the HIV infected brain. Front Biosci. 2008;13:1294–307.
23. Byrd DA, Fellows RP, Morgello S, Franklin D, Heaton RK, Deutsch R, Atkinson JH, Clifford DB, Collier AC, Marra CM, et al. Neurocognitive impact of substance use in HIV infection. J Acquir Immune Defic Syndr. 2011;58:154–62.
24. Martin-Thormeyer EM, Paul RH. Drug abuse and hepatitis C infection as comorbid features of HIV associated neurocognitive disorder: neurocognitive and neuroimaging features. Neuropsychol Rev. 2009;19: 215–31.
25. Bell JE, Arango JC, Anthony IC. Neurobiology of multiple insults: HIV-1-associated brain disorders in those who use illicit drugs. J NeuroImmune Pharmacol. 2006;1:182–91.
26. Rogers TJ, Peterson PK. Opioid G protein-coupled receptors: signals at the crossroads of inflammation. Trends Immunol. 2003;24:116–21.
27. El-Hage N, Gurwell JA, Singh IN, Knapp PE, Nath A, Hauser KF. Synergistic increases in intracellular Ca^{2+}, and the release of MCP-1, RANTES, and IL-6 by astrocytes treated with opiates and HIV-1 Tat. Glia. 2005;50:91–106.
28. El-Hage N, Wu G, Wang J, Ambati J, Knapp PE, Reed JL, Bruce-Keller AJ, Hauser KF. HIV-1 Tat and opiate-induced changes in astrocytes promote chemotaxis of microglia through the expression of MCP-1 and alternative chemokines. Glia. 2006;53:132–46.
29. El-Hage N, Bruce-Keller AJ, Yakovleva T, Bazov I, Bakalkin G, Knapp PE, Hauser KF. Morphine exacerbates HIV-1 Tat-induced cytokine production in astrocytes through convergent effects on $[Ca^{2+}]_i$, NF-κB trafficking and transcription. PLoS One. 2008;3:e4093.
30. Zou S, Fitting S, Hahn YK, Welch SP, El-Hage N, Hauser KF, Knapp PE. Morphine potentiates neurodegenerative effects of HIV-1 Tat through actions at μ-opioid receptor-expressing glia. Brain. 2011;134:3616–31.
31. Sorce S, Myburgh R, Krause KH. The chemokine receptor CCR5 in the central nervous system. Prog Neurobiol. 2011;93:297–311.
32. Kelder W, McArthur JC, Nance-Sproson T, McClernon D, Griffin DE. β-chemokines MCP-1 and RANTES are selectively increased in cerebrospinal fluid of patients with human immunodeficiency virus-associated dementia. Ann Neurol. 1998;44:831–5.
33. McManus CM, Weidenheim K, Woodman SE, Nunez J, Hesselgesser J, Nath A, Berman JW. Chemokine and chemokine-receptor expression in human glial elements: induction by the HIV protein, Tat, and chemokine autoregulation. Am J Pathol. 2000;156:1441–53.
34. Martin-Blondel G, Brassat D, Bauer J, Lassmann H, Liblau RS. CCR5 blockade for neuroinflammatory diseases--beyond control of HIV. Nat Rev Neurol. 2016;12:95–105.
35. Dragic T, Litwin V, Allaway GP, Martin SR, Huang Y, Nagashima KA, Cayanan C, Maddon PJ, Koup RA, Moore JP, Paxton WA. HIV-1 entry into CD4+ cells is mediated by the chemokine receptor CC-CKR-5. Nature. 1996;381:667–73.
36. Dean M, Carrington M, Winkler C, Huttley GA, Smith MW, Allikmets R, Goedert JJ, Buchbinder SP, Vittinghoff E, Gomperts E, et al. Genetic restriction of HIV-1 infection and progression to AIDS by a deletion allele of the CKR5 structural gene. Hemophilia growth and development study, multicenter AIDS cohort study, multicenter hemophilia cohort study, San Francisco City cohort, ALIVE study. Science. 1996;273:1856–62.
37. Ioannidis JP, Rosenberg PS, Goedert JJ, Ashton LJ, Benfield TL, Buchbinder SP, Coutinho RA, Eugen-Olsen J, Gallart T, Katzenstein TL, et al. Effects of CCR5-Δ32, CCR2-64I, and SDF-1 3'A alleles on HIV-1 disease progression: an international meta-analysis of individual-patient data. Ann Intern Med. 2001; 135:782–95.
38. Levine AJ, Singer EJ, Shapshak P. The role of host genetics in the susceptibility for HIV-associated neurocognitive disorders. AIDS Behav. 2009;13:118–32.
39. Llibre JM, Rivero A, Rojas JF, Garcia Del Toro M, Herrero C, Arroyo D, Pineda JA, Pasquau J, Masia M, Crespo M, et al. Safety, efficacy and indications of prescription of maraviroc in clinical practice: factors associated with clinical outcomes. Antivir Res. 2015;120:79–84.

40. Kelly KM, Beck SE, Metcalf Pate KA, Queen SE, Dorsey JL, Adams RJ, Avery LB, Hubbard W, Tarwater PM, Mankowski JL. Neuroprotective maraviroc monotherapy in simian immunodeficiency virus-infected macaques: reduced replicating and latent SIV in the brain. AIDS. 2013;27:F21–8.

41. Gates TM, Cysique LA, Siefried KJ, Chaganti J, Moffat KJ, Brew BJ. Maraviroc-intensified combined antiretroviral therapy improves cognition in virally suppressed HIV-associated neurocognitive disorder. AIDS. 2016;30:591–600.

42. Ndhlovu LC, Umaki T, Chew GM, Chow DC, Agsalda M, Kallianpur KJ, Paul R, Zhang G, Ho E, Hanks N, et al. Treatment intensification with maraviroc (CCR5 antagonist) leads to declines in CD16-expressing monocytes in cART-suppressed chronic HIV-infected subjects and is associated with improvements in neurocognitive test performance: implications for HIV-associated neurocognitive disease (HAND). J Neuro-Oncol. 2014;20:571–82.

43. Guo CJ, Li Y, Tian S, Wang X, Douglas SD, Ho WZ. Morphine enhances HIV infection of human blood mononuclear phagocytes through modulation of β-chemokines and CCR5 receptor. J Investig Med. 2002;50:435–42.

44. Miyagi T, Chuang LF, Doi RH, Carlos MP, Torres JV, Chuang RY. Morphine induces gene expression of CCR5 in human CEMx174 lymphocytes. J Biol Chem. 2000;275:31305–10.

45. El-Hage N, Bruce-Keller AJ, Knapp PE, Hauser KF. CCL5/RANTES gene deletion attenuates opioid-induced increases in glial CCL2/MCP-1 immunoreactivity and activation in HIV-1 Tat-exposed mice. J NeuroImmune Pharmacol. 2008;3:275–85.

46. Avdoshina V, Garzino-Demo A, Bachis A, Monaco MC, Maki PM, Tractenberg RE, Liu C, Young MA, Mocchetti I. HIV-1 decreases the levels of neurotrophins in human lymphocytes. AIDS. 2011;25:1126–8.

47. Bachis A, Avdoshina V, Zecca L, Parsadanian M, Mocchetti I. Human immunodeficiency virus type 1 alters brain-derived neurotrophic factor processing in neurons. J Neurosci. 2012;32:9477–84.

48. Masvekar RR, El-Hage N, Hauser KF, Knapp PE. Morphine enhances HIV-1SF162-mediated neuron death and delays recovery of injured neurites. PLoS One. 2014;9:e100196.

49. Fitting S, Knapp PE, Zou S, Marks WD, Bowers MS, Akbarali HI, Hauser KF. Interactive HIV-1 Tat and morphine-induced synaptodendritic injury is triggered through focal disruptions in Na$^+$ influx, mitochondrial instability, and Ca^{2+} overload. J Neurosci. 2014;34:12850–64.

50. Nath A, Conant K, Chen P, Scott C, Major EO. Transient exposure to HIV-1 Tat protein results in cytokine production in macrophages and astrocytes. A hit and run phenomenon. J Biol Chem. 1999;274:17098–102.

51. Kruman II, Nath A, Mattson MP. HIV-1 protein Tat induces apoptosis of hippocampal neurons by a mechanism involving caspase activation, calcium overload, and oxidative stress. Exp Neurol. 1998;154:276–88.

52. Bruce-Keller AJ, Turchan-Cholewo J, Smart EJ, Geurin T, Chauhan A, Reid R, Xu R, Nath A, Knapp PE, Hauser KF. Morphine causes rapid increases in glial activation and neuronal injury in the striatum of inducible HIV-1 Tat transgenic mice. Glia. 2008;56:1414–27.

53. Wiley CA, Baldwin M, Achim CL. Expression of HIV regulatory and structural mRNA in the central nervous system. AIDS. 1996;10:843–7.

54. Weiss JM, Nath A, Major EO, Berman JW. HIV-1 Tat induces monocyte chemoattractant protein-1-mediated monocyte transmigration across a model of the human blood-brain barrier and up-regulates CCR5 expression on human monocytes. J Immunol. 1999;163:2953–9.

55. Ostrowski MA, Justement SJ, Catanzaro A, Hallahan CA, Ehler LA, Mizell SB, Kumar PN, Mican JA, Chun TW, Fauci AS. Expression of chemokine receptors CXCR4 and CCR5 in HIV-1-infected and uninfected individuals. J Immunol. 1998;161:3195–201.

56. Bokhari SM, Yao H, Bethel-Brown C, Fuwang P, Williams R, Dhillon NK, Hegde R, Kumar A, Buch SJ. Morphine enhances Tat-induced activation in murine microglia. J Neuro-Oncol. 2009;15:219–28.

57. Gonek M, McLane VD, Stevens DL, Lippold K, Akbarali HI, Knapp PE, Dewey WL, Hauser KF, Paris JJ. CCR5 mediates HIV-1 Tat-induced neuroinflammation and influences morphine tolerance, dependence, and reward. Brain Behav Immun. 2018;69:124–38.

58. Maung R, Hoefer MM, Sanchez AB, Sejbuk NE, Medders KE, Desai MK, Catalan IC, Dowling CC, de Rozieres CM, Garden GA, et al. CCR5 knockout prevents neuronal injury and behavioral impairment induced in a transgenic mouse model by a CXCR4-using HIV-1 glycoprotein 120. J Immunol. 2014;193:1895–910.

59. Sun S, Chen D, Lin F, Chen M, Yu H, Hou L, Li C. Role of interleukin-4, the chemokine CCL3 and its receptor CCR5 in neuropathic pain. Mol Immunol. 2016;77:184–92.

60. Victoria ECG, de Brito Toscano EC, de Sousa Cardoso AC, da Silva DG, de Miranda AS, da Silva Barcelos L, Sugimoto MA, Sousa LP, de Assis Lima IV, de Oliveira ACP, et al. Knockdown of C-C chemokine receptor 5 (CCR5) is protective against cerebral ischemia and reperfusion injury. Curr Neurovasc Res. 2017;14:125–31.

61. Barber TJ, Imaz A, Boffito M, Niubo J, Pozniak A, Fortuny R, Alonso J, Davies N, Mandalia S, Podzamczer D, Gazzard B. CSF inflammatory markers and neurocognitive function after addition of maraviroc to monotherapy darunavir/ritonavir in stable HIV patients: the CINAMMON study. J Neuro-Oncol. 2018;24:98–105.

62. Parkhurst CN, Yang G, Ninan I, Savas JN, Yates JR 3rd, Lafaille JJ, Hempstead BL, Littman DR, Gan WB. Microglia promote learning-dependent synapse formation through brain-derived neurotrophic factor. Cell. 2013;155:1596–609.

63. Elkabes S, DiCicco-Bloom EM, Black IB. Brain microglia/macrophages express neurotrophins that selectively regulate microglial proliferation and function. J Neurosci. 1996;16:2508–21.

64. Bredesen DE, Rabizadeh S. p75NTR and apoptosis: Trk-dependent and Trk-independent effects. Trends Neurosci. 1997;20:287–90.

65. Glazner GW, Mattson MP. Differential effects of BDNF, ADNF9, and TNFalpha on levels of NMDA receptor subunits, calcium homeostasis, and neuronal vulnerability to excitotoxicity. Exp Neurol. 2000;161:442–52.

66. Chao MV, Bothwell M. Neurotrophins: to cleave or not to cleave. Neuron. 2002;33:9–12.

67. Miguez-Burbano MJ, Espinoza L, Bueno D, Vargas M, Trainor AB, Quiros C, Lewis JE, Asthana D. Beyond the brain: the role of brain-derived neurotrophic factor in viroimmune responses to antiretroviral therapy among people living with HIV with and without alcohol use. J Int Assoc Provid AIDS Care. 2014;13:454–60.

68. Angelucci F, Ricci V, Pomponi M, Conte G, Mathe AA, Attilio Tonali P, Bria P. Chronic heroin and cocaine abuse is associated with decreased serum concentrations of the nerve growth factor and brain-derived neurotrophic factor. J Psychopharmacol. 2007;21:820–5.

69. Bachis A, Campbell LA, Jenkins K, Wenzel E, Mocchetti I. Morphine withdrawal increases brain-derived neurotrophic factor precursor. Neurotox Res. 2017;32:509–17.

70. Nosheny RL, Ahmed F, Yakovlev A, Meyer EM, Ren K, Tessarollo L, Mocchetti I. Brain-derived neurotrophic factor prevents the nigrostriatal degeneration induced by human immunodeficiency virus-1 glycoprotein 120 in vivo. Eur J Neurosci. 2007;25:2275–84.

71. Bachis A, Major EO, Mocchetti I. Brain-derived neurotrophic factor inhibits human immunodeficiency virus-1/gp120-mediated cerebellar granule cell death by preventing gp120 internalization. J Neurosci. 2003;23:5715–22.

72. Yang K, Perez-Polo JR, Mu XS, Yan HQ, Xue JJ, Iwamoto Y, Liu SJ, Dixon CE, Hayes RL. Increased expression of brain-derived neurotrophic factor but not neurotrophin-3 mRNA in rat brain after cortical impact injury. J Neurosci Res. 1996;44:157–64.

73. Oyesiku NM, Evans CO, Houston S, Darrell RS, Smith JS, Fulop ZL, Dixon CE, Stein DG. Regional changes in the expression of neurotrophic factors and their receptors following acute traumatic brain injury in the adult rat brain. Brain Res. 1999;833:161–72.

74. Lebrun-Julien F, Bertrand MJ, De Backer O, Stellwagen D, Morales CR, Di Polo A, Barker PA. ProNGF induces TNFα-dependent death of retinal ganglion cells through a p75NTR non-cell-autonomous signaling pathway. Proc Natl Acad Sci U S A. 2010;107:3817–22.

75. Kiprianova I, Freiman TM, Desiderato S, Schwab S, Galmbacher R, Gillardon F, Spranger M. Brain-derived neurotrophic factor prevents neuronal death and glial activation after global ischemia in the rat. J Neurosci Res. 1999;56:21–7.

76. Roux PP, Colicos MA, Barker PA, Kennedy TE. p75 neurotrophin receptor expression is induced in apoptotic neurons after seizure. J Neurosci. 1999;19:6887–96.

77. Dowling P, Ming X, Raval S, Husar W, Casaccia-Bonnefil P, Chao M, Cook S, Blumberg B. Up-regulated p75NTR neurotrophin receptor on glial cells in MS plaques. Neurology. 1999;53:1676–82.

78. Goutan E, Marti E, Ferrer I. BDNF, and full length and truncated TrkB expression in the hippocampus of the rat following kainic acid excitotoxic damage. Evidence of complex time-dependent and cell-specific responses. Brain Res Mol Brain Res. 1998;59:154–64.

79. Mahajan SD, Schwartz SA, Shanahan TC, Chawda RP, Nair MP. Morphine regulates gene expression of alpha- and beta-chemokines and their receptors on astroglial cells via the opioid mu receptor. J Immunol. 2002;169:3589–99.

80. Szabo I, Chen XH, Xin L, Adler MW, Howard OM, Oppenheim JJ, Rogers TJ. Heterologous desensitization of opioid receptors by chemokines inhibits chemotaxis and enhances the perception of pain. Proc Natl Acad Sci U S A. 2002;99:10276–81.

81. Hahn YK, Paris JJ, Lichtman AH, Hauser KF, Sim-Selley LJ, Selley DE, Knapp PE. Central HIV-1 Tat exposure elevates anxiety and fear conditioned responses of male mice concurrent with altered mu-opioid receptor-mediated G-protein activation and β-arrestin 2 activity in the forebrain. Neurobiol Dis. 2016;92:124–36.

82. Chen C, Li J, Bot G, Szabo I, Rogers TJ, Liu-Chen LY. Heterodimerization and cross-desensitization between the μ-opioid receptor and the chemokine CCR5 receptor. Eur J Pharmacol. 2004;483:175–86.

83. Szabo I, Wetzel MA, Zhang N, Steele AD, Kaminsky DE, Chen C, Liu-Chen LY, Bednar F, Henderson EE, Howard OM, et al. Selective inactivation of CCR5 and decreased infectivity of R5 HIV-1 strains mediated by opioid-induced heterologous desensitization. J Leukoc Biol. 2003;74:1074–82.

84. Arnatt CK, Falls BA, Yuan Y, Raborg TJ, Masvekar RR, El-Hage N, Selley DE, Nicola AV, Knapp PE, Hauser KF, Zhang Y. Exploration of bivalent ligands targeting putative mu opioid receptor and chemokine receptor CCR5 dimerization. Bioorg Med Chem. 2016;24:5969–87.

85. Yuan Y, Arnatt CK, El-Hage N, Dever SM, Jacob JC, Selley DE, Hauser KF, Zhang Y. A bivalent ligand targeting the putative mu opioid receptor and chemokine receptor CCR5 heterodimers: binding affinity versus functional activities. Medchemcomm. 2013;4:847–51.

86. El-Hage N, Dever SM, Podhazer EM, Arnatt CK, Zhang Y, Hauser KF. A novel bivalent HIV-1 entry inhibitor reveals fundamental differences in CCR5-μ-opioid receptor interactions between human astroglia and microglia. AIDS. 2013;27:2181–90.

16

Analyses of gene expression profiles in the rat dorsal horn of the spinal cord using RNA sequencing in chronic constriction injury rats

Hui Du[1†], Juan Shi[2†], Ming Wang[2], Shuhong An[2], Xingjing Guo[3] and Zhaojin Wang[2*] (iD)

Abstract

Background: Neuropathic pain is caused by damage to the nervous system, resulting in aberrant pain, which is associated with gene expression changes in the sensory pathway. However, the molecular mechanisms are not fully understood.

Methods: Wistar rats were employed for the establishment of the chronic constriction injury (CCI) models. Using the Illumina HiSeq 4000 platform, we examined differentially expressed genes (DEGs) in the rat dorsal horn by RNA sequencing (RNA-seq) between CCI and control groups. Then, enrichment analyses were performed for these DEGs using Gene Ontology (GO) function, Kyoto Encyclopedia of Genes and Genomes (KEGG) pathway, Hierarchical Cluster, and protein-protein interaction (PPI) network.

Results: A total of 63 DEGs were found significantly changed with 56 upregulated (e.g., Cxcl13, C1qc, Fcgr3a) and 7 downregulated (e.g., Dusp1) at 14 days after CCI. Quantitative reverse-transcribed PCR (qRT-PCR) verified changes in 13 randomly selected DEGs. GO and KEGG biological pathway analyses showed that the upregulated DEGs were mostly enriched in immune response-related biological processes, as well as 14 immune- and inflammation-related pathways. The downregulated DEGs were enriched in inactivation of mitogen-activated protein kinase (MAPK) activity. PPI network analysis showed that Cd68, C1qc, C1qa, Laptm5, and Fcgr3a were crucial nodes with high connectivity degrees. Most of these genes which have previously been linked to immune and inflammation-related pathways have not been reported in neuropathic pain (e.g., Laptm5, Fcgr3a).

Conclusions: Our results revealed that immune and defense pathways may contribute to the generation of neuropathic pain after CCI. These mRNAs may represent new therapeutic targets for the treatment of neuropathic pain.

Keywords: Dorsal horn, Chronic constriction injury, RNA sequencing, Differentially expressed genes

Background

Neuropathic pain is a chronic pain and may result from primary damage, disease or dysfunction of the peripheral or central nervous system, which is characterized by an increased responsiveness of nociceptive neurons in the nervous system [1]. The molecular mechanisms of neuropathic pain remain poorly understood, but it is known to involve nerve injury, inflammatory cytokine release, anatomical remodeling, and nociceptive receptors. [2, 3]. Thus, an improved understanding of pathogenesis from gene interactions in neuropathic pain is crucial for the development of the genetic and various neurobiological base therapeutic strategies to prevent neuropathic pain and improve the treatment effect.

The chronic constriction injury (CCI) rat model which simulates the symptoms of chronic nerve compression has been used as a model of neuropathic pain because rats subjected to CCI behave analogously to humans with neuropathic pain [4, 5]. Reportedly, CCI

* Correspondence: zjwang@tsmc.edu.cn
†Hui Du and Juan Shi contributed equally to this work.
2Department of Human Anatomy, Taishan Medical University, Taian 271000, China
Full list of author information is available at the end of the article

is highly associated with inflammation [6, 7]. Activation of immune and immune-like glial cells in the injured nerve, dorsal root ganglia, and spinal cord could generate a variety of mediators such as cytokines, chemokines, and other inflammatory mediators [8]. Interestingly, some of these mediators, such as cytokines and chemokines, can directly activate or sensitize nociceptors, contributing to the development of neuropathic pain [9].

Gene expression profile studies can be used to provide understanding of the molecular mechanisms underlying the development and maintenance of neuropathic pain [10–12]. Some studies using microarray and RNA sequencing (RNA-seq) analysis have been conducted to investigate the mechanism underlying the generation of neuropathic pain in spared nerve injury (SNI) model [13, 14]. Although they identified several crucial differentially expressed genes (DEGs) and different immune actions in SNI models, the alteration of gene expression and mechanisms on neuropathic pain are still unclear. Therefore, the present study was carried out to compare the different gene expression profiles of the dorsal horn of CCI rats and controls using the Illumina Hiseq 4000 to reveal the underlying regulatory mechanism of CCI rat models. Moreover, the molecular and cellular functions of the predicted mRNAs as well as the signaling pathways involved based on the present experiment will be further investigated.

Methods
Animals
Adult male Wistar rats weighing 200–250 g were obtained from the Animal Center of Taishan Medical University. All experimental procedures followed the guidelines of the Taishan Medical University Institutional Animal Care and Use Committee. Efforts were made to minimize the number of animals used and their sufferings.

CCI models
CCI to the sciatic nerve of the right hind limb in rats was performed based on previous description [15]. Briefly, animals were anesthetized with 4% chloral hydrate (10 ml/kg; i.p.). The sciatic nerve of the right hind limb was exposed at the middle of the thigh by blunt dissection. To prevent the interruption of blood circulation through the epineural vasculature, four chromic gut ligatures were loosely tied (4.0 silk) around the nerve with spacing at ∼ 1 mm. In the control group, the right sciatic nerve was exposed for 2–3 min, but was not ligated. Following surgery, the skin was closed with a single suture, and the animals were allowed to recover for various period of time before behavioral testing.

Mechanical withdrawal threshold (MWT)
All behavioral tests were performed in a blinded manner. Mechanical allodynia and thermal hyperalgesia are reproducible and sensitive behavioral readouts of neuropathic pain. Behavioral testing was conducted prior to surgery and on days 1, 3, 7, 10, and 14 following surgery. Animals were allowed to acclimate to elevated cages (20 × 14 × 16 cm) with a wire mesh bottom. MWT was measured by assessing hind paw sensitivity to innocuous mechanical stimulation. Von Frey filaments (0.41–15.1 g; North Coast, Gilroy, CA) were applied to the plantar aspect of the right hind paw. Lifting, licking the paw, and running away were all considered as positive responses. The maximum applied pressure was recorded. The MWT of each animal was the average of six measurements taken at 5 min intervals.

Thermal withdrawal latency (TWL)
In this assay, rats were placed in a transparent, square, bottomless acrylic box (17 × 11.5 × 14 cm) and allowed to adapt for 20 min. Responses to thermal stimulation were evaluated using a 37,370 plantar test apparatus as a source of radiant heat. A beam of focused light set at 60 °C was directed towards the plantar surface of the hind paw, and the maximum latency time was recorded. The time to purposeful withdrawal of the foot from the beam of light was measured. A cutoff time was set at 40 s to prevent tissue damage. Every hind paw was tested alternately at 5 min intervals. The results obtained for each rat were expressed in second as the mean of six withdrawal latencies. Finally, the average value was used for statistical analysis.

Tissue collection, RNA isolation, cDNA library preparation, and sequencing
Animals were deeply anesthetized with isoflurane (3%) at 14 days after surgery and perfused through the ascending aorta with normal saline (100 ml, 4 °C). The L4–5 spinal cord segments that correspond to L4–5 spinal nerve roots and match L1 vertebral level were dissected. The dorsal horns of L4–5 spinal cord were collected. Total RNA was extracted from the dorsal horn tissue using Trizol reagent (Invitrogen, Carlsbad) according to the manufacturer's protocol. RNA quantity and quality were measured using a NanoDrop ND-1000. The cDNA library was constructed using KAPA Stranded RNA-Seq Library Preparation Kit (Illumina) following the manufacturer's protocol. Briefly, poly-(A) mRNA was isolated from total RNA using the NEB-Next Oligo d(T) magnetic beads. Under an elevated temperature, mRNA was fragmented into small pieces after the fragmentation buffer was added. Using the mRNA fragments as templates, the first-strand cDNA

was synthesized with random primers. Then, the second-strand cDNA was obtained using DNA polymerase I and RNase H. The synthetic cDNAs were end-repaired by polymerase and ligated with "A-tailing" base adaptors. Suitable fragments were selected for PCR amplification to construct the final cDNA library. The final double-stranded cDNA samples were verified with an Agilent 2100 Bioanalyzer (Agilent Technologies). After cluster generation (TruSeq SR Cluster Kit v3-cBot-HS, Illumina), sequencing was performed on an Illumina HiSeq 4000 sequencing platform.

RNA-seq data processing

Image analysis, base calling, and error estimation were performed using Illumina/Solexa Pipeline version 1.8 (Off-Line Base Caller software, version 1.8). Quality control was checked on the raw sequence data using FastQC (https://en.wikipedia.org/wiki/FASTQ_format). Raw data were pre-processed using Solexa CHASTITY and Cutadapt to remove adaptor sequences, ribosomal RNA, and other contaminants that may interfere with clustering and assembly. The trimmed reads are mapped to the corresponding reference genome using HISAT2 (version 2.0.4) for RNA-seq, and StringTie (version 1.2.3) was used to reconstruct the transcriptome [16, 17]. Then, Ballgown software was applied to calculate the fragments per kilobase of exon per million fragments mapped (FPKM) in RNA-seq data and analyze DEGs [18, 19], with the FPKM ≥ 0.5 (Cuffquant) considered statistically significant.

Bioinformatics analysis

The Gene Ontology (GO) functional and Kyoto Encyclopedia of Genes and Genomes (KEGG) pathway enrichment analysis were performed for DEGs using the Database for Annotation, Visualization and Integrated Discovery (DAVID) and KEGG Orthology-Based Annotation System (KOBAS) online tools (http://www.geneontology.org and http://www.genome.jp/kegg). Hierarchical cluster analysis was performed for enriched genes by Cluster 3.0 software. The protein-protein interaction (PPI) network of the proteins encoded by the DEGs was searched using STRING online software (http://string-db.org/).

Quantitative reverse transcription-PCR (qRT-PCR) analysis

Thirteen DEGs (11 regulated and 2 downregulated genes) were randomly selected and detected by qRT-PCR. The expression of β-actin mRNA was also determined as an internal control. Total RNA was extracted from the dorsal horn tissue using Trizol reagent (Invitrogen) according to the manufacturer's protocol. RNA concentration was determined spectrophotometrically. cDNA was synthesized using a cDNA synthesis kit (Invitrogen) according to the manufacturer's instructions. Primer sequences are listed in the Table 1. qRT-PCR was performed in triplicates by

using a 7300 real-time PCR system (Applied Biosystems, Foster City, CA) according to the manufacturer's instructions. A comparative cycle of threshold fluorescence (ΔCt) method was used, and the relative transcript amount of target gene was normalized to that of β-actin using the $2^{-\Delta\Delta Ct}$ method. The final results of qRT-PCR were expressed as the ratio of test mRNA to control.

Statistical analysis

Data are presented as the means $\pm$ SEM. The results from the behavioral study were statistically analyzed using repeated measures analysis of variance. qRT-PCR results were analyzed using one-way analysis of variance (ANOVA) followed by Tukey's multiple comparison test. Significance was set at $p < 0.05$.

Results

Model identification of neuropathic pain

The neuropathic pain rat model was established by CCI to the sciatic nerve of the right hind limb in rats. Both mechanical allodynia and thermal sensitivity were determined in all CCI model rats at 0, 1, 3, 7, and 14 days after surgery, respectively. CCI rats exhibited higher sensitivity to mechanical and thermal stimuli from days 1 to 14. Both MWT and TWL reached a steady peak at day 14 after surgery (Fig. 1).

Differential gene expression in the spinal cord

To determine genes that are involved in the pathological process of neuropathic pain, the dorsal horn of L4–5 spinal cord of rats was analyzed using an Illumina HiSeq 4000 sequencing technique at 14 days after CCI surgery. Using the FPKM of ≥ 0.5, abundant expression levels were compared to those of CCI-induced neuropathic pain with control. We identified a total of 17,912 mRNA transcripts corresponding to 14,546 genes in CCI-induced neuropathic pain rat models after 14 days (Additional file 1: Table S1; Additional file 2: Table S2). Sixty-three genes were differentially expressed between CCI-induced neuropathic pain and control tissues (Table 2; Additional file 3: Table S3) using two criteria: a greater than 1.5 fold expression level change and p value ≤ 0.05 from ANOVA test. The related gene expression frequency and abundance in the dorsal horn of the CCI rat were showed in Fig. 2a. These 63 genes included 56 upregulated genes (e.g., Cxcl13, C1qc, Cgr3a) and 7 downregulated genes (e.g., Urgcp, Usp1) as shown in the volcano plot (Fig. 2b).

GO functional analysis of DEGs

According to the functional annotation in GO database, the upregulated DEGs were mostly enriched in biological processes (BP) related to immune and defense responses (Additional file 4: Table S4), cellular component (CC)

Table 1 The primers used in real-time PCR

Primers	Forward	Reverse	Amplicon size (bp)
Cxcl13	GGCCACGGTATTCTGGAGAC	CCATCTGGCAGTAGGATTCACA	192
Reg3b	GTCCTGGATGCTGCTCTCCT	GGCAACTAATGCGTGCAGAG	92
Plac8	AGGCAGCAACAGTTATCGTGAC	CTCATCGCCACCGTTGTTCC	196
C1qc	GTCAAGTTCAATTCCGCCATCAC	TGTGGTGGACGAAGTAGTAGAGG	103
Ccl2	CCTGCTGCTACTCATTCACTGG	TTCTGATCTCACTTGGTTCTGGTC	197
C1qa	TGTCTGTCTATCGTGTCCTCCTC	GATGCTGTCGGCTTCAGTACC	192
C3	TGTGAGCCTGGAGTGGACTAC	CTGAGCCTGACTTGATGACCTG	112
C1qb	AGGTGGCTCTGGAGACTACAAG	GAACTGGCGTGGTAGGTGAAG	198
C4a	CCAGACTCACATCTCCATCTCAAG	CCTCCAGGTCTCCGATCTCAG	80
Ngfr	CCTGCCTGGACAGTGTTACATTCTC	CAGTCTCCTCGTCCTGGTAGTAGC	132
Aif1	CCAACAGGAAGAGAGGTTGGA	CAGCATTCGCTTCAAGGACA	169
Urgcp	ACGTCAGCAGCAACTCCAAG	GGATTCGTGCCTAAGTTGAGGT	106
Dusp1	AGATATGCTCGACGCCTTGG	TGTCTGCCTTGTGGTTGTCC	122
β-actin	TGTCACCAACTGGGACGATA	GGGGTGTTGAAGGTCTCAAA	165

terms such as endocytic vesicle and phagocytic cup (Additional file 5: Table S5), and molecular function (MF) terms related to IgG binding and chemokine activity (Additional file 6: Table S6). The GO enrichment terms of BP, CC, and MF for upregulated DEGs are shown in Fig. 3a.

Meanwhile, the downregulated DEGs were enriched in BP terms such as regulation of spindle checkpoint and inactivation of mitogen-activated protein (MAP) kinase (MAPK) activity (Additional file 7: Table S7), CC terms such as Cul3-RING ubiquitin ligase complex (Additional file 8: Table S8), and MF terms such as MAP kinase phosphatase (MKP) kinase activity (Additional file 9: Table S9). The GO enrichment terms of BP, CC, and MF for downregulated DEGs are shown in Fig. 3b.

KEGG pathway enrichment analysis of DEGs

The DEGs between CCI model and control were subjected to KEGG pathway enrichment analysis using the software KOBAS. The p value < 0.05 was set as the threshold of significant enrichment. Based on the KEGG pathway enrichment analysis, the upregulated DEGs were significantly enriched in 14 signaling pathways, such as complement and coagulation cascades, B cell receptor signaling pathway, cytokine-cytokine receptor interaction, and Fc gamma R-mediated phagocytosis signaling pathway, which were mostly related to immune and inflammatory responses (Fig. 4a, Additional file 10: Table S10). However, none of the downregulated gene was significantly enriched in any KEGG pathway.

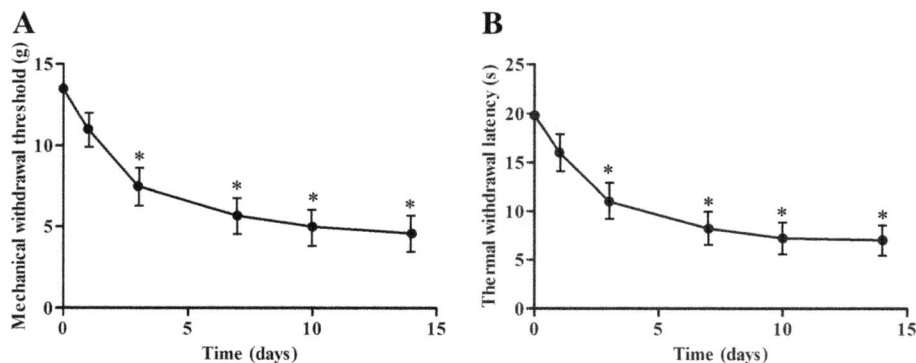

Fig. 1 Nociceptive behavior developed in chronic constriction injury (CCI) model rats. Mechanical withdrawal threshold (MWT) in each time point (**a**) and thermal withdrawal latency (TWL) in each time point (**b**). $n = 6$, *$p < 0.05$ compared with controls

Table 2 The upregulated and downregulated genes in rat neuropathic pain model

Gene name	Locus	Fold change	p value	Biological process
Cxcl13	chr14:15253125-15258207	6.426350091	0.001461007	Chemokine-mediated signaling pathway
Reg3b	chr4:109467272-109470510	4.596165659	0.00238738	Negative regulation of cell death
Plac8	chr14:10692764-10714524	2.75098502	0.02157393	Negative regulation of apoptotic process
C1qc	chr5:155255005-155258392	2.72105301	0.003170161	Innate immune response
Ccl2	chr10:69412017-69413870	2.696533508	0.000586007	Glial cell migration
C1qa	chr5:155261250-155264143	2.585336373	0.001012602	Innate immune response
C3	chr9:9721105-9747167	2.470300657	0.007779142	Complement activation
C1qb	chr5:155246447-155252003	2.318601492	0.004223697	Innate immune response
C4a	chr20:4302347-4508214	2.268474076	0.003906162	Complement activation
C4a	chr20:2651599-2678141	2.117474349	0.002292613	Complement activation
Fcer1g	chr13:89601896-89606326	1.897610848	0.009152089	Innate immune response
Ngfr	chr10:83389847-83408061	1.889723015	0.012534711	Sensory perception of pain
Fcgr3a	chr13:89385859-89396051	1.846156689	0.020151454	Regulation of sensory perception of pain
Fyb	chr2:55835151-55983804	1.841013316	0.003152222	Immune response
Fcgr1a	chr2:198430530-198458041	1.820562407	0.032185553	Regulation of immune response
LOC103691423	chr2:23260651-23260965	1.812907143	0.032394733	
Cd22	chr1:89314558-89329418	1.806446581	0.027087834	Cell adhesion
Gapt	chr2:41869556-41871858	1.801373741	0.01683096	Innate immune response
Ly86	chr17:28104589-28191436	1.801122811	0.029526635	Innate immune response
Cd33	chr1:98398660-98402968	1.787375322	0.005028128	Regulation of immune response
Pld4	chr6:137323713-137331231	1.78323674	0.008341961	Phagocytosis
Ltc4s	chr10:35737664-35739625	1.774305996	0.014581973	Response to axon injury
Cd53	chr2:209489279-209537087	1.752658145	0.009085537	Cell surface receptor signaling pathway
Ctsz	chr3:172527107-172537877	1.750656844	0.009448762	Regulation of neuron death
Clec4a1	chr4:155947453-155959993	1.73513319	0.007661068	Adaptive immune response
Rpe65	chr2:266141581-266169197	1.717980882	0.005397693	Cellular response to electrical stimulus
Irf8	chr19:54314865-54336640	1.713827049	0.025622097	Phagocytosis
Atf3	chr13:109817728-109849632	1.667935639	0.005824841	Positive regulation of cell proliferation
Apobec1	chr4:155386711-155401480	1.665506432	0.016894935	Regulation of cell proliferation
Tmem176a	chr4:78458625-78462423	1.661562833	0.01247483	Cell differentiation
Cyp4b1	chr5:134508730-134526089	1.656053246	0.040180738	Cell differentiation
Gpr31	chr1:53519829-53520788	1.649462641	0.019751159	signal transduction
Aoah	chr17:45872414-46115004	1.639719248	0.031572447	Inflammatory response
LOC102557117	chr5:187312-187688	1.636194027	0.027745501	
Clec7a	chr4:163216163-163227334	1.629244213	0.022249116	Innate immune response
Bin2	chr7:142273833-142300382	1.625336862	0.00919119	Cell chemotaxis
Gpr34	chrX:10023489-10031167	1.618400204	0.007940879	Signal transduction
Mx1	chr11:37891156-37914983	1.613580093	0.003770887	Innate immune response
Gpr183	chr15:108364701-108376221	1.613459608	0.003571085	Adaptive immune response
AABR07001573.2	chr1:53220397-53284319	1.605472328	0.042391557	
Cd68	chr10:56268720-56270640	1.59862216	0.025231623	Neutrophil degranulation
AC115371.1	chr15:33606124-33611579	1.597574602	0.016091626	
Oosp1	chr1:228032983-228053645	1.593938444	0.009835678	Response to stimulus
Tmem176b	chr4:78450724-78458179	1.581317379	0.012542608	Cell differentiation

Table 2 The upregulated and downregulated genes in rat neuropathic pain model *(Continued)*

Gene name	Locus	Fold change	p value	Biological process
Adgre1	chr9:9431860-9585865	1.578724864	0.04691516	Adaptive immune response
Fcgr2b	chr13:89327794-89433815	1.569218908	0.024948119	Immune response
Cyth4	chr7:119820537-119845003	1.56917098	0.047508716	Regulation of molecular function
Aif1	chr20:5161333-5166448	1.565044457	0.027459054	Response to axon injury
Plek	chr14:100151210-100217913	1.548834783	0.020475153	Integrin-mediated signaling pathway
Wipf3	chr4:84597323-84676775	1.545203106	0.024900292	Cell differentiation
Itgad	chr1:199495298-199623960	1.537780288	0.044440601	Microglial cell activation
RGD1309350	chr1:213577122-213580542	1.527740296	0.000267242	Purine nucleobase metabolic process
Anxa3	chr14:14364008-14426437	1.51105029	0.043685994	Phagocytosis
Laptm5	chr5:149047681-149069719	1.508262862	0.03919455	Transport
Tmem154	chr2:183674522-183711812	1.504875551	0.034809815	
Csf1r	chr18:56414488-56458300	1.503532191	0.008357977	Cytokine-mediated signaling pathway
Urgcp	chr14:85957716-85991211	0.32013414	0.002977579	Cell cycle
LOC500300	chr4:148782479-148784562	0.58414901	0.0290017	Regulation of autophagy
Klhdc7a	chr5:158436757-158439078	0.594907041	0.026052604	Protein ubiquitination
AABR07026893.1	chr17:3729421-3729810	0.620034111	0.041049018	
Dusp1	chr10:16970626-16973418	0.627386061	0.031077843	Inactivation of MAPK activity
Plac9	chr16:3851270-3866008	0.633314755	0.03114494	
AABR07042903.1	chr19:14345993-14346891	0.666129407	0.046588447	

Hierarchical cluster analysis of DEGs

To elucidate the role of DEGs in CCI model tissues, DEGs were hierarchically clustered dependent on the gene enrichment features of control against CCI model tissues (Fig. 4b). The most prominently upregulated genes consisted of families of chemokines (Cxcl13 and Ccl2), complement components (C1qc, Ccl2, C1qa, C3, C1qb, and C4a), Fc fragment receptors (Fcer1g, Fcgr3a, Fcgr1a, and Fcgr2b), cluster of differentiations (Cd22, Cd33, Cd53, and Cd68), and G protein-coupled receptors (Gpr31, Gpr34, and Gpr183). Strikingly, chemokine genes showed the greatest upregulation such as Cxcl13

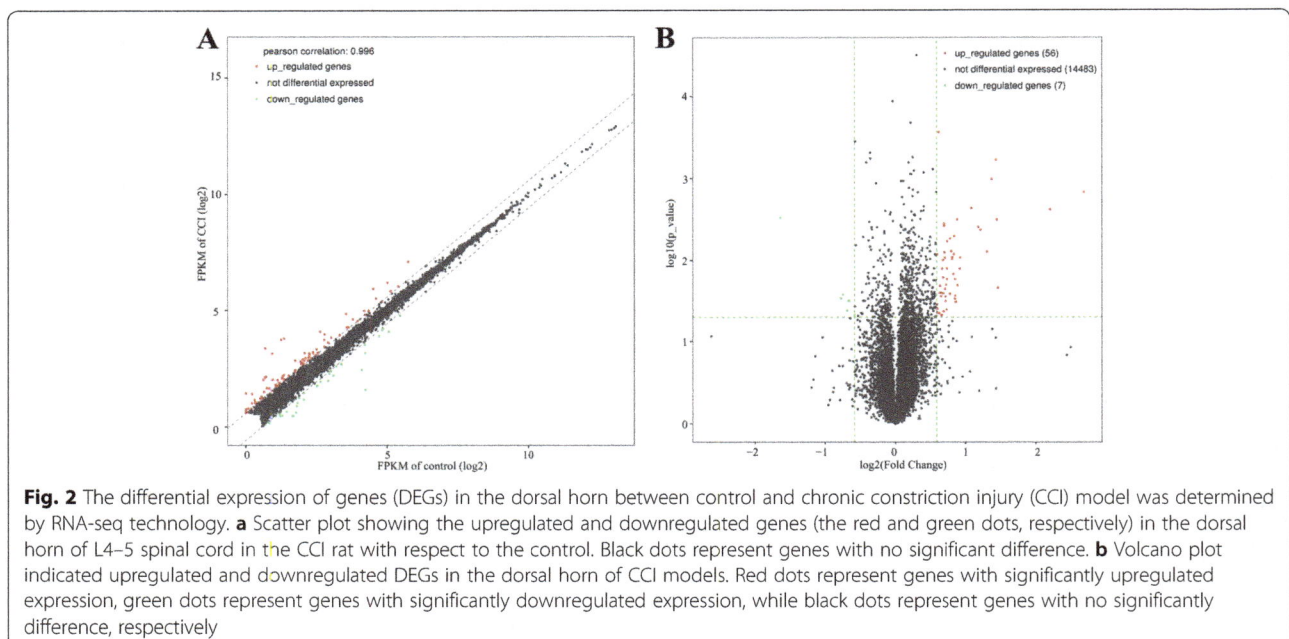

Fig. 2 The differential expression of genes (DEGs) in the dorsal horn between control and chronic constriction injury (CCI) model was determined by RNA-seq technology. **a** Scatter plot showing the upregulated and downregulated genes (the red and green dots, respectively) in the dorsal horn of L4–5 spinal cord in the CCI rat with respect to the control. Black dots represent genes with no significant difference. **b** Volcano plot indicated upregulated and downregulated DEGs in the dorsal horn of CCI models. Red dots represent genes with significantly upregulated expression, green dots represent genes with significantly downregulated expression, while black dots represent genes with no significantly difference, respectively

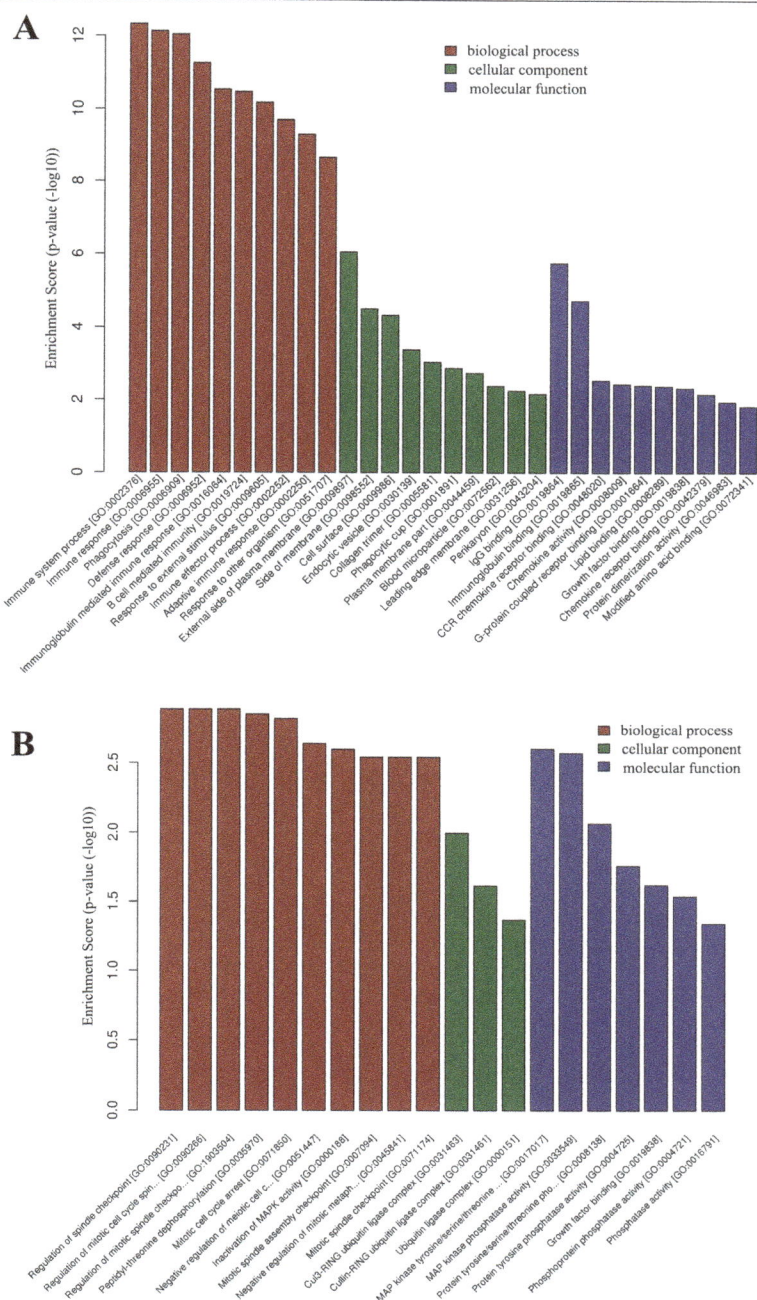

Fig. 3 The Gene Ontology (GO) analysis of differentially expressed genes (DEGs) in the dorsal horn of chronic constriction injury (CCI) rats. GO annotation of upregulated DEGs (**a**) and downregulated DEGs (**b**) of CCI model versus control. Bar plots show the top ten enrichment score ($-\log_{10}(p$ value)) values of the significant enrichment terms of DEGs involving biological process, cellular component, and molecular function

(6.426 fold increase). Most of these genes which have previously been linked to immune and inflammation-related pathways have not been reported in neuropathic pain; and only 20 genes (e.g., Cxcl13, C1qc, Ccl2, C1qa, Fcer1g, Ngfr, Cd53, Cd68, Dusp1) have been demonstrated to be involved in this pathogenesis. This clustering analysis of RNA-seq data will indicate that the DEGs in CCI model are closely associated with the development of neuropathic pain.

PPI network analysis

To investigate the interaction and hub genes of DEGs involved in pathogenesis of neuropathic pain, the DEGs PPI network were constructed using STRING. The results

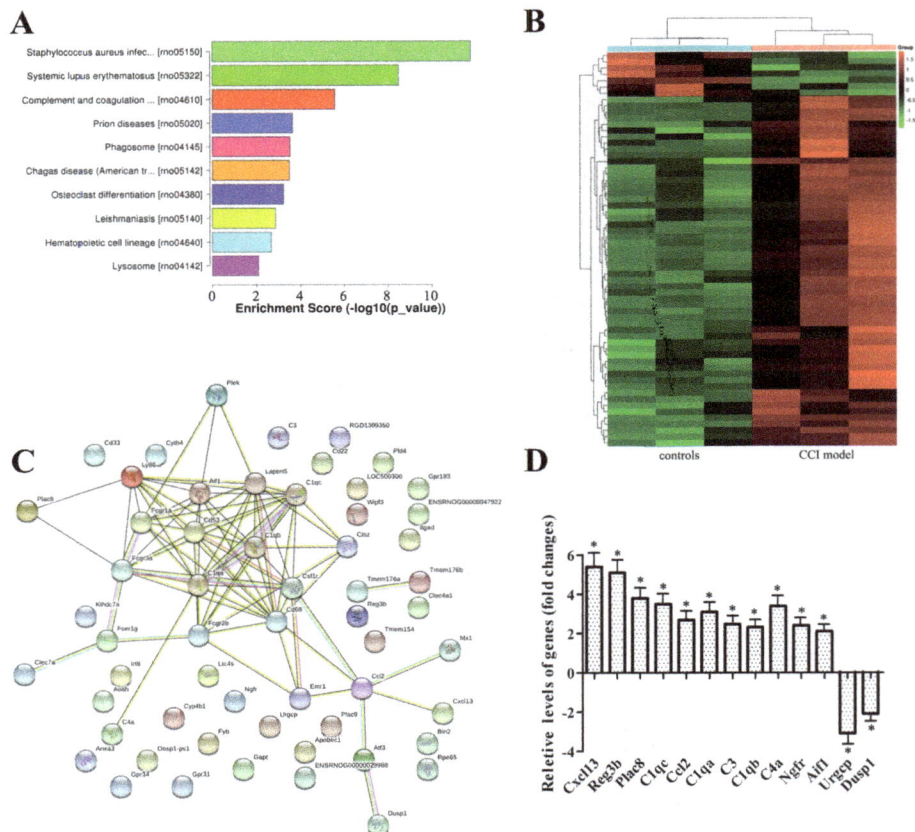

Fig. 4 Kyoto Encyclopedia of Genes and Genomes (KEGG), hierarchical clustering, and protein-protein interaction (PPI) network analysis of differentially expressed genes (DEGs) in the dorsal horn of chronic constriction injury (CCI) rats. **a** Histogram of KEGG pathway enrichment distribution of DEGs. The bar plot shows the top ten enrichment score ($-\log_{10}(p$ value)) value of the significant enrichment pathway. **b** Heat map of DEGs showing hierarchical clustering of changed DEGs of rats in CCI group compared with control group. In clustering analysis, upregulated and downregulated genes are colored in red and green, respectively. **c** STRING analysis for biological interactions within DEGs of RNA-seq datasets, involved in immune and inflammatory function. The line color indicates the type of interaction evidence, and line thickness indicates the strength of data support. **d** Quantitative reverse transcription-PCR (qRT-PCR) analysis for differences in expression levels of DEGs in the dorsal horn between CCI models and controls. Results were calculated by normalizing to β-actin in the same sample with the ΔCt method. Changes in relative levels of gene mRNAs expressed as folds of controls. All values were mean ± SEM. *$p < 0.05$ ($n = 3$)

demonstrated that the predicted PPI in CCI rats were driving the complex interaction network at 14 days after CCI (Fig. 4c). The established PPI network (PPI enrichment p value < 1.0e−16) contained 58 nodes (hub genes) and 77 edges (interactions). Five of the top genes with relatively high connectivity degrees (≥ 11) were high lighted: Cd68 (degree = 14), C1qc (degree = 12), C1qa (degree = 11), Laptm5 (degree = 11), and Fcgr3a (degree = 11). Many novel DEGs that we screened may play an important role through regulation of protein expression in neuropathic pain, but future in-depth studies are required.

Validation by qRT-PCR
To evaluate the reliability of the Illumina sequencing technology, 13 DEGs (11 upregulated and 2 downregulated genes) were randomly selected and detected by qRT-PCR. Figure 4d shows that the upregulation or

downregulation trend of candidate genes between CCI-induced model and control group revealed by the qRT-PCR data is congruent with that revealed by RNA-seq method. The result of qRT-PCR analyses provides evidence that the RNA-seq method for the large-scale gene expression quantification was reliable.

Discussion
In this study, we profiled gene expression in the dorsal horn following CCI-induced neuropathic pain, using RNA-seq method. Sixty-three DEGs were identified in CCI rat model, including 56 upregulated and 7 downregulated genes. We also predicted potential functions of DEGs using GO, KEGG pathway, and PPI network analysis in the CCI model. These findings prompted the proposal that DEGs played a significant role in neuropathic pain processing,

and sequencing analysis revealed a potential therapeutic target of neuropathic pain.

Accumulating evidence showed that Cxcl13 and Ccl2 are known to be involved in pathogenesis of neuropathic pain via different forms of neuron-glia interaction in the spinal cord [20, 21]. The chemokines by binding to the G protein-coupled receptors play an essential role in pathological pain conditions triggered by either peripheral inflammation or nerve injury [23, 24]. Our results demonstrated that chemokine genes showed the greatest upregulation, such as Cxcl13 (6.426 fold increase), suggesting that chemokines play a crucial role in the development of neuropathic pain. Furthermore, complements, a key component of the innate immune system and potentially important trigger of some types of neuropathic pain, have been associated with neuroinflammation [22, 25, 26]. Previous study showed that C1qc, C1qa, and Fcer1g might contribute to the generation of neuropathic pain after SNI via immune and defense pathways [26]. Activation of Cd68, the inflammatory microglia-dominant molecule, could result in neuropathic pain in mice with peripheral nerve injury [27]. Cd53, the inflammation-related gene, is chronically upregulated after spinal cord injury [28, 29]. The up-expression of nerve growth factor (NGF) and the NGF receptor is involved in regulating the function of sensory and the development of neuropathic pain [30]. In the present study, upregulated genes included chemokines, complement components, Fc fragment receptors, cluster of differentiations, G protein-coupled receptors, and NGF receptor. Most of the genes are well known in neuropathic pain (e.g., Cxcl13, C1qc, Ccl2) [20–30], suggesting DEGs with the differential functions in diverse cellular pathways, and many are involved in neuropathic pain development and progression.

Previous study demonstrated that Urgcp plays a critical role in glial cell cycle and cell proliferation [31]. Dusp1, a MKP-1, plays a pivotal role in controlling MAPK-dependent inflammatory responses [32]. In the present study, we found that Urgcp and Dusp1 displayed obvious down-expression in CCI rats, which would provide a better understanding of immune and glia cell proliferation, as well as MAPK-dependent inflammatory response abnormalities involved in the neuropathic pain of CCI rats.

In order to obtain insights into DEGs function, GO analysis annotation was applied to the DEG gene pool. GO terms for biological process categories included immune system process, phagocytosis, defense response, and response to external stimulus. Several studies using SNI rat model have reported that key higher expressed genes included those associated with immune and inflammatory pathways in neuropathic pain [20–30], similar to those in CCI model we observed. GO functional analysis showed that downregulated DEGs might associate with inactivation

of MAPK activity in CCI models. Inhibition of MAPKs results in downregulation of downstream molecules (cytokines, chemokines, nitric oxide, etc.) in immunocompetent cells and depresses the excitability of neurons in the spinal cord [33, 34]. Therefore, spinal MAPK signaling pathway, such as p38-MAPK (p38) or extracellular receptor-activated kinases (ERKs), may play an important role in the development of chronic allodynia in CCI [35].

PPI network analysis showed that Cd68, C1qc, C1qa, Laptm5, and Fcgr3a were crucial nodes with high connectivity degrees. Laptm5 and Fcgr3a which have previously been linked to immune and inflammation-related pathways have not been reported in neuropathic pain [36, 37]; and other three genes (Cd68, C1qc, and C1qa) have been demonstrated to be involved in this pathogenesis [26, 27]. Previous study showed that Laptm5 is involved in the dynamics of lysosomal membranes associated with microglial activation after nerve injury [36]. Upregulation of Fcgr3a increased the microglial phagocytic capacity in neuroinflammation [37]. It might be inferred that Laptm5 and Fcgr3a are neuroinflammation-related genes that influence neuropathic pain behavior after CCI.

Conclusions

In conclusion, our results suggest that genes involved in immune and defense responses are affected most significantly after CCI. Genes like Cxcl13, Cd68, C1qc, Laptm5, and Fcgr3a are crucial for neuropathic pain after CCI in rat models. These genes could be used as novel diagnostic and therapeutic targets against CCI-induced neuropathic pain. However, the predicted expressions and interactions need to be further validated by extensive experiments.

Additional files

Additional file 1: Table S1. All expressed transcripts in chronic constriction injury (CCI) model rats. (XLSX 3674 kb)

Additional file 2: Table S2. All expressed genes in chronic constriction injury (CCI) model rats. (XLSX 2944 kb)

Additional file 3: Table S3. Differentially expressed genes (DEGs) in chronic constriction injury (CCI) model rats. (XLSX 19 kb)

Additional file 4: Table S4. Biological processes (BP) result of the upregulated differentially expressed genes (DEGs) in chronic constriction injury (CCI) model rats. (XLS 162 kb)

Additional file 5: Table S5. Cellular component (CC) result of the upregulated differentially expressed genes (DEGs) in chronic constriction injury (CCI) model rats. (XLS 34 kb)

Additional file 6: Table S6. Molecular function (MF) result of the upregulated differentially expressed genes (DEGs) in chronic constriction injury (CCI) model rats. (XLS 33 kb)

Additional file 7: Table S7. Biological processes (BP) result of the downregulated differentially expressed genes (DEGs) in chronic constriction injury (CCI) model rats. (XLS 52 kb)

Additional file 8: Table S8. Cellular component (CC) result of the downregulated differentially expressed genes (DEGs) in chronic constriction injury (CCI) model rats. (XLS 28 kb)

Additional file 9: Table S9. Molecular function (MF) result of the downregulated differentially expressed genes (DEGs) in chronic constriction injury (CCI) model rats. (XLS 29 kb)

Additional file 10: Table S10. Kyoto Encyclopedia of Genes and Genomes (KEGG) result of the upregulated differentially expressed genes (DEGs) in chronic constriction injury (CCI) model rats. (XLS 35 kb)

Abbreviations

BP: Biological processes; CC: Cellular component; CCI: Chronic constriction injury; DAVID: Database for Annotation, Visualization and Integrated Discovery; DEGs: Differentially expressed genes; ERKs: Extracellular receptor-activated kinases; FPKM: Fragments per kilobase of exon per million fragments mapped; GO: Gene Ontology; KEGG: Kyoto Encyclopedia of Genes and Genomes; KOBAS: KEGG Orthology-Based Annotation System; MAPK: Mitogen-activated protein (MAP) kinases; MF: Molecular function; MKP: MAP kinase phosphatase; MWT: Mechanical withdrawal threshold; NGF: Nerve growth factor; PPI: Protein-protein interaction; qRT-PCR: Quantitative reverse transcription-PCR; RNA-seq: RNA sequencing; SNI: Spared nerve injury; TWL: Thermal withdrawal latency

Acknowledgements

The authors would like to thank Dr. Zhen Ye for skillful assistance in protein-protein interaction (PPI) network analysis. RNA-seq experiments were performed by KangChen Bio-tech, Shanghai, China.

Funding

This work was supported by the National Natural Science Foundation of China (31871215) and Scientific Research Projects of Colleges and Universities in Shandong Province (J15LK07).

Authors' contributions

ZW, HD, and JS designed the overall project. JS, MW, SA, and XG performed the experiments. ZW, HD, and JS were responsible for the analysis and interpretation of the data and drafted the manuscript. All authors revised and approved the final manuscript.

Competing interests

The authors declare that they have no competing interests.

Author details

[1]Department of Histology and Embryology, Taishan Medical University, Taian 271000, China. [2]Department of Human Anatomy, Taishan Medical University, Taian 271000, China. [3]Department of Physiology, Taishan Medical University, Taian 271000, China.

References

1. Baron R, Binder A, Wasner G. Neuropathic pain: diagnosis, pathophysiological mechanisms, and treatment. Lancet Neurol. 2010;9:807–19. https://doi.org/10.1016/S1474-4422(10)70143-5.
2. Hayashi Y, Kawaji K, Sun L, Zhang X, Koyano K, Yokoyama T, Kohsaka S, Inoue K, Nakanishi H. Microglial Ca(2+)-activated K(+) channels are possible molecular targets for the analgesic effects of S-ketamine on neuropathic pain. J Neurosci. 2011;31:17370–82. https://doi.org/10.1523/JNEUROSCI.4152-11.2011.
3. Leng C, Chen L, Gong X, Ma B, Gan W, Si Y, Xiao H, Li C. Upregulation of P2X2 and P2X3 receptors in rats with hyperalgesia induced by heroin withdrawal. Neuroreport. 2018;29:678–84. https://doi.org/10.1097/WNR.0000000000001018.
4. Sumizono M, Sakakima H, Otsuka S, Terashi T, Nakanishi K, Ueda K, Takada S, Kikuchi K. The effect of exercise frequency on neuropathic pain and pain-related cellular reactions in the spinal cord and midbrain in a rat sciatic nerve injury model. J Pain Res. 2018;11:281–91. https://doi.org/10.2147/JPR.S156326.
5. Da Silva JT, Evangelista BG, Venega RAG, Oliveira ME, Chacur M. Early and late behavioral changes in sciatic nerve injury may be modulated by nerve growth factor and substance P in rats: a chronic constriction injury long-term evaluation. J Biol Regul Homeost Agents. 2017;31:309–19.
6. Zhang Y, Chi D. Overexpression of SIRT2 alleviates neuropathic pain and neuroinflammation through deacetylation of transcription factor nuclear factor-kappa B. Inflammation. 2018;41:569–78. https://doi.org/10.1007/s10753-017-0713-3.
7. Ghasemzadeh Rahbardar M, Amin B, Mehri S, Mirnajafi-Zadeh SJ, Hosseinzadeh H. Anti-inflammatory effects of ethanolic extract of Rosmarinus officinalis L. and rosmarinic acid in a rat model of neuropathic pain. Biomed Pharmacother. 2017;86:441–9. https://doi.org/10.1016/j.biopha.2016.12.049.
8. Austin PJ, Moalem-Taylor G. The neuro-immune balance in neuropathic pain: involvement of inflammatory immune cells, immune-like glial cells and cytokines. J Neuroimmunol. 2010;229:26–50. https://doi.org/10.1016/j.jneuroim.2010.08.013.
9. Cook AD, Christensen AD, Tewari D, McMahon SB, Hamilton JA. Immune cytokines and their receptors in inflammatory pain. Trends Immunol. 2018;39:240–55. https://doi.org/10.1016/j.it.2017.12.003.
10. Liu H, Xia T, Xu F, Ma Z, Gu X. Identification of the key genes associated with neuropathic pain. Mol Med Rep. 2018;17:6371–8. https://doi.org/10.3892/mmr.2018.8718.
11. Kummer KK, Kalpachidou T, Kress M, Langeslag M. Signatures of altered gene expression in dorsal root ganglia of a Fabry disease mouse model. Front Mol Neurosci. 2018;10:449. https://doi.org/10.3389/fnmol.2017.00449.
12. Chen CJ, Liu DZ, Yao WF, Gu Y, Huang F, Hei ZQ, Li X. Identification of key genes and pathways associated with neuropathic pain in uninjured dorsal root ganglion by using bioinformatic analysis. J Pain Res. 2017;10:2665–74. https://doi.org/10.2147/JPR.S143431.
13. Vallejo R, Tilley DM, Cedeño DL, Kelley CA, DeMaegd M, Benyamin R. Genomics of the effect of spinal cord stimulation on an animal model of neuropathic pain. Neuromodulation. 2016;19:576–86. https://doi.org/10.1111/ner.12465.
14. Hong H, Hong Q, Liu J, Tong W, Shi L. Estimating relative noise to signal in DNA microarray data. Int J Bioinforma Res Appl. 2013;9:433–48. https://doi.org/10.1504/IJBRA.2013.056085.
15. Fox A, Kesingland A, Gentry C, McNair K, Patel S, Urban L, James I. The role of central and peripheral cannabinoid1 receptors in the antihyperalgesic activity of cannabinoids in a model of neuropathic pain. Pain. 2001;92:91–100.
16. Kim D, Langmead B, Salzberg SL. HISAT: a fast spliced aligner with low memory requirements. Nat Methods. 2015;12:357–60. https://doi.org/10.1038/nmeth.3317.
17. Pertea M, Pertea GM, Antonescu CM, Chang TC, Mendell JT, Salzberg SL. StringTie enables improved reconstruction of a transcriptome from RNA-seq reads. Nat Biotechnol. 2015;33:290–5. https://doi.org/10.1038/nbt.3122.
18. Frazee AC, Pertea G, Jaffe AE, Langmead B, Salzberg SL, Leek JT. Ballgown bridges the gap between transcriptome assembly and expression analysis. Nat Biotechnol. 2015;33:243–6. https://doi.org/10.1038/nbt.3172.
19. Mortazavi A, Williams BA, McCue K, Schaeffer L, Wold B. Mapping and quantifying mammalian transcriptomes by RNA-Seq. Nat Methods. 2008;5:621–8. https://doi.org/10.1038/nmeth.1226.
20. Zhang ZJ, Jiang BC, Gao YJ. Chemokines in neuron-glial cell interaction and pathogenesis of neuropathic pain. Cell Mol Life Sci. 2017;74:3275–91. https://doi.org/10.1007/s00018-017-2513-1.
21. Al-Mazidi S, Alotaibi M, Nedjadi T, Chaudhary A, Alzoghaibi M, Djouhri L. Blocking of cytokines signaling attenuates evoked and spontaneous neuropathic pain behaviours in the paclitaxel rat model of chemotherapy-induced neuropathy. Eur J Pain. 2018;22:810–21. https://doi.org/10.1002/ejp.1169.
22. Xu J, Zhang L, Xie M, Li Y, Huang P, Saunders TL, Fox DA, Rosenquist R, Lin F. Role of complement in a rat model of paclitaxel-induced peripheral neuropathy. J Immunol. 2018;200:4094–101. https://doi.org/10.4049/jimmunol.1701716.
23. Martínez-Muñoz L, Villares R, Rodríguez-Fernández JL, Rodríguez-Frade JM, Mellado M. Remodeling our concept of chemokine receptor function: from monomers to oligomers. J Leukoc Biol. 2018;104:323–31. https://doi.org/10.1002/JLB.2MR1217-503R.

24. Silva RL, Lopes AH, Guimarães RM, Cunha TM. CXCL1/CXCR2 signaling in pathological pain: role in peripheral and central sensitization. Neurobiol Dis. 2017;105:109–16. https://doi.org/10.1016/j.nbd.2017.06.001.

25. Kallio-Laine K, Seppänen M, Lokki ML, Lappalainen M, Notkola IL, Seppälä I, Koskinen M, Valtonen V, Kalso E. Widespread unilateral pain associated with herpes simplex virus infections. J Pain. 2008;9:658–65. https://doi.org/10.1016/j.jpain.2008.02.003.

26. Wang J, Ma SH, Tao R, Xia LJ, Liu L, Jiang YH. Gene expression profile changes in rat dorsal horn after sciatic nerve injury. Neurol Res. 2017;39: 176–82. https://doi.org/10.1080/01616412.2016.1273590.

27. Kiguchi N, Kobayashi D, Saika F, Matsuzaki S, Kishioka S. Inhibition of peripheral macrophages by nicotinic acetylcholine receptor agonists suppresses spinal microglial activation and neuropathic pain in mice with peripheral nerve injury. J Neuroinflammation. 2018;15:96. https://doi.org/10.1186/s12974-018-1133-5.

28. Giardini AC, Dos Santos FM, da Silva JT, de Oliveira ME, Martins DO, Chacur M. Neural mobilization treatment decreases glial cells and brain-derived neurotrophic factor expression in the central nervous system in rats with neuropathic pain induced by CCI in rats. Pain Res Manag. 2017;2017: 7429761. https://doi.org/10.1155/2017/7429761.

29. Byrnes KR, Washington PM, Knoblach SM, Hoffman E, Faden AI. Delayed inflammatory mRNA and protein expression after spinal cord injury. J Neuroinflammation. 2011;8:130. https://doi.org/10.1186/1742-2094-8-130.

30. Patel MK, Kaye AD, Urman RD. Tanezumab: therapy targeting nerve growth factor in pain pathogenesis. J Anaesthesiol Clin Pharmacol. 2018;34:111–6. https://doi.org/10.4103/joacp.JOACP_389_15.

31. Dodurga Y, Seçme M, Eroğlu C, Gündoğdu G, Avcı ÇB, Bağcı G, Küçükatay V, Lale Şatıroğlu-Tufan N. Investigation of the effects of a sulfite molecule on human neuroblastoma cells via a novel oncogene URG4/URGCP. Life Sci. 2015;143:27–34. https://doi.org/10.1016/j.lfs.2015.10.005.

32. Kim H, Woo JH, Lee JH, Joe EH, Jou I. 22(R)-hydroxycholesterol induces HuR-dependent MAP kinase phosphatase-1 expression via mGluR5-mediated Ca(2+)/PKCα signaling. Biochim Biophys Acta. 2016; 1859:1056–70. https://doi.org/10.1016/j.bbagrm.2016.05.008.

33. Monneau YR, Luo L, Sankaranarayanan NV, Nagarajan B, Vivès RR, Baleux F, Desai UR, Arenzana-Seisdedos F, Lortat-Jacob H. Solution structure of CXCL13 and heparan sulfate binding show that GAG binding site and cellular signalling rely on distinct domains. Open Biol. 2017;7. pii: 170133. https://doi.org/10.1098/rsob.170133.

34. Landry RP, Martinez E, DeLeo JA, Romero-Sandoval EA. Spinal cannabinoid receptor type 2 agonist reduces mechanical allodynia and induces mitogen-activated protein kinase phosphatases in a rat model of neuropathic pain. J Pain. 2012;13:836–48. https://doi.org/10.1016/j.jpain.2012.05.013.

35. Kawasaki Y, Kohno T, Zhuang ZY, Brenner GJ, Wang H, Van Der Meer C, Befort K, Woolf CJ, Ji RR. Ionotropic and metabotropic receptors, protein kinase A, protein kinase C, and Src contribute to C-fiber-induced ERK activation and cAMP response element-binding protein phosphorylation in dorsal horn neurons, leading to central sensitization. J Neurosci. 2004;24:8310–21.

36. Origasa M, Tanaka S, Suzuki K, Tone S, Lim B, Koike T. Activation of a novel microglial gene encoding a lysosomal membrane protein in response to neuronal apoptosis. Brain Res Mol Brain Res. 2001;88:1–13.

37. Sivagnanam V, Zhu X, Schlichter LC. Dominance of E. coli phagocytosis over LPS in the inflammatory response of microglia. J Neuroimmunol. 2010;227: 111–9. https://doi.org/10.1016/j.jneuroim.2010.06.021.

Permissions

The contributors of this book come from diverse backgrounds, making this book a truly international effort. This book will bring forth new frontiers with its revolutionizing research information and detailed analysis of the nascent developments around the world.

We would like to thank all the contributing authors for lending their expertise to make the book truly unique. They have played a crucial role in the development of this book. Without their invaluable contributions this book wouldn't have been possible. They have made vital efforts to compile up to date information on the varied aspects of this subject to make this book a valuable addition to the collection of many professionals and students.

This book was conceptualized with the vision of imparting up-to-date information and advanced data in this field. To ensure the same, a matchless editorial board was set up. Every individual on the board went through rigorous rounds of assessment to prove their worth. After which they invested a large part of their time researching and compiling the most relevant data for our readers.

The editorial board has been involved in producing this book since its inception. They have spent rigorous hours researching and exploring the diverse topics which have resulted in the successful publishing of this book. They have passed on their knowledge of decades through this book. To expedite this challenging task, the publisher supported the team at every step. A small team of assistant editors was also appointed to further simplify the editing procedure and attain best results for the readers.

Apart from the editorial board, the designing team has also invested a significant amount of their time in understanding the subject and creating the most relevant covers. They scrutinized every image to scout for the most suitable representation of the subject and create an appropriate cover for the book.

The publishing team has been an ardent support to the editorial, designing and production team. Their endless efforts to recruit the best for this project, has resulted in the accomplishment of this book. They are a veteran in the field of academics and their pool of knowledge is as vast as their experience in printing. Their expertise and guidance has proved useful at every step. Their uncompromising quality standards have made this book an exceptional effort. Their encouragement from time to time has been an inspiration for everyone.

The publisher and the editorial board hope that this book will prove to be a valuable piece of knowledge for researchers, students, practitioners and scholars across the globe.

List of Contributors

M. S. Unger, P. Schernthaner, J. Marschallinger, H. Mrowetz and L. Aigner
Institute of Molecular Regenerative Medicine, Paracelsus Medical University, Strubergasse 21, 5020 Salzburg, Austria
Spinal Cord Injury and Tissue Regeneration Center Salzburg (SCI-TReCS), Paracelsus Medical University, Salzburg, Austria

J. Marschallinger
Department of Neurology and Neurological Sciences, Stanford University School of Medicine, Stanford, USA

Tianjiao Duan, Alex J. Smith and Alan S. Verkman
Departments of Medicine and Physiology, University of California, 1246 Health Sciences East Tower, 513 Parnassus Ave, San Francisco, CA 94143-0521, USA

Tianjiao Duan
Department of Neurology, Second Xiangya Hospital of Central South University, Changsha 410011, Hunan, People's Republic of China

Sunny Malhotra, Carme Costa, Luciana Midaglia, Nicolás Fissolo, Jordi Río, Joaquín Castilló, Xavier Montalban and Manuel Comabella
Servei de Neurologia-Neuroimmunologia, Centre d'Esclerosi Múltiple de Catalunya (Cemcat), Institut de Recerca Vall d'Hebron (VHIR), Hospital Universitari Vall d'Hebron, Universitat Autònoma de Barcelona, Barcelona, Spain

Luisa M. Villar, Silvia Medina and José C. Álvarez-Cermeño
Departments of Neurology and Immunology, Hospital Universitario Ramón y Cajal, Instituto Ramón y Cajal de Investigacion Sanitaria, Madrid, Spain

Marta Cubedo
Departament d'Estadística, Facultat de Biologia, Universitat de Barcelona, Barcelona, Spain

Alex Sánchez
Unitat d'Estadística i Bioinformàtica, Institut de Recerca, HUVH, Barcelona, Spain

Genetics, Microbiology and Statistics Department, Universitat de Barcelona, Barcelona, Spain

V. Alexandra Moser, Mariana F. Uchoa and Christian J. Pike
Neuroscience Graduate Program, University of Southern California, 3641 Watt Way, HNB 120, Los Angeles, CA 90089, USA

Christian J. Pike
Leonard Davis School of Gerontology, University of Southern California, 3715 McClintock Avenue, Los Angeles, CA 90089-0191, USA

Yao-Jun Cai, Fen Wang, Zhang-Xiang Chen, Li Li, Hua Fan, Zhang-Bi Wu and De-Fa Zhu
Department of Endocrinology, Anhui Geriatric Institute, the First Affiliated Hospital of Anhui Medical University, Hefei 230032, China

Jin-Fang Ge
Anhui Key Laboratory of Bioactivity of Natural Products, School of Pharmacy, Anhui Medical University, Hefei 230032, China

Wen Hu
Department of Pathology, Anhui Provincial Hospital Affiliated to Anhui Medical University, Hefei 230032, China

Qu-Nan Wang
Department of Toxicology, School of Public Health, Anhui Medical University, Hefei 230032, China

Yuan Tang, Fariborz Soroush, Jordan C. Langston, Qingliang Yang and Mohammad F. Kiani
Department of Mechanical Engineering, College of Engineering, Temple University, Philadelphia, PA 19122, USA

Shuang Sun and Laurie E. Kilpatrick
Center for Inflammation, Clinical and Translational Lung Research, Lewis Katz School of Medicine, Temple University, Philadelphia, PA 19140, USA

Elisabetta Liverani
Sol Sherry Thrombosis Research Center, Lewis Katz School of Medicine, Temple University, Philadelphia, PA 19140, USA

Mohammad F. Kiani
Department of Radiation Oncology, Lewis Katz School of Medicine, Temple University, Philadelphia, PA 19140, USA

Peter L. P. Smith, Amin Mottahedin, Pernilla Svedin, Carl-Johan Mohn, Henrik Hagberg, Joakim Ek and Carina Mallard
Institute of Neuroscience and Physiology, Department of Physiology, Sahlgrenska Academy, University of Gothenburg, SE-405 30 Gothenburg, Sweden

Henrik Hagberg
Institute of Clinical Sciences, Department of Obstetrics and Gynaecology, Sahlgrenska Academy, University of Gothenburg, Gothenburg, Sweden

Tanja Blume, Carola Focke, Maximilian Deussing, Nathalie L. Albert, Simon Lindner, Franz-Josef Gildehaus, Barbara von Ungern-Sternberg, Peter Bartenstein, Axel Rominger and Matthias Brendel
Department of Nuclear Medicine, University Hospital, LMU Munich, Marchioninistraße 15, 81377 Munich, Germany

Tanja Blume, Finn Peters and Jochen Herms
German Center for Neurodegenerative Diseases (DZNE) Munich, Feodor-Lynen-Str. 17, 81377 Munich, Germany

Laurence Ozmen and Karlheinz Baumann
Roche, Pharma Research and Early Development, NORD DTA / Neuroscience Discovery, Roche Innovation Center Basel, F. Hoffmann-La Roche Ltd., Grenzacherstrasse 124, CH-4070 Basel, Switzerland

Axel Rominger
Department of Nuclear Medicine, Inselspital, University Hospital Bern, Freiburgstrasse 4, 3010 Bern, Switzerland

Jochen Herms
Center of Neuropathology and Prion Research, Feodor-Lynen-Straße 23, 81377 Munich, Germany

Jochen Herms, Axel Rominger and Matthias Brendel
Munich Cluster for Systems Neurology (SyNergy), Munich, Germany

Soraya Wilke Saliba, Hannah Jauch, Brahim Gargouri, Albrecht Keil and Bernd L. Fiebich
Neuroimmunology and Neurochemistry Research Group, Department of Psychiatry and Psychotherapy, Medical Center - University of Freiburg, Faculty of Medicine, University of Freiburg, Freiburg, Germany

Thomas Hurrle, Nicole Volz, Florian Mohr and Stefan Bräse
Institute of Organic Chemistry, Karlsruhe Institute of Technology (KIT), Karlsruhe, Germany

Thomas Hurrle and Stefan Bräse
Institute of Toxicology and Genetics, Karlsruhe Institute of Technology (KIT), Hermann-von-Helmholtz-Platz 1, 76344 Eggenstein-Leopoldshafen, Germany

Florian Mohr
Department of Molecular Physiology, Leiden Institute of Chemistry, Leiden University, Leiden, the Netherlands

Bernd L. Fiebich
Department of Psychiatry and Psychotherapy, Laboratory of Translational Psychiatry, University Hospital Freiburg, Hauptstr. 5, 79104 Freiburg, Germany

Ju-Young Lee, Jin Han Nam, Youngpyo Nam, Hye Yeon Nam, Gwangho Yoon, Jeongyeon Kim and Hyang-Sook Hoe
Department of Neural Development and Disease, Korea Brain Research Institute (KBRI), 61 Cheomdan-ro, Dong-gu, Daegu 41068, South Korea

Eunhwa Ko, Sang-Bum Kim and Hwan Geun Choi
New Drug Development Center, Daegu-Gyeongbuk Medical Innovation Foundation, 80 Cheombok-ro, Dong-gu, Daegu 41061, South Korea

Mahealani R Bautista, Christina C Capule, Takaoki Koyanagi, Geoffray Leriche and Jerry Yang
Department of Chemistry and Biochemistry, University of California, San Diego, La Jolla, CA 92093-0358, USA

Raj Putatunda, Yonggang Zhang, Fang Li, Xiao-Feng Yang and Wenhui Hu
Center for Metabolic Disease Research, Temple University Lewis Katz School of Medicine, 3500 N Broad Street, Philadelphia, PA 19140, USA

Raj Putatunda, Yonggang Zhang, Fang Li and Wenhui Hu
Department of Pathology and Laboratory Medicine, Temple University Lewis Katz School of Medicine, 3500 N Broad Street, Philadelphia, PA 19140, USA

Mary F Barbe
Department of Anatomy and Cell Biology, Temple University Lewis Katz School of Medicine, 3500 N Broad Street, Philadelphia, PA 19140, USA

Xiao-Feng Yang
Department of Pharmacology, Temple University Lewis Katz School of Medicine, 3500 N Broad Street, Philadelphia, PA 19140, USA

Patrick P. Lowe, Benedek Gyongyosi, Abhishek Satishchandran, Arvin Iracheta-Vellve, Yeonhee Cho, Aditya Ambade and Gyongyi Szabo
Department of Medicine, University of Massachusetts Medical School, 364 Plantation Street, Worcester, MA 01605, USA

Jiawen Qian, Chen Wang, Bo Wang, Yuedi Wang, Junying Xu, Ronghua Liu and Yiwei Chu
Department of Immunology, School of Basic Medical Sciences, and Institute of Biomedical Sciences, Fudan University, No. 138, Yi Xue Yuan Rd., Mail Shanghai 200032, People's Republic of China

Jiawen Qian, Chen Wang, Bo Wang, Yuedi Wang, Feifei Luo, Junying Xu and Yiwei Chu
Biotherapy Research Center, Fudan University, Shanghai 200032, China

Jiao Yang
Jiangsu Key Lab of Medical Optics, Suzhou Institute of Biomedical Engineering and Technology, Chinese Academy of Sciences, Suzhou 215000, China

Chujun Zhao
Northfield Mount Hermon School, Mount Hermon, MA 01354, USA

Kristi Henjum and Lars N. G. Nilsson
Department of Pharmacology, Institute of Clinical Medicine, University of Oslo and Oslo University Hospital, Blindern, 0316 Oslo, Norway

Else Quist-Paulsen
Department of Infectious Diseases, Oslo University Hospital, Ullevaal Hospital, Nydalen, N-0450 Oslo, Norway
Institute of Clinical Medicine, University of Oslo, Blindern, 0318 Oslo, Norway

Henrik Zetterberg and Kaj Blennow
Department of Psychiatry and Neurochemistry, Institute of Neuroscience and Physiology, The Sahlgrenska Academy at University of Gothenburg, SE-431 80 Mölndal, Sweden
Clinical Neurochemistry Laboratory, Sahlgrenska University Hospital, SE-431 80 Mölndal, Sweden

Henrik Zetterberg
Department of Degenerative Disease, UCL Institute of Neurology, Queen Square, Gower Street, London WC1E 6BT, UK
UK Dementia Research Institute at UCL, Gower Street, London WC1E 6BT, UK

Leiv Otto Watne
Oslo Delirium Research Group, Department of Geriatric Medicine, Oslo University Hospital, Nydalen, N-0424 Oslo, Norway
Institute of Basic Medical Sciences, University of Oslo, Domus Medica, Sognsvannsveien 9, N-0372 Oslo, Norway

Sarah Kim, Yun Kyung Hahn, Shiping Zou, Kurt F Hauser and Pamela E Knapp
Department of Anatomy and Neurobiology, Virginia Commonwealth University School of Medicine, 1217 E. Marshall St, Richmond, VA 23298-0709, USA

Elizabeth M Podhaizer, Virginia D McLane, Kurt F Hauser and Pamela E Knapp
Department of Pharmacology and Toxicology, Virginia Commonwealth University, Richmond, VA 23298, USA

Kurt F Hauser and Pamela E Knapp
Institute for Drug and Alcohol Studies, Virginia Commonwealth University, Richmond, VA 23298, USA

Shiping Zou
BioLegend, Inc., 210 Rustcraft Rd., Dedham, MA
02026, USA

Hui Du
Department of Histology and Embryology, Taishan
Medical University, Taian 271000, China

**Juan Shi, Ming Wang, Shuhong An and Zhaojin
Wang**
Department of Human Anatomy, Taishan Medical
University, Taian 271000, China

Xingjing Guo
Department of Physiology, Taishan Medical
University, Taian 271000, China

Index